Decision Making, Affect, and Learning

Attention and Performance

Decision Making, Affect, and Learning
Attention and Performance XXIII

Edited by

Mauricio R. Delgado
Department of Psychology
Rutgers University
Newark, NJ USA

Elizabeth A. Phelps
Department of Psychology and
Center for Neural Science
New York University
New York, NY USA

Trevor W. Robbins
Department of Experimental Psychology
University of Cambridge
Cambridge, UK

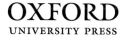
OXFORD
UNIVERSITY PRESS

OXFORD

UNIVERSITY PRESS

Great Clarendon Street, Oxford, OX2 6DP,
United Kingdom

Oxford University Press is a department of the University of Oxford.
It furthers the University's objective of excellence in research, scholarship,
and education by publishing worldwide. Oxford is a registered trade mark of
Oxford University Press in the UK and in certain other countries

Published in the United States of America by Oxford University Press
198 Madison Avenue, New York, NY 10016, United States of America

British Library Cataloguing in Publication Data
Data available

Library of Congress Cataloguing in Publication Data
Data Available

ISBN 978-0-19-960043-4

Whilst every effort has been made to ensure that the contents of this book are as
complete, accurate and up-to-date as possible at the date of writing, Oxford
University Press is not able to give any guarantee or assurance that such is the case.
Readers are urged to take appropriately qualified medical advice in all cases. The
information in this book is intended to be useful to the general reader, but should
not be used as a means of self-diagnosis or for the prescription of medication.

Preface

The study of decision making is a truly multi-disciplinary endeavor, subsuming investigations in disciplines as disparate as behavioral and cognitive neuroscience, economics, ethology, experimental psychology, mathematical modeling, psychiatry and psychopharmacology. Most of these approaches are represented in this volume, which grew out of a Workshop conference convened in Stowe, Vermont on July 13-17th 2008, as part of the *Attention and Performance* (A&P) series, enabling us to convey the vibrancy and excitement of this rapidly developing field.

In order to understand the complexities of efficient decision making leading to adaptive outcomes, we believe it is necessary to pursue a theoretically-motivated, behavioral economic approach to decision making that takes into account the individual heuristic biases and idiosyncrasies of affective processing of the individual human operator. The neural analysis of affect also encompasses neurochemically defined 'reward' and 'punishment' systems which drive the fundamental processes of associative learning through which experience comes to influence decision making. There is no doubt that the considerable advances made in the neuroscience of reinforcement learning and affective processing described here have contributed enormously to our evolving understanding of the neural basis of decision making. The organization of this book reflects four interacting facets described below. Three of them begin with special Tutorial Essays that set the scene for the succeeding chapters.

Following a comprehensive and valuable Tutorial Review by Daw on the computational methods now available for both learning and neural modeling, Section 1 provides four essays on the interface between behavioral economics and basic psychological processes. Camerer directly poses the question of how conditioning and emotional processes bear on economic decisions. McClure and van den Bos ask how a well-known typical violation of economic rationality ('the winner's curse') can be explained through an interaction between modeling reinforcement theory and neuroscience. Chater and Vlaev ponder the psychological factors that contribute to value instability through a combination of modeling reinforcement learning and cognitive choice. Kalentscher and Pennartz provide obvious problems for decision-making principles based on value by considering phenomena and mechanisms of intransitive choice.

Section II on neural mechanisms of decision making begins with a salutary Tutorial Review in which Hayden and Platt illustrate the difficulties of bringing together studies on decision making under uncertainty using behavioral studies with single-unit recording in monkeys and fMRI in human volunteers. The rest of this Section nonetheless emphasizes the considerable advances that have been made in identifying neural correlates of decision making processes. Thus, Venkatraman et al use functional magnetic resonance imaging in studies of risky decision making to show how specific neural systems in the cerebral cortex support variability in human choice and strategy, for example, the use of compensatory trade-offs and simplifications of decision rules. Doya and colleagues use mathematical models of decision making, in order to inform their human fMRI studies of temporal discounting, as affected by dietary manipulations of the central serotonin system. Sakagami and colleagues also combine human fMRI and monkey electrophysiology to study neural mechanisms underlying value-based choice. The last two chapters of this Section focus on the central role of the orbitofrontal cortex in decision making. Thus, Clarke and Roberts examine the role of the orbitofrontal cortex in coordinating behavioral and autonomic activity in choice situations in marmoset monkeys, its interactions with other systems such as the amygdala and striatum, and its neurochemical modulation, for example, by serotonin. Walton and colleagues compare the functions of the anterior cingulate cortex and orbitofrontal cortex in choice behavior over time, mainly on the basis of lesion studies in monkeys, but substantiated by studies using human fMRI. These contributions confirm that the orbitofrontal cortex has important functions in decision-making cognition which are being illuminated by studies in experimental animals, as well as in humans.

The chapters in Section III have a slightly different theme, being especially implicated in underlying striatal-based reward and aversive processes. Roesch and Schoenbaum's Tutorial Review surveys their electrophysiological investigations of reinforcement learning, in terms of possible interactions of the rat orbitofrontal cortex in outcome processing with the amygdala, and also with attentional and prediction error mechanisms of the dopaminergic mid-brain. Four subsequent chapters focus on the basal ganglia, directly addressing the issues of how these structures (somewhat implicitly) mediate appetitive and aversive learning (Pessiglione et al) and are modulated by cognitive control centers that regulate affect and decision making (Martin and Delgado). Through studies of normal volunteers and patients with Parkinson's disease, Cools examines the contribution of striatal and prefrontal dopamine modulation to component processes for human decision making, using probabilistic reversal learning as the main behavioral choice paradigm. Wimmer and Shohamy also investigate the striatal role in learning in humans via Parkinson's disease but pose the question that the possible importance of dopamine-dependent memory processing in hippocampus may previously have been underestimated. It is instructive that Niewehnhuis and Jepma's chapter concerns instead the role of a different ascending chemical neurotransmitter system, noradrenaline, in modulating attentional processes relevant to the 'explore or exploit' model. Typical of the multidisciplinarity in evidence at this Workshop, they show how a theoretical approach fed by behavioral electrophysiological data from monkeys can be used to make predictions about psychopharmacological manipulations of the noradrenergic system in studies of human decision making and performance. Finally, utilizing both mathematical modeling and functional neuroimaging in humans, Paulus focuses on the role of the insular cortex in mediating interoceptive cues, whether aversive or rewarding, in "homeostatic" decision making and relates their abnormal processing to particular psychiatric disturbances, including anxiety and addiction.

The concluding Section IV goes on to describe three main neuropsychiatric or developmental applications of research into decision-making cognition. Chapters by Ernst (using mainly functional resonance imaging paradigms to simulate gambling scenarios) and by Casey et al (with a focus on neural mechanisms of inhibitory control) elucidate the neural basis of risky and impulsive decision making in adolescents. The chapters by Goldstein and by Ersche provide contrasting neuropsychological analyses of decision-making cognition in substance abusers. Sahakian and Morein-Zamir review evidence of affective bias in decision making cognition in patients with depression, using an approach that combines neuropsychological and functional neuroimaging techniques. These chapters well exemplify the scope of the field and its potential for clinical application.

We hope our readers enjoy reading these contributions to the prestigious 'A&P' series as much as we have; it was a truly memorable meeting and we hope to have captured some of its most exciting elements. We are most grateful to Martin Baum and his colleagues at Oxford University Press for their understanding and support in bringing this project to fruition. Thanks also to Sandra Yoshida for excellent assistance. Finally, we acknowledge support for the A&P conference that led to this Volume from the National Institute on Drug Abuse (NIDA), the National Institute on Aging (NIA), Wyeth Inc., and the James S. McDonnell Foundation, who supported both the conference and a collaborative network between New York University and the University of Cambridge that inspired this venture.

M.R. Delgado,
E.A. Phelps, and T.W. Robbins,
New York and Cambridge U.K.
October 2010

Contents

Section III **Neural systems of emotion, reward, and learning**

Section IV **Neurodevelopmental and clinical aspects**

The Attention and Performance Symposia

Since the first was held in The Netherlands in 1966, the Attention and Performance Symposia have become an established and highly successful institution. They are now held every 2 years, in a different country. The original purpose remains: to promote communication among researchers in experimental cognitive psychology and cognate areas working at the frontiers of research on 'attention, performance and information processing'. The format is an invited workshop-style meeting, with plenty of time for papers and discussion, leading to the publication of an edited volume of the proceedings.

The International Association for the Study of Attention and Performance exists solely to run the meetings and publish the volume. Its Executive Committee selects the organizers of the next meeting, and develops the program in collaboration with them, with advice on potential participants from an Advisory Council of up to 100 members. Participation is by invitation only, and the Association's Constitution requires participation from a wide range of countries, a high proportion of young researchers, and a substantial injection of new participants from meeting to meeting.

Held usually in a relatively isolated location, each meeting has four and a half days of papers presented by a maximum of 26 speakers, plus an invited Association Lecture from a leading figure in the field. There is a maximum of 65 participants (including the current members of the executive committee and the organizers). There are no parallel sessions, and all participants commit themselves to attending all the sessions. There is thus time for substantial papers followed by extended discussion, both organized and informal, and opportunities for issues and ideas introduced at one point in the meeting to be returned to and developed later. Speakers are encouraged to be provocative and speculative, and participants who do not present formal papers are encouraged to contribute actively to discussion in various ways, for example as formal discussants, by presenting a poster, or as contributors to scheduled discussion sessions. This intensive workshop atmosphere has been one of the major strengths and attractions of these meetings. Manuscript versions of the papers are refereed anonymously by other participants and external referees and published in a high-quality volume edited by the organizers, with a publication lag similar to many journals. Unlike many edited volumes, the Attention and Performance series reaches a wide audience and has considerable prestige. Although not a journal, it is listed in journal citation indices with the top dozen journals in experimental psychology. According to the Constitution, 'Papers presented at meetings are expected to describe work not previously published, and to represent a substantial contribution . . .' Over the years, contributors have been willing to publish original experimental and theoretical research of high quality in the volume, and this tradition continues. A and P review papers have also been much cited. The series has attracted widespread praise in terms such as 'unfailingly presented the best work in the field' (S. Kosslyn, Harvard), 'most distinguished series in the field of cognitive psychology' (C. Bundesen, Copenhagen), 'held in high esteem throughout the field because of its attention to rigor, quality and scope . . . indispensable to anyone who is serious about understanding the current state of the science' (M. Jordan, MIT), 'the books are an up to the minute tutorial on topics fundamental to understanding mental processes' (M. Posner, Oregon).

In the early days of the Symposium, when the scientific analysis of attention and performance was in its infancy, thematic coherence could be generated merely by gathering together the most active researchers in the field. More recently, experimental psychology has ramified, 'cognitive science' has been born, and converging approaches to the issues we study have developed in neuroscience. Participation has therefore become interdisciplinary, with neuroscientists, neuropsychologists, and computational modelers joining the experimental psychologists. Each meeting now focuses on a restricted theme under the general heading of 'attention and performance'. Recent themes include: Synergies in Experimental Psychology: Artificial Intelligence and Cognitive Neuroscience (USA, 1990); Conscious and Unconscious Processes (Italy, 1992); Integration of Information (Japan, 1994); Cognitive Regulation of Performance: Interaction of Theory and Application (Israel, 1996); and Control of Cognitive Processes (UK, 1998); Common Processes in Perception and Actions (Germany, 2000); Functional Brain Imaging of Visual Cognition (Italy, 2002); Processes of Change in Brain and Cognitive Development (USA, 2004); Sensorimotor Foundations of Higher Cognition (France, 2006); and Decision Making, Affect, and Learning (USA 2008).

Contributors

Timothy E. J. Behrens
Department of Experimental Psychology
University of Oxford
South Parks Road
Oxford OX1 3UD
UK

Colin F. Camerer
Division of Humanities and
Social Sciences
Caltech
1200 E. California Blvd.
Pasedena, CA 91125
USA
Camerer@hss.caltech.edu

B.J. Casey
Sackler Institute
Weill Medical College of Cornell
University
1300 York Ave., Box 140
New York, NY 10065
USA
bjc2002@med.cornell.edu

Nick Chater
Behavioural Science Group
Warwick Business School
University of Warwick
Covertry, CV4 7AL
UK
Nick.Chater@wbs.ac.uk

H. F. Clarke
Department of Experimental Psychology
University of Cambridge
Downing Street
Cambridge, CB2 3EB
UK
hfc23@cam.ac.uk

Roshan Cools
Donders Institute for Brain, Cognition
and Behaviour
Radboud University Nijmegen
Centre for Cognitive Neuroimaging
P.O. Box 9101
6500 HB Nijmegen
The Netherlands
roshan.cools@donders.ru.nl;
roshan.cools@gmail.com

Nathaniel D. Daw
Center for Neural Science and
Department of Psychology
New York University
4 Washington Place, Room 809
New York, NY 10003
USA
daw@cns.nyu.edu

Mauricio R. Delgado
Department of Psychology
101 Warren St., 340 Smith Hall
Rutgers University
Newark, NJ 07102
USA
delgado@psychology.rutgers.edu

Kenji Doya
Neural Computation Unit
Okinawa Institute of Science and
Technology
1919-1 Tancha, Onna
Okinawa, 904-0412
Japan
doya@oist.jp

Monique Ernst
Neurodevelopment of Reward Systems/
Mood and Anxiety 15K North Drive
Bethesda MD 20892
USA
ernstm@mail.nih.gov

Karen D. Ersche
University of Cambridge
School of Clinical Medicine
Department of Psychiatry
Brain Mapping Unit, Herchel Smith
Building,
Cambridge, UK
ke220@cam.ac.uk

Chris D. Frith
Wellcome Trust Centre for
Neuroimaging
University College London
UK
Center for Functional Integrative
Neuroscience
University of Aarhus
Aarhus, Denmark

Adriana Galván
Department of Psychology
University of California Los Angeles
1285 Franz Hall
Los Angeles, LA 90095
USA

Rita Z. Goldstein
Brookhaven National Laboratory
PO Box 5000
Upton, NY, 11973
USA
rgoldstein@bnl.gov

Todd A. Hare
Department of Computation and
Neural Systems
California Institute of Technology
HSS 228–77
Pasadena, CA 91125
USA

Benjamin Y. Hayden
Department of Neurobiology
Duke University Medical School
Durham, NC 27710
hayden@neuro.duke.edu

Scott A. Huettel
Center for Cognitive Neuroscience
Duke University, Box 90999
Durham, NC 27710
USA
scott.huettel@duke.edu

Makoto Ito
Neural Computation Unit
Okinawa Institute of Science and
Technology
1919-1 Tancha, Onna
Okinawa, 904-0412
Japan
ito@oist.jp

Marieke Jepma
Leiden University
Institute of Psychology
Cognitive Psychology Unit
Wassenaarseweg 52
2333 AK Leiden
The Netherlands
mjepma@fsw.leidenuniv.nl

Tobias Kalenscher
Swammerdam Institute for Life Sciences
(SILS)
University of Amsterdam
Science Park 904
1098 XH, Amsterdam
The Netherlands
Tobias.Kalenscher@gmail.com

Samuel M. McClure
Department of Psychology
Stanford University
Jordan Hall, Bldg. 420
450 Serra Mll Stanford, CA 94305
USA
smcclure@stanford.edu

Sharon Morein-Zamir
University of Cambridge
Department of Psychiatry
Box 189, Level 4C
Addenbrooke's Hospital
Hills Road
Cambridge CB2 2QQ
UK
sm658@cam.ac.uk

Laura N. Martin
Department of Psychology
101 Warren St.
Smith Hall
Rutgers University
Newark, NJ 07102
USA
lnmartin@psychology.rutgers.edu

Sander Nieuwenhuis
Leiden University
Institute of Psychology
Cognitive Psychology Unit
Wassenaarseweg 52
2333 AK Leiden
The Netherlands
snieuwenhuis@fsw.leidenuniv.nl

Kensaku Nomoto
Brain Science Institute
Tamagawa University
Tamagawagakuen 6-1-1
Machida, Tokyo
Japan

Stefano Palminteri
Institut du Cerveau et de la Moelle
épinière (ICM)
INSERM UMRS 975
Paris, France

Xiaochuan Pan
Brain Science Institute
Tamagawa University
Tamagawagakuen 6-1-1
Machida, Tokyo
Japan

Martin P. Paulus
Department of Psychiatry
Laboratory of Biological Dynamics and
Theoretical Medicine
University of California San Diego
8950 Villa La Jolla Dr. Suite C213
La Jolla CA 92037-0985
USA
mpaulus@ucsd.edu

John W. Payne
Center for Cognitive Neuroscience
Duke University, Box 90999
Durham, NC 27710
USA
jpayne@duke.edu

Cyriel M.A. Pennartz
Swammerdam Institute for Life Sciences
(SILS)
University of Amsterdam
Science Park 904
1098 XH, Amsterdam
The Netherlands
c.m.a.pennartz@uva.nl

Mathias Pessiglione
Institut du Cerveau et de la Moelle
épinière (ICM)
INSERM UMRS 975
Paris,
France
m.pessiglione@filion.ucl.ac.uk

Michael L. Platt
Department of Neurobiology
Duke University Medical School
Durham, NC 27710
platt@neuro.duke.edu

Trevor W. Robbins
Department of Experimental
Psychology
University of Cambridge
Downing Street
CB2 3EB Cambridge, UK
twr2@cam.ac.uk

A.C. Roberts
Department of Physiology
Development and Neuroscience
University of Cambridge
Downing Street
Cambridge, CB2 3DY
UK
acr4@cam.ac.uk

Matthew R. Roesch
Department of Psychology and Program
in Neuroscience and Cognitive Science
University of Maryland
College Park, MD 20742
USA
mroes001@umaryland.edu

Peter H. Rudebeck
Department of Experimental
Psychology
University of Oxford
South Parks Road
Oxford OX1 3UD
UK
peter.rudebeck@psy.ox.ac.uk

Matthew F. S. Rushworth
Department of Experimental Psychology
University of Oxford
South Parks Road
Oxford OX1 3UD
UK

Barbara J. Sahakian
University of Cambridge
Department of Psychiatry and MRC/
Wellcome Trust Behavioural and Clinical
Neuroscience Institute
Addenbrooke's Hospital, Box 189
Cambridge CB2 2QQ
UK
Bjs-sec@medschl.com.ac.uk

Masamichi Sakagami
Brain Science Institute
Tamagawa University
6-1-1 Tamagawagakuen
Machida, Tokyo
Japan
sakagami@lab.tamagawa.ac.jp

Kazuyuki Samejima
Brain Science Institute
Tamagawa University
6-1-1 Tamagawagakuen
Machida, Tokyo
Japan

Liane Schmidt
Department of Psychology
Columbia University
1190 Amsterdam Avenue
406 Schermerhorn Hall
New York, NY 10027
USA

Geoffrey Schoenbaum
Department of Anatomy and
Neurobiology
University of Maryland School
of Medicine
20 Penn St, HSF-2 S251
Baltimore, MD 21201
USA
schoenbg@schoenbaumlab.org

Daphna Shohamy
Department of Psychology
Columbia University
1190 Amsterdam Ave, MC5501
406 Schermerhorn Hall
New York, NY 10027
USA
shohamy@psych.columbia.edu

Wouter van den Bos
Department of Psychology
Leiden University
Pieter de la Court gebouw
Wasseraarseweg J2
2333 AK Leiden
wbos@fsw.leidenuniv.nl

Ivo Vlaev
Faculty of Medicine
Imperial College London
St Mary's Campus, 10th Flooor
QEQM building
London, W2 INY
UK
ivlaev@imperial.ac.uk

Vinod Venkatraman
Center for Cognitive Neuroscience
Duke University, Box 90999
Durham, NC 27710
USA
vinod@biac.duke.edu

Mark E. Walton
Department of Experimental Psychology
University of Oxford
South Parks Road
Oxford OX1 3UD
UK
mark.walton@psy.ox.ac.uk

G. Elliott Wimmer
Department of Psychology
Columbia University
1190 Amsterdam Ave, MC5501
406 Schermerhorn Hall
New York, NY 10027
USA
gew2105@columbia.edu

Manami Yamamoto
Brain Science Institute
Tamagawa University
6-1-1 Tamagawagakuen
Machida, Tokyo,
Japan

Abbreviations

ACC	anterior cingulate cortex	I-RISA	impaired response inhibition and salience attribution
ADHD	attention-deficit/hyperactivity disorder	LC	locus coeruleus
AMPT	alpha-mehtylparatyrosine	LFP	local field potential
APTD	acute phenylalanine and tyrosine depletion	LPFC	lateral prefrontal cortex
		LTP	long-term plasticity
ATD	acute tryptophan depletion	MDD	major depressive disorder
BA	Brodmann area	MLE	maximum likelihood estimate
BD	bipolar disorder	mOFC	medial orbitofrontal cortex
BIS-11	Barratt impulsiveness scale, version 11	mPFC	medial prefrontal cortex
		MRI	magnetic resonance imaging
BLNG	basolateral nuclear group	MTL	medial temporal lobe
BOLD	blood-oxygen-level-dependent	MUA	multi-unit recording
BP	binding potential	NAC	nucleus accumbens
CANTAB	Cambridge neuropsychological test automated battery	NE	norepinephrine
		OCD	obsessive-compulsive disorder
CBT	cognitive behavioral therapy	OFC	orbitofrontal cortex
CDF	cumulative distribution function	OPT	original prospect theory
CEA	central extended amygdalae	PD	Parkinson's disease
CGp	posterior cingulate cortex	PET	positron emission tomography
CGT	Cambridge gamble task	PFC	prefrontal cortex
CPT	cumulative prospect theory	POMPD	partially observable Markov decision problem
DA	dopamine		
DBS	deep brain stimulation	PPC	posterior parietal cortex
DDM	drift diffusion model	PT	prospect theory
dmPFC	dorsomedial prefrontal cortex	RL	reinforcement learning
DTI	diffusion tensor imaging	RNNE	risk neutral Nash equilibrium
ERPs	event-related potentials	SCR	skin conductance response
EU	expected utility theory	SPATs	sequential paired association trials
fMRI	functional magnetic resonance imaging	SSRI	serotonin selective reuptake inhibitors
FMT	6-[^{18}F]fluoro-L-m-tyrosine	STRAP-R	sensitivity to reinforcement of addictive and other primary rewards
FRN	feedback-related negativity		
FTM	fractal triadic model	SUA	single-unit activity
IAPS	International Affective Picture System	TD	temporal difference
		VMPFC	ventromedial prefrontal cortex
IDED	intra-dimensional/extra-dimensional set-shifting test	VStr	ventral striatum
		VTA	ventral tegmental area
IGT	Iowa Gambling Task	WCST	Wisconsin Card Sorting Test
ITI	inter-trial interval		

Psychological processes underlying decision making

Chapter 1

Trial-by-trial data analysis using computational models

(Tutorial Review)

Nathaniel D. Daw

Abstract

Researchers have recently begun to integrate computational models into the analysis of neural and behavioral data, particularly in experiments on reward learning and decision making. The present chapter aims to review and rationalize these methods. We expose these tools as instances of broadly applicable statistical techniques, consider the questions they are suited to answer, provide a practical tutorial and tips for their effective use, and, finally, suggest some directions for extension or improvement. The techniques are illustrated with fits of simple models to simulated datasets. Throughout, we flag interpretational and technical pitfalls of which we believe authors, reviewers, and readers should be aware.

1.1 Introduction

In numerous and high-profile studies, researchers have recently begun to integrate computational models into the analysis of data from experiments on reward learning and decision making (Platt and Glimcher, 1999; O'Doherty et al., 2003; Barraclough et al., 2004; Sugrue et al., 2004; Samejima et al., 2005; Daw et al., 2006; Li et al., 2006; Frank et al., 2007; Kable and Glimcher, 2007; Lohrenz et al., 2007; Schonberg et al., 2007; Tom et al., 2007; Hampton et al., 2008; Hare et al., 2008; Plassmann et al., 2008; Wittmann et al., 2008). As these techniques are spreading rapidly, but have been developed and documented somewhat sporadically alongside the studies themselves, the present review aims to clarify the toolbox (see also O'Doherty et al., 2007). In particular, we discuss the rationale for these methods and the questions they are suited to address. We then offer a relatively practical tutorial about the basic statistical methods for their answer and how they can be applied to data analysis. The techniques are illustrated with fits of simple models to simulated datasets. Throughout, we flag interpretational and technical pitfalls of which we believe authors, reviewers, and readers should be aware. We focus on cataloging the particular, admittedly somewhat idiosyncratic, combination of techniques frequently used in this literature, but also on exposing these techniques as instances of a general set of tools that can be applied to analyze behavioral and neural data of many sorts.

A number of other reviews (Daw and Doya, 2006; Dayan and Niv, 2008) have focused on the scientific conclusions that have been obtained with these methods, an issue we omit almost entirely here. There are also excellent books that cover statistical inference of this general sort with much greater generality, formal precision, and detail (MacKay, 2003; Gelman et al., 2004; Bishop, 2006; Gelman and Hill, 2007).

1.2 **Background**

Much work in this area grew out of the celebrated observation (Barto, 1995; Schultz et al., 1997) that the firing of midbrain dopamine neurons (and also the BOLD signal measured via fMRI in their primary target, the striatum; Delgado et al., 2000; Knutson et al., 2000; McClure et al., 2003; O'Doherty et al., 2003) resembles a "prediction error" signal used in a number of computational algorithms for reinforcement learning (RL, i.e., trial-and-error learning in decision problems; Sutton and Barto, 1998). Although the original empirical articles reported activity averaged across many trials, and the mean behavior of computational simulations was compared to these reports, in fact, a more central issue in learning is how behavior (or the underlying neural activity) changes trial by trial in response to feedback. In fact, the computational theories are framed in just these terms, and so more recent work on the system (O'Doherty et al., 2003; Bayer and Glimcher, 2005) has focused on comparing their predictions to raw data time series, trial by trial: measuring, in effect, the theories' goodness of fit to the data, on average, rather than their goodness of fit to the averaged data.

This change in approach represents a major advance in the use of computational models for experimental design and analysis, which is still unfolding. Used this way, computational models represent exceptionally detailed, quantitative hypotheses about how the brain approaches a problem, which are amenable to direct experimental test. As noted, such trial-by-trial analyses are particularly suitable to developing a more detailed and dynamic picture of learning than was previously available.

In a standard experiential decision experiment, such as a "bandit" task (Sugrue et al., 2004; Lau and Glimcher, 2005; Daw et al., 2006), a subject is offered repeated opportunities to choose between multiple options (e.g. slot machines) and receives rewards or punishments according to her choice on each trial. Data might consist of a series of choices and outcomes (one per trial). In principle, any arbitrary relationship might obtain between the entire list of past choices and outcomes, and the next choice. Computational theories constitute particular claims about some more restricted function by which previous choices and feedback give rise to subsequent choices. For instance, standard RL models (such as "Q learning"; Watkins, 1989) envision that subjects track the expected reward for each slot machine, via some sort of running average over the feedback, and it is only through these aggregated "value" predictions that past feedback determines future choices.

This example points to another important feature of this approach, which is that the theories purport to quantify, trial-by-trial, variables such as the reward expected for a choice (and the "prediction error," or difference between the received and expected rewards). That is, the theories permit the estimation of quantities (expectations, expectation violations) that would otherwise be *subjective*; this, in turn, enables the search for neural correlates of these estimates (Platt and Glimcher, 1999; Sugrue et al., 2004).

By comparing the model's predictions to trial-by-trial experimental data, such as choices or BOLD signals, it is possible, using a mixture of Bayesian and classical statistical techniques, to answer two sorts of questions about a model, which are discussed in Sections 1.3 and 1.4 below. The art is framing questions of scientific interest in these terms.

The first question is *parameter estimation*. RL models typically have a number of free parameters—measuring quantities such as the "learning rate," or the degree to which subjects update their beliefs in response to feedback. Often, these parameters characterize (or new parameters can be introduced so as to characterize) factors that are of experimental interest. For instance, Behrens et al. (2007) tested predictions about how particular task manipulations would affect the learning rate.

The second type of question that can be addressed is *model comparison*. Different computational models, in effect, constitute different hypotheses about the learning process that gave rise to the data. These hypotheses may be tested against one another on the basis of their fit to the data. For example, Hampton et al. (2008) use this method to compare which of different approaches subjects use for anticipating an opponent's behavior in a multiplayer competitive game.

1.2.1 Learning and observation models

In order to appreciate the extent to which the same methods may be applied to different sets of data, it is useful to separate a computational theory into two parts. The first, which we will call the *learning model*, describes the dynamics of the model's internal variables, such as the reward expected for each slot machine. The second part, which we will call the *observation model*, describes how the model's internal variables are reflected in observed data: for instance, how expected values drive choice or how prediction errors produce neural spiking. Essentially, the observation model regresses the learning model's internal variables onto the observed data; it plays a similar role as (and is often, in fact, identical to) the "link function" in generalized linear modeling. In this way, a common learning process (a single *learning model*) may be viewed as giving rise to distinct observable data streams in a number of different modalities (e.g., choices and BOLD, through two separate *observation models*). Thus, although we describe the methods in this tutorial primarily in terms of choice data, they are directly applicable to other modalities simply by substituting a different observation model.

Crucially, whereas the learning model is typically deterministic, the observation models are *noisy*: that is, given the internal variables produced by the learning model, an observation model assigns some *probability* to any possible observations. Thus the "fit" of different learning models, or their parameters, to any observed data can be quantified statistically in terms of the probability they assign to the data, a procedure at the core of the methods that follow.

1.3 Parameter estimation

Model parameters can characterize a variety of scientifically interesting quantities, from how quickly subjects learn (Behrens et al., 2007) to how sensitive they are to different rewards and punishments (Tom et al., 2007). Here we consider how to obtain statistical results about parameters' values from data. We first consider the general statistical rationale underlying the problem; then develop the details for an example RL model, before considering various pragmatic factors of actually performing these analyses on data. Finally, having discussed these details in terms of choice data, we discuss how the same methods may be applied to other sorts of data.

Suppose we have some model M, with a vector of free parameters $\boldsymbol{\theta}_M$. The model (here, the composite of our learning and observation models) describes a probability distribution, or likelihood function: $P(D|M, \boldsymbol{\theta}_M)$ over possible datasets D. Then, Bayes' rule tells us that having observed a dataset D:

$$P(\boldsymbol{\theta}_M|D, M) \propto P(D|M, \boldsymbol{\theta}_M) \cdot P(\boldsymbol{\theta}_M|M). \tag{1.1}$$

That is, the posterior probability distribution over the free parameters, given the data, is proportional to the product of two factors: (1) the likelihood of the data, given the free parameters, and (2) the prior probability of the parameters. This equation famously shows how to start with a theory of how parameters (noisily) produce data, and invert it into a theory by which data (noisily) reveal the parameters that produced it. Classically, we seek a point estimate of the parameters $\boldsymbol{\theta}_M$ rather than a posterior distribution over all possible values; if we neglect (or treat as flat) the prior over the parameters $P(\boldsymbol{\theta}_M|M)$, then the most probable value for $\boldsymbol{\theta}_M$ is the maximum likelihood estimate: the setting of the parameters that maximizes the likelihood function: $P(D|M, \boldsymbol{\theta}_M)$. We denote this $\hat{\boldsymbol{\theta}}_M$.

1.3.1 Maximum likelihood estimation for reinforcement learning (RL)

1.3.1.1 An RL model

We may see how the general ideas play out in a simple reinforcement learning setting. Consider a simple game in which on each trial t, a subject makes a choice c_t (= L or R) between a left and a right slot-machine, and receives a reward r_t (= \$1 or \$0) stochastically. According to a simple Q-learning model (Watkins, 1989), on each trial, the subject assigns an expected value to each machine: $Q_t(L)$ and $Q_t(R)$. We initialize these values to (say) 0, and then on each trial, the value for the chosen machine is updated as:

$$Q_{t+1}(c_t) = Q_t(c_t) + \alpha \cdot \delta_t \tag{1.2}$$

where $0 \leq \alpha \leq 1$ is a free learning-rate parameter, and $\delta_t = r_t - Q_t(c_t)$ is the prediction error. Equation 1.2 is our learning model. To explain the choices in terms of the values, we assume an observation model. In RL, it is often assumed that subjects choose probabilistically according to a softmax distribution:

$$P(c_t = L \mid Q_t(\mathrm{L}), Q_t(\mathrm{R})) = \frac{\exp(\beta \cdot Q_t)(\mathrm{L}))}{\exp(\beta \cdot Q_t)(\mathrm{R})) + \exp(\beta \cdot Q_t)(\mathrm{L}))}. \tag{1.3}$$

Here, β is a free parameter known in RL as the inverse temperature parameter. However, note that eqn. 1.3 is also equivalent to standard logistic regression, where the dependent variable is the binary choice variable c_t and there is one predictor variable, the difference in values $Q_t(L) - Q_t(R)$.

Therefore, β can also be viewed as the regression weight connecting the Q s to the choices. More generally, when there are more than two choice options, the softmax model corresponds to a generalization of logistic regression known as conditional logit regression (McFadden, 1974).

The model of eqns. 1.2 and 1.3 is only a representative example of the sorts of algorithms used to study reinforcement learning. Since our focus here is on the methodology for estimation given a model, a full review of the many candidate models is beyond the scope of the present chapter (for exhaustive treatments see: Bertsekas and Tsitsiklis, 1996; Sutton and Barto, 1998). That said, most models in the literature are variants on the example shown here. Another commonly used (Daw et al., 2006; Behrens et al., 2007) and seemingly rather different family of learning methods is Bayesian models such as the Kalman filter (Kakade and Dayan, 2002). In fact, the Q-learning rule of eqn. 1.2 can be seen as a simplified case of the Kalman filter: the Bayesian model uses the same learning rule but has additional machinery that determines the learning rate parameter α on a trial-by-trial basis (Kakade and Dayan, 2002; Behrens et al., 2007; Daw et al., 2008).

1.3.1.2 Data likelihood

Given the model described above, the probability of a whole dataset D (i.e., a whole sequence of choices $c = c_{1...\tau}$ given the rewards $r = r_{1...\tau}$) is just the product of their probabilities from Equation 1.3:

$$\prod_t P(c_t = L \mid Q_t(L), Q_t(R)). \tag{1.4}$$

Note that the terms Q_t in the softmax are determined (via eqn. 1.2) by the rewards $r_{1...t-1}$ and choices $c_{1...t-1}$ on trials prior to t.

Together, eqns. 1.2 and 1.3 constitute a full likelihood function $P(D|M, \boldsymbol{\theta}_M)$, and we can estimate the free parameters ($\boldsymbol{\theta}_M = \langle \alpha, \beta \rangle$) by maximum likelihood. Figure 1.1 illustrates the process: 1000 choice trials were simulated according to the model (with parameters $\alpha = 0.25$ and $\beta = 1$, marked with x). The likelihood of the observed data was then computed for a range of parameters, and plotted (with brighter shading for higher likelihood) on a 2-D grid. In this case, the maximum likelihood point ($\hat{\alpha} = 0.34$ and $\hat{\beta} = 0.93$, marked with circle) was near the true parameters.

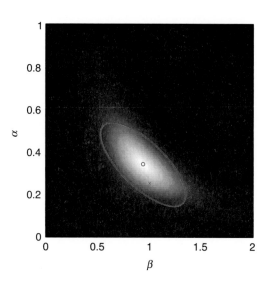

Fig. 1.1 Likelihood surface for simulated reinforcement learning data, as a function of two free parameters. Lighter shading denotes higher data likelihood. The maximum likelihood estimate is shown as an "o" surrounded by an ellipse of one standard error (a region of about 90% confidence); the true parameters from which the data were generated are denoted by an "x."

1.3.1.3 Confidence intervals

Of course, in order actually to test a hypothesis about the parameters' values, we need to be able to make statistical claims about the quality of the estimate $\hat{\boldsymbol{\theta}}_M$. Intuitively, the degree to which our estimate can be trusted depends on how much better it accounts for the data than other nearby parameter estimates; that is, on how sharply peaked is the "hill" of data likelihoods in the space of parameters. Such peakiness is characterized by the second derivative (the Hessian) of the likelihood function with respect to the parameters. The Hessian is a square matrix (here, 2×2) with a row and column for each parameter. Evaluated at the peak point $\hat{\boldsymbol{\theta}}_M$, the elements of the Hessian are larger the more rapidly the likelihood function is dropping off away from it in different directions, which corresponds to a more reliable estimate of the parameters. Conversely, the matrix inverse of the Hessian (like the reciprocal of a scalar) is larger for poorer estimates, like error bars. More precisely, if H is the Hessian of the negative log of the likelihood function at the maximum likelihood point $\hat{\boldsymbol{\theta}}_M$, then a standard estimator for the covariance of the parameter estimates is its matrix inverse H^{-1} (MacKay, 2003).

The diagonal terms of H^{-1} correspond to variances for each parameter separately, and their square roots measure one standard error on the parameter. Thus, for instance, 95% confidence intervals around the maximum likelihood estimate may be estimated as $\hat{\boldsymbol{\theta}}$ plus or minus 1.96 standard errors.

1.3.1.4 Covariance between parameters

The off-diagonal terms of H^{-1} measure *covariance* between the parameters, and are useful for diagnosing model fit. In general, large off-diagonal terms are a symptom of a poorly specified model or some kinds of bad data. In the worst case, two parameters may be redundant, so that there is no unique optimum. The Q-learning model has a more moderate coupling between the parameters. As can be seen by the elongated, tilted shape of the "ridge" in Fig. 1.1, estimates of α and β tend to be inversely coupled in this model. By increasing β while decreasing α (or vice versa: moving northwest or southeast in the figure), a similar likelihood is obtained. This is because the reward r_t is multiplied by both α (in eqn. 1.2 to update Q_t) and then by β (in eqn. 1.3) before affecting the choice likelihood on the next trial. As a result of this, either parameter individually cannot be estimated so tightly by itself (the "ridge" is a bit wide if you cross it horizontally in β or vertically in α), but their product is well-estimated (the hill is most narrow when crossed from northeast to southwest). The large oval in the figure traces out a one-standard error ellipse in the two parameters jointly, derived from H^{-1}; its tilt follows the contour of the ridge.

Often in applications such as logistic regression, a corrected covariance estimator is used that is thought to be more robust to problems such as mismatch between the true and assumed models. This "Huber–White" or "sandwich" estimator (Huber, 1967; Freedman, 2006) is $H^{-1}BH^{-1}$ where $B = \sum_t g(c_t)^{\mathrm{T}} g(c_t)$, and $g(c_t)$, in turn, is the gradient (vector of first partial derivatives with respect to the parameters) of the negative log likelihood of the t th data point c_t, evaluated at $\hat{\boldsymbol{\theta}}_M$. This is harder to compute in practice, since it involves keeping track of g, which is laborious. However, as discussed below, g can also be useful when searching for the maximum likelihood point.

1.3.2 **Pragmatics**

Above, we developed the general equations for maximum likelihood parameter estimation in an RL model; how can these be implemented in practice for data analysis?

First, although we have noted an equivalence between eqn. 1.3 and logistic regression, it is not possible simply to use an off-the-shelf regression package to estimate the parameters. This is because, although the observation stage of the model represents a logistic regression from values Q_t to choices c_t, the values are not fixed but themselves depend on the free parameters (here, α) of the learning process. As these do not enter the likelihood linearly they cannot be estimated by a generalized linear model. Thus, we must search for the full set of free parameters that optimize the likelihood function.

1.3.2.1 Likelihood function

At the heart of optimizing the likelihood function is computing it. It is straightforward to write a function that takes in a dataset (a sequence of choices and rewards) and a candidate setting of the free parameters, loops over the data computing eqns. 1.2 and 1.3, and returns the aggregate likelihood of the data. Importantly, the product in eqn. 1.4 is often an exceptionally small number; it is thus numerically more stable to compute its log, i.e., the *sum* over trials of the log of the choice probability from eqn. 1.3, which is:
$$\beta \cdot Q_t(c_t) - \log\left(\exp(\beta \cdot Q_t(L)) + \exp(\beta \cdot Q_t(R))\right).$$

Since log is a monotonic function, this quantity has the same optimum but is less likely to underflow the minimum floating point value representable by a computer. (Another numerical trick is to note that eqn. 1.3 is invariant to the addition or subtraction of any constant to all of the Q values. The chance of the exponentials under- or overflowing can thus be reduced by evaluating the log probability for Q values after first subtracting their mean.)

How, then, to find the optimal likelihood? In general, it may be tempting to cover the space of parameters with a discrete grid, compute the likelihood everywhere, and simply search for the best, much as is illustrated in Fig. 1.1. We recommend against this approach. First, most models of interest have more than two parameters, and exhaustively testing all combinations in a higher dimensional space becomes intractable. Second, and not unrelated, discretizing the parameters too coarsely, or searching within an inappropriate range, can lead to poor results; worse yet, since the parameters are typically coupled (as in Fig. 1.1), a poor search on one will also corrupt the estimates for other parameters.

1.3.2.2 Nonlinear optimization

To avoid errors related to discrete grid search, one may use routines for nonlinear function optimization that are included in many scientific computing languages. These functions do not discretely grid the parameter space, but instead search continuously over candidate values. In Matlab, for instance, this can be accomplished by functions such as `fmincon` or `fminsearch`; similar facilities exist in such packages as R and the SciPy toolbox for Python. Given a function to compute the likelihood and also starting settings for the free parameters, these functions search for the optimal parameter settings (the parameters that minimize the function, which means that the search must be applied to the negative log likelihood). Because these functions conduct a local search—e.g., variants on hill climbing—and because in general, likelihood surfaces may not be as well-behaved as the one depicted in Fig. 1.1, but may instead have multiple peaks, these optimizers are not guaranteed to find a global optimum. A solution to this problem is to call them many times from different starting points (e.g., randomly chosen or systematically distributed on a grid), and use the best answer (lowest negative log likelihood) found. It is important to remember that the goal is to find the single best setting of the parameters, so it is only the best answer (and not, for instance, some average) that counts.

1.3.2.3 Gradients and Hessians

Nonlinear optimization routines, such as `fmincon`, are also, often, able to estimate the Hessian of the log likelihood function numerically, and can return this matrix for use in computing confidence intervals. Alternatively, it is possible (albeit laborious) to compute both the Hessian H and the gradient g of the likelihood analytically alongside the likelihood itself. This involves repeatedly using the chain rule of calculus to work out, for instance, the derivative of the log likelihood of the data with respect to α (the first element of g) in terms of the derivatives of the log likelihoods for each choice,

$$\frac{\partial \log(P(c_t))}{\partial \alpha},$$

which in turn depend, through eqn. 1.3 on c_+,

$$\frac{\partial P(c_t)}{\partial Q_t}$$

and

$$\frac{\partial Q_t}{\partial \alpha}.$$

The last of these is vector valued,

$$\left[\frac{\partial Q_t(L)}{\partial \alpha}, \frac{\partial Q_t(R)}{\partial \alpha}\right],$$

and depends through the derivative of eqn. 1.2 on r_t and recursively on

$$\frac{\partial Q_{t-1}}{\partial \alpha}$$

and so on back to r_1 and

$$\frac{\partial Q_1}{\partial \alpha} = [0,0].$$

(It is easier to envision computing this forward, alongside the data likelihood: i.e., computing

$$\frac{\partial \log(P(c_t))}{\partial \alpha}$$

along with $\log(P(c_t))$ and

$$\frac{\partial Q_t}{\partial \alpha}$$

along with Q_t at each step, while looping through each trial's data in order.) If g is computed, it can be provided to the optimization function so as to guide the search; this often markedly improves the optimizer's performance.

1.3.2.4 Boundaries

With some function optimizers (e.g. Matlab's `fmincon`), it is possible to place boundaries on the free parameters. We suggest that these be used with caution. On one hand, some free parameters have semantics according to which values outside some range appear senseless or may be unstable. For instance, the learning rate α in eqn. 1.2 is a fractional stepsize and thus naturally ranges between zero and one. Moreover, for $\alpha > 1$, the Qs can grow rapidly and diverge. Thus, it makes some sense to constrain the parameter within this range. Similarly, negative values of β seem counterproductive, while very large values of β lead to large exponentiated terms in computing the log of eqn. 1.3, and ultimately program crashes due to arithmetic overflow. Also, for some subjects in this model, the maximum likelihood parameter estimates can occur at a very large β and a very small α (Schonberg et al., 2007). For reasons like these, it can be tempting to constrain β also to stay within some range.

However, if optimal parameters rest at these boundaries, this is cause for concern, since it indicates that the true optima lie outside the range considered and the estimates found depend rather arbitrarily on the boundary placement. Also, note again that, since the parameters are often interrelated, constraining one will impact the others as well. Although fits outside a sensible range can be simply due to noise, this can also suggest a problem with the model, a bad dataset, or a programming bug. There may, for instance, be features of the data that can only be captured within the model in question by adopting seemingly nonsensical parameters. (For instance, the issue with abnormally large α and small β, mentioned above, arises for a subset of subjects whose choices aren't well explained by this model.) It should also be noted that most of the statistical inference techniques discussed in this chapter—including the use of the inverse Hessian to estimate error bars, and the model comparison techniques discussed in Section 1.4—are ultimately based on approximating the likelihood function around $\hat{\boldsymbol{\theta}}_M$ by a Gaussian "hill." Thus, none of these methods is formally justified when estimated parameters lie on a boundary, since the hill will be severely truncated, and the point being examined may not even actually be its peak.

To the extent that inadmissible parameter estimates arise not due to poor model specification, but instead simply due to the inherent noise of maximum likelihood estimation, one possible alternative to a hard constraint on parameters is a prior. In particular, eqn. 1.1 suggests that prior information about the likely range of the parameters could enter via the term $P(\boldsymbol{\theta}_M|M)$ and would serve to regularize the estimates. In this case we would use a maximum a posteriori estimator for $\hat{\boldsymbol{\theta}}_M$; i.e., optimize the (log) product of both terms on the right hand side of eqn. 1.1, rather than only the likelihood function. Apart from the change of objective function, the process of estimation remains quite similar. Indeed, hard constraints, such as $0 \le \alpha \le 1$, are equivalent to a uniform prior over a fixed range, but soft constraints (which assign, say, decreasing prior likelihood to larger parameter values in a graded manner) are equally possible in this framework. Of course, it is hard to know how to select a prior in an objective manner. One empirical source for a prior at the level of the individual is the behavior of others in the population from which the individual was drawn, a point to which we return in the next section.

In summary, parameter estimation via nonlinear function approximation is feasible but finicky. Program crashes and odd parameter estimates are common due to issues such as numerical stability and parameter boundaries. We have discussed a number of practical suggestions for minimizing problems, but the most important point is simply that the process is not as automatic as it sounds: it requires ongoing monitoring and tuning.

1.3.3 Intersubject variability and random effects

Typically, a dataset will include a number of subjects. Indeed, often questions of scientific interest involve characterizing a population—do students, on average, have nonzero learning rates in a subliminal learning task (Pessiglione et al., 2008)?—or comparing two populations—for instance, do Parkinson's disease patients exhibit a lower learning rate than healthy controls (Frank et al., 2004)? How do we extend the methods outlined above to incorporate multiple subjects and answer population-level questions?

1.3.3.1 Fixed-effects analysis

One obvious approach, which we generally do not advocate, is simply to aggregate likelihoods not just across trials, but also across subjects, and to estimate a single set of parameters $\hat{\theta}_M$ that optimize the likelihood of the entire dataset. Such an analysis treats the data from all subjects as though they were just more data from a single subject. That is, it treats the estimated parameters as fixed effects, quantities that do not vary across subjects (Fig. 1.2a). Of course, this is unlikely to be the case. Indeed, the variability between subjects in a population is precisely what is relevant to answering statistical questions about the population. (Do college students have a nonzero learning rate? Do Parkinson's patients learn slower than controls?) For population-level questions, treating parameters as fixed effects, and thereby conflating within- and between-subject variability, can lead to serious problems such as overstating the true significance of results. This issue is familiar in fMRI data analysis (Holmes and Friston, 1998; Friston et al., 2005) but less so in other areas of psychology and neuroscience.

1.3.3.2 Summary statistics approach

An often more appropriate, but equally simple procedure, is for n subjects separately to estimate a set of maximum likelihood parameters for each subject. Then we may test the mean value of a parameter or compare groups using (e.g.) a one- or two-sample t-test on the estimates. Intuitively, such a procedure seems reasonable. It treats each parameter estimate as a random variable (a random effect), and essentially asks what value one would expect to estimate if one were to draw a new subject from the population, then repeat the entire experiment and analysis. This summary statistics procedure is widely used, and this use is at least partly justified by a formal relationship with the more elaborate statistical model laid out next (Holmes and Friston, 1998; Friston et al., 2005). However, note one odd feature of this procedure: it ignores the within-subject error bars on each subject's parameter estimates.

1.3.3.3 Hierarchical model of population

We can clarify these issues by extending our approach of modeling the data-generation process explicitly to incorporate a model of how parameters vary across the population

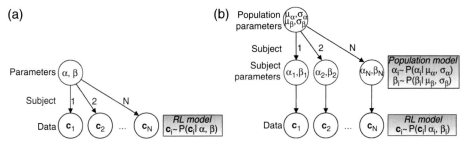

Fig. 1.2 Models of population data. (a) Fixed effects: model parameters are shared between subjects. (b) Random effects: each subject's parameters are drawn from a common population distribution.

(Fig. 1.2b; Penny and Friston, 2004). Suppose that when we recruit a subject i from a population, we also draw a set of parameters (e.g., α_i and β_i) according to some statistical distributions that characterize the distribution of parameters in the population. Perhaps β_i is Gaussian-distributed with some mean μ_β and standard deviation σ_β. We denote this Gaussian as: $P(\beta_i | \mu_\beta, \sigma_\beta)$.

Similarly α_i would be given by some other probability distribution. In the examples below, we also assume that $P(\alpha_i | \mu_\alpha, \sigma_\alpha)$ is also Gaussian. An alternative reflecting the (potentially problematic) assumption of bounds on α (i.e., $0 < \alpha < 1$) is instead to assume a distribution with support only in this range. The parameter might be distributed, for instance, as a beta distribution or as a Gaussian: $x_i \sim N(\mu_\alpha, \sigma_\alpha)$ transformed through a logistic function,

$$\alpha_i = \frac{1}{1 + \exp(-x_i)}.$$

Structural questions about which sort of distribution to use are ultimately *model selection* questions, which can be addressed through the methods discussed in Section 1.4.

Adopting a model of the parameters in the population gives us a two-level *hierarchical* model of how a full dataset is produced (Fig. 1.2): Each subject's parameters are drawn from population distributions, then the Q values and the observable choice data are generated, as before, according to an RL model with those parameters. Usually, the parameters of interest are those characterizing the population (e.g. μ_α, σ_α, μ_β, and σ_β); for instance, it is these that we would like to compare between different populations to study whether Parkinson's disease affects learning. The full equation that relates these population-level parameters to a particular subject's choices, c_i, is then the probability given to them by the RL model, here abbreviated: $P(c_i | \alpha_i, \beta_i)$, averaged over all possible settings of the individual subject's parameters according to their population distribution:

$$P(c_i | \mu_\alpha, \mu_\beta, \sigma_\alpha, \sigma_\beta) = \int d\alpha_i \, d\beta_i P(\alpha_i | \mu_\alpha, \sigma_\alpha) P(\beta_i | \mu_\beta, \sigma_\beta) P(c_i | \alpha_i, \beta_i) \quad (1.5)$$

This formulation emphasizes that individual parameters α_i and β_i intervene between the observable quantity and the quantity of interest, but from the perspective of drawing inferences about the population parameters, they are merely nuisance variables to be averaged out. The probability of a full dataset consisting of choice sets $c_1 \ldots c_N$ for N subjects is just the product over subjects:

$$P(c_1 \ldots c_N | \mu_\alpha, \mu_\beta, \sigma_\alpha, \sigma_\beta) = \prod_i P(c_i | \mu_\alpha, \mu_\beta, \sigma_\alpha, \sigma_\beta) \quad (1.6)$$

We can then use Bayes' rule to recover the population parameters in terms of the full dataset:

$$P(\mu_\alpha, \mu_\beta, \sigma_\alpha, \sigma_\beta | c_1 \ldots c_N) \propto P(c_1 \ldots c_N | \mu_\alpha, \mu_\beta, \sigma_\alpha, \sigma_\beta) P(\mu_\alpha, \mu_\beta, \sigma_\alpha, \sigma_\beta) \quad (1.7)$$

1.3.3.4 Estimating population parameters in a hierarchical model

Equation 1.7 puts us in a position, in principle, to estimate the population parameters from the set of all subjects' choices, using maximum likelihood or maximum a posteriori methods, exactly as discussed for individual subjects in the previous section. Confidence intervals on these parameters (from the inverse Hessian) allow between-group comparisons. This would require programming a likelihood function that returns the (log) probability of given choices over a population of subjects, given the four population-level parameters (eqn. 1.6). This, in turn, requires averaging, for each individual subject, over possible sets of values for that subject's parameters according to eqn. 1.5 and then aggregating results over subjects. Such a function could then be optimized as before, using a nonlinear function optimizer, such as `fmincon`.

The difficulty with this approach, in practice, is that the integral in eqn. 1.5 is intractable, so it must be approximated in some way to compute the likelihood. One possibility is via sampling, e.g., by drawing k (say, 10,000) settings of the parameters for each subject according to the distributions $P(\alpha_i|\mu_\alpha, \sigma_\alpha)$ and $P(\beta_i|\mu_\beta, \sigma_\beta)$, then averaging over these samples to approximate the integral as:

$$\frac{1}{k} \cdot \sum_{j=1}^{k} P(c_i | \alpha_j, \beta_j).$$

One practical issue here is that optimization routines, such as `fmincon`, require the likelihood function to change smoothly as they adjust the parameters. Sampling a set of individual subject parameters anew for each setting of the population parameters the optimizer tries can therefore cause problems, but this can generally be addressed by using the same underlying random numbers at each evaluation (i.e., resetting the random seed to the same value each time the likelihood function is evaluated; Ng and Jordan, 2000; Bhat, 2001).

1.3.3.5 Estimating population parameters via summary statistics

Suppose that we know the true values of the individual subject parameters α_i and β_i: for instance, suppose we could estimate these perfectly from the choices. In this case, we could estimate the population parameters directly from the subject parameters, since eqn. 1.7 reduces to: $P(\mu_\alpha, \sigma_\alpha | \alpha_1...\alpha_N) \propto \prod_i [P(\alpha_i | \mu_\alpha, \sigma_\alpha)] \cdot P(\mu_\alpha, \sigma_\alpha)$, and similarly for β_i. Moreover, assuming the distributions $P(\alpha_i|\mu_\alpha, \sigma_\alpha)$ and $P(\beta_i|\mu_\beta, \sigma_\beta)$ are Gaussian, then finding the population parameters for these expressions is just the familiar problem of estimating a Gaussian distribution from samples. In particular, the population means and variances can be estimated in the normal way by the sample statistics. Importantly, we could then compare the estimated mean parameters between groups or (within a group) against a constant using standard t-tests. Note that in this case, since the parameter estimates arise from an average of samples, confidence intervals can be derived from the sample standard deviation divided by the square root of the number of samples, i.e., the familiar standard error of the mean in Gaussian estimation. We need not use the Hessian of the underlying likelihood function in this case.

We can thus interpret the two-stage summary statistics procedure discussed above, as an approximate estimation strategy for the hierarchical model of Fig. 1.2b, and an alternative to the strategy of direct maximum likelihood estimation discussed above. In particular, the procedure would be correct for Gaussian distributed parameters, if the uncertainty about the within-subject parameters were negligible. What is the effect of using this as an approximation when this uncertainty is instead substantial, as when the parameters were estimated from individual subject model fits? Intuitively, the within-subject estimates will be jittered with respect to their true values due to estimation noise. We might imagine (and in some circumstances, it is indeed the case) that in computing the population means, μ_α and μ_β, this jitter will average out and the resulting estimates will be unbiased. However, the estimation noise in the individual parameter estimates will *inflate* the estimated population variances beyond their true values (Fig. 1.3).

What mostly matters for our purposes is the validity of t-tests and confidence intervals on the estimated population means. For some assumptions about the first-level estimation process, Holmes and Friston (1998) demonstrate that for t-tests and confidence intervals, the inflation in the population variance is expected to be of just the right amount to compensate for the unaccounted uncertainty in the subject-level parameters. While this argument is unlikely to hold exactly for the sorts of computational models considered here, it also seems that this procedure is relatively insensitive to violations of

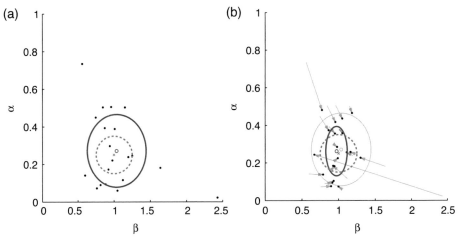

Fig. 1.3 (a) Estimating population parameters via summary statistics. Learning parameters for 20 simulated subjects from the bivariate Gaussian distribution with mean shown with "×" and standard deviation shown as a dotted ellipse. 1000 choice trials for each subject were simulated, and the model fit to each individual by maximum likelihood. The individual fits are shown as dots, and their summary statistics are shown with an "o" (mean) and a solid ellipse (standard deviation). Here, the population mean is well estimated, but the population variance is inflated. (b) Parameters for the simulated subjects were re-estimated by maximum a posteriori taking the population summary statistics from part a (thin, gray ellipse) as a prior. Estimates are pulled toward the population mean. Summary statistics for the new estimates are shown with an "o" and a solid ellipse.

the assumptions (Friston et al., 2005). Thus, these considerations provide at least partial justification for use of the summary statistics procedure.

1.3.3.6 Estimating individual parameters in a hierarchical model

Though we have so far treated them as nuisance variables, in some cases, the parameter values for an individual in a population may be of interest. The hierarchical model also provides insight into estimating these, while taking into account the characteristics of the population from which the individual was drawn (Friston and Penny, 2003). Assuming we know the population level parameters, Bayes' rule specifies that:

$$P(\alpha_i, \beta_i \mid c_i, \mu_\alpha, \mu_\beta, \sigma_\alpha, \sigma_\beta) \propto P(c_i \mid \alpha_i, \beta_i) P(\alpha_i, \beta_i \mid \mu_\alpha, \mu_\beta, \sigma_\alpha, \sigma_\beta). \tag{1.8}$$

Here again, we might make use of this equation as an approximation, even if we have only an estimate of the population parameters, ignoring the uncertainty in that estimate.

Equation 1.8 takes the form of eqn. 1.1: $P(c_i \mid \alpha_i, \beta_i)$ is just the familiar likelihood of the subject's choice sequence given the parameters, but playing the role of the prior is $P(\alpha_i, \beta_i \mid \mu_\alpha, \mu_\beta, \sigma_\alpha, \sigma_\beta) = P(\alpha_i \mid \mu_\alpha, \sigma_\alpha) P(\beta_i \mid \mu_\beta, \sigma_\beta)$, the population distribution of the parameters. This equation thus suggests a procedure for determining a prior over a subject's parameters from other, empirical data: the distribution of the parameters in the population from which the subject was drawn.

If we estimate (or re-estimate) the subject's parameters by maximizing eqn. 1.8, then the estimated parameters will be drawn toward the group means, reflecting the fact that the data for other subjects in a population are also relevant to estimating a subject's parameters (Fig. 1.3b). Thus, in the context of a hierarchical model, the combination of prior and likelihood in Bayes' rule specifies exactly how to balance this population information with data about the individual in estimating parameters.

1.3.4 Summary and recommendations

For most questions of interest, it is important to treat model parameters as random effects, so as to enable statistical conclusions about the population from which the subjects were drawn. Given such a model, the easy way to estimate it is the summary statistics procedure, and since this is so simple, transparent, and fairly well-behaved, we recommend it as a starting point. The more complex alternative—the fit of a full hierarchical model based on an approximation to eqn. 1.5—is better justified and seems a promising avenue for improvement.

1.3.5 Extensions

The basic procedures outlined above admit of many extensions. Of particular importance is how they may be applied to types of data other than choices.

1.3.5.1 Other types of data

We have conducted the discussion so far in terms of choice data. But an entirely analogous process can be (and has been) applied to many other data sources, such as neural spiking (Platt and Glimcher, 1999; Barraclough et al., 2004; Sugrue et al., 2004) or fMRI measurements (O'Doherty et al., 2003; Wittmann et al., 2008). All that is required, in principle, is to replace the observation model of eqn. 1.3 with one appropriate to the data modality. The viewpoint is that a common learning model (here, eqn. 1.2), may be observed, indirectly, through many different sorts of measurements that it impacts. The observation model provides a generative account of how a particular sort of measurement may be impacted by the underlying learning.

For instance, it is natural to assume that spike rates (or perhaps log spike rates) taken from an appropriate window reflect model variables such as δ_t corrupted by Gaussian noise, e.g.,

$$S_t = \beta_0 + \beta_1 \delta_t + N(0, \sigma) \qquad (1.9)$$

or similarly for value variables, e.g., $Q_t(L)$ or $Q_t(c_t)$. This replaces the logistic regression of model values on to choices with *linear* regression of model values on to spike rates, and unifies the learning model-based approach here with the ubiquitous use of regression to characterize spike responses. Thus, here again, we could estimate not just the magnitude and significance of spiking correlates (β_1 in eqn. 1.9), but also the underlying learning rate parameter α that best explains a time series of per-trial spike rates. Analogous to the case of choice data, while the observation stage of this model terminates in linear regression, parameters in the learning model (here, α) affect the data nonlinearly, so the entire model cannot be fit using a standard regression routine, but instead a nonlinear search must be used. This model of spiking could also be extended hierarchically, analogously to the discussion above, to reason about the characteristics of a population of neurons recorded from a particular region; or even, through another level of hierarchy, regions in multiple animals.

The same linear (or log-linear) observation model can also be used to examine whether reaction times or other behavioral data, such as pupilometry, are modulated by reward expectancy, and if so, to examine the underlying learning process. Approaches of this sort can be used to model learning in behavioral data obtained from Pavlovian experiments (i.e., those involving reward or punishment expectancy without choices; O'Doherty et al., 2003; Seymour et al., 2007). Finally, by fitting a model through both behavioral and neural modalities, it is possible to conduct a neurometric/psychometric comparison (Kable and Glimcher, 2007; Tom et al., 2007; Wittmann et al., 2008).

1.3.5.2 fMRI

A very similar observation model is also common in analyzing fMRI data. This typically involves assuming an underlying time series with impulses of height given by the variable of interest (e.g., δ_t) at appropriate times (e.g., when reward is revealed, with $\delta_t = 0$ otherwise). To produce the BOLD time series measured in a voxel, it is assumed that this impulse time series is convolved with a hemodynamic response filter, and finally scaled and corrupted by additive Gaussian noise, as in eqn. 1.9. The full model might be written:

$$b_t = \beta_0 + \beta_1(\text{HRF} * \delta_t) + N(0, \sigma) . \qquad (1.10)$$

In fact, this observation model (augmented with a hierarchical random effects model over the regression weights, such as β_1, across the population) is identical to the general linear model used in standard fMRI analysis packages, such as SPM. Thus, a standard approach is simply to enter model-predicted time series (e.g., δ or Q) as parametric regressors in such a package (O'Doherty et al., 2003, 2007).

Since these packages implement only the linear-regression stage of the analysis, inference in fMRI tends to focus on simply testing the estimated regression weights (e.g., β_1 from eqn. 1.10) against a null hypothesis of 0, to determine *whether* and *where in the brain* a variable like δ_t is significantly reflected in BOLD time series. Thus, the predictor time series are typically generated with the parameters of the underlying learning model (here, the learning rate α) fixed, e.g., having previously been fit to behavior.

One practical point is that, in our experience (Daw et al., 2006; Schonberg et al., 2007), multisubject fMRI results from analyses of this sort are, in practice, more robust if a single α (and a single set of any other parameters of the learning model) is used to generate regressors for all subjects. A single set of parameters might be obtained from a fixed effect analysis of behavior, or from the population-level parameter means in a random effects analysis. This issue may arise because maximum likelihood parameter estimates are relatively noisy, or because differences in learning model parameters can effectively produce differences between subjects in the scaling of predictor time series, which inflate the variability in their regression weights across the population and suppress the significance of population-level fMRI results.

The approach of using fixed learning parameters rather than fitting them to BOLD data is mandated by efficiency: for whole-brain analyses, a linear regression to estimate β_1 for fixed α is feasible, but conducting a laborious *nonlinear* estimate of α at each of hundreds of thousands of voxels in the brain is computationally infeasible. Of course, if a BOLD time series for a particular voxel or area of interest were isolated, then a full model could be estimated from it using nonlinear optimization, much as described above for spikes, reaction times, or choices.

1.3.5.3 Linearized parameter estimation

Short of a nonlinear fit to a targeted area, it is also possible to use a whole-brain linear regression approach to extract at least some information about the learning model parameters that best explain the BOLD signal (Wittmann et al., 2008). Suppose we compute the prediction error time series δ_t for some relevant choice of α, such as that found from behavior, say 0.5. Denote this $\delta_t(0.5)$. Now we may also compute a second time series $\frac{\partial \delta_t}{\partial \alpha}$: the partial derivative of the prediction error time series with respect to α. For any choice of α, this is another time series. We evaluate it at the same point, here $\alpha = 0.5$ and denote the result as $\delta_t'(0.5)$.

The partial derivative measures how the original regressor time series would change as you move the parameter α infinitesimally away from its starting value of 0.5. Indeed, one can approximate the partial derivative as the difference,

$$\frac{\delta_t(0.5 + \Delta) - \delta_t(0.5)}{\Delta},$$

between the original regressor and that recomputed for a slightly larger learning rate, $\alpha = (0.5 + \Delta)$ for some small Δ; or equivalently, express the regressor for a larger α, $\delta_t (0.5 + \Delta)$ as $\delta_t(0.5)+\Delta\delta_t'(0.5)$.

(The true derivative is just the limit of the difference as $\Delta \to 0$, and can also be computed exactly with promiscuous use of the chain rule of calculus, in a similar manner to the gradient of the likelihood function discussed above.)

We can now approximate $\delta_t(\alpha)$ for any learning rate α as:

$$\delta_t(\alpha) \approx \delta_t(0.5)+(\alpha{-}0.5)\delta_t'(0.5) \qquad (1.11)$$

This *linear* approximation of $\delta_t(\alpha)$ is, formally, the first two terms of a Taylor expansion of the function. Since this approximation is linear in α, we can estimate it using linear regression, e.g., using a standard fMRI analysis package. In particular, if we include the partial derivative as an additional regressor in our analysis, so that we are modeling the BOLD time series in a voxel as $b_t = \beta_0 + \beta_1(\mathrm{HRF} * \delta_t(0.5)) + \beta_2(\mathrm{HRF} * \delta_t'(0.5)) + N(0,\sigma)$, then the estimate of β_2—the coefficient for the partial derivative of the regressor—is an estimate of α under the linearized approximation, since it plays the same role as $(\alpha - 0.5)$ in eqn. 1.11. Normalizing by the overall effect size, the estimate of α is:

$$\frac{\hat{\beta}_2}{\hat{\beta}_1} + 0.5$$

However, since the linear approximation is poor, it would be unwise to put too much faith in the particular numerical value estimated by this method. Instead, this approach is most useful for simply testing whether the α that best explains the data is greater or less than the chosen value (here, 0.5), by testing whether β_2 is significantly positive or negative. It can also be used for testing whether neural estimates of α covary, across subjects, with some other factor (Wittmann et al., 2008).

A very similar approach is often used in fMRI to capture the (nonlinear) effects of intersubject variation in the hemodynamic response filter (Friston et al., 1998).

1.3.5.4 Other learning models

Clearly, the learning model itself (eqn. 1.2) could also be swapped with another as appropriate to a task or hypothesis; for instance, one with more free parameters or a different learning rule. Again the basic strategy described above is unchanged. In Section 1.4, we consider the question of comparing which of several candidate models is a better account for data.

1.3.5.5 Other population models

Above, we assumed that individual subject parameters followed simple distributions, such as a unimodal Gaussian, $P(\beta_i | \mu_\beta, \sigma_\beta)$.

This admits of many extensions. First, subjects might cluster into several types. This can be captured using a multimodal *mixture model* of the parameters (Camerer and Ho, 1998), e.g., in the two-type case: $\pi_1 N(\mu_{\alpha 1}, \sigma_{\alpha 1})N(\mu_{\beta 1}, \sigma_{\beta 1})+(1-\pi_1)N(\mu_{\alpha 2}, \sigma_{\alpha 2})N(\mu_{\beta 2}, \sigma_{\beta 2})$.

Parameters μ_{α_1} and so on can be estimated to determine what the modes are that best fit the data; π_1 controls the predominance of subject type 1; and the question how many types of subjects do the data support is a model selection question, answerable by the methods discussed in Section 1.4.

A separate question is whether intersubject parametric variability can be explained or predicted via factors other than random variation (Wittmann et al., 2008). For instance, perhaps IQ predicts learning rate. If we have separately measured each subject's IQ, IQ_i, then we might test this hypothesis by estimating a hierarchical model with additional IQ effects in the generation of learning rates, such as: $P(\alpha_i \mid \mu_\alpha, \sigma_\alpha, \kappa_{IQ}, IQ_i) = N(\mu_\alpha + \kappa_{IQ} IQ_i, \sigma_\alpha)$.

Here, the parameter κ_{IQ} controls the strength of the hypothesized linear effect. This parameter can be estimated (and the null hypothesis that it equals zero can be tested) using the same methods discussed above.

1.3.5.6 Parametric nonstationarity

Finally, we have assumed that model parameters are stationary throughout an experimental session, which is unlikely actually to be the case in many experiments. For instance, in a two-armed bandit problem in which one option pays off 40% of the time and the other pays off 60% of the time, subjects may figure out which option is better and then choose it more or less exclusively. In the model we have considered, a constant setting of the parameters often cannot account for such behavior—for instance, a high learning rate promotes rapid acquisition but subsequent instability; a learning rate slow enough to explain why subjects are asymptotically insensitive to feedback would also predict slow acquisition. In all, fast acquisition followed by stable choice of the better option might be modeled with a decrease over trials in the learning rate, perhaps combined with an increase in the softmax temperature. (This example suggests that, here again, the interrelationship between estimated parameters introduces complexity, here in characterizing and analyzing their separate change over time.)

Three approaches have been used to deal with parametric nonstationarity. The approach most consistent with the outlook of this review is to specify a computational theory of the dynamics of free parameters, perhaps itself parameter-free or expressed in terms of more elementary parameters that are expected to be stationary (Behrens et al., 2007). Such a theory can be tested, fit, and compared using the same methods discussed here. For instance, as already mentioned, the Kalman filter model (Kakade and Dayan, 2002) generalizes the model of eqn. 1.2 and specifies a particular learning rate for each trial. The coupling between softmax temperature and learning rate is one pitfall in testing such a theory, since if we treat the temperature as constant in order to test the model's account of variability in the learning rate, then changes in the temperature will not be accounted for and may masquerade as changes in the learning rate.

In lieu of a bona fide theory from first principles of a parameter's dynamics, one can specify a more generic parametrized account of changing parameters (Camerer and Ho, 1998). Note, of course, that we can't simply fit a separate free temperature β_t for each trial, since that would involve as many free parameters as data points. But we can specify some functional form for change using a few parameters. For instance, perhaps β ramps up or down linearly, so that:

$$\beta_t = \beta_{start} + \frac{(\beta_{end} - \beta_{start})t}{T}.$$

Here, the constant parameter β is replaced with two parameters, which can be fit as before. Another possibility (Samejima et al., 2004) is to use a Gaussian random walk, e.g., $\beta_{t=1} = \beta_{start}$; $\beta_{t+1} = \beta_t + \varepsilon_t$; ε_t: $N(0, \sigma_\varepsilon)$, which also has two free parameters, β_{start} and σ_ε. Note, however, that this model is difficult to fit. Given only a setting for the free parameters, β_t is not determined, since its dynamics are probabilistic. Thus, computing the data likelihood for any individual subject requires averaging over many different possible random trajectories of $\beta_1 \ldots \beta_T$, much as we did for different subject-specific parameters in eqn. 1.5.

A final approach to dealing with parametric nonstationarity is to design tasks in an attempt to minimize it (Daw et al., 2006). Returning to the example of the bandit problem, if the payoff probabilities for the two bandits were not fixed, but instead diffused slightly and randomly from trial to trial, then, ideally, instead of settling on a machine and ceasing to learn, subjects would have to continue learning about the value of the machines on each trial. Intuitively, if the speed of diffusion is constant from trial to trial, this might motivate relatively smooth learning, i.e., a nearly constant learning rate. Formally, ideal observer models such as the Kalman filter (Kakade and Dayan, 2002) predict that learning rates should be asymptotically stable in tasks similar to this one.

1.4 Model comparison

So far, we have assumed a fixed model of the data and sought to estimate its free parameters. A second question that may be addressed by related methods is to what extent the data support different candidate models.

In neural studies, model comparisons have often played a supporting role for parametric analyses of the sort discussed in Section 1.3, since comparing a number of candidate models can help to validate or select the model whose parameters are being estimated. More importantly, many questions of scientific interest are themselves naturally framed in terms of model selection. In particular, models like that of eqn. 1.2 and its alternatives constitute different hypotheses about the mechanisms or algorithms that the brain uses to solve RL problems. These hypotheses can be compared against one another based on their fit to data.

Such an analysis can formally address questions about methods of valuation: for instance, do subjects really make decisions by directly learning a net value for each action, in the manner of eqn. 1.2, or do they instead evaluate actions indirectly by learning more fundamental facts about the task and reasoning about them? (In RL, the latter approach is known as "model-based" learning; Daw et al., 2005.) They can also assess refinements to a model or its structure: for instance, are there additional influences on action choice above the effect of reward posited by eqn. 1.2? Analogous analyses may also be applied to assess parts of the data model other than the learning itself; for instance the observation model (are spike counts well described as linear or do they saturate?) or the population model (are there multiple subtypes of subject or a single cluster?).

How well a model fits data depends on the settings of its free parameters; moreover, blindly following the approach to parameter optimization from the previous section will not produce a useful answer to the model-selection question, since, in general, the more free parameters a model has, the better will be its fit to data at the maximum likelihood point. The methods discussed below address this problem.

In some cases, questions of interest might be framed either in terms of parameter estimation or model selection, and thus addressed using either the methods of the previous or the current situation. For instance, categorical structural differences can sometimes be recast as graded parametric differences (as in "automatic relevance determination"; MacKay, 2003). In general, since the methods in both sections all arise from basically similar reasoning (mainly, the fanatical use of Bayes' rule) in a common framework, similar questions framed in both ways should yield similar results.

1.4.1 Examples from reinforcement learning (RL)

We illustrate the issues of model selection using some simple alternatives to the model of choice behavior discussed thus far. In fact, the practical ingredients for model evaluation are basically the same as those for parameter estimation; as before, what is needed is simply to compute data likelihoods under a model, optimize parameters, and estimate Hessians.

1.4.1.1 Policy and value models

One fundamental issue in RL is the representational question, what is actually learned that guides behavior? In this respect, one important distinction is between value-based models, such as eqn. 1.2 that learn about the values of actions, vs. another family of policy-based algorithms that learn directly about what choice strategies work best (Dayan and Abbott, 2001). In the simple choice setting here, the latter replaces eqn. 1.2 with an update such as:

$$\pi_{t+1}(c_t) = \pi_t(c_t) + (r_t - \bar{r}) \tag{1.12}$$

then chooses as before with

$$P(c_t = L \mid \pi_t(L), \pi_t(R)) = \frac{\exp(\beta \cdot \pi_t(L))}{\exp(\beta \cdot \pi_t(R)) + \exp(\beta \cdot \pi_t(L))} .$$

The learning equation tracks a new variable π_t measuring preference over the alternatives ($\bar{r}$ is a comparison constant often taken to be an average over all received rewards; for simplicity, in the simulations below we took it to be fixed at 0.5, which was the true average). The latter equation is just the softmax choice rule of eqn. 1.3, rewritten in terms of π_t instead of Q_t.

Equation 1.12 hypothesizes a different learning process (that is, a differently constrained form for the relationship between feedback and subsequent choices) than does eqn. 1.2. The interpretation of this difference may seem obscure in this particular class of tasks, where the difference is indeed subtle. The key point is that the model of the previous section estimates the average reward Q expected for each choice, and chooses actions based on the comparison between these value estimates; whereas a model like eqn. 1.12 is obtained by treating the parameters π as generic "knobs" controlling action choice, and then attempts to set the knobs so as to attain as much reward as possible. (See Dayan and Abbott, 2001, chapter 9, for a full discussion.)

One prominent observable difference arising from this distinction is that the policy-based algorithm will ultimately tend to turn the action choice "knobs" as far as possible toward exclusive choice of the richer option ($\pi \to \infty$ for a better than average option), whereas the values Q in the value model asymptote at the true average reward (e.g., 60 cents for an option paying off a dollar 60% of the time). Depending on β (assumed to be fixed), these asymptotic learned values may imply less-than-complete preference for the better option over the worse. This particular prediction is only one aggregate feature of what are, in general, different trial-by-trial hypotheses about learning dynamics. Thus, while it might be possible simply to examine learning curves for evidence that choices asymptote short of complete preference, the difference between models can be assessed more robustly and quantitatively by comparing their fit to raw data in the manner advocated here.

1.4.1.2 Choice autocorrelation

Note also that these models contain different numbers of free parameters: the Q-learning model has two (α and β), while the policy model has only β (treating $\bar{r}$ as given or determined by the received rewards). As already noted, this introduces some difficulty in comparing them. This difficulty is illustrated more obviously by another simple alternative to the Q-learning model, which can be expressed by replacing the softmax rule of eqn. 1.3 with:

$$P(c_t = L \mid Q_t(L), Q_t(R), L_{t-1}, R_{t-1}) = \frac{\exp(\beta \cdot Q_t(L) + \kappa \cdot L_{t-1})}{\exp(\beta \cdot Q_t(R) + \kappa \cdot R_{t-1}) + \exp(\beta \cdot Q_t(L) + \kappa \cdot L_{t-1})} \tag{1.13}$$

Here, L_{t-1} and R_{t-1} are binary indicator variables that take on the values 1 or 0 according to whether the choice on trial $t - 1$ was L or R. The motivation for models of this sort is the observation that, whereas the Q-learning model predicts that choice is driven only by reward history, in choice datasets, there is often significant additional choice autocorrelation (e.g., switching or perseveration) not attributable to the rewards (Lau and Glimcher, 2005). Equation 1.13 thus includes a simple effect of the previous choice, scaled by the new free parameter, κ, for which positive values promote sticking and negative values promote alternation.

1.4.2 Classical model comparison

How can we determine how well each model fits the data? By analogy with parameter fitting, we might consider the probability of the data for some model M_1, evaluated at the maximum likelihood parameters: $P(D|M_1, \hat{\boldsymbol{\theta}})$.

The upside of this is that this is a quantity we know how to compute (it was the entire focus of Section 1.3); the downside is that it provides an inflated measure of how well a model predicts a dataset.

To see this, consider comparing the original Q-learning model (M_1: eqns. 1.2 and 1.3) with the version that includes previous-choice effects (M_2: eqns. 1.2 and 1.13). Note that M_1 is actually a special case of M_2, for $\kappa = 0$. (The models are known as nested.) Since every setting of parameters in M_1 is available in M_2, the maximum likelihood point for M_2 is necessarily at least as good as that for M_1. In particular, even for a dataset that is actually generated according to M_1 (i.e., with $\kappa = 0$), it is highly likely that, due to noise in any particular set of choices (eqn. 1.3) there will be some accidental bias toward perseveration or switching, and thus that the data will be slightly better characterized with a positive or negative κ, producing a higher likelihood for M_2 (Fig. 1.4). This phenomenon is known as overfitting: in general, a more complex model will fit data better than a simpler model, by capturing noise in the data. Of course, we could fit a 300-choice dataset perfectly and trivially with a 300-parameter "model" (one parameter for each choice), but clearly such a model is a poor predictive account of the data.

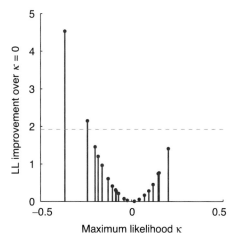

Fig. 1.4 Overfitting: 300 trials each from 20 subjects were simulated using the basic Q-learning model, then fit with the model including an additional parameter κ capturing choice autocorrelation. For each simulated subject, the maximum likelihood estimate for κ is plotted against the difference in log-likelihood between this model and the best fit of the true model with $\kappa = 0$. These differences are always positive, demonstrating overfitting, but rarely exceed the level expected by chance (95% significance level from likelihood ratio test, gray dashed line).

1.4.2.1 Cross-validation

But in what sense is an overfit model worse, if it actually assigns a higher probability to the fit data? One way to capture the problem is to fit a model to one dataset, then compute the likelihood under the previously fit parameters for a *second* dataset generated independently from the same distribution as the original. Intuitively, to the extent a model fit is simply capturing noise in the original dataset, this will hurt rather than help in predicting the second ("holdout," "cross-validation") dataset: by definition, the noise is unlikely to be the same from one dataset to the next. Conversely, a model fits well exactly to the extent that it captures the repeatable aspects of the data, allowing good predictions of additional datasets. This procedure allows models with different numbers of parameters to be compared on equal footing, on the basis of the likelihood of the holdout data: the holdout likelihood score is not inflated by the number of parameters in the model, since in any case *zero* parameters are fit to the second dataset.

In some areas of neuroscience—notably multivoxel fMRI pattern analyses (Norman et al., 2006)—this "cross-validation" procedure is the predominant method to assess and compare model fit. In contrast, it has rarely been used in studies of reinforcement learning (though see Camerer and Ho, 1999). We do not recommend it in this area, mainly because it is difficult in time series data to define a second dataset that is truly independent of the first. Additionally, there are concerns about whether split datasets (e.g., train on early trials and test on late trials) are really identically distributed due to the possibility that subjects' parameters are changing.

1.4.2.2 Likelihood ratio test

Let us consider again the likelihood of a single dataset, using best-fitting parameters. It turns out that while this metric is inflated, it is still useful, because the degree of inflation can in some cases be quantified. Specifically, it is possible to assess how likely is a particular level of improvement in a model's fit to data, if this were due to adding only superfluous parameters and fitting noise (Fig. 1.4, dashed line). For the particular case of nested models, this allows us to estimate the probability of the observed data under the null hypothesis that the data are actually due to the simpler model, and thus (if this P-value is low) reject simpler model with confidence. The resulting test is called the likelihood ratio test, and is very common in regression analysis. To carry it out, fit both a complex model, M_2, and a simpler nested model, M_1, to the same dataset, and compute twice the difference in log likelihoods, $d = 2 \cdot [\log P(D|M_2, \hat{\boldsymbol{\theta}}_{M_2}) - \log P(D|M_1, \hat{\boldsymbol{\theta}}_{M_1})]$. (Since M_2 nests M_1, this difference will be positive or zero.) The probability of a particular difference d arising under M_1 follows a chi-square distribution with a number of degrees of freedom equal to the number, n, of additional parameters in M_2; so the P-value of the test (a difference d or larger arising due to chance) is one minus the chi-square cumulative distribution at d. (In Matlab, the P-value is `1-chi2cdf(d,n)` and the critical d value for 95% significance is `chi2inv(.95,n)`.)

This test cannot be used to compare models that are not nested in one another, such as the value and policy RL models of eqns. 1.2 and 1.12. For this application, and to develop more intuition for the problems of overfitting and model comparison, we turn to Bayesian methods.

1.4.3 Bayesian model comparison in theory

1.4.3.1 Model evidence

In general, we wish to determine the posterior probability of a model M, given data D. By Bayes' rule:

$$P(M|D) \propto P(D|M)P(M) \tag{1.14}$$

The key quantity here is $P(D|M)$, known as the *model evidence*: the probability of the data under the model. Importantly, this expression does not make reference to any particular parameter settings, such as $\hat{\boldsymbol{\theta}}_M$, since in asking how well a model predicts data we are not given any particular parameters. This is why the score examined above, $P(D|M,\hat{\boldsymbol{\theta}}_M)$, is inflated by the number of free parameters: it takes as *given* parameters that are in fact *fit* to the data. That is, in asking how well a model predicts a dataset, it is a fallacy, having seen the data, to retrospectively choose the parameters that would have best fit it. This overstates the ability of the model to predict the dataset. Comparing models according to $P(D|M)$, instead, avoids overfitting.

Instead, the possible values of the model parameters are in this instance (as in others we have seen before) nuisance quantities that must be averaged out according to their probability *prior to examining the data*, $P(\boldsymbol{\theta}_M | M)$.

That is:

$$P(D|M) = \int d\boldsymbol{\theta}_M P(D|M,\boldsymbol{\theta}_M)P(\boldsymbol{\theta}_M | M) \tag{1.15}$$

1.4.3.2 The "automatic Occam's razor"

Another way to see that comparing models according to eqn. 1.14 is immune to overfitting, is to note that this equation incorporates a preference for simpler models. One might assume that this could be incorporated by simply assuming such a preference in $P(M)$, the prior over models, but in fact, it arises automatically due to the other term, $P(D|M)$ (MacKay, 2003). $P(D|M)$ is a probability distribution, so over all possible datasets, it must sum to 1: $\int dD \cdot P(D|M) = 1$.

This means that a more flexible model (one with more parameters that is able to achieve good fit to many datasets with different particular parameter settings) must correspondingly assign lower $P(D|M)$ to all of them since a fixed probability of 1 is divided among them all. Conversely, an inflexible model will fit only a few datasets well, and $P(D|M)$ will be higher for those datasets. Effectively, the normalization of $P(D|M)$ imposes a penalty on more complex and flexible models (MacKay, 2003).

1.4.3.3 Bayes factors

The result of a Bayesian model comparison is a statistical claim about the relative fit of one model over another. When comparing two models, a standardized measure of their relative fit is the Bayes factor, defined as ratio of their posterior probabilities (Kass and Raftery, 1995):

$$\frac{P(M_1 \mid D)}{P(M_2 \mid D)} = \frac{P(D \mid M_1)P(M_1)}{P(D \mid M_2)P(M_2)}. \tag{1.16}$$

(Here the denominator from Bayes rule, which we have anyway been ignoring, actually cancels out.) The log of the Bayes factor is symmetric: positive values favor M_1 and negative values favor M_2. Although Bayes factors are not the same as classical P values, they can loosely be interpreted in a similar manner. A Bayes factor of 20 (or a log Bayes factor of about 3) corresponds to 20:1 evidence in favor of M_1, which is similar to $P = 0.5$. Kass and Raftery (1995) present a table of conventions for interpreting Bayes factors; note that their logs are taken in base-10 rather than base-e.

1.4.4 Bayesian model comparison in practice

The theory of Bayesian model selection is a very useful conceptual framework; for instance, it clarifies why the maximum likelihood score is an inappropriate metric for model comparison. However, actually using these methods in practice poses two problems. The first is one we have already encountered repeatedly: the integral in eqn. 1.15 is intractable, and it must be approximated, as discussed below.

1.4.4.1 Priors

The second problem, which is different here, is the centrality of the prior over parameters, $P(\boldsymbol{\theta}_M|M)$ to the analysis. We have mostly ignored priors thus far, because their subjective nature arguably makes them problematic in the context of objective scientific communication. However, in the analysis above, the prior over parameters controls the average in eqn. 1.15. What it means, on the view we have described, to ask how well a model predicts data, parameter-free, is to ask how well it predicts data, averaged and weighted over the possible parameter settings. For this purpose, specifying a model necessarily includes specifying the admissible range of parameters for this average and their weights, i.e., the prior. The choice also affects the answer: the "spread" of the prior controls the degree of implicit penalty for free parameters that the automatic Occam's razor imposes (see MacKay, 2003, chapter 28, for a full discussion). For instance, a fully specified parameter (equivalent to a prior with support at only one value) is not free and does not contribute a penalty; as the prior admits of more possible parameter settings, the model becomes more complex. Moreover, because we are taking a weighted average over parameter settings, and not simply maximizing over them, simply ignoring the prior as before is often not mathematically well behaved.

Thus, most of the methods discussed below do require assuming a prior over parameters. Only the simplest method, BIC, ignores this.

1.4.4.2 Sampling

One approach to approximating the integral of 15 is, as before, by sampling. In the simplest case, one would draw candidate parameter settings according to $P(\boldsymbol{\theta}_M|M)$; compute the data likelihood $P(D|M,\boldsymbol{\theta}_M)$ for each, and average. This process does not involve any optimization, only evaluating the likelihood at randomly chosen points. Naive sampling of this sort can perform poorly if the number of model parameters is large. See MacKay (2003) and Bishop (2006) for discussion of more elaborate sampling techniques that attempt to cope with this situation.

1.4.4.3 Laplace approximation

A very useful shortcut for the integral of eqn. 1.15 is to approximate the function being integrated with a Gaussian, for which the integral can then be computed analytically. In particular, we can characterize the likelihood surface around the maximum a posteriori parameters $\hat{\boldsymbol{\theta}}_M$ as a Gaussian centered on that point. (This is actually the same approximation that motivates the use of the inverse Hessian H^{-1} for error bars on parameters in Section 1.3.)

This *Laplace approximation* results in the following expression:

$$\log(P(D|M)) \approx \log(P(D|M,\hat{\boldsymbol{\theta}}_M)) + \log(P(\hat{\boldsymbol{\theta}}_M|M)) + \tfrac{n}{2}\log(2\pi) - \tfrac{1}{2}\log|H| \qquad (1.17)$$

where n is the number of parameters in the model and $|H|$ is the determinant of the Hessian (which captures the covariance of the Gaussian). The great thing about this approximation is that we already know how to compute all the elements; they are just what we used in Section 1.3. One bookkeeping issue here is that this equation is in terms of the MAP parameter estimate (including the prior), rather than the maximum likelihood. In particular, here $\hat{\boldsymbol{\theta}}_M$ refers to the setting of parameters that maximizes the first two terms of eqn. 1.17, not just the first one. Similarly, H is the Hessian of the function being optimized (minus the sum of the first two terms of eqn. 1.17), evaluated at the MAP point, not the Hessian of just the log likelihood.

Equation 1.17 can thus be viewed as the maximum (actually MAP) likelihood score, but penalized with an additional factor (the last two terms) that corrects for the inflation of this quantity that was discussed in Section 1.4.2.

1.4.4.4 BIC and cousins

A simpler approximation, which can be obtained from eqn. 1.17 in a limit of large data, is the Bayesian Information Criterion (BIC; Schwarz, 1978). This is:
$\log(P(D|M)) \approx \log(P(D|M,\hat{\boldsymbol{\theta}}_M)) - \tfrac{n}{2}\log m,$

where m is the number of datapoints (e.g., choices). This is also a penalized likelihood score (the penalty is given by the second term), but it does not depend on the prior over parameters and can instead be evaluated for $\hat{\boldsymbol{\theta}}_M$ being the maximum likelihood parameters. The neglect of a prior, while serendipitous from the perspective of scientific communication, seems also somewhat dubious given the entirely crucial role of the prior discussed above. Also, counting datapoints m and particularly free parameters n can be subtle; importantly, the fit of a free parameter should really only be penalized to the extent it actually contributes to explaining the data (e.g., a parameter that has no effect on observable data is irrelevant; other parameters may be only loosely constrained by the data; MacKay, 2003). The last term of the Laplace approximation accounts properly for this by factoring in the uncertainty in the posterior parameter estimates, while parameter-counting approaches like BIC or the likelihood ratio test do not. This can produce notably better results (Fig. 1.5).

Finally, other penalized scores for model comparison exist. The most common is the Akaike Information Criterion (AIC; Akaike, 1974): $\log(P(D|M,\hat{\boldsymbol{\theta}}_M))-n$.

Although this has a similar form to BIC, we do not advocate its use since it does not arise from an approximation to $\log(P(D|M))$, and thus cannot be used to approximate Bayes factors (eqn. 1.16), which seem the most reasonable and standard metric to report.

1.4.5 Summary and recommendations

Models may be compared to one another on the basis of the likelihood they assign to data; however, if this likelihood is computed at parameters chosen to optimize it, the measure

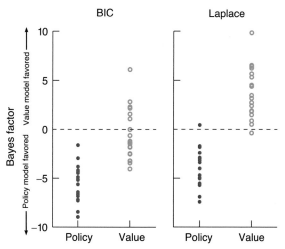

Fig. 1.5 Model comparison with complexity penalties: 300 choice trials each from 20 subjects were simulated using the one-parameter policy model (solid dots) and the two-parameter value model (open dots); the choices were then fit with both models and Bayes factors comparing the two models were computed according to both BIC and Laplace approximations to the model evidence. (For Laplace, the prior over parameters were taken as uniform over a large range.) BIC (left) overpenalizes the value model for its additional free parameter, and favors the simpler policy model even for many of the simulated value model subjects (open dots below the dashed line); the Laplace approximation not only sets the penalty more appropriately, but it also separates the two sets of subjects more effectively because it takes into account not just the raw number of parameters but also how well they were actually fit for each subject.

must be corrected for overfitting to allow a fair comparison between models with different numbers of parameters. In practice, when models are nested, we suggest using a likelihood ratio test, since this permits reporting a classical *P*-value and is well accepted. When they are not, an approximate Bayes factor can be computed instead; BIC is a simple and widely accepted choice for this, but its usage rests more on convention than correctness. If one is willing to define a prior, and defend it, we suggest exploring the Laplace approximation, which is almost as simple but far better founded.

One important aspect of the Laplace approximation, compared to BIC (and also the likelihood ratio test), is that it does not rely simply on counting parameters. Even if two candidate models have the same number of parameters—and thus scores like BIC are equivalent to just comparing raw likelihoods—the complexity penalty implied by eqn. 1.15 may not actually be the same between them if the two sets of parameters are differently constrained, either a priori or by the data. As in Fig. 1.5, this more accurate assessment can have salutary effects.

1.4.6 Model comparison and populations

So far we have described model comparison mostly in the abstract, with applications to choice data at the single-subject level. But how can we extend them to multisubject data of the sort discussed in Section 1.3.3? There are a number of possibilities, of which the simplest will often suffice.

A first question is whether we treat the choice of model as itself a fixed or random effect. Insofar as the model is a categorical claim about how the brain works, it may often seem natural to assume that there is no variability across subjects in the model identity (as opposed to in its parameters). Thus, model identity is often taken as a fixed effect across subjects. (Note that even if we assume a lack of variability in the true model underlying subjects' behavior, because of noise in the parameters and the choices, every subject might not always appear to be using the same model when analyzed individually.) By Bayes' rule:

$$P(M \mid c_1 ... c_N) \propto P(c_1 ... c_N \mid M)P(M). \tag{1.18}$$

Then one simple approach is to neglect the top level of the subject parameter hierarchy of Fig. 1.2, and instead assume that individual parameters are drawn independently according to some fixed (known or ignored) prior. In this case, the right-hand side of eqn. 1.18 decomposes across subjects, and inference can proceed separately, similar to the summary statistics procedure for parameter estimation:

$$\log[P(c_1 ... c_N \mid M)P(M)] = \sum_i [\log P(c_i \mid M)] + \log P(M).$$

That is, we can just aggregate the probability of the data given the model over each subject's fit (single-subject BIC scores or Laplace-approximated model evidence, for instance: not raw data likelihoods) to compute the model evidence for the full dataset. These aggregates can then be compared between two models to compute a Bayes factor over the population. In this case, it is useful also to report the number of subjects for whom the individual model comparison would give the same answer as that for the population, in order to help verify the assumption that the model is a fixed effect.

The more involved approach to population variability discussed in Section 1.3.3 was to integrate out single-subject parameters according to eqn. 1.5 (e.g., by sampling them), in order to estimate the top-level parameters using the full model of Fig. 1.2. In principle, it is possible to combine this approach with model selection—indeed, this is the only possibility if the models in question are at the population level (e.g., if one is asking how many clusters of subjects there are). In this case, $P(c_1...c_N | M) = \int d\boldsymbol{\theta}_{pop} P(c_1...c_N | M, \boldsymbol{\theta}_{pop}) P(\boldsymbol{\theta}_{pop} | M)$, where $\boldsymbol{\theta}_{pop}$ are the population-level parameters, $\langle \mu_\alpha, \mu_\beta, \sigma_\alpha, \sigma_\beta \rangle$. This integral has the form of eqn. 1.14 and can be approximated in the same way, e.g., with BIC or a Laplace approximation; this, in turn, will involve also computing $P(c_1...c_N | M, \boldsymbol{\theta}_{pop})$, which by eqns. 1.6 and 1.5 involves another integral (over the individual subject parameters) whose approximation was discussed in Section 1.3.3. Note that in this case, the prior that must be assumed is over the population parameters, not directly over the individual parameters.

Finally, one could take the identity of the model as varying over subjects, i.e., as a random effect (Stephan et al., 2009). This involves adding another level to the hierarchy of Fig. 1.2, according to which, for each subject, one of a set of models is drawn with some according to a multinomial distribution (given by new free parameters) and then the model's parameters and the data are drawn as before. Inference about the probability could then proceed analogously to that for other population-level parameters.

Note that one alternative sometimes observed in the literature (Stephan et al., 2009) is summary statistics reported and tested for individual-subject Bayes factors (e.g., "across subjects, model M_1 is favored over M_2 by an average log Bayes factor of 4.1, which is significantly different from zero by a t-test"). Such an approach does not appear to have an obvious analogy with summary statistics for *parameter inference* that would justify its use in terms of a hierarchical population model like that of Fig. 1.2. (The difference is that the hierarchical model of parameters directly specifies intersubject variation over the parameters, which can then be directly estimated by summary statistics on parameter estimates. A hierarchical model parameterizing intersubject variability in *model identity* would imply variability over estimated Bayes factors only in a complex and indirect fashion; thus, conversely, the summary statistics on the Bayes factors don't seem to offer any simple insight into the parameters controlling intersubject variability in model identity.)

1.5 Pitfalls and alternatives

We close this tutorial by identifying some pitfalls, caveats, and concerns with these methods that we think it is important for readers to appreciate.

1.5.1 Why not assess models by counting how many choices they predict correctly?

We have stressed the use of a probabilistic observation model to connect models to data. For choice behavior, an approach that is sometimes used and that may initially seem more intuitive is to optimize parameters (and compare model fit) on the basis of the number of choices correctly predicted (Brandstätter et al., 2006). For instance, given the learning model of eqn. 1.2, we might ask, on each trial, whether the choice c_t is the one with the maximal Q value, and if so score this trial as "correctly predicted" by the model. We might then compare parameters or models on the basis of this score, summed over all trials.

This approach is poor in a number of respects. Because it eschews the use of an overt statistical observation model of the data, this scoring technique forgoes obvious connections to statistical estimation, which are what, we have stressed, permit actual statistical conclusions to be drawn. Similarly, whereas the use of observation models clarifies how the same underlying learning model might be applied in a consistent manner to multiple data modalities, there is no obvious extension of the trial-counting scoring technique to BOLD or spiking data.

Finally, even treated simply as a score for evaluating models or parameters, and not as a tool for statistical estimation, the number of "correctly predicted" choices is still evidently inferior to the probabilistic data likelihood. In particular, because the data likelihood admits the possibility of noise in the choices, it considers a model or a set of parameters to be better when they come closer to predicting a choice properly (for instance, if they assign that choice 45% rather than 5% probability, even when the other choice is nevertheless viewed as more likely). Counting "correct" predictions does not distinguish between these cases.

1.5.2 How can we isolate between-group differences in parameters if parameter estimates are correlated?

As mentioned, even if learning parameters, such as temperature and learning rate, are actually independent from one another (i.e., in terms of their distribution across a population), the estimates of those parameters from data may be correlated due to their having similar expected effects on observable data (Fig. 1.1). This may pose interpretational difficulty for comparing populations, as when attempting to isolate learning deficits due to some neurological disease. For instance, if Parkinson's disease patients actually have a lower learning rate than controls but a normal softmax temperature, and we estimate population distributions for both parameters as discussed in Section 1.3.3, it is possible that their deficit might also partly masquerade as a decreased softmax temperature. However, the question what subset of parameters is fixed or varying across groups is more naturally framed as a structural, model-selection question, which may also be less prone to ambiguities in parameter estimation. Such an analysis would ask whether the pattern of behavior across both populations can best be explained by assuming only one or the other parameter varies (on average) between groups while the other one is shared. In this case, three models (shared mean learning rate, shared mean softmax temperature, neither shared) might be compared.

1.5.3 How well does the model fit?

This is a common question. One suspects it is really meant as another way of asking the question discussed next—is there some other, better model still to be found?—to which there is really no answer. Nevertheless, there are a number of measures of model performance that may be useful to monitor and report. Although it is difficult to conclude much in absolute terms from these measures, if this reporting becomes more common, the field may eventually develop better intuitions about their interpretation.

Data likelihoods (raw or BIC-corrected) are often reported, but these measures are more interpretable if standardized in various ways. First, it is easy to compute the log data likelihood under pure chance. This allows reporting the fractional reduction in this measure afforded by the model (toward zero, i.e., $P(D \mid \theta_M, M) = 1$ or perfect prediction), a statistic known as "pseudo-r^2"(Camerer and Ho, 1999). If R is the log data likelihood under chance (e.g., for 100 trials of a two-choice task, $100 \cdot \log(.5)$) and L is the log likelihood under the fit model, then pseudo-r^2 is $1 - \frac{L}{R}$.

Second, since likelihood measures are typically aggregated across trials, it can be more interpretable to examine the average log likelihood per trial, i.e., $\frac{L}{T}$ for T trials. For choice data, exponentiating this average log likelihood, $\exp(\frac{L}{T})$ produces a probability that is easily interpreted relative to the chance level.

Finally, it is easy to conduct a simple statistical verification that a model fits better than chance. Since every model nests the 0-parameter empty model (which assumes all data are due to chance) a likelihood ratio test can be used to verify that any model exceeds the performance of this one. Better still is to compare the full model against a submodel that contains only any parameters modeling mean response tendencies, nuisance variables, or biases. This is commonly done in regression analysis.

1.5.4 Is there another explanation for a result?

There certainly could be. We may conclude that a model fits the data better than another model (or, assuming a particular model, estimate its parameters) but it seems impossible entirely to rule out the possibility that there is yet another model so far unexamined that would explain the data still better (though see Lau and Glimcher, 2005, for one approach). Although this issue is certainly not unique to this style of analysis, in our experience, authors and readers may be less likely to appreciate it in the context of a model-based analysis, perhaps because of the relatively novel and technical nature of the process.

In fMRI, particularly, the problem of correlated regressors is extremely pernicious. As discussed, many studies have focused on testing whether, and where in the brain, time series generated from computational models correlate significantly with BOLD time series (O'Doherty et al., 2007). These model-generated regressors are complicated and rather opaque objects and may very well be correlated with other factors (for instance, reaction time, time on task, or amount won), which might, in turn, suffice to explain the neural activity.

It is thus important to identify possible confounds and exclude them as factors in explaining the neural signal (e.g., by including them as nuisance regressors). Also, almost certainly, a model-generated signal will be correlated with similar time series that might be generated from other similar models. This points again to the fact that these methods are suited to drawing *relative* conclusions comparing multiple hypotheses (the data support model A over model B). It is tempting to instead employ them in more confirmatory fashion (e.g., interpreting a finding that some model-generated signal loads significantly on BOLD as evidence supporting the correctness of model A in an absolute sense). Sadly, confirmatory reasoning of this sort is common in the literature, but it should be treated with suspicion.

There is no absolute answer to these difficulties, other than paying careful attention to identifying and ruling out confounds in designing and analyzing studies, rather than adopting a confirmatory stance. We also find it particularly helpful, in parallel, to analyze our data using more traditional (non-model-based) methods such as averaging responses over particular kinds of trials, and also to fit more generic models such as pure regression models to test the assumptions of our more structured models (Lau and Glimcher, 2005). Although these methods all have their own serious limitations, they are in some sense more transparent and visualizable; they are rooted in rather different assumptions than model-based analyses and so provide a good double-check; and the mere exercise of trying to identify how to test a model and visualize data by traditional means is useful for developing intuitions about what features of the data a model-based analysis may be picking up.

Ultimately, in our view, the methods of computational model fitting discussed here are exceptionally promising and flexible tools for asking many novel questions at a much more detailed and quantitative level than previously possible. The preceding review aimed to provide readers the tools to apply these methods to their own experimental questions. But like all scientific methods, they are most useful in the context of converging evidence from a range of approaches.

Acknowledgments

This work was supported by a Scholar Award from the McKnight Foundation and Human Frontiers Science Program Grant RGP0036/2009-C. I am very grateful to Peter Dayan, John O'Doherty, Yael Niv, Aaron Bornstein, Sam Gershman, Dylan Simon, and Larry Maloney for many helpful conversations about the issues covered here.

References

Akaike, H. (1974). A new look at the statistical model identification. *IEEE transactions on automatic control*, **19**(6): 716–23.

Barraclough, D.J., Conroy, M.L., and Lee, D. (2004). Prefrontal cortex and decision-making in a mixed-strategy game. *Nature Neuroscience*, **7**(4): 404–10.

Barto, A.G. (1995). Adaptive critics and the basal ganglia. In Houk, J.C., Davis, J.L., and Beiser, D.G. (eds), *Models of information processing in the basal ganglia*, pp. 215–32. MIT Press, Cambridge, MA.

Bayer, H.M. and Glimcher, P.W. (2005). Midbrain dopamine neurons encode a quantitative reward prediction error signal. *Neuron*, **47**: 129–41.

Behrens, T.E.J., Woolrich, M.W., Walton, M.E., and Rushworth, M.F.S. (2007). Learning the value of information in an uncertain world. *Nature Neuroscience*, **10**(9): 1214–21.

Bertsekas, D.P. and Tsitsiklis, J.N. (1996). *Neuro-dynamic programming*. Athena Scientific, Belmont, MA.

Bhat, C. (2001). Quasi-random maximum simulated likelihood estimation of the mixed multinomial logit model. *Transportation Research Part B*, **35**(7): 677–93.

Bishop, C. (2006). *Pattern recognition and machine learning*. Springer, New York.

Brandstätter, E., Gigerenzer, G., and Hertwig, R. (2006). The priority heuristic: making choices without trade-offs. *Psychological Review*, 113(2): 409–32.

Camerer, C. and Ho, T. (1998). Experience-weighted attraction learning in coordination games: probability rules, heterogeneity, and time-variation. *Journal of Mathematical Psychology*, 42(2–3): 305–26.

Camerer, C. and Ho, T. (1999). Experience-weighted attraction learning in games: a unifying approach. *Econometrica*, 67(4): 827–74.

Daw, N.D. and Doya, K. (2006). The computational neurobiology of learning and reward. *Current Opinion in Neurobiology*, 16: 199–204.

Daw, N.D., Niv, Y., and Dayan, P. (2005). Uncertainty-based competition between prefrontal and dorsolateral striatal systems for behavioral control. *Nature Neuroscience*, 8: 1704–11.

Daw, N.D., O'Doherty, J.P., Dayan, P., Seymour, B., and Dolan, R.J. (2006). Cortical substrates for exploratory decisions in humans. *Nature*, 441(7095): 876–9.

Daw, N.D., Courville, A.C., and Dayan, P. (2008). Semi-rational models: The case of trial order. In Chater, N. and Oaksford, M. (eds), *The probabilistic mind*. Oxford University Press.

Dayan, P. and Abbott, L.F. (2001). *Theoretical neuroscience: computational and mathematical modeling of neural systems*. MIT Press, Cambridge, MA.

Dayan, P. and Niv, Y. (2008). Reinforcement learning: the good, the bad and the ugly. *Current Opinion in Neurobiology*, 18(2): 185–96.

Delgado, M.R., Nystrom, L.E., Fissell, C., Noll, D.C., and Fiez, J.A. (2000). Tracking the hemodynamic responses to reward and punishment in the striatum. *Journal of Neurophysiology*, 84: 3072–7.

Frank, M.J., Moustafa, A.A., Haughey, H.M., Curran, T., and Hutchison, K.E. (2007). Genetic triple dissociation reveals multiple roles for dopamine in reinforcement learning. *Proceedings of the National Academy of Sciences of the United States of America*, 104(41): 16311–6.

Frank, M.J., Seeberger, L.C., and O'Reilly, R.C. (2004). By carrot or by stick: cognitive reinforcement learning in Parkinsonism. *Science*, 306(5703): 1940–3.

Freedman, D. (2006). On the so-called "Huber sandwich estimator" and "robust standard errors." *American Statistician*, 60(4): 299–302.

Friston, K.J. and Penny, W. (2003). Posterior probability maps and SPMs. *Neuroimage*, 19(3): 1240–9.

Friston, K.J., Fletcher, P., Josephs, O., Holmes, A., Rugg, M.D., and Turner, R. (1998). Event-related fMRI: characterizing differential responses. *Neuroimage*, 7(1): 30–40.

Friston, K.J., Stephan, K.E., Lund, T.E., Morcom, A., and Kiebel, S. (2005). Mixed-effects and fMRI studies. *Neuroimage*, 24(1): 244–52.

Gelman, A., Carlin, J., and Stern, H. (2004). *Bayesian data analysis*. CRC Press Boca Raton.

Gelman, A. and Hill, J. (2007). *Data analysis using regression and multilevel/hierarchical models*. Cambridge University Press, New York.

Hampton, A.N., Bossaerts, P., and O'Doherty, J.P. (2008). Neural correlates of mentalizing-related computations during strategic interactions in humans. *Proceedings of the National Academy of Sciences of the United States of America*, 105(18): 6741–6.

Hare, T.A., O'Doherty, J., Camerer, C.F., Schultz, W., and Rangel, A. (2008). Dissociating the role of the orbitofrontal cortex and the striatum in the computation of goal values and prediction errors. *Journal of Neuroscience*, 28(22): 5623–30.

Holmes, A. and Friston, K. (1998). Generalisability, random effects and population inference. *Neuroimage*, 7: s754.

Huber, P. (1967). The behavior of maximum likelihood estimates under nonstandard conditions. In *Proceedings of the fifth Berkeley symposium in mathematical statistics*, vol. 1, pp. 221–33.

Kable, J.W. and Glimcher, P.W. (2007). The neural correlates of subjective value during intertemporal choice. *Nature Neuroscience*, 10(12): 1625–33.

Kakade, S. and Dayan, P. (2002). Acquisition and extinction in autoshaping. *Psychological Review*, **109**: 533–44.

Kass, R.E. and Raftery, A.E. (1995). Bayes factors. *Journal of the American Statistical Association*, **90**: 7730–95.

Knutson, B., Westdorp, A., Kaiser, E., and Hommer, D. (2000). FMRI visualization of brain activity during a monetary incentive delay task. *NeuroImage*, **12**: 20–27.

Lau, B. and Glimcher, P.W. (2005). Dynamic response-by-response models of matching behavior in rhesus monkeys. *Journal of the Experimental Analysis of Behavior*, **84**: 555–79.

Li, J., McClure, S.M., King-Casas, B., and Montague, P.R. (2006). Policy adjustment in a dynamic economic game. *PLoS One*, **1**: e103.

Lohrenz, T., McCabe, K., Camerer, C.F., and Montague, P.R. (2007). Neural signature of fictive learning signals in a sequential investment task. *Proceedings of the National Academy of Sciences of the United States of America*, **104**(**22**): 9493–8.

MacKay, D. (2003). *Information theory, inference, and learning algorithms*. Cambridge University Press.

McClure, S.M., Berns, G.S., and Montague, P.R. (2003). Temporal prediction errors in a passive learning task activate human striatum. *Neuron*, **38**(**2**): 339–46.

McFadden, D. (1974). Conditional logit analysis of qualitative choice behavior. In Zarembka, P., (ed.), *Frontiers in econometrics*, pp. 105–42. Academic Press, New York.

Ng, A. and Jordan, M. (2000). PEGASUS: A policy search method for large MDPs and POMDPs. In *Proceedings of the sixteenth Conference on Uncertainty in Artificial Intelligence*, pp. 406–415.

Norman, K.A., Polyn, S.M., Detre, G.J., and Haxby, J.V. (2006). Beyond mind-reading: multi-voxel pattern analysis of fMRI data. *Trends in Cognitive Science*, **10**(**9**): 424–30.

O'Doherty, J.P., Dayan, P., Friston, K., Critchley, H., and Dolan, R.J. (2003). Temporal difference models and reward-related learning in the human brain. *Neuron*, **38**(**2**): 329–37.

O'Doherty, J.P., Hampton, A., and Kim, H. (2007). Model-based fMRI and its application to reward learning and decision-making. *Annuals of the New York Academy of Sciences*, **1104**: 35–53.

Penny, W. and Friston, K. (2004). Hierarchical models. *Human brain function* (2nd edn), pp. 851–63. Elsevier, London.

Pessiglione, M., Petrovic, P., Daunizeau, J., Palminteri, S., Dolan, R.J., and Frith, C.D. (2008). Subliminal instrumental conditioning demonstrated in the human brain. *Neuron*, **59**(**4**): 561–7.

Plassmann, H., O'Doherty, J., Shiv, B., and Rangel, A. (2008). Marketing actions can modulate neural representations of experienced pleasantness. *Proceedings of the National Academy of Sciences of the United States of America*, **105**(**3**): 1050–4.

Platt, M.L. and Glimcher, P.W. (1999). Neural correlates of decision variables in parietal cortex. *Nature*, **400**(*6741*): 233–8.

Samejima, K., Doya, K., Ueda, Y., and Kimura, M. (2004). Estimating internal variables and parameters of a learning agent by a particle filter. *Advances in Neural Information Processing Systems*, **16**, 1335–42.

Samejima, K., Ueda, Y., Doya, K., and Kimura, M. (2005). Representation of action-specific reward values in the striatum. *Science*, **310**(*5752*): 1337–40.

Schonberg, T., Daw, N.D., Joel, D., and O'Doherty, J.P. (2007). Reinforcement learning signals in the human striatum distinguish learners from nonlearners during reward-based decision-making. *Journal of Neuroscience*, **27**(*47*): 12860–7.

Schultz, W., Dayan, P., and Montague, P.R. (1997). A neural substrate of prediction and reward. *Science*, **275**: 1593–99.

Schwarz, G. (1978). Estimating the dimension of a model. *Annals of Statistics*, **6**: 461–4.

Seymour, B., Daw, N., Dayan, P., Singer, T., and Dolan, R. (2007). Differential encoding of losses and gains in the human striatum. *Journal of Neuroscience*, **27**(*18*): 4826–31.

Stephan, K.E., Penny, W.D., Daunizeau, J., Moran, R.J., and Friston, K.J. (2009). Bayesian model selection for group studies. *Neuroimage*, **46**: 1004–17.

Sugrue, L.P., Corrado, G.S., and Newsome, W.T. (2004). Matching behavior and the representation of value in the parietal cortex. *Science*, **304**: 1782–7.

Sutton, R.S. and Barto, A.G. (1998). *Reinforcement learning: an introduction*. MIT Press, Cambridge, MA.

Tom, S.M., Fox, C.R., Trepel, C., and Poldrack, R.A. (2007). The neural basis of loss aversion in decision-making under risk. *Science*, **315**(*5811*): 515–8.

Watkins, C.J.C.H. (1989). *Learning from delayed rewards*. PhD thesis, Cambridge University, Cambridge, England.

Wittmann, B.C., Daw, N.D., Seymour, B., and Dolan, R.J. (2008). Striatal activity underlies novelty-based choice in humans. *Neuron*, **58**(6): 967–73.

Chapter 2

Psychological influences on economic choice: Pavlovian cuing and emotional regulation

Colin F. Camerer

Abstract

In the simplest economic theory, choices depend only on stable preferences among goods, prices and information about those goods, and budgets of money and time. However, many studies show that other factors influence choices through psychological processes that can be understood using different cognitive and neural measures. One factor is a Pavlovian consummatory process, which experimentally increases expressed prices for food objects when the objects are physically proximate. Inserting a plexiglass screen between the subject and the food deactivates the process and reduces value. Another factor is deliberate regulation of emotional reactions to financial outcomes (extending emotional regulation research to economic value). Down-regulating emotional reactions to losing money appears to reliably reduce the expressed "loss-aversion" parameter that accounts for choice patterns. The reduction in loss-aversion inferred from behavior is correlated with changes in skin-conductance response upon loss, compared to gain, which links anticipated aversion to loss and experienced reaction.

Economic theories of choice typically assume three components: (1) people have stable preferences encoded by a utility function; (2) people have information and form beliefs; and (3) people face constraints (typically income, but also money and attention). The predominant paradigm combines these three elements in the form of mathematical constrained optimization: People are assumed to choose a combination of goods that maximize overall utility, given their information, and subject to an income constraint. This paradigm usually produces sharp predictions about relationships that can be tested using field or experimental data. It is sometimes called the "rational actor" or "revealed preference" approach.[1]

The approach is useful because it points to key variables that are likely to influence choices—viz., prices, information, and income. Which variables influence choice is important to describe behavior and to implement changes. If a government wanted to reduce obesity, for example, in the rational actor approach it can only do so by supplying better information about the consequences of eating, taxing unhealthy food or subsidizing healthy food, or changing constraints or (somehow) preferences. Furthermore, there is little doubt that choices do respond to changes in prices, usually in empirically predictable ways.

This chapter is about how other kinds of psychological variables can influence choices. This theme is illustrated with two examples: (1) physical proximity of goods that induces "Pavlovian cuing" and increases economic value of foods; and (2) emotional regulation, which influences choices among risky gambles with possible gains and losses.

The influence of psychological variables is important both for practical reasons (such as discovering a wider variety of ways to change to behavior) and because they provide an empirical tool to develop a mechanistic theory of how exactly the brain is making choices. Developing a mechanistic, behavioral, and mathematical theory of choice and exchange is the goal of "neuroeconomics." This is an unusual and ambitious synthesis because neuroscience has focused mostly on linking behavior and mechanism, and economic theory has focused mostly on linking behavior and mathematical theory. Adding mathematical representation to neuroscience, and adding mechanism to economics are, therefore, big departures from previous practice, which have obvious potential.

The study of psychological influences on choice in economics was invigorated by the "behavioral economics" approach in the 1980s (e.g. Camerer et al., 2004). Behavioral economists imported ideas and methods from psychology to show how limits on rationality, willpower, and greed could make different predictions than the rational actor model and could be integrated into extended models of boundedly rational choice.

The value of behavioral economics comes from the fact that, in practical and empirical applications, economic analyses rest on some hidden assumptions, which are often psychologically implausible.

One assumption is "description-dependence" (no framing effects): what goods people prefer is assumed to be invariant to how those goods are described (unless the description can be considered information, or requires constrained resources to process). For example, describing a medical treatment as having a "90% survival rate" or a "10% mortality rate" should not make any difference, since the information contained in the two

---

[1] Economists stick with the highly simplified rational actor approach because they are generally not interested in individual choices per se, but rather are interested in aggregate behavior among certain groups, or in localized markets. Having a precise model of human nature (such as constrained optimization) is helpful as a "microfoundation" that can be used to construct models of larger scale behavior.

descriptions is equivalent, and it does not take fancy calculation to convert one rate into the other.

Another assumption is "procedure-dependence:" the procedure by which choices are made should not matter (unless, again, the procedures change information or require more resources). A remarkable example is default or status quo bias. Suppose a new employee at one firm is told that a portion of their salary will be invested in a tax-deferred 401-k plan unless they "opt out" by checking a box saying they don't want to make that investment. Employees at another firm are told the salary will only be invested if they check a box and "opt in." If checking a box does not take much time or money, and the company's choice of whether the default is opt-out or opt-in does not provide information about what is best to do, then the percentages of employees who invest should be the same in the two firms. However, several studies with large samples show that switching the default makes a very large difference, in savings behavior (Benartzi and Thaler, 1995; Carroll et al., 2009) and also in organ donation (Goldstein and Johnson, 2003).

These types of psychological effects both present a challenge to the rational-choice theory and show the importance of "choice architecture" for implementing large-scale choices (e.g., Sunstein and Thaler, 2008). Behavioral economics has now generated a large number of studies showing how descriptive and procedural variables that are psychologically important can actually influence behavior in many settings (health, asset markets, housing, gambling, consumer choice, etc.; see DellaVigna, 2009).

Many studies have shown a long list of variables that could influence choice: attention, anchoring, sensory properties, attitude-like associations or construal, contrast and relative-scaling effects (e.g., Chater, this volume), Pavlovian cues, and cognitive appraisal. This list is not a complete alternative theory but is being actively used to search for more general principles in neuroeconomic theorizing.

In this chapter I will describe two classes of phenomena in some detail: Pavlovian descriptive cues in food valuation; and emotional regulation in risky choice. To cognitive neuroscientists, these effects are hardly surprising. However, to economists, these are startling effects that are not predicted by the preference–information–constraint paradigm and for which economic theory has no ready language. They can, therefore, serve as small examples of how cognitive neuroscience ideas and economic choice paradigms can be put together.

2.1 Physical-proximity effects in consumer choice

A central principle in economics is that only the consequences of choices should be considered in deciding what to choose (provided the trading frictions and costs of making the choice are low compared to the likely consequences). A corollary implication of this principle is that small differences in how choices are described, displayed, or made should not matter.

Psychology and neuroscience, however—as well as marketing practices and the attention lavished on them by firms, consumer advocates, and regulators—suggest that small effects of display and proximity can have large effects. Displays can activate associations, emotions, and Pavlovian consummatory responses (i.e., enhancement of appetite by cues either innately associated or learned to be associated with later consumption), all of which could affect choice.

An example is a recent study (Bushong et al., 2010; hereafter BKCR) on experimental choices of simple familiar foods. BKCR compare three conditions (between subjects): a text display, a picture display, and putting the actual items in front of subjects. These conditions are compared because they are archetypes of situations in which consumers often find themselves. Consider, for example, choosing a meal in a restaurant by reading a text-based menu, looking at a picture-based menu (as is common in some countries), or being exposed to a buffet table, or rolling dessert tray, where the foods are physically available.

Two separate experiments suggest that, in comparison to text or picture displays, the physical presentation of a food item or a trinket has a sizable effect on its value. This presents a puzzle for the behavioral sciences, and especially for the emerging field of neuroeconomics: why do the brain's valuation systems treat these three types of displays so differently?

BKCR propose and test three different explanations of the real-exposure effect based on recent research in psychology and neuroscience. They suggest that Pavlovian consummatory mechanisms, which are unfamiliar to economists but have been well established in behavioral neuroscience, might be at work (Balleine et al., 2008, Rangel et al., 2008, Seymour et al., 2007). The function of these mechanisms is to deploy behaviors that lead to the consumption of appetitive items when physically exposed to them. Furthermore, these processes appear to influence behavior by changing the value that the brain assigns to particular items.

In the first experiment, $N = 57$ subjects were recruited who had normal eating habits. They were told to eat, and then fast for three hours before the experiment. They were given a \$3 endowment that they could keep or spend on food. The food items were 80 familiar snack foods. They first rated how much they liked the foods by answering the question: "How much would you like to eat this item at the end of the experiment?" on a scale of –7 ("not at all") to 7 ("very much"), with 0 denoting indifference. They then gave monetary bids for how much of their endowment they would pay to buy the foods. To make their bidding incentive-compatible, we used a Becker–DeGroot–Marschak procedure, in which the subject competes with a random computerized bidder and pays the computer's bid if her own bid is higher (and otherwise does not get the food). It is easy to show algebraically that in this system a person should bid just what the food is worth to them. Bidding more risks overpaying and bidding less risks missing the chance to buy the food at a price they would pay.

Figure 2.1 shows the results. First, as can be seen in the top panel, the average dollar bid in the text condition (68 cents, SD = 0.52) is approximately equal to the average bid in the picture condition (71 cents, SD = 0.53, t-test, $P = 0.88$, two-tailed). Both averages are significantly smaller than the average bid in the real condition (113 cents, SD = 0.61 two-sided t-test, $P<0.004$). As the bottom panel illustrates, a random effects linear model with random intercepts and slopes showed no significant differences between the slopes of the bidding curves (i.e., bids as a linear function of liking-rating) in any of the three conditions.

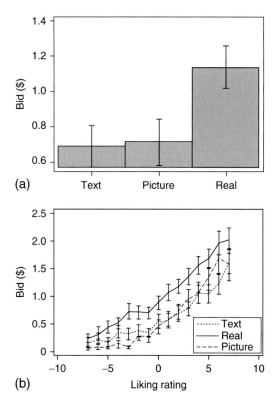

Fig. 2.1 Results for King et al (in press) experiment 1: Consumer's willingness-to-pay for a food item is larger when it is physically present. a) Average bids and standard error bars in the three treatments: text, image, and physically proximal presentation. There was no significant difference between the text and picture conditions, but both were significantly lower than bids in the real condition ($P<0.004$). b) Bids as a function of self-reported liking ratings for each of the treatments. There was no statistically significant change in the linear slope of these curves across conditions.

Two natural explanations quickly spring to mind. One is that some sensory cue, such as smell, is activating Pavlovian-conditioned processes and ramping up expectations of value. This is ruled out by a subsequent experimental condition in which the goods are trinkets (e.g. keychains) that do not uniformly have a smell, sound, or other sensory property shared with foods.

The second natural explanation is that physical presentation of the foods activates some gustatory process that enhances value. However, in another control experiment, subjects see a picture of the food on their computer screen, *do not* see the entire food package physically presented (as in the first experiment), but are given small tastes of the food in a paper cup. Somewhat surprisingly, this "taste" condition does *not* enhance value like the physical presentation of the entire food package does. Thus, it appears to be necessary to have the food physically present to activate Pavlovian responses.

Is it possible for a *different* consummatory cue—an anti-cue, really—to erase the response to physical proximity? To see, BKCR did another experiment that is almost identical to the first, except that a fully transparent plexiglass wall was placed between the subject and the physically proximate food (see Fig. 2.2 for a picture).[2] Our hypothesis was

2 In addition, only the computer picture and real food conditions were run, along with the new plexiglass plus real food condition, and the text condition was dropped.

that, if consummatory cues are at work, then the presence of a physical barrier would decrease the likelihood that the processes would be activated (because the subjects instinctively knew that the barrier made the items unavailable) and would reduce expressed values. Our intuition was confirmed in discussions with primatologists (Rob Boyd, personal communication) who say that lab-raised monkeys are quite sensitive to physical and social cues that regulate access. Keep in mind that the plexiglass is very clear, so that any "information" about the quality of the foods, which is increased by their physical proximity in the Fig. 2.1 results, is also present in the plexiglass condition. If information is describing the display effect, then the plexiglass should have no effect on values.

$N = 30$ Caltech students participated in this experiment. Only 20 foods were used, and a fully transparent plexiglass wall (dimensions 8 ft by 8 ft by ¼ in) was placed midway between the subject and the experimenter. The barrier was high enough so that the subjects could not reach over the barrier, and clear enough that the features of the food package were clearly visible.

Figure 2.3 summarizes bids in this new plexiglass condition with the previous picture and real food condition bids (from Fig. 2.1). The average bid in the plexiglass condition (81 cents, SD = 0.53) is substantially smaller than the average bid in the real condition (114 cents, SD = 0.53, two-sided t-test, $P<0.042$). Note that the average liking rating happened to be slightly higher (but insignificantly so) in the plexiglass condition (mean = 1.62), than in the real condition (mean = 1.16), which implies that the effect cannot be attributed to differences in the underlying liking-rating value of the food items. A random effects linear model with random intercepts and slopes showed no significant differences between the slopes of the bidding curves (i.e., bids as a linear function of liking-rating) in any of the three conditions. (The plexiglass seems to entirely wipe out the consumatory effect of physical proximity of food.)

We emphasize three aspects of the Pavlovian consummatory processes theory that we posit as a potential explanation for our findings. First, the text and picture of the stimuli are more weakly reinforced Conditioned Stimuli (CS's) triggering the consummatory response because people see many more pictures of food, in advertisements, magazines, etc., than they actually consume. So, they learn that simply seeing a picture won't be followed by eating that often. (This claim could be tested in small-scale cultures where food is rarely depicted visually or verbally, or in other cultures—if they exist—in which food is stored away until just before consumption, so that physical proximity is very strongly associated with immediate consumption.) Second, the Pavlovian consummatory processes are not activated when the organism knows that the stimuli cannot be acquired because it is behind the plexiglass. Third, the Pavlovian consummatory processes are triggered by all appetitive items, which is necessary to explain why we get similar results for foods and trinkets.

These results also provide insight into other studies of economics goods. Many studies have shown an apparent "endowment effect" (Kahneman et al., 1990, Knetsch and Sinden, 1984), in which subjects' valuations for items depend on whether or not they own them. In a typical paradigm, half the subjects are randomly endowed with a good they are told they own (e.g., a nice coffee mug) and asked how much they would have to

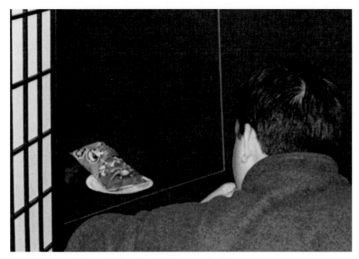

Fig. 2.2 Display of a food item behind transparent plexiglass.

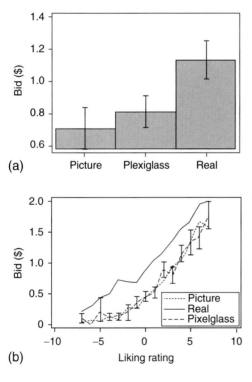

Fig. 2.3 Results from Bushong et al (2010) experiment 3: The introduction of a transparent plexiglass barrier between the subjects and the foods eliminates the difference between the real and picture conditions. a) A comparison of average bids and standard error bars in the picture, real with plexiglass, and real without plexiglass conditions. There was no significant difference between the picture and plexiglass conditions, but the bids in the plexiglass case were lower than in the real condition ($P<0.042$). b) Bids as a function of self-reported liking ratings for each of the treatments. There was no statistically significant change in the linear slope of these curves across conditions.

be paid to sell it. The other half are randomly endowed with no good (and are sometimes given extra money to compensate for the value of the good that the other group got and they did not) and asked how much they would pay to buy one. The endowment effect refers to the empirical regularity that selling prices are larger than buying prices, by a ratio of 1.3 to 2 or more.

The endowment effect is sensitive to whether the actual items are physically present at the time of the experiment. Plott and Zeiler (2005) find no endowment effect for goods and conclude that the effect is an artifact of previously-used experimental procedures. However, in their experiment *all* subjects had a coffee mug placed in front of them, which is a departure from previous procedures in which only "owner" subjects had a mug physically present. Knetsch and Wong (2009) found no endowment effect when two goods were simply passed around and inspected by subjects (but not physically proximate at the time of decision) and they found a strong effect when an endowed good was in front of a subject. Reb and Connolly (2007) also found that effects of possession (touch) were generally stronger than endowed ownership. The observed influence of the physical presence or touch of the goods across both studies is consistent with the effect of Pavlovian consummatory mechanisms. Valuations for small toys (e.g, a slinky) increase when subjects are allowed to touch them (Peck and Shu, 2009).

Marketing practices seem to anticipate these types of effects. Stores often display real products to consumers and encourage physical contact and tasting samples (e.g., test-driving cars).

However, producing consummatory effects (and later sales) is especially challenging for other marketing channels, such as telephone and online sales. Those sellers, by definition, are restricted to image, text, and sound displays. Presumably successful sellers find ways to activate consummatory mechanisms without true physical proximity (using particularly vivid images, sound, and so forth).

While marketing practices evolve to get consumers to buy, governments are often interested in some degree of regulation of packaging and displays of items that are associated with unhealthy consumption, such as addictive substances and junk foods, to help consumers self-regulate (Wertenbroch, 1998). Indeed, some large stores display cigarettes and expensive alcohol behind plastic cases. The plastic may be designed to prevent shoplifting, but could also be a treatment variable (like the plexiglass in our experiments), which conceivably reduces purchase.

These effects might also extend to social bargaining situations. A common legal practice is to present a plaintiff with a signed check when making an offer for a settlement. Our results suggest that this practice might increase the likelihood that the settlement offer is accepted.[3]

---

[3] In a sequential trust game, Solnick (2007) found that subjects in the second-mover trustee role returned only half as much actual cash as other subjects who were asked to return play money or make a numerical statement of the intended cash return. Since money is a highly conditioned stimulus, the results of this experiment can also be explained through our mechanism. Under this explanation, the physical presence of money triggers approach responses that makes it hard to transfer it to the other player.

The BKCR results are related to several other findings about the effects of displays and environmental cues on decision making. Next I discuss their similarities and differences with the Pavlovian consummatory mechanisms.

First, a series of experiments have studied the impact of display mode on self-control (Mischel and Moore, 1973, Mischel and Underwood, 1974, Shiv and Fedorikhin, 1999, Wertenbroch, 1998). These studies show that subjects are less likely to choose a tempting option when it is represented symbolically (e.g., in a picture) than when it is put in front of the subjects. Previous interpretations of the experiments have emphasized the tempting nature of the goods, but a mechanistic explanation has not been provided. The results in this paper suggest that Pavlovian consummatory processes could be at work in these studies, and that this might contribute to self-control problems when the tempting good is present. In fact, choosing between immediate and delayed rewards sometimes confounds an actual physical display of the immediate reward with a symbolic or imagined delayed reward. It follows that some aspects of preference for immediacy may be intimately related with the real-exposure effect we document.

Second, several studies have found that cues associated with being watched by others seem to increase pro-sociality in simple economic games. For example, Haley and Fessler (2005) demonstrated the effect of subtle social cues on the dictator game by using a pair of eyes (to cue a sense of being watched) and noise-muffling headphones (to cue a sense of being alone). They found that the eyes cue increased giving, but the headphones did not decrease it. Bateson et al. (2006) found that eye pictures increased voluntary payments for coffee in an office. Rigdon et al. (2008) demonstrated that three small dots at the top of a piece of paper, when oriented in a way that mimics a face, increases giving in a dictator game for males (but not for females). All of these are examples of how social cues can affect behavior, perhaps through highly-evolved responses to the presence of others (which the brain might "detect" equally well through the perception of real or artificial faces). Note, however, that the types of cues and mechanisms at work are different from the real-exposure effect. In our case, the triggering cue is the food itself and the mechanisms at work are Pavlovian consummatory processes.

Third, cues have also been shown to have strong effects in drug cravings and consumption. Addicts often experience a craving, and are more likely to consume, when cues associated with previous drug use are present. This often leads to relapse, even after years of abstinence (for a review of the evidence see Bernheim and Rangel, 2004). Although direct exposure to a drug of choice is thought to trigger the type of Pavlovian consummatory mechanisms discussed in this paper, other drug cues can trigger cravings and recidivism, even if the actual drug is not present. Such cues include seeing a place or friend associated with drug use, or watching films showing the use of drug paraphernalia. This is thought to operate through at least two separate mechanisms. First, drug cues trigger physiological "opponent process," which causes unpleasant withdrawal-like symptoms (Laibson, 2001; Siegel, 1976). This is thought to increase the marginal utility of consuming the substance. Second, cues are also thought to trigger habitual behavioral responses that promote drug-seeking behaviors, even if utility maximization calculations suggest that this is not the optimal course of behavior (Bernheim and Rangel, 2004; Rangel et al., 2008; Redish, 2004).

Finally, cues can also affect behavior through a mechanism known in behavioral economics as "projection bias" (Loewenstein et al., 2003). Projection bias occurs when environmental states that change the current predicted utility of consuming an item (e.g., the current level of hunger or weather) can affect choices, even if the environmental state will be different when consumption occurs. Pavlovian cuing is like projection bias in which the cue's presence is a "state." Because such states or cues do not affect eventual consequences, their effects on choice violate the "consequentialist view" of idealized choice described in the introduction. For example, Gilbert et al. (2002) showed that shoppers who were given a muffin to eat before entering a supermarket were more likely to restrict their purchases to the items in their shopping list, rather than adding unplanned impulse purchases. This finding shows that the value assigned to foods that won't be eaten until much later depended on the level of hunger at the time of decision, which is presumably uncorrelated with the hunger state at the time of consumption (for a closely related result, see also Read and van Leeuwen, 1998). Conlin et al. (2007) report field evidence for a similar effect of weather: unusually cold weather at the time of ordering cold-weather clothes from a catalog predicts whether goods are later returned. Note that projection bias is quite distinct from the real-exposure effect that we have identified in this paper. In projection bias, cues affect behavior because subjects overestimate the extent to which the future experience utility of consuming an item will be equal to the experienced utility of consuming it now. Thus, it is due to a cognitive bias. In addition, the cues at work may have nothing to do with the physical presence of the good itself.

2.2 Emotional regulation in risky choice

Making good risky choices requires animals to weigh likelihoods of outcomes, the values of different outcomes, and combines those likelihoods and values in some way. In decision theory, a variety of models have been proposed. The most popular is expected utility theory (EU). In EU, outcomes have numerical utilities, and outcome utilities are weighted by the objective probabilities of the outcomes occurring.[4]

In 1979, Kahneman and Tversky published an influential alternative to EU, called "prospect theory" (PT). PT is the most widely-cited empirical paper published since 1970 in a leading economics journal (Kim et al., 2006). Part of its large influence is because the theory has gotten attention and been applied in a wide range of social sciences, and, to some extent, in decision neuroscience.

PT is different from EU in two important ways: nonlinear weighting of probabilities, and reference-dependence.

---

[4] In a related theory, probabilities are not objective but are instead "subjective" (or "personal"). In that theory, subjective probabilities can be inferred from choices, just as utilities are.

Nonlinear weighting of probabilities: in PT, probabilities P are thought to be transformed by a psychophysical function $\pi(p)$ into "decision weights." Evidence for such a function $\pi(p)$ comes from fitting functions to experimental choices among monetary gambles (see Hsu et al., 2009). The most prominent property of typical empirical estimates of $\pi(p)$ is overweighting of low probabilities, with dramatic increase in proportional overweighting as probabilities become very small (i.e., $\pi(p)/p$ gets large as p falls). For example, the values estimated by Hsu et al. (2009) imply that a one-in-a-million chance of winning a lottery is given a weight of 1 in 500. This overweighting is thought to play a role in explaining some kinds of gambling (e.g., Lottery) and overreactions to rare threats (like plane crashes).

Hsu et al. (2009) report evidence of nonlinear $\pi(p)$ in ventral striatum, and cross-subject variation in the degree of nonlinearity appears to be reflected in differential activity as well. However, Wu et al. (2009) compare choices based on objective stated probabilities (as in most economics experiments) with implicit choices during a motor reach task. In their task, subjects must touch a narrow bar within 700 ms to win a large prize. Since reaching accurately under such time pressure is difficult, the reach is essentially a risky choice with a small chance of yielding a large prize and a larger chance of a smaller prize (if they miss the narrow main target). A slower reach will be more accurate but will risk missing the 700 ms deadline; so the decision of how quickly to reach is like choosing a probability of winning. They find that the implicit weights associated with prize probabilities, as revealed by frequencies of reach success, exhibit a shape that is closer to linear $\pi(p)$. It is not known why this effect occurs. It could be due to an attentional overreaction to low probabilities when presented abstractly in typical choice paradigms ("a 0.001 chance of winning a lottery…"), which is not present when probability is implicitly encoded in motor control.

Reference-dependence: the most interesting and rich property of prospect theory is the hypothesis that the carriers of value are perceived gains and losses relative to a point of reference, rather than only net consequences that result from a decision. Koszegi and Rabin (2006 a, b) combine the reference-dependent part with consequence evaluation.

Reference-dependence has three important potential implications.

First, the way in which consequences are described or "framed" can shift the point of reference and change what choices are made.

Second, it is psychophysically natural to think that there are comparable degrees of diminishing marginal sensitivity to increased gains and to increased losses, which implies a convex disutility of loss function (i.e., losing $100 is bad, losing $100 more is not quite as bad, etc.).

Third, and most important for the purposes of this chapter, there appears to be a sharp distinction between losses and gains, a property called "loss-aversion." People are loss averse if they choose as if losses are substantially more painful than equal-sized gains are pleasurable. Field data on economic decisions suggest a role for loss-aversion in stock markets (Barberis and Huang 2007; Benartzi and Thaler, 1995), the pricing and purchasing of consumer goods (Hardie et al., 1993; Putler, 1992) and condominiums (Genesove and Mayer, 2001), the choice of labor supply hours by cabdrivers (Camerer et al., 1997; Crawford and Meng, in press), and the tendency for professional golfers to leave putts too short of the hole (Pope and Schweitzer, in press).

Whether there is a neural basis to the elements of prospect theory is currently being investigated. There have been many confirmatory results and some new surprises. Fox and Poldrack (2008) describe several such studies. Since their review, there have been several studies of the nonlinear weighting function, some noted above.[5] There is also clear evidence of reference-dependence framing effects (De Martino et al., 2006). Interestingly, these effects are weaker in autistic subjects (De Martino et al., 2008) and are modulated by 5HTT alleles (Roiser et al., 2009).

Importantly, loss-aversion is thought to have the biggest effect when combined with a natural "myopia" or isolation of single decisions from a temporal stream or portfolio of similar decisions (Camerer, 2000). The myopic loss-aversion often observed in the lab and field can be surprising. Figure 2.4 shows an example that is particularly visually striking. The data come from an experiment (Brown et al., 2009) in which subjects are given stochastic "income" units in a series of 30 periods, which they can save for future periods or use to buy consumption units.[6] Each point is one period for one subject ($N = 14,228$). The x-axis plots the value of the conditionally optimal amount of consumption (which comes from a complex two-state dynamic program). Note that this conditional value is negative in many periods (i.e., there are a lot of points on the left half of the graph) because, when the income in a period is low, there is no sensible way to avoid negative value. The y-axis shows the value of the consumption units that subjects actually chose. There is a strong correlation between conditional values and actual values, but there is also a clear reluctance to choose actual values that are negative (i.e., there is a visible pile-up of points at small positive values on the y-axis and comparably fewer points with small negative values). The effect is striking because subjects know that their 210 separate decisions will later be added together to determine their earnings. So a few, small losses will be netted against many gains, and there is no sensible reason to avoid a single loss so myopically.

---

[5] For an insightful commentary see: Berns et al., 2008; Boorman and Sallet, 2009; Hsu et al., 2009; Tobler et al., 2008.

[6] The consumption units are either money which is accumulated across the periods and paid at the end of the experiment, or small sips of a beverage. Dynamic programming shows that there is an optimal amount to save or consume in each period. The optimal amounts depend on the amount of savings that has been accumulated, the amount that has been consumed in previous periods, and the number of periods remaining. Computing the optimal solution and subjects learn to do it surprisingly well through trial-and-error, or by imitating others.

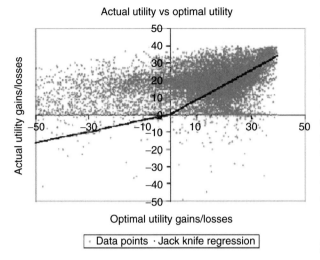

Fig. 2.4 Actual point values (y-axis) plotted against optimal condition point values (x-axis) from consumption choices in a dynamic simulated savings experiment (Brown, Chua, Camerer 2009). Note how few actual point values are negative even when optimal point values are negative (i.e., points are piled up at a "shelf" in the positive y-axis).

2.2.1 Emotional regulation

One experimental tool for understanding the nature of loss-aversion is emotional regulation (Sokol-Hessner et al., 2009; hereafter SH). Research on emotion regulation suggests there is some degree of control over affective states. This control can reduce (down-regulate) or enhance (up-regulate) the emotional impact of a given stimulus in real time.

Several studies suggest a role for emotion in the construction of preference and in economic behavior (e.g., Loewenstein, 1996). A field study with stock market data showed that stocks tend to go up when it is sunnier where stocks are traded (Hirshleifer and Shumway, 2003). In the endowment effect, mentioned above, people demand more to sell goods to which they feel attached, compared to how much they pay for good to which they aren't attached. One study showed two interesting effects of emotion induction: one selling and buying prices (Lerner et al., 2004). When disgust was induced by watching a clip from *Trainspotting*, both selling and buying prices fell. When sadness was induced by watching a tear-jerking clip from *The Champ*, buying prices went up and selling prices went down (reversing the typical endowment effect). The authors theorized that when feeling sad, people desire a change, which means buying a good you don't have (as in "retail therapy") and trading what you do have for money. The combination of the two effects—more buying and less selling—appears to reverse the endowment effect.

Emotional regulation is both a tool for modulating emotional effects (with potential practical applications, such as cognitive therapy), and a scientific tool for illuminating the circuitry that links cognition, emotion, and behavior. When people regulate emotional reactions, they report decreased negative affect and also show signs of decreased physiological responding, and decreased activity in brain areas that are closely linked to emotions and affect. Most emotion-regulation research has used pictures (which are calibrated to produce reliable strong emotions), but in principle any stimulus that results in an emotional response could be the target of regulation.

Loss-aversion appears to exist across many domains and cultures (Tanaka et al., 2010) and species (Chen et al., 2006). SH therefore sought to explore the role of intentional-regulation strategies on emotion-related aspects of risky choices involving potential loss. SH focuses on intentional-emotion regulation using stimulus reinterpretation (often termed "reappraisal") (Gross 1998; Ochsner et al., 2002; Ochsner et al., 2004). Reinterpretation means thinking about properties of the stimulus differently, to alter their emotional content. For example, a photograph of people crying can be interpreted to be either joyful or grieving. In the context of monetary decisions, reinterpretation of a particular outcome could include putting it in a greater context as one of many outcomes (Read et al., 1999), or taking a different perspective on a choice, perhaps imagining that oneself is an experienced professional trader, rather than an excitable amateur investor. These kinds of strategies are sometimes recommended to investors in articles or investment guides (Scherer 2005). For example, one investment company reminded their clients that: "These reinterpretations do not encourage denial; instead, they focus on the affect-inducing individual stock returns and attempt to influence the affect they induce."

In the experiment, SH et al., used the following regulation instruction: "Note that this instruction confounds different features which could all play a distinct role—one's 'identity' as a trader, investing someone else's money, and 'broad bracketing' in which losses are combined with past or likely future gains ('you win some and lose some')." In this initial study, SH et al. did not try to disentangle the different effects of these instructional features; they simply wanted to see if there was a regulation effect from the combination of features.

SH et al. examined the effect of emotional regulation in both indirect and direct ways. The indirect way is to use a mathematical model of how gains and losses appear to be weighted and combined during choice, to infer the weight placed on losses ("loss-aversion"), and how it is modulated by regulation. The direct way is measurement of skin conductance in response to actual gains and losses that result from gambles played for money. The prediction in both cases is that regulation will decrease aversion to loss (as exhibited by choices) and reaction to losses (as exhibited by skin conductance response; SCR). By combining the above variables and individual-level behavioral and physiological analyses, we can explore subtle effects within-subjects, and can speak directly to the effects of our strategy on a given individual, rather than being limited to group analysis.

Importantly, it is not well-understood whether aversion to loss is simply a reflection of a type of "decision utility" manifested in choices—decisions are made anticipating a disproportionately unpleasant reaction to loss—or whether losses actually are experienced as more painful than equivalent gains are pleasurable ("experienced utility," e.g., Camerer 2005; Novemsky and Kahneman, 2005). By measuring both apparent anticipation of loss, revealed by choices, and actual hedonic (skin conductance) reaction to losses, we can provide some insight into whether decision and experienced utilities are closely linked or not.

Participants made a series of forced monetary choices between a binary gamble in which winning G and losing L are equally likely, and a guaranteed amount. All choice outcomes were realized immediately after decision and displayed on a screen. Altogether 140 choices constituted a "set," from which we quantified three aspects of behavior: the weighting of losses relative to gains (loss-aversion, λ), attitudes towards chance (risk aversion, r), and consistency over choices (logit sensitivity, m).

The gain, loss, and certain values in the choice set were selected a priori to allow accurate estimation of a range of possible values of λ, r, and m. The participants completed two full sets of choices: one while using the "Attend" strategy, which emphasized each choice in isolation from any context, "as if it was the only one," and the other using the "Regulate" strategy, emphasizing choices in their greater context, "as if creating a portfolio" (complete instructions included in the supplementary material). This allowed separate quantification of "Attend" and "Regulate" behavior for each subject. Trials were grouped into 10-trial alternating Attend and Regulate blocks. This is a challenging design because it requires subjects to voluntarily turn the regulation on and off, and hence understates how strong these effects could be with more controlled involuntary exogeneous treatments.

In the first study, participants were initially endowed with $30 and were paid this sum plus actual gains or losses from 10% of the trials selected at random and played for real money upon completion of the study. Study 2 had an identical behavioral session and participants also returned for a separate session in which their skin conductance response (SCR, a measure of sympathetic nervous system activity) was measured. These SCRs are used to measure arousal in response to actual gains and losses when gamble results were shown to subjects (trial-by-trial) after their choices.

The value of gains (x) and losses (y) were assumed to be reflected by "utility functions" $u(x) = x^r$ for gains and $u(x) = -((-x)r$ for losses. The expected utility of the gamble is assumed to be:

$$.5x^r - .5\lambda(-y)^r$$

The logit probability of choosing the gamble is $p(6)=1/(1+e^{-mu(6)})$

Note that when $\lambda=1$, gains and losses are valued equally ("gain-loss neutral"). A value of $\lambda>1$ indicates overvaluation of losses ("loss averse"), and $\lambda<1$ indicates gains are overvalued relative to losses ("gain-seeking").

The parameter r represents risk aversion due to the presence of diminishing sensitivity to changes in value as the absolute value increases. The parameter m refers to the sensitivity of the participant's choices to changes in the difference between subjective values of the gamble and the guaranteed amount.

For all participants SH et al. separately estimated "Attend" and "Regulate" λ, r, and m values using maximum likelihood estimation. The emotional regulation hypothesis is that parameter values that are inferred from choices, particularly for λ values, will be different in the Attend and Regulation conditions.

In fact, mean parameter estimates in the Attend condition were $\lambda= 1.40$ (SE 0.15), $r = 0.83$ (0.04), and $m = 2.57$ (0.29). In the Regulate condition, mean parameter estimates

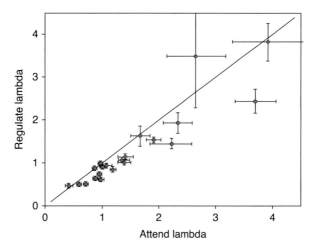

Fig 2.5 Values of loss-aversion coefficient lambda λ during attend trials (x-axis) and regulate trials (y-axis). Each point is an estimate for one subject. Standard error crosses represent 2-standard errors of estimates in the two conditions (attend and regulate). Crosses which do not intersect the 45-degree line indicate statistically significant decreases in loss aversion due to emotional regulation.

were λ = 1.17 (0.15), r = 0.87 (.04), and m = 2.39 (0.29). A paired t-test using the differences in coefficients between Attend and Regulate conditions across subjects shows a significant effect for ((t(29) = 3.64, $P < 0.0011$), but not for the other parameters.

Most of the subjects (26 of 30) subjects showed decreases in loss-aversion when using the Regulate strategy but there was variability across individuals in the size of the decrease (Fig. 2.5). Overall, individuals' loss-aversion, as measured during the attend instruction ($\lambda_{\text{"Attend"}}$), was reduced by an average of 16% (SE 3.09%) during the regulate instruction ($\lambda_{\text{"Regulate"}}$) (see Fig. 2.2).

The subjects' instructions and task in the second study was the same as the first, except that subjects' SCR was measured throughout. The goal of this study was to see if loss-aversion was evident in biological reactions recorded by SCR, particularly in response to actual losses and gains. Do subjects literally "sweat the losses?"

The behavioral parametric results replicate the first study. Mean Attend and Regulate parameter estimates inferred from gamble choice were λ = 1.31 (SE = 0.13) and λ = 1.15 (0.12). Within-subject paired t-tests between the "Attend" and "Regulate" conditions show a strong reduction in the loss-aversion coefficient λ (t(28) = 6.91, $P < 1.6 \times 10^{-7}$) and no effects for the other two parameters.

Skin conductance responses (SCR) after the outcome of the gamble were announced are measured in units of microsiemens (mS, square-root transformed to reduce skewness) and were normalized by the amount of money won or lost on a given trial. The normalized measures create an average Gain SCR score and average Loss SCR score, for each subject, with units of:

$$\sqrt{\mu S} / \$$$

(that is, skin conductance change per dollar). Using these Gain and Loss SCR scores, we created an SCR difference score of Loss SCR–Gain SCR as a physiological measure of

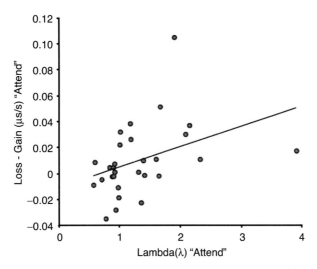

Fig. 2.6 Across-subject correlation between subject-specific measurement of loss-aversion parameters inferred from risky gamble choices during baseline "attend" condition (x-axis), and subject-specific measurement of the difference in galvanic skin response (GSR) to actual losses minus gains (normalized by dollar size of loss or gain) (y-axis). The positive correlation (r =0.39, P<0.035) implies that subjects who valued gambles as if they disliked possible losses more strongly also had stronger GSR responses to actual losses than to actual gains (dollar-for-dollar) when gamble outcomes were revealed. This graph therefore links "decision utility" (inferred from choices) and "experienced utiity" (proxied by GSR).

loss-aversion—how much more strongly SCR reacts to losses (dollar-for-dollar) compared to equivalent gains, compared to an overall baseline.

In the Attend condition, the SCR difference score is modestly correlated positively with the behavioral loss-aversion coefficient λ inferred from choices (r(27) = 0.394, P<0.035) (see Fig. 2.6). The comparable correlation in the "Regulate" condition is about the same (r(27) = 0.403, P<0.031).

These results support the idea that taking a perspective similar to that of a trader can alter choices and arousal responses related to loss-aversion.

SH Study 1 showed that an intentional reinterpretive regulation strategy decreased loss-aversion (as inferred from behavior), without affecting other parameters. Study 2 demonstrated that behavioral loss-aversion was correlated with a physiological arousal measure, per-dollar skin conductance response to loss outcomes relative to gain outcomes.

One goal of this study was to find an ecologically plausible reinterpretive strategy that could lead to a change in the emotional significance of some of the components of decision making. In this context, it appears that "thinking like a trader" may reduce the anticipatory and actual (psychophysiological) emotional impact of loss outcomes.

Other studies have shown treatment effects that could be interpreted as effecting perspective-taking, and hence loss-averse behavior. For example, a study by Thaler et al. (1997) applied an ecologically plausible situational manipulation (based on the frequency of feedback for risky investments) in a between-subjects design. They showed that temporally bracketing choices decreased the occurrence of behavior consistent with loss-aversion. Other studies have hypothesized that emotional attachment and cognitive perspective might modulate loss-aversion, perhaps through changes in a "reference point," which in turn affect anticipated gain and loss valuations (Koszegi and Rabin, 2007 a, b; Novemsky and Kahneman, 2005 a, b).

In addition, our demonstration of changes in arousal due to the intentional regulation strategy coincides with evidence from studies of the cognitive regulation of emotion illustrating significant behavioral, physiological (Eippert et al., 2007), and neural changes associated with the intentional use of regulation strategies to reappraise emotional stimuli (e.g., Ochsner et al., 2002). Because the "trader perspective," or portfolio approach, that our regulation strategy encourages also involves reinterpretation of outcomes, it is possible that a related mechanism is at work. In that context, this study may provide some insight into what separates professional traders and gamblers from amateurs. It is possible that professionals and amateurs are fundamentally different people from the start, but it is also possible that professionals have learned not just facts about investments, but strategies for addressing the normal emotional responses that might prevent amateurs from making the same decisions, given the same information (Lo et al., 2005; Lo and Repin, 2002). Indeed, professional sports card dealers (Camerer 2005), condominium investors (rather than owners) (Genesove and Mayer, 2001) and experienced cab drivers (Camerer et al., 1997) show less apparent response to loss than less experienced agents. A related interpretation is that these experienced economic agents have an expectation of trade, so there is no distaste of "losing" something that was not yours to begin with. Studies with these groups combining behavioral, cognitive, and emotional measures would adjudicate between these types of explanations.

Our results also shed light on the debate noted earlier, about whether losses hurt as much as our decisions to avoid them suggest, or whether we are overzealous at the time of decision in predicting that losses will hurt disproportionately, when in fact they aren't any worse than gains are good. In other words, is loss-aversion due to a basic hedonic property of our reaction to losses, as are simple basic preferences for food, sleep, sex, and warmth? Or is it a kind of error in judgment caused by an exaggerated fear of losses relative to their actual impact (as suggested by Kermer et al., 2006), perhaps due to an under-appreciation of the capacity of our "emotional immune system" to adapt to negative events (Wilson and Gilbert, 2005)?

These results support the former, "hedonic," interpretation. Losses appear to reflect both decision utility and experienced utility, because differential physiological arousal responses occur in response to actual feedback about loss and gain, and are correlated with the degree of loss-aversion inferred from behavior. This correlation suggests that loss-aversion is not entirely a judgment error. However, our results also support the general hypothesis that cognitive strategies can systematically reduce loss-aversion behaviorally and physiologically; so whatever "fear of loss" may exist is not so basic as to be immutable, but is instead subject to short-run emotional regulation. Finally, note that a recent study finds that two patients with focal bilateral amygdala damage exhibit no aversion to loss (compared to matched controls) in similar simple gamble choices (De Martino et al., 2010). This is more evidence that fear of loss is an emotional reaction, perhaps transmitted by amygdala to cortical integration systems in normal people.

2.3 Conclusion

The economic theory of choice has proved to be useful in explaining aggregate choices and guiding policy using just three moving parts—stable preferences, information, and constraints.

Cognitive science and neuroscience can supplement this model by showing how attention, emotion, cognitive difficulty, and other variables, also influence choices. This chapter described two "case studies" of these effects. The first part showed that the way familiar choices are described or presented can dramatically influence bidding prices. Bids are higher when a package of food is physically present, but the increase is "switched off" when a plexiglass barrier disables the appetitive process cued by physical proximity. The second part showed that emotional regulation of the fear of loss could lower the behavioral tendency toward overweighting losses compared to gains (loss-aversion), and is also manifested in autonomic responses to feedback about actual losses when chosen gambles are immediately played for money.

These two particular experimental paradigms are not closely related. However, they show two ways in which the standard choice–belief–constraint paradigm in economics must be complicated. The effects of physical proximity show that appetitive processes subtly influenced by display and availability—and turned off by a mere sheet of plexiglas—can affect what people seem to prefer. These effects suggest choices are not driven by immutable preferences, but are instead the end result of a complex biological chain of events in which immediate food access can play a substantial role. Similarly, the effects of emotional regulation suggest that aversion to loss (and subsequent reaction when gambles are played and lost) is not a stable preference but can instead results from a biological process that involves emotion and can be consciously regulated (just as a dieter can conceivably "will" self-control—albeit perhaps only temporarily and erratically—through various tricks).

Interestingly, the idea that emotional regulations, not unlike those used to downregulate loss-aversion, could influence the entire economy has received an interesting endorsement. In July 2009, an anonymous donor in Rhode Island financed a billboard campaign called "Recession 101" to post billboards with slogans reminding people that severe economic recessions don't last forever (Los Angeles Times, 2009). Billboard slogans included:

"Interesting fact about recessions… they end"

"Self worth is greater than net worth"
"This will end long before those who caused it are paroled"

Most economists (and Rhode Islanders quoted in the article as well) are skeptical that such regulation-inducing thoughts will have much effect. But perhaps they do, or some regulatory treatments work sometimes for some people. Whether they do, and how, might someday be understood by progress in neuroeconomics and related disciplines.

References

Balleine, B.W., Daw, N., and O'Doherty, J. (2008). Multiple forms of value learning and the function of dopamine. In P.W. Glimcher, E. Fehr, C. Camerer and R.A. Poldrack (eds), *Neuroeconomics: decision-making and the brain* (pp. 367–88). New York: Elsevier.

Barberis, N. and Huang, M. (2007). The loss-aversion / narrow framing approach to the equity premium puzzle. In R. Mehra (ed.), *Handbook of the equity risk premium* (pp. 199–229). North Holland, Amsterdam: Elsevier Science.

Bateson, M., Nettle, D., and Roberts, G. (2006). Cues of being watched enhance cooperation in a real-world setting. *Biology Letters, 2(3)*, 412–4.

Benartzi, S. and Thaler, R.H. (1995). Myopic loss-aversion and the equity premium puzzle. *Quarterly Journal of Economics,* 110, 73–92.

Bernheim, B.D. and Rangel, A. (2004). Addiction and cue-triggered decision processes. *American Economic Review,* 94(5), 1558–90.

Berns G.S., Capra C.M., Chappelow, J., Moore, S., and Noussair, C. (2008) Nonlinear neurobiological probability weighting functions for aversive outcomes. *Neuroimage,* 39, 2047–57.

Boorman, E.D. and Sallet, J. (2009) Mean–variance or prospect theory? The nature of value representations in the human brain. *Journal of Neuroscience,* 29(25), 7945–7.

Bray, S., Rangel, A., Shimojo, S., Balleine, B., and O'Doherty, J.P. (2008) The neural mechanisms underlying the influence of Pavlovian cues on human decision making. *Journal of Neuroscience,* 28(22), 5861–66.

Brown, A.L., Chua, Z.E., and Camerer, C. (2009). Learning and visceral temptation in dynamic saving experiments. *Quarterly Journal of Economics,* 124(1), 197–231.

Bushong, B., King, L.M., and Camerer, C. F., Rangel, A. (2010). Pavlovian processes in consumer choice: the physical presence of a good increases willingness-to-pay. *American Economic Review,* 100(4), 1556–71.

Camerer, C. (2000). Prospect theory in the wild: evidence from the field. In D. Kahneman and A. Tversky (eds), *Choices, values, and frames* (pp. 288–300). Cambridge University Press.

Camerer, C. (2005). Three cheers—psychological, theoretical, empirical—for loss-aversion. *Journal of Marketing Research,* 42, 129–33.

Camerer C., Babcock L, Loewenstein G., and Thaler R.H. (1997). Labor supply of New York City cab-drivers: one day at a time. *Quarterly Journal of Economics,* 112, 407–41.

Camerer, C., Loewenstein, G., and Rabin M. (2004). *Advances in behavioral economics.* Princeton University Press.

Carroll, G. et. al. (2009). Optimal defaults and active decisions. *Quarterly Journal of Economics,* 124(4), 1639–74.

Chen, M.K,. Lakshminarayanan, V., and Santos, L. (2006). How basic are behavioral biases? Evidence from capuchin monkey trading behavior. *Journal of Political Economy,* 114, 517–37.

Colander, D. (2007). Retrospectives: Edgeworth's hedonimeter and the quest to measure utility. *Journal of Economic Perspectives,* 21, Spring, 215–25.

Conlin, M., O'Donoghue, T., and Vogelsang, T.J. (2007). Projection bias in catalog orders. *American Economic Review, 97(4)*, 1217–49.

Crawford, V. and Meng, J. (2009). New York City cabdrivers' labor supply revisited: reference-dependent preferences with rational-expectations targets for hours and income. Working paper.

De Martino, B. et. al. (2006). Frames, biases, and rational decision-making in the human brain. *Science,* 313, 684–7.

De Martino, B. et. al. (2008). Explaining enhanced logical consistency during decision making in autism. *Journal of Neuroscience, 28(42)*, 10746–50.

De Martino, B., Colin, C., and Adolphs R. (2010). Amygdala damage abolishes loss-aversion. *PNAS,* 107(8), 3788–92.

DellaVigna, S. (2009). Psychology and economics: evidence from the field. *Journal of Economic Literature,* 47, 315–72.

Eippert F. et al., (2007) Regulation of emotional responses elicited by threat-related stimuli. *Hum Brain Mapp* 28, 409–23.

Fox, C.R. and Poldrack, R.A. (2008). Prospect theory on the brain: studies on the neuroeconomics of decision under risk. In **Glimcher, P., Camerer, C., Fehr, E.** and **Poldrack, R.** (eds), *Handbook of neuroeconomics.* New York: Elsevier, pp. 145–74.

Genesove, D. and Mayer, C. (2001). Loss-aversion and seller behavior: evidence from the housing market. *Quarterly Journal of Economics,* 116, 1233–60.

Gilbert, D.T., Gill, M.J., and Wilson, T.D. (2002). The future is now: temporal correction in affective forecasting. *Organizational Behavior and Human Decision Processes, 88(1),* 430–44.

Gross, J.J. (1998). Antecedent- and response-focused emotion regulation: divergent consequences for experience, expression, and physiology. *Journal of Personality and Social Psychology,* 74, 224–37.

Haley, K.J. and Fessler, D.M.T. (2005). Nobody's watching?: subtle cues affect generosity in an anonymous economic game. *Evolution and Human Behavior, 26(3),* 245–56.

Hardie, B.G.S., Johnson, E.J., and Fader, P.S. (1993). Modeling loss-aversion and reference dependence effects on brand choice. *Marketing Science,* 12, 378–94.

Hirshleifer, D. and Shumway, T. (2003). Good day sunshine: stock returns and the weather. *Journal of Finance, 58(3),* 1009–32.

Hsu, M., Krajbich, I., Zhao, C., and Camerer, C. (2009). Neural response to anticipated reward under risk is nonlinear in probabilities. *Journal of Neuroscience,* 29, 2231–7.

Johnson, E.J. and Goldstein, G. (2003). Do defaults save lives? *Science,* 302, 1338–9.

Kahneman, D. and Tversky, A. (1979). Prospect theory—analysis of decision under risk. *Econometrica,* 47(2), 263–91.

Kahneman, D. and Tversky, A. (eds) (2000). *Choices, values and frames.* New York: Cambridge University Press.

Kahneman, D., Knetsch, J.L., and Thaler, R.H. (1990). Experimental tests of the endowment effect and the coase theorem. *Journal of Political Economy,* 98, 1325–48.

Kermer, D.A., Driver-Linn, E., Wilson, T.D., and Gilbert, D.T. (2006). Loss-aversion is an affective forecasting error. *Psychological Science,* 17, 649–53.

Kim, E.H., Morse, A., and Zingales, L. (2006). What has mattered to economics since 1970? *Journal of Economic Perspectives, 20(4),* 189–202.

Knetsch, J.L. and Sinden, J.A. (1984). Willingness to pay and compensation demanded: experimental evidence of an unexpected disparity in measures of value. *Quarterly Journal of Economics,* 99, 507–21.

Knetsch, J.L. and Wong, W.K. (2009). The endowment effect and the reference state: evidence and manipulations. *Journal of Economic Behavior and Organization, 71(2),* 407–13.

Koszegi, B. and Rabin, M. (2006a). A model of reference-dependent preferences. *Quarterly Journal of Economics*, **121**(4), 1133–66.

Koszegi, B. and Rabin, M. (2006b). Reference-dependent risk attitudes. *American Economic Review*, **97**(4), 1047–73.

Laibson, D. (2001). A cue-theory of consumption. *Quarterly Journal of Economics*, **116**(1), 81–119.

Lerner, J.S., Small, D.A., and Loewenstein, G. (2004). Heart strings and purse strings: carryover effects of emotions on economic decisions. *Psychological Science*, **15**, 337–41.

Lo, A.W. and Repin, D.V. (2002). The psychophysiology of real-time financial risk processing. *Journal of Cognitive Neuroscience*, **14**, 323–39.

Lo, A.W., Repin, D.V., and Steenbarger, B.N. (2005). Fear and greed in financial markets: a clinical study of day-traders. *American Economic Review*, **95**, 352–9.

Loewenstein, G. (1996). Out of control: visceral influences on behavior. *Organizational Behavior and Human Decision Processes*, **65**(3), 272–92.

Loewenstein, G., O'Donoghue, T., and Rabin, M. (2003). Projection bias in predicting future utility. *Quarterly Journal of Economics*, **118**(4), 1209–48.

Los Angeles Times. (2009). Signs of the times: "Recession 101" billboard try to put perspective on trouble economy. *July 16 (AP wire story)*.

Mischel, W. and Moore, B. (1973). Effects of attention to symbolically presented rewards on self-control. *Journal of Personality and Social Psychology*, **28**(2), 172–79.

Mischel, W. and Underwood, B. (1974). Instrumental ideation in delay of gratification. *Child Development*, **45**(4), 1083–88.

Novemsky, N. and Kahneman, D. (2005a). The boundaries of loss-aversion. *Journal of Marketing Research*, **42**, 119–28.

Novemsky, N. and Kahneman, D. (2005b). How do intentions affect loss-aversion?. *Journal of Marketing Research*, **42**, 139–40.

Ochsner, K.N., Bunge, S.A., Gross, J.J., and Gabrieli, J.D.E. (2002). Rethinking feelings: an fMRI study of the cognitive regulation of emotion. *Journal of Cognitive Neuroscience*, **14**, 1215–29.

Ochsner, K.N. et. al. (2004). For better or for worse: neural systems supporting the cognitive down- and up-regulation of negative emotion. *NeuroImage*, **23**, 483–99.

Peck, J. and Shu, S.B. (2009). The effect of mere touch on perceived ownership. *Journal of Consumer Research*, **36**(3), 434–47.

Plott, C.R. and Zeiler, K. (2005). The willingness to pay–willingness to accept gap, the "endowment effect," subject misconceptions, and experimental procedures for eliciting valuations. *American Economic Review*, **95**(3), 530–45.

Pope, D. and Schweitzer, M. (in press). Is Tiger Woods loss averse? Persistent bias in the face of experience, competition, and high stakes. *American Economic Review*.

Putler, D.S. (1992). Incorporating reference price effects into a theory of consumer choice. *Marketing Science*, **11**, 287–309.

Rangel, A., Camerer, C., and Montague, P. R. (2008) A framework for studying the neurobiology of value-based decision making. *Nature Reviews Neuroscience*, **9**(7), 545–56.

Read, D., and van Leeuwen, B. (1998). Predicting hunger: the effects of appetite and delay on choice. *Organizational Behavior and Human Decision Processes*, **76**(2), 189–205.

Read, D., Loewenstein, G., and Rabin, M. (1999). Choice bracketing. *Journal of Risk and Uncertainty*, **19**, 171–97.

Reb, J. and Connolly, T. (2007). Possession, feelings of ownership and the endowment effect. *Judgment and Decision Making*, **2**, 107–114.

Redish, A.D. (2004). Addiction as a computational process gone awry. *Science*, **306**(5703), 1944–7.

Rigdon, M., Ishii, K., Watabe, M., and Kitayama, S. (2009). Minimal social cues in the dictator game. *Journal of Economic Psychology, 30(3)*, 358–67.

Roiser, J. et. al. (2009). A genetically mediated bias in decision-making driven by failure of amygdala control. *Journal of Neuroscience, 29(18)*, 5985–91.

Scherer, K.R. (2005). What are emotions? And how can they be measured? *Social Science Information, 44*, 695–729.

Seymour, B., Singer, T., and Dolan, R. (2007). The neurobiology of punishment. *Nature Reviews Neuroscience, 8(4)*, 300–11.

Shiv, B. and Fedorikhin, A. (1999). Heart and mind in conflict: the interplay of affect and cognition in consumer decision making. *Journal of Consumer Research, 26(3)*, 278–92.

Siegel, S. (1976). Morphine analgesic tolerance: its situation specificity supports a Pavlovian conditioning model. *Science, 193*, 323–25.

Sokol-Hessner, P., Delgado, M., Hsu, M., Camerer, C., and Phelps, E. (2009) Thinking like a trader: cognitive re-appraisal and loss-aversion. *Proceedings of the National Academy of Sciences, 106(13)*, 5035–40.

Solnick, S. (2007). Cash and alternate methods of accounting in an experimental game. *Journal of Economic Behavior and Organization, 62(2)*, 316–21.

Sunstein, C. and Thaler, R. (2008). *Nudge: improving decisions about health, wealth, and happiness.* Yale University Press, New Haven, CT, USA.

Tanaka, T., Camerer, C., and Nguyen, Q. (2010). Risk and time preferences: linking experimental and household survey data from Vietnam. *American Economic Review, 100(1)*, 557–71.

Thaler, R.H., Tversky, A., Kahneman, D., and Schwartz, A. (1997). The effect of myopia and loss aversion on risk taking: an experimental test. *Quarterly Journal of Economics, 112(2)*, 647–61.

Tobler, P.N. et al. (2008). Neuronal distortions of reward probability without choice. *Journal of Neuroscience, 28(45)*, 11703–11.

Wertenbroch, K. (1998). Consumption self-control by rationing purchase quantities of virtue and vice. *Marketing Science, 17(4)*, 317–37.

Wilson, T.D. and Gilbert, D.T. (2005). Affective forecasting—knowing what to want. *Current Directions Psychological Science, 14*, 131–34.

Wu, S.W., Delgado, M.R., and Maloney, L.T. (2009). Economic decision-making compared with an equivalent motor task. *Proceedings of the National Academy of Sciences, 196(15)*, 6088–93.

Chapter 3

The psychology of common value auctions

Samuel M. McClure and Wouter van den Bos

Abstract

One of the most interesting but unresolved phenomena in auction behavior is the winner's curse—the strong tendency of participants to bid more than rational agent theory prescribes, often at a significant loss. To address this, we propose an approach that uses neuroscience as a means to determine the nature of the mechanisms at play as people learn to bid. We begin by conceptualizing auctions as competitive social environments in which decisions are made on the basis of information acquired over time. This formulation yields novel predictions about the origins and persistence of the winner's curse. First, we hypothesized that there is an intrinsic social value in winning or losing the auctions, and we show that, indeed, the level of social competition in auctions does predict the magnitude of the winner's curse. Second, adding these social value parameters to a reinforcement learning model, we are able to predict the behavior of naïve auction participants. Finally, we confirm that neural systems implicated in reinforcement learning are active as predicted by the developed learning model. The fusion of neuroscience and modeling provides direct support for this model of bidding, differentiating our account from others with similar behavioral predictions. Overall, this analysis illustrates the value of neuroscience methodologies in developing and testing theories of decision making.

3.1 Introduction

The winner's curse is a well-recognized behavioral anomaly observed in a form of auctions known as common value auctions. This structure of auction encompasses a broad range of transactions, including all situations in which people are bidding on an item with a fixed inherent value about which they have only imperfect information. The winner's curse was first described in relation to auctions for off-shore oil-drilling rights (Capen et al., 1971). Since both the amount of oil in some regions, as well as the market price for oil, have some true value that can only be approximated, then this qualifies as a prototypical common value auction. Furthermore, since estimates of the value of oil in any particular region are subject to error, individual companies may have relatively optimistic or pessimistic estimates at the time of auction. If and when companies bid close to their estimated values, then the winner will generally be that company with the highest estimate, since bids can only be determined on the basis of idiosyncratic estimated values. However, the highest estimate from a group of independent bidders is likely to be an overestimate. If bids are submitted that are close to estimated values, then when revenues have been tallied, net losses will be discovered and the winner will "curse" their poor investment—hence the winner's curse. Since this original publication on the winner's curse phenomenon, the curse has been observed in a variety of markets, including baseball free agency (Blecherman and Camerer, 1996; Cassing and Douglas, 1980), book publishing (Dessauer, 1981), construction (Dyer and Kagel, 1996), and corporate takeovers (Roll, 1986). The winner's curse is therefore prevalent and of practical importance.

There are several hypotheses addressing the origin of the winner's curse. Avoiding the curse requires recognizing that winning the auction provides information about your estimate for the value of the good being auctioned relative to the other auction participants' estimates. That is, the winner is likely to have a higher estimate than the fellow bidders. The consequence of this is that, while estimates may be correct on average, the estimated value *conditional on winning* is too high and so bids must be reduced. The maths required to solve the optimal bid, given this statistical fact, is rather involved and is more than can be accomplished with mental calculation. So, one argument for the cause of the winner's curse is based on bounded rationality and suggests that people are simply unable to accurately perform the computation (e.g., Crawford and Iriberri, 2007; Eyster and Rabin, 2005). There are other favored explanations as well, including the idea that the curse arises from risk aversion (Lind and Plott, 1991) or that a systematic bias is introduced by a pure "joy of winning" (Goeree and Offerman, 2003).

In this chapter, we conceptualize common value auctions as competitive social environments in which decisions are made primarily on the basis of evidence accrued from previous bidding experience. Two lines of evidence support this framing of the problem. First, the social nature of the problem is recognized to be critical. The joy of winning, purely for the sake of winning, is a prevalent theory for systematic biases in bids (Goeree and Offerman, 2003). We will argue that this "joy" is derived from social comparison, and increases with competitiveness. Second, previous work has also shown that experience in the auction environment is strongly correlated with performance. Participants begin by performing very poorly and slowly learn to correct for the curse through time (although the correction is generally never complete; Kagel and Levin, 2002). We propose that people learn bid strategies using a type of error-based reinforcement learning (RL). This way of framing the auction environment yields interesting novel predictions about the origins of the winner's curse and the neural mechanisms supporting auction behavior.

Numerous theories have been proposed to explain why the winner's curse persists, even with lots of experience and high stakes. It is beyond the scope of this chapter to describe these in greater detail than what is written above. Traditionally, theories are critiqued on the basis of parsimony and the ability to describe a range of related phenomena. Here we propose a different criterion for establishing a theory that is based in neuroscience. With the rise of non-invasive functional brain imaging and progress in understanding the functional organization of the brain, the involvement of computational processes proposed by different theories may be directly observed (or not) in support of the hypothesis. We employ this approach here and discuss its implications for decision science.

The remainder of the chapter maintains a continuous narrative in laying out several related results. For the sake of clarity, we divide the argument into five remaining sections. In Section 3.2 we define the winner's curse formally and outline the (optimal) Nash equilibrium bidding strategy. Section 3.3 includes experiments demonstrating that social context is a critical factor underlying the winner's curse, above and beyond the influence of other explanations, such as risk aversion. We begin building a complete model of bidding behavior by accounting for learning in the task with a reinforcement learning model developed in Section 3.4. The validity of this learning model is established with functional brain imaging in Section 3.5. We conclude in the final Section 3.6.

3.2 **Experimental common value auctions and the winner's curse**

We begin by defining a number of terms that we will use throughout to establish a theory of bidding behavior. To this end, in a common value auctions we refer to the fixed, but unknown, value of the item for bid as x_0. Participants bid on the basis of private estimates, x_i, that are imperfect signals of value correlated with x_0. For the studies described below, we borrow from the experimental procedures developed by Kagel and Levin due to the large prior literature establishing and validating the winner's curse using these methods (Kagel and Levin, 2002). In these tasks, subjects are told the maximum and minimum possible values of x_0: x_L and x_H, respectively. Private estimates, x_i, are taken from a uniform distribution around x_0 with error ε (Fig. 3.1). The error is also known by all auction participants.

Under these conditions the optimal, Nash equilibrium bidding strategy can be determined. The solution is given by:

$$b_i = x_i - \varepsilon + Y \tag{3.1}$$

where

$$Y = \frac{2\varepsilon}{n+1} \exp\left(-\frac{n}{2\varepsilon}[x_i - (x_L + \varepsilon)]\right) \tag{3.2}$$

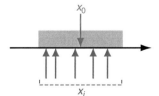

Fig. 3.1 The winner's curse. Common value auctions involve bidding on an item with a fixed, unknown value (arrow, x_0) based on estimates (arrows, x_i for each bidder i). The winner is likely to be the bidder with the highest estimate of value (rightmost arrow). If bids are not made sufficiently below estimates then net losses are likely to occur.

and n is the number of bidders (Milgrom and Weber, 1982). This function assumes that participants are risk neutral. When estimates are farther than ε from the bounds on x_0, then Y is very close to zero and can be ignored (as it has been elsewhere; Garvin and Kagel, 1994).

Participants almost always bid above the Nash equilibrium bidding strategy. One possibility for why this occurs is that people adopt a "naïve" bidding strategy by assuming that bidding their estimates will match the expected value of the auctioned item and give zero profits on average. A continuum can be generated between this strategy and the optimal strategy by expressing bids according to:

$$b_i = x_i - (1 - \kappa)\varepsilon, \tag{3.3}$$

where κ captures the degree to which bids exceed the optimal strategy. The Nash equilibrium and naïve bidding strategies fall conveniently at $\kappa = 0$ and $\kappa = 1$, respectively. We call κ the "bid factor" in subsequent discussion. It is generally observed that κ begins very high (near 1) for bidders with no experience and reduces significantly with repeated bidding sessions, although it generally never converges to 0 even after a lot of experience (Kagel and Levin, 2002). The consequence of this is that participants lose money in laboratory common value auctions, with a fair number of participants going bankrupt (i.e., lose all of their endowment) during the course of an experiment.

Numerous control experiments have been done to ensure that the laboratory winner's curse is robust to trivial explanations (Cox et al., 1998; Lind and Plott, 1991). These findings, plus the pervasiveness of the curse for professional auction bidders (Dyer et al., 1989), indicate that the winner's curse may be reliably studied in the laboratory.

In all experiments to be discussed, the same basic task structure is used. Participants in all experiments were instructed that private estimates are given to each person and are drawn randomly and with equal probability from a range of values all within an error range of the true value of the good, x_0. During the experiment they are given private estimates and told the size of the error. The error range was always drawn from the set {$4, $5, $6, $7, $8} and true values were in the range of [$14, $42]. At the beginning of the experiment participants were endowed with $30. Auction winners paid the value of their bid for the item, so that the highest bidder's revenue changed an amount given by $x_0 - b_1$ (b_1 is the size of the largest bid). All other bidders' revenue remained unchanged.[1] People were only ever aware of their bids and private estimates; we did not provide any additional information at the end of an auction round except personal winnings (or losses). Individual experiments lasted 50 rounds and were composed of 5 or 6 bidders. For functional imaging experiments, all bidders were scanned simultaneously.

---

[1] Roughly one-fifth of naïve participants lost their entire endowment during the course of the 50 round experiments. We elected to allow people to continue bidding, even with negative revenue. Other experimenters have removed bankrupt bidders, or had them pay off negative ending revenues (Cox et al., 1998; Lind and Plott, 1991). These manipulations had insignificant effects on the size of the observed winner's curse (Kagel and Levin, 2002).

3.3 **Social influences on bidding**

One intriguing and unexplained finding in research on the winner's curse is the effect of modifying the degree of competition. To date this has been accomplished by changing the number of bidders in the auctions. The predicted effect of this manipulation, on the basis of rational behavior, is clear: with more participants, bidding should become more conservative, since winning provides more information that one's signal is an overestimate (Kagel and Levin, 1986). However, the behavioral effect of increasing the number of bidders is opposite to this prediction. The winner's curse increases and people bid more aggressively.

Despite the clear social nature of the auction environment, very little work has explored social context as a mediating factor in the winner's curse. However, there are some suggestions that social manipulations will affect bidding, as they influence performance in other economic games (e.g., Miller et al., 1998). Furthermore, social factors, such as perceived relative social status, are known to have strong effects on motivation (Walton and Cohen, in press). If losing an auction is interpreted to be negative information about social status (and winning as positive), then the "joy of winning" is a natural consequence. Indeed, recent work suggests that signals about social rank activate the ventral striatum equivalently to signals about monetary gain (Zink et al., 2008).

The purpose of this section is to demonstrate that social context influences perceived value of outcomes in auctions and consequently biases bids to produce a winner's curse. More formally, for the remainder of the chapter we assume a working hypothesis that social factors create value for winning and losing that is independent of the monetary outcomes of the task. Winning becomes more valuable by some factor r_{win} and losing is aversive by an amount r_{loss}, so that the outcomes of the auction become:

$$r = \begin{cases} x_0 - b_i + r_{win} & \text{if } b_i = b_1 \\ -r_{loss} & \text{otherwise} \end{cases} \qquad (3.4)$$

where b_1 indicates the largest bid.

3.3.1 **Social basis for the winner's curse**

In order to establish that the winner's curse reflects social influences of valuation (and not cognitive limitations of the participants), we conducted a set of experimental common value auctions (originally reported in van den Bos et al., 2008). First we had naïve participants perform in an auction. Auction winners were told the outcome of the auction in net winning or loss. In order to increase the salience of the social aspects of the auction, we displayed the name and a photo of the winning bidder to all auction participants after each round. As shown in Fig. 3.2, the winner's curse was evident under these conditions. We call this the "Human Naïve" condition (Fig. 3.3A).

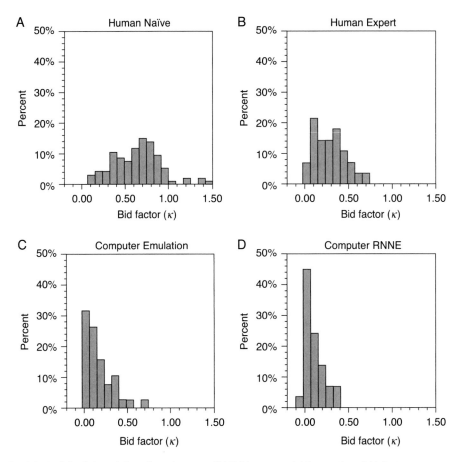

Fig. 3.2 Social origins of the winner's curse. (A) With no special instruction, bid factors are widely distributed as a result of learning during the course of the task. (B) When recalled and instructed on how to play the Nash equilibrium strategy (i.e., $\kappa = 0$), bidding was stable over the 50 rounds of the experiments. However, bids were still significantly above the optimal strategy generally resulting in net losses for subjects. (C) Under identical training and experimental conditions as in (B), people playing against computer opponents now bid significantly closer to the Nash equilibrium strategy. The computer opponent in this case simulated bids so as to match the distribution of bid factors in (B). (D) If the computer instead bids the Nash equilibrium strategy, bidding is only modestly changed relative to (C). It was only against the computer opponents that participants made net profits during the course of the experiment.

Participants were subsequently recalled after a 2-week period. For the follow-up experiment, the "Human Expert" condition, participants were first instructed as to the cause of the winner's curse and told what the rational strategy is (i.e., $b_i = x_i - \varepsilon$). This instruction included an oral presentation by the experimenter, as well as written instructions and a quiz to demonstrate comprehension. The written instructions and quiz are included in the appendix of van den Bos et al. (2008). The oral presentation followed the written

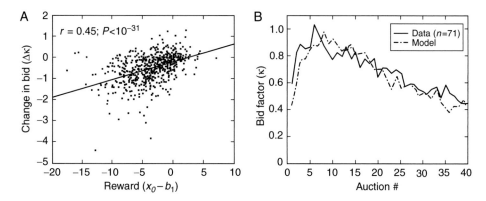

Fig. 3.3 Learning in common value auctions. (A) Changes in bidding after winning an auction are proportional to the size of loss or gain. (B) With repeated play, learning causes bidding to converge toward the rational strategy given by the Nash equilibrium. However, the bid factor asymptotes above zero.

instructions closely and will not be discussed further. The quiz was used to ensure that people could compute and implement the risk neutral Nash equilibrium (RNNE) bidding strategy and was completed without error by all participants.

Following this instruction, participants played with the same task design as in the Human Naïve experiment. We observed that, even though participants were fully competent in their ability to implement the rational strategy, they continued to bid with a positive bid factor (Fig. 3.3B). In fact, bids were indistinguishable from those submitted at the end of the original experiment (Mann-Whitney U-test, $z = -0.866$, $P = 0.195$, one-sided; comparison with median κ in final five rounds of Human Naïve experiment). This finding does not completely rule out cognitive limitations as an important factor in auctions; however, the fact that the magnitude of the winner's curse was not affected when cognitive demands were lifted suggests that cognitive constraints are not necessary to explain the size of bidding errors.

Following the Human Expert experiment, we had participants complete a questionnaire that asked them why they bid above the Nash equilibrium solution, if they had. Answers generally indicated that they wished to win more often than the instructed strategy allowed. There are two ways to interpret these responses. First, it may be assumed that people are implementing a strategy that they believe will prevail against other people who perform in accord with RNNE. It is certainly true that bidding slightly above this optimal bid increases the odds of submitting the highest bid. However, bidding above RNNE is necessarily costly; even though more auctions will be won, an increased percentage of these wins will incur a loss of revenue. The expectation is that, if this type of strategizing occurred, then people should soon abandon it, since they were recently instructed on how to maximize earnings. Instead, participants maintained bidding above RNNE for 50 rounds of auctions, indicating that this in an equilibrium point. This leads to a second interpretation of the participants' responses:

people value being the high bidder and are averse to not winning the auctions. It is this interpretation that is captured by eqn. 3.4 and for which we provide empirical support below.

To investigate the influence of social factors on bidding, we tested what effect removing social factors has on behavior in the expert condition. To keep everything else the same as in the Human Expert condition, we once again had participants first complete the task naïve and subsequently recalled them after a 2-week period. They were then instructed about the rational strategy, as before, only now they played against computer opponents.

Bidding against overly aggressive competitors changes the Nash equilibrium solution. We, therefore, first had the computer simulate other bidders by drawing from the distribution of bid factors (κ) that people submitted in the Human Expert experiment (Fig. 3.3B). We refer to this manipulation as the "Computer Emulation" condition. Despite playing against equivalent opponents, the median bid in this experiment was very close to rational (median $\kappa = 0.10$, Fig. 3.3C). Bids in this condition were significantly more conservative than against human opponents (Mann-Whitney U-test, $z = -2.674$, $P = 0.003$, one-sided). Also, for the first time, participants made net profits in the experiment ($t(1,37) = -5.407$, $P<0.001$).

A final group of subjects completed the same testing and training procedure and then played against computer opponents who bid the Nash equilibrium strategy: "Computer RNNE" (risk neutral Nash equilibrium). Bids in this condition were only modestly different than when the computer emulated human bidding (median $\kappa = 0.07$, Fig. 3.3D). The final two computer experiments strongly suggest that the winner's curse that persists after initial experiences with auctions has its origins in social valuations.

While these experiments demonstrate that social context is critical for explaining the winner's curse, it is important to point out that "social value" is intentionally used vaguely. The social value driving the winner's curse is certain to be a complex notion and our current results only implicate that something about our limited social context is an essential underlying factor. There are, admittedly, many more specific theories suggested by these findings. For example, is social value determined by the desire to establish social status? Is it sensitive to manipulations that allow or disallow reputation building? There are numerous experiments suggested by these findings that remain for future work. However, the finding that social context is a critical component of the winner's curse, and that cognitive limitations are not, is a significant advance and is all we aim to establish here.

These results offer similar conclusions to a recent publication by Mauricio Delgado and colleagues (2008). In their experiments, participants were informed of the exact value of the item under auction and had to determine how much below this value to bid in order to maximize profits. In this situation, people also bid above what is appropriate for maximizing revenue. Using function brain imaging, Delgado et al. concluded that losing in a social context is associated with a reduction in activity in brain areas associated with reward. The degree to which this was true predicted individual differences in bidding so that people bid more if losing had a greater negative impact on brain activity. These results are additional strong evidence supporting a role for socially derived value from winning an auction. The fact that these results were found in a very different style of auction indicates the generality of the effects.

3.3.2 Risk aversion

A common explanation for the winner's curse is that people are averse to risk, or, equivalently, evince a biased utility function based on lower probability of winning money. If utility is skewed with reference to the probability of outcomes, then increasing bids (and the winner's curse) follow naturally (Lind and Plott, 1991). Prior work has aimed to directly contrast "joy of winning" with risk aversion, and have generally sided with risk aversion as the better explanation of observed data (e.g., Goeree and Offerman 2003). There are several limitations of this previous work that we avoid. First, many studies have suggested that even subtle changes in the social setting can have large effects on the behavior of the participants (e.g., Miller, 1998). Importantly, as we show with these experiments, the social setting in which the experiment takes place also has a significant influence on bidding strategies. Thus the advantage of our study over previous studies is that we now carefully control for social factors. Second, previous studies compared the difference in goodness of fit for different econometric models, such as risk aversion or "joy of winning" (e.g., Goeree and Offerman, 2003). This approach is very theory-sensitive; that is, the outcome is dependent on how these different processes are formalized. As a result it could happen that an alternative hypothesis is ruled out because of the way it was expressed. In contrast with this approach, we are able to directly test the behavioral predictions in a theory-free fashion by controlling for the social setting of our experiments. Using this method we are able to show that, even when the probabilities of winning are exactly the same (Human Expert versus Computer Emulation conditions), participants still show variability in bidding as a function of social context. This effect cannot be explained by risk or loss aversion, regardless of the assumed functional form. The finding further suggests the necessity that models incorporate social value as well (e.g., eqn 3.4 as our working model).

It should also be pointed out that, even though the effects of our experimental manipulations cannot be explained by risk aversion, our results indicate that the probability of winning does influence bidding strategies to a small degree (computer emulation versus computer RNNE). We consider it likely that the risk attitude of the participants may explain the small but significant increase in bid factor in our final experiment in which neither social factors nor learning plays a role.

3.4. Towards a complete model of bidding: an analysis of learning

We have presented data indicating that the winner's curse does not depend on cognitive limitations, as has been commonly supposed. Additionally, we have shown that overbidding is critically dependent on social context. This leaves a mechanistic void about how bids are determined. The winner's curse phenomenon is universally presented in a way that suggests that solutions to the bidding problem must be solved deliberatively. That is, participants must realize that winning the auction is indicative of a high estimate and reduce bids accordingly. In the remainder of the chapter we challenge this formulation and propose instead that, at least in laboratory experiments, people adjust bids in a much more automatic fashion that is well described by a reinforcement-driven trial-and-error process.

There are two broad classes of cognitive processes that come into play when formulating judgments and arriving at decisions (e.g., Kahneman, 2003). These classes have been referred to by many different names but we refer to them here as deliberative and automatic. The reinforcement learning-driven process that we aim to establish is clearly an automatic process. Furthermore, the neural systems that are known to underlie reinforcement learning, and that are involved in bidding as well (Section 3.5), are an evolutionary older system that are believed to produce automatic motivational drives.

3.4.1 Learning what to bid

When challenged to discover a bidding strategy in a common value auction, participants show clear evidence of improvement over time. They begin by bidding at, or close to, their private value estimate x_i and then gradually reduce their bids with time (see Fig. 3.3B).[2] This finding strongly suggests that participants use an error-based updating mechanism to develop a stable bidding strategy (cf. Armantier, 2004). Use of an error-based updating mechanism is further supported by our findings, below, that changes in bidding are directly correlated with the amount won or lost on the auction (Fig. 3.3A).

There is a wealth of recent work in psychology and neuroscience using error-based reinforcement learning (RL) algorithms to model human decision making and associated neural responses (e.g., Li et al., 2007; McClure et al., 2003a; Montague et al., 1996). In terms of understanding auction behavior, this recent work allows us to develop models of learning in the auction environment that build on established models. Additionally, insofar as our models predict brain activity in neural systems known to be involved in reinforcement learning, then functional brain imaging can validate the use of these models.

Auctions are a challenging environment for RL methods. This is particularly true since the outcome of the auction depends both on how aggressively one bids, as well as how aggressively the other auction participants bid. (Where aggressiveness corresponds to higher bidding relative to one's private estimate.) Since it is impossible to ever know other bidders' behavior, the state properties that produce a reward outcome are only partially defined. Formally, the auction environment is a partially observable Markov decision problem (POMPD). There are no general algorithms for solving POMDPs (e.g., White, 1991). To reduce the problem to a fully observable problem, our algorithm assumes each participant behaves as though other bidders play with the same bid factor in each round as that which they themselves employ.

Another challenge for developing a learning model is the fact that learning occurs very quickly in common value auctions. Generally, RL methods decompose a problem into a number of discrete states, s, and actions, a, and learn the value for each state-action pair independently. As long as the task allows each state to be visited infinitely often, then learning

---

[2] Behavior actually initially becomes more aggressive in the mean before improvement is apparent; this observation is explained by our hypotheses, but discussion is reserved until later.

algorithms are guaranteed to converge to the true expected value for each state. For auctions, this method is inadequate since participants use different bid factors on nearly each round of the auction and the number of states is very large. In order to converge to a stable strategy in 50 trials, as is observed behaviorally, learning *must* generalize across states.

3.4.2 Reinforcement learning algorithm

In developing a learning algorithm we allow learning to generalize to unsampled bid factors based on two assumptions.

3.4.2.1 Assumption 1: when losing an auction, participants assume that all bids less than what they submitted would have also lost

The reward outcome when losing an auction is zero. If $V(\kappa t)$ is the predicted value of bidding κt at time t, then a reward prediction error signal for all states is produced according to

$$\delta(\kappa) = \begin{cases} -V(\kappa), & \kappa \leq \kappa_t \\ 0, & \kappa > \kappa_t \end{cases} \tag{3.5}$$

3.4.2.2 Assumption 2: when winning an auction, participants assume that larger bids would have also won the auction

Since auction winners are informed of the true value (x_0) of the item, then the outcome that would have been obtained for larger bids is also known. The reward earned for bidding b_i is given by $x_0 - b_i$. We take the action space to be given by bid factors, κ, which relate to b_i according to eqn 3.3. Thus, the potential outcomes for more aggressive bids can be known and compared to expectation, giving reward prediction errors according to:

$$\delta(\kappa) = \begin{cases} 0, & \kappa < \kappa_t \\ x_0 - (x_i - (\kappa - 1)\varepsilon) - V(\kappa), & \kappa \geq \kappa_t \end{cases} \tag{3.6}$$

Learning based on reward prediction errors is modeled as in most RL methods, with a learning rate α determining the influence of δ on new values of $V(\kappa)$:

$$V(\kappa) \leftarrow V(\kappa) + \alpha\delta(\kappa) \tag{3.7}$$

This global update mechanism suffers from problems related to the fact that the probability of winning with a given bid factor changes over time. For the modeling results shown, we scale α so that updating only occurs within a limited range of the bid factor employed on any trial t. This was implemented by creating an effective learning rate that decreases inversely with distance from κ_t:

$$\alpha_\kappa = \frac{\alpha}{1 + \kappa - \kappa_t} \tag{3.8}$$

Decisions were then generated by the model using a soft-max decision function, with a parameter m that modifies the likelihood of selecting sub-optimal bids:

$$P(\kappa) = \frac{\exp(mV(\kappa))}{\sum_{\kappa'} \exp(mV(\kappa'))} \tag{3.9}$$

The value function, V, was initialized to zero for all values of κ. We also experimented with randomized initial values of κ, which is commonly used in RL algorithms to encourage initial exploration of strategies. However, random initialized values did not affect the performance of the model significantly. The results here are reported for V initialized to zero.

3.4.3 Experimental test of reinforcement learning in auctions

We implemented the above learning algorithm with the modified reward functions based on the above results on social valuations (eqn 3.4). Overall, this model has four free parameters (r_{win}, r_{loss}, α, m). We estimated the parameters using a simplex optimization algorithm in Matlab. The model simulated the performance of five bidders and average bid factors were calculated over 50 auction rounds with 1000 runs of the model to reduce variance. Best-fitting model parameters were determined so as to minimize the sum-squared error between average model performance and the average performance of all 71 participants that have completed the task in the Human Naïve condition against human opponents. The best fitting model parameters were $r_{win} = 0.65$, $r_{loss} = 0.63$, $\alpha = 0.145$, and $m = 10$. Average bid factors produced with these parameters are plotted against time in Fig. 3.3B.

Importantly, the learning model captured an interesting property of the behavioral data that is apparent in Fig. 3.3B as two phases of adaptation. Average bids start initially at a mean κ of approximately 0.5, subsequently rise to near 1.0, and finally decline to an asymptote near 0.3. The initial increase in average bids is easily explained with our model. Bids are initially random, so that while the average bid factor is 0.5, the winning bids during the first several rounds occur near $\kappa = 1.0$. The rise in the mean bid towards 1.0 is driven by the increased aggressiveness of bidders who lose in initial rounds (driven by punishments dependent on r_{loss}). The behavioral data support this account. Variance in bid factors begins very high and falls off rapidly as participants all begin to play with a bid factor of 1.0 after approximately five rounds. Losses incurred with large bid factors eventually drive mean bids downwards.

Losses in initial rounds are punishing by an amount equal to $-r_{loss}$ to model the cost of viewing another participant win the auction. Since learning from losses is generalized to more conservative bets, as well as the action taken, increased competitiveness follows naturally. Based on this account, the initial rise in bidding aggressiveness is evidence for the aversive effect of losing the auction.

3.5 Neural correlates of reinforcement learning in common value auctions

A reinforcement learning account of the winner's curse differs dramatically from most prior work on the phenomenon. It is generally assumed that reductions in bids reflect recognition of the statistical problem that underlies the curse. The persistence of the curse is taken as an indication of sub-optimal reasoning to overcome the statistical challenge.

By contrast, a reinforcement learning explanation implies that participants need not ever understand the causes of their recurring losses. Instead, they simply must adjust bids on the basis of round-by-round earnings. To further support this explanation of the winner's curse, we turn to neuroscience. There has been a tremendous amount of recent research relating the midbrain dopamine system to reinforcement learning. The seed for all of this work is the single neuron recording experiments performed by Wolfram Schultz and colleagues in macaque (reviewed in Schultz, 1998).

In a wonderful progression of studies, Schultz found that dopamine neurons respond robustly to reward receipt, but only when it is unpredicted based on prior events. For example, if a door opening consistently precedes reward, then dopamine responses shift to the time of the door opening and are nonexistent at the time of reward receipt (Mirenowicz and Schultz, 1994). Montague and colleague (1996) formalized these results using RL models. The models explained the shift in timing of responses and also predicted the reduction in firing observed following the absence of anticipated reward. Through these RL models, the phasic firing of dopamine neurons has been equated to the reward prediction error signal used to update the expected value of different actions and environmental stimuli.

The prediction error theory of dopamine firing has been tested in impressive detail. The theory predicts that dopamine should facilitate changes in synaptic strength at target neurons. This has been observed directly at cortico-striatal synapses (Reynolds et al., 2001). Postsynaptic changes in gene expression are also consistent with this prediction. Dopamine has been directly linked to increased expression of AMPA glutamate receptors, e.g., Sun et al., 2005. The value function, which is the target of the prediction error signal, has been related to responses of striatal neurons that are directly targeted by dopamine neurons (Hikosaka et al., 2000). There is now uniform consensus that dopamine-mediated changes in the striatum forms the basis for many types of reward-based decisions (Frank et al., 2004; Hikosaka et al., 2000; McClure et al., 2003b). Current research investigates details of this theory, such as what form of RL the dopamine system implements (Daw and Touretzky, 2002; McClure et al., 2003a; O'Doherty et al., 2004) and how the reward prediction error signal is used in other cognitive function such as memory (Lisman and Grace, 2005) and cognitive control (Braver and Cohen, 2000).

This work on dopamine and RL has been extended to humans through the use of functional magnetic resonance imaging (fMRI). The first efforts along these lines aimed to study blood flow (through blood-oxygen-level-dependent, BOLD) responses in targets of the midbrain dopamine system. The reasons behind this were twofold: (1) the fMRI-BOLD response is thought to be generated in large part by synaptic currents, and thus signals from dopaminergic neurons may be expected to be greatest in terminal brain regions; and (2) dopaminergic nuclei are technically difficult to study using fMRI, although recent work has developed methods to allow for direct study of these nuclei (D'Ardenne et al., 2008).

fMRI studies have consistently found that the BOLD response mirrors the prediction error signal evident in animal studies (Berns et al., 2001; McClure et al., 2003a; O'Doherty et al., 2003). Prediction error signals are particularly prominent in the striatum where the majority of dopamine terminals exists, but are also apparent through the ventromedial prefrontal and orbitofrontal cortex. Some aspects of the prediction error signal observed in the striatum are not replicated when imaging is focused on dopaminergic nuclei (D'Ardenne et al., 2008). In particular, when reward is less than expected, a negative prediction error signal is observed in the striatum but not in the midbrain. This supports the emerging hypothesis that the striatum is a convergence point for multiple reinforcement learning signals that separately represent different components of the prediction error (Daw et al., 2002; Seymour et al., 2004, 2007).

To date, the majority of experiments investigating reward processing have studied learning in simple contexts such as Pavlovian or instrumental conditioning. Some work has aimed to extend these findings to decision making, but this work is still just emerging. Notably, there is some conflicting data about how dopamine neurons represent future actions (Morris et al., 2006; Roesch et al., 2007). These discrepancies have not hindered identification of prediction error signals in simple repeated-play decision tasks, in which prediction error signals estimated by learning models have been found to correlate with BOLD responses in the striatum (Daw et al. 2006; Li et al., 2007).

By assuming that error-based reinforcement learning underlies the development of bidding strategies in common value auctions, this work leads to the strong hypothesis that prediction error signals should predict fMRI BOLD responses in the striatum and/or the ventromedial prefrontal cortex (VMPFC).

3.5.1 fMRI evidence in support of reinforcement learning in auctions

Using the reinforcement learning model from above, we generated individual trial-by-trial estimates of reward prediction error for the submitted bid. Since imaging experiments were limited by time to a total of 40 auction rounds, fits were determined using the aggregate behavior for all subjects. With the best-fitting model parameters, estimates of prediction errors were produced by entering the bid factor submitted by the subject, and calculating the difference between the outcome during the experiment with the model estimate of V at the submitted bid. Updates to V were then made using best fitting values for α.

A general linear model analysis was then performed using SPM5 (Wellcome Trust Center for Neuroimaging, London, UK). A regressor was included for the time periods during which participants viewed their private estimates and error information and entered their bid. For the effect of interest, we generated a regressor that scaled linearly with prediction error at the time when the outcome of the auction was presented. All regressors were convolved with a hemodynamic response function to account for the temporal dynamics inherent to brain blood flow responses. Details about the timing of events in the experiment are shown in Fig. 3.4.

A random effects analysis was completed by taking a one-sample t-test over regression coefficients across the 13 subjects that completed the experiment and had usable data. The results of this analysis are shown in Fig. 3.5. We find that the prediction error

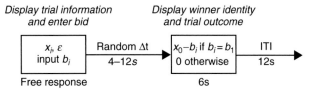

Display trial information and enter bid

Display winner identity and trial outcome

x_i, ε input b_i | Random Δt 4–12s | $x_0 - b_i$ if $b_i = b_1$ 0 otherwise | ITI 12s

Free response

6s

Fig. 3.4 fMRI experiment design. The fMRI analyses will focus on the response to feedback. The random time between bid input and feedback allows this response to be isolated statistically in a general linear model. The long inter-trial interval (ITI) is chosen to allow the BOLD response to return to baseline between trials.

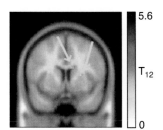

Fig. 3.5 Neural correlates of reinforcement learning in common value auctions. Trial-by-trial estimates of reward prediction errors were produced by a learning algorithm fit across all participants. A whole-brain analysis was then performed to identify voxels that correlated with prediction errors. Clusters of activation were observed in the striatum (dorsal caudate and putamen; $P<0.005$, uncorrected), which has been shown previously to be important for instrumental learning.

correlates with responses in the dorsal striatum (with activations in the head of the caudate as well as the putamen) at a threshold of $P<0.005$ (uncorrected for multiple comparisons). Activations in the dorsal striatum have been seen repeatedly in simple learning tasks and are characteristic of reward prediction errors during instrumental learning. This is therefore direct evidence indicating that reinforcement learning occurs in the brain as anticipated while participants learn to bid.

3.6 **Conclusions**

The lure of neuroscience methods is the possibility of producing quantitative data that directly relate to the processes that underlie decision making. To be effective in testing and establishing theories, our understanding of brain function must be sufficiently precise to make alternative explanations implausible. Currently, the number of specific hypotheses that can be produced according to this criterion is rather limited. This is illustrated clearly at two points in this chapter.

First, we believe that we can establish social factors as playing a central role in producing a persistent winner's curse (that remains even after extensive learning). There is a vibrant field in cognitive neuroscience that investigates the neural basis for social cognition and several recent findings are directly relevant here. Berns and colleagues (2005) explored social influences on visual perception and found that social conformity was a powerful influence on accuracy in mental rotation problems (cf. Asch, 1952). Additionally, information about others' decisions had pronounced effects on activity in cortical areas related to mental rotation. Other work has explored the brain areas involved in social processes such as theory of mind (Saxe et al., 2004). One area of particular interest arising from this work is the medial prefrontal cortex, which has emerged as a brain area almost universally activated when making social attributions (Frith and Frith, 2006; Harris and Fiske, 2006). Activity in the VMPFC is modulated by reward as well as social context (Harris et al., 2007; van den Bos et al., 2007), suggesting that this may be a region of particular interest for auctions. It is an intriguing hypothesis that activity in the VMPFC will be modulated by the experimental manipulations of social context (e.g., increased competition by increasing number of subjects or changing nature of opponents). However, future research will be necessary to test these predictions. More critically for the point here, the best prediction that we can make on the basis of these results is that social factors should influence behavior at a locus somewhere in the medial prefrontal cortex. This is a large region of cortex that is only roughly understood. In this instance, the balance of power is more on the side of behavioral theories that may provide an opportunity to improve our understanding of this region of the brain.

Second, and by contrast, understanding of the neural basis of reinforcement learning is very advanced. We can make specific predictions about the location of activity and its magnitude trial-by-trial. By confirming the predicted signals, our hypothesis has withstood a very strong test indicating that reinforcement learning processes underlie bidding in common value auctions. This is a clear demonstration of the power of neuroscience (and fMRI) in advancing decision science. Previous work has been limited to inferring mechanism from behavior without the possibility of disproving competing hypotheses with very similar behavioral predictions.

The value added by neuroscience methodologies in decision science is still just slowly becoming evident. We feel that the style of argument presented here, using reverse inference as the science permits, represents a class that will become ever more common as cognitive neuroscience continues to mature.

References

Armantier, O. (2004). Does observation influence learning? *Games Econ Beh,* **46**, 221–39.

Asch, S,E.(1952). *Social Psychology.* Prentice-Hall, New York.

Axelrod, R. (1980). Effective choice in the Prisoner's Dilemma. *J. Conflict Resolution,* **24**, 3–25.

Bajari, P., and Hartacsu, A. (2003). The winner's curse, reserve prices and endogenous entry: empirical insights from eBay auctions. *RAND J Econ,* **34**, 329–55.

Berns, G.S., McClure. S.M., Pagnoni, G, and Montague, P.R. (2001). Predictability modulates human brain responses to reward. *J Neurosci,* **21**, 2793–98.

Berns, G.S., Chappelow, J., Zink, C.F., Pagnoni, G., Martin-Skurski, M.E., and Richards, J. (2005). Neurobiological correlates of social conformity and independence during mental rotation. *Biol Psychiatry,* **58**, 245–53.

Blecherman, B., and Camerer, C.F. (1996). Is there a winner's curse in the market for baseball players? *Evidence from the field.* Social science working paper 966, California Institute of Technology.

Braver, T.S., and Cohen, J.D. (2000). On the control of control: The role of dopamine in regulating prefrontal function and working memory. In *Attention and Performance XVIII: Control of cognitive processes* (Monsell S and Driver J, eds), pp.713–37. Oxford University Press, Oxford.

Capen, E,C., Clapp, R.V., Campbell, and WM. (1971). Competitive bidding in high risk situations. *J Petroleum Tech,* **23**, 641–53.

Cassing, J., and Douglas, R.W. (1980). Implications of the auction mechanism in baseball's free agent draft. *Southern Econ Rev, 47*, 110–21.

Clark, K., and Sefton, M. (2001). The sequential Prisoner's Dilemma: evidence on reciprocation. *Econ J, 111*, 51–68.

Cox, J.S., Dinkin, S.H., and Smith, V.L. (1998) *Endogenous entry and exit in common value auctions.* Mimeograph, University of Arizona, Tucson.

Crawford, V., and Iriberri, N. (2007). Level-k auctions: can a nonequilibrium model of strategic thinking explain the winner's curse and overbidding in private-value auctions. *Econometrica, 75*, 1721–70.

D'Ardenne, K., McClure, S.M., Nystrom, L.E., and Cohen, J.D. (2008). BOLD responses reflecting dopaminergic signals in the human ventral tegmental area. *Science, 319*, 1264–67.

Daw, N.D., and Touretzky, D.S. (2002). Long-term reward prediction in TD models of the dopamine system. *Neural Comput, 14*, 2567–83.

Daw, N.D., Kakade, S., and Dayan, P. (2002). Opponent interactions between serotonin and dopamine. *Neural Netw, 15*, 603–616.

Daw, N.D., O'Doherty, J.P., Dayan, P., Seymour, B., and Dolan, R.J. (2006). Cortical substrates for exploratory decisions in humans. *Nature, 441*, 876–79.

Delgado, M.R., Schotte, A., Ozbay, E.Y., Phelps, E.A. (2008). Understanding overbidding: Using the neural circuitry of reward to design economic auctions. *Science, 321*, 1849–1852.

Dessauer, J.P. (1981). *Book publishing.* Bowker, New York.

Dyer, D., and Kagel, J.H. (1996). Bidding in common value auctions: How the commercial construction industry corrects for the winner's curse. *Management Sci,42*, 1463–75.

Dyer, D., Kagel, J.H., and Levin, D. (1989). A comparison of naïve and experienced bidders in common value offer auctions: a laboratory analysis. *Econ J, 99*, 108–115.

Eyster, E., and Rabin, M. (2005). Cursed equilibrium. *Econometrica, 73*, 1623–72.

Frank, M.J., Seeberger, L.C., and O'Reilly, R.C. (2004). By carrot or by stick: cognitive reinforcement learning in parkinsonism. *Science, 306*, 1940–43.

Frith, C.D., and Frith, U. (2006). The neural basis of mentalizing. *Neuron, 50*, 531–34.

Garvin, S., and Kagel, J. (1994). Learning in common value auctions: some initial observations. *J Econ Behav Organ, 25*, 351–72.

Goeree, J.K., and Offerman, T. (2003) Winner's curse without overbidding. *Eur Econ Rev, 47*, 625–44.

Harris, L.T., and Fiske, S.T. (2006). Dehumanizing the lowest of the low: neuro-imaging responses to extreme outgroups. *Psych Sci, 17*, 847–54.

Harris, L.T., McClure, S.M., Van den Bos, W., Fiske, S.T., and Cohen, J.D. (2007). MPFC as an affective region especially tuned to social stimuli. *Cogn Affect Behav Neurosci, 7*, 309–316.

Hikosaka, O., Takikawa, Y., and Kawagoe, R. (2000). Role of the basal ganglia in the control of purposive saccadic eye movements. *Physiol Rev, 80*, 953–78.

Kagel, J.H., and Levin, D. (1986). The winner's curse and public information in common value auctions. *Am Econ Rev, 76*, 894–920.

Kagel, J.H., and Levin, D. (2002). Bidding in common value auctions: a survey of experimental research. In: *Common value auctions and the winner's curse* (JH Kagel and D Levin, eds), pp. 1–84. Princeton University Press, Princeton.

Kahneman, D. (2003). A perspective on judgment and choice: mapping bounded rationality. *Am Psychol, 58*, 697–720.

Li, J, McClure, S.M., King-Casas, B., and Montague, P.R. (2006). Policy adjustment in a dynamic economic game. *PLoS One 1*, e103.

Lind, B., and Plott, C.R. (1991). The winner's curse: experiments with buyers and sellers. *Am Econ Rev, 81*, 335–46.

Lisman, J.E., and Grace, A.A. (2005). The hippocampal-VTA loop: controlling the entry of information into long-term memory. *Neuron, 46*, 703–713.

Maunsell, J.H. (2004). Neuronal representation of cognitive state: reward or attention? *Trends Cogn Sci*, **8**, 261–65.

McClure, S.M., Berns, G.S., and Montague, P.R. (2003a). Temporal prediction errors in a passive learning task active human striatum. *Neuron*, **38**, 339–46.

McClure, S.M., Daw, N.D., and Montague, P.R. (2003b). A computational substrate for incentive salience. *Trends Neurosci*, **26**, 423–28.

Milgrom, P.R., and Weber, R.J. (1982). A theory of auctions and competitive bidding. *Econometrica*, **50**, 1485–527.

Miller, D.T., Downs, J.S., and Prentice, D.A. (1998). Minimal conditions for the creation of a unit relationship: the social bond between birthdaymates. *Er J Soc Psychol*, **28**, 475–81.

Mirenowicz, J., and Schultz, W. (1994). Importance of unpredictability for reward responses in primate dopamine neurons. *J Neurophysiol*, **72**, 1024–27.

Montague, P.R., Dayan, P., and Sejnowski, T.J. (1996) A framework for mesencephalic dopamine systems based on predictive Hebbian learning. *J Neurosci*, **16**, 1936–47.

Morris, G., Nevet, A., Arkadir, D., Vaadia, E., and Bergman, H. (2006). Midbrain dopamine neurons encode decision for future actions. *Nat Neurosci*, **9**, 1057–63.

Oda, R. (1997). Biased face recognition in the Prisoner's Dilemma game. *Evolution Hum Behav*, **18**, 309–315.

O'Doherty, J., Dayan, P., Friston, K., Critchley, H., and Dolan, R.J. (2003). Temporal difference models and reward-related learning in the human brain. *Neuron*, **38**, 329–37.

O'Doherty, J., Dayan, P., Schultz, J., Deichmann, R., Friston, K., and Dolan, R.J. (2004). Dissociable roles of ventral and dorsal striatum in instrumental conditioning. *Science*, **304**, 452–54.

Reynolds, J.N., Hyland, B.I., and Wickens, J.R. (2001) A cellular mechanism for reward-related learning. *Nature*, **413**, 67–70.

Roesch, M.R., Calu, D.J., and Schoenbaum, G. (2007). Dopamine neurons encode the better option in rats deciding between differently delayed or sized rewards. *Nat Neurosci*, **10**, 1615–24.

Roll, R. (1986). The hubris hypothesis of corporate takeovers. *J Business*, **59**, 197–216.

Saxe, R., and Carey, S., Kanwisher, N. (2004) Understanding other minds. *Annu Rev Psychol*, **55**, 87–124.

Schultz, W. (1998). Predictive reward signal of dopamine neurons. *J Neurophysiol*, **80**, 1–27.

Seymour, B., O'Doherty, J.P., Dayan, P., Kolzenburg, M., Jones, A.K., Dolan, R.J. et al. (2004). Temporal difference models describe higher-order learning in humans. *Nature*, **429**, 664–67.

Seymour, B., Daw, N.D., Dayan, P., Singer, T., and Dolan, R.J. (2007). Differential encoding of losses and gains in the human striatum. *J Neurosci*, **27**, 4826–31.

Sun, X., Zhao, Y., and Wolf, M.E. (2005). Dopamine receptor stimulation modulates AMPRA receptor synaptic insertion in prefrontal cortex neurons. *J Neurosci*, **25**, 7342–51.

Tajfel, H. (1970). Experiments in intergroup discrimination. *Sci Am*, **223**, 96–102.

Van den Bos, W., McClure, S.M., Harris, L.T., Fiske, S.T., Cohen, J.D. (2007). Dissociating affective evaluation and social cognitive processes in ventral medial prefrontal cortex. *Cogn Affect Behav Neurosci*, **7**, 337–46.

Van den Bos, W., Li, J., Lau, T., Maskin, E., Cohen, J.D., Montague, P.R., and McClure, S.M. (2008). The value of victory: social origins of the winner's curse in common value auctions. *Judg Dec Making*, **3**, 483–92.

Walton, G.M., and Cohen, G.L. (2007) A question of belonging: Race, social fit, and achievement. *J Pers Soc Psychol*, **92**, 82–96.

White, C.C. (1991). A survey of solution techniques for the partially observed Markov decision process. *Ann. Operations Res*, **32**, 215–30.

Zink, C.F., Tong, Y., Chen, Q., Bassett, D.S., Stein, J.L., and Meyer-Lindenberg, A. (2008). Know your place: neural processing of social hierarchy in humans. *Neuron*, **58**, 273–83.

Chapter 4

The instability of value

Nick Chater and Ivo Vlaev

Abstract

Rational theories of decision making under risk typically assume that outcomes can be associated, either directly or implicitly, with utilities; and that decision makers choose options with the greatest utility. That is, the different choice options are assigned a value, independent of comparison with each other, and higher value options are chosen preferentially. We argue that, descriptively, people lack internal scales for utility, even for immediate subjective experiences, such as pain, or indeed other key economic variables, such as probability and time, a view consistent with evidence from psychophysics, cognitive psychology, and neuroscience. Instead, we consider the process of local comparison as fundamental. The sugary candy is preferred because it is more sugary than the other candy; water is preferred because it quenches thirst better than food. Such comparisons are local, because the evaluation of the individual features of an item depends on the features of other available options. We call this a local comparative theory of decision, as opposed to the traditional value-based theories of decision. We also describe a theory of decision making, decision by sampling (Stewart et al., 2006), which operates in purely relative, and hence highly unstable, terms, and captures various decision-making anomalies. We also draw some implications for neuroscience, psychology, economics, and ethics.

It is often easy to determine which of two options to chose. For a hungry rat, two food pellets is better than one; a pellet with high sugar content is preferable to a pellet with low sugar content. For a rat that is thirsty but not hungry, water is preferable to food. But what underlies such preferences?

Two types of viewpoint are possible. One sees the process of *comparison* as fundamental. The sugary pellet is preferred because it is *more* sugary than the other pellet; water is preferred by a thirsty rat because it quenches thirst *better* than food. Let us call this the *comparative* theory of decision.

The alternative view sees comparison as mediated by a computation of internal *value*. That is, the different choice options are assigned a value, independent of comparison with each other; and higher value options are chosen preferentially. So the hungry rat assigns a value of 4 to the non-sugary pellet; and assigns a value of 6 to the sugary pellet—and makes these assessments independently, without comparing between the available options. The sugary pellet is typically chosen, because 6 is larger than 4. Now, of course, a value-based theory of decision making need not be grounded in explicitly represented *numbers*—strength of activity in a population of neurons might, for example, suffice. Let us call this the *value-based* theory of decision. For the moment, we leave open the question of whether the significance of the numbers, which stand for these values, is merely their order (i.e., all that matters is that 6 is greater than 4), or has some richer interpretation. The *value-based* approach is indirect, because it does not compare options themselves, but computes and compares their values. But it is also potentially much more powerful. Whereas comparative theories of decision making have, in principle, to deal with every set of choice options afresh, indirect theories have the potential to make a spectacular simplification. Once we know the agent's value for each item, it should be possible to predict its preferences between sets of items (whether all sets of items, or just some sets, depends on the strength of our additional theoretical assumptions). The agent should choose, always or at least most frequently, the highest value set of items. Indeed, once we know the value of each item, all choices are, in principle at least, easy: just as two food pellets is clearly better than one, an option with high value is clearly better than an option with lower value. Of course, in practice, things may not be so easy, e.g., because it may be difficult to calculate the value of a complex choice. But if such values can be determined, the process of choice itself is easy—choose the highest.

A comparative view of choice may allow that comparisons are determined, in part, by local context—including, crucially, the other available options. Specifically, whether A or B is preferred may depend on other options C, D,..., E. This will occur, in particular, if the features of A and B are evaluated in the light of the features of C, D, and E; and hence the tradeoff between the relative strengths and weaknesses of A and B may be shifted. According to a value-based account, this cannot happen. Each of A and B is assigned a value, independent of other options, and the item with the highest value is preferred. We shall see that such *local comparison* effects are, however, widespread in the empirical literature—and are consequences of basic properties of the cognitive system.

Value-based theories of decision making are embodied in utilitarianism and early economic theory (although, as we shall see, later economic thinking took a different turn). Utility (or, in the utilitarian ethical framework, happiness) was taken to be an internal, psychological, entity that could be numerically measured and, potentially, optimized. Psychological accounts of individual choice have also postulated that people compute values for options, and choose on the basis of those values (Kahneman and Tversky, 1979; Loomes and Sugden, 1982; Quiggin, 1993; Tversky and Kahneman, 1992). Finally, recent work in neuroscience, especially in the framework of neuroeconomics, has been widely interpreted as promising a *direct* neural measure of value, in terms of levels of activity in key brain regions (Camerer et al., 2005; Padoa-Schioppa and Assad, 2008; Plassmann et al., 2007).

While many theories in psychology and neuroscience are based on internal representations of value, economics has stepped back from such theoretical claims, and taken comparison as basic: people are assumed to have binary preferences between pairs of options (which can, by extension, yield preferences over many, indeed continuously many, options, as in choosing how to allocate a budget across several possible goods). Depending on the properties of the preference relation (completeness, transitivity, reflexivity, and continuousness), it is sometimes possible to string together pair-wise preferences into a scale, so that items at one end of the scale are preferred more than items at the other. In this way, a notion of utility can be reconstructed. But, according to this "revealed preference" interpretation, utility is viewed as a purely instrumental notion—it is simply a highly convenient way of compactly representing binary preferences (Samuelson, 1937). Utility is not assumed to have any neural or psychological basis. In particular, there is no assumption of a cognitive or neural representation of a scale of value. But, crucially, taking an instrumental stance with respect to utility requires that comparisons are stable. That is, which of two options, A or B, is preferred is independent of the potential availability of any other options, C, D, E. This is because the choice between A and B follows "as if" the choice is determined by assessing which of A or B is assigned a higher utility; and the utility of any item (and, specifically, of A and B) cannot depend on what other items might be available.

In this paper, we argue for a *local comparative* theory of choice, and against value-based approaches (whether value or utility is interpreted psychologically or instrumentally), in the light of current psychological and neuroscientific data. We argue that local comparison, not valuation, is a cognitively fundamental operation. Options can be compared with respect to each other, in the light of a specific local choice context; but not valued individually, on an internal utility scale.

Section 4.1 explores what can be learned from related debates in psychophysics: specifically, we consider the debate concerning the existence of internal scales for perceptual magnitudes. Section 4.2 outlines a specific theory of choice (Stewart et al., 2006). Section 4.3 and 4.4 briefly consider the behavioral and neuroscientific evidence for comparative vs. value-based accounts. In Section 4.5, we briefly consider the relevance of these issues for wider issues in neuroscience, psychology, economics, and ethics.

4.1 The representation of magnitudes: the view from psychophysics

Value-based theories of choice require that people and animals can map options into an internal scale, which represents that value, so that which of two options is most highly valued is independent of the presence of other "irrelevant" options. That is, value-based theories assume that the representation of each option is independent of comparison with other options—because, in such theories, valuation is used to explain comparison, rather than vice versa.

From the instrumentalist perspective on value, which, as we noted above, is widespread in economics, all that matters is whether people behave "as if" their choices are governed by such scales (as we shall return to such explanation later). But, from the point of view of the brain and cognitive sciences it is natural to focus on underlying mechanisms: Do such internal psychological scales exist? Is there a neural implementation of such scales of value? Rather than approach this question directly, we begin by considering a related question from psychophysics, where the empirical data are much more extensive and better understood.

A founding concern of psychophysics, since Weber and Fechner, has been the relationship between physical inputs to the senses, which can be measured in well-defined physical units (frequency, sound pressure level, luminance, force) and their consequences for subjective experience. And a natural assumption has been that internal subjective experience should, like the external physical world, be captured by measuring scales, i.e., the assumption is that there are internal scales of sensation. According to this viewpoint, it is natural to search for the *function* that maps from outer, physical, dimensions on to inner, subjective experience. Initial investigations led to the postulation of Fechner Law's, that subjective experience is a logarithmic function of the corresponding physical input (Fechner, 1966). In the light of a monumental series of empirical studies, S.S. Stevens argued, instead, for a power law relationship between physical magnitudes and subjective experience (e.g., Stevens, 1957).

However, a range of considerations suggest that there is no such function: indeed, that there are no internal scales on to which physical magnitudes are mapped (e.g., Laming, 1997). Note, first, that sensory judgments are almost entirely *comparative* rather than absolute. For example, consider the subjective judgments of different shades of gray, ranging between pure white and pure black. The grayness of a patch is determined not by any function of its degree of luminance, but instead, to a good approximation, by the ratio of its luminance, to the luminance of the brightest patch in the scene (this is Wallach's ratio rule, 1948). This observation yields the prediction that, if what is normally a dull gray patch (when viewed in the context of natural scenes), is presented against a background of even duller patches, so that it is the brightest element of the visual field, it will be perceived as a pure, brilliant white. This striking consequence empirically observed (Wallach, 1948). More generally, subjective sensory experience appears to be a function of the comparison of each stimulus, rather than involving a separate evaluation of each element of the sensory input. Moreover, the neurophysiology of the sensory pathway confirms this picture—even from the earliest stages of sensory processing, the system typically "normalizes" absolute sensory values, possibly to increase information coding efficiency (e.g., Barlow, 1961).

One possible reaction to this type of consideration is to propose that there *is* an underlying internal scale, but that it is highly flexible. For example, perhaps the internal scale captures the relative, rather than the absolute, values of magnitudes. Even such an unstable internal scale seems difficult to defend, however. Consider the task of absolute identification (Miller, 1956). People are asked to identify n magnitudes on a sensory dimension (e.g., loudness or brightness), with the numbers $1 \ldots n$, where 1 is the smallest magnitude and n is the largest. On each trial, one of a small set of magnitudes is presented (say 5 or 7). The participant attempts to identify it by labelling it with a number indicating its original position in the set of distinct magnitudes (where, typically, the smallest magnitude is labelled as "1" and the largerst might be, say, "5" or "7" as appropriate. After each trial, the participant is then given immediate feedback concerning the "correct" label. Remarkably, it turns out that the limit of human performance on most sensory continua is about five items, a limit that seems to be utterly resistant to practice (Shiffrin and Nosofsky, 1994; see also: Stewart et al., 2005, for a recent review).

This extraordinarily severe limit contrasts sharply with the limits of discrimination in most sensory systems. For example, the range of human hearing runs over about 100 just noticeable differences. That is, 100 different loudnesses could be arranged in series, such that a listener could accurately distinguish one from the next. If perception involved mapping external inputs into an internal scale, then it would be natural to assume that the internal scale is able to discriminate 100 loudness. Then, by "reading" off the relevant internal scales, we might expect that people would be able to identify large numbers of loudnesses.

Yet this is precisely what people cannot do—so, if there is an internal scale, people seem to be unable to access it. Moreover, the limits on identification performance are largely invariant to the *range* of items to be identified, and the particular magnitude that is being judged (Brown et al., 2007; Garner, 1962; Laming, 1984; Miller, 1956). Finally, note that, if the internal scale were relative, then it should be possible to dramatically enhance performance by comparing against a fixed "reference" stimulus (e.g., such a stimulus could, for example, be alternated with variable stimuli). There is no evidence that any such manipulation produces any improvement in performance in absolute identification. These considerations, while not decisive, may, at minimum, be viewed as raising the possibility that people do not possess stable, absolute, internal scales for values—or, more modestly, if such scales exist, people seem to have very little ability to access them in judgment tasks, and, we might suspect, in making choices.

If external sensory inputs are not mapped into an internal scale, then how are they represented? One possibility falls back on comparison, as mentioned above. Thus, while people may not have an absolute representation of magnitudes, they may, nonetheless, be able to compare which of two items is brighter or louder. The ability to make only a small number of such comparisons (relating the present item to the previous one or two items) automatically leads to a drastically reduced ability to identify stimuli correctly. Moreover, the ability to make binary comparisons can apply across any sensory magnitude—including *changes* in sensory magnitudes. Hence, if the stimuli move from very quiet (1), to fairly quiet (3), to very loud (7), then, the participant may judge that the final stimulus is louder than both of previous stimuli (and hence is at least 4); but may also judge that the final jump is larger than the prior jump (from 1 to 3)—and hence the participant may decide that, if the items are assumed to be evenly spaced, that the next magnitude should be labeled as either a 6 or a 7. According to this viewpoint, *comparison*, rather than representation on an internal scale, is basic (see Laming, 1984; see also: Stewart et al., 2005, for a slightly different model of absolute identification, which assumes that people have no absolute internal scales).

The case of psychophysical magnitudes raises the possibility that comparison, rather than representation on an internal scale, may be cognitively basic. Now, if each loudness or brightness could be compared with a large sample of (or, in the limit, all previously encountered) loudnesses or brightnesses, then it would be possible for a person to construct a fairly accurate scale. If, for example, a person had a sample of 100 distinct comparison brightnesses that they could conjure up and accurately compare against, it should be possible to distinguish roughly 100 different brightnesses, depending on how many of those brightnesses are exceeded by the current stimulus.

So, it is at least arguable that in psychophysics, comparison, rather than internal scales, is basic; and that people are only able to compare the item under consideration against a small number of other items. Here, we consider the possibility of extending this conclusion from psychophysics to decision making.

The focus on binary comparison, rather than value, is, in itself, rather conducive to modern economic thinking. The "ordinalist revolution" in economics (see Cooter and Rappoport, 1984, for a historical discussion) was, after all, precisely an attempt to move away from a psychological or neural interpretation of value, and view value as a purely instrumental notion that can be derived from patterns of preferences.

Notice, though, that the present psychophysical observations are crucially not readily compatible with this move: because in perceptions comparisons are *local*. Thus, for example, which of two objects is judged to be largest, or which of two patches is judged as brightest, can be reversed, simply by changing the set of other objects in the visual stimulus. Thus, a medium-brightness patch against a light, local background is judged to be lighter than a medium-brightness patch against a dark, local background. A medium-sized circle next to small circles appears larger than a medium-sized circle next to large circles. Such effects are ubiquitous throughout perception, and are often extremely powerful (Laming, 1997). Such local contrast effects, if they also apply to choice, will lead to preference reversals, depending on irrelevant options available, and hence are incompatible with a global, ordinal scale. As we shall see, such effects appear to be widespread in decision making, raising the possibility that theories of decision making need to adopt a *local* ordinal perspective, rather than attempting to specify a global preference order.

4.2 A comparative theory of choice: decision by sampling

Let us take the comparative view of choice at face value—in its purest form, the decision-maker has no representation of value whatever but, instead, a set of comparative preferences concerning options. So a decision maker might, for example, have no stable sense of sweetness, but by comparing a particular item with other items retrieved from memory or available in the current situation, he or she can infer that the item under consideration is mid-way in the rank order of all other items (it was sweeter than half the items and less sweet than the other half). The decision maker will judge that the product in question is of average sweetness. The same conclusion will be reached if the perceived sweetness was first translated on an internal scale, the range of which is established by the range of previously experienced sweetness magnitudes—but no such internal scale is postulated.

This example illustrates our key cognitive claim: that people are not able to represent absolute magnitudes of stimuli of any kind (including attributes like utilities, payoffs, and probabilities). Instead, they represent magnitudes ordinally—in relation to other magnitudes that they can sample from memory or from the current environment. This framework was described in the *decision-by-sampling* theory proposed by Stewart et al. (2006), who also argued that, when people represent a magnitude, they can only do so on the basis of whether it is *larger* or *smaller* than other magnitudes sampled from memory or from the immediate context. Note that such sampling of knowledge implies that stimuli are judged only relative to each other and, therefore, that the utility of an option is dependent on the other options that can be retrieved from memory. As a consequence, there is no ability to represent on any cardinal scale the absolute value of a magnitude of any kind. The best a decision maker can do is to rank-order the available choice options on each dimension for judgment (i.e., constructing an ordinal scale) and then simply average (or take some other function of) the attribute values of an option, in order to reach an overall valence.

Note, however, that we do not even need to postulate the existence of a stable, internal, ordinal scale, because the decision maker's evaluation of an item's value on some dimension is derived from binary comparisons between a small number of choice alternatives available in the working memory (perceived from the environment or retrieved from memory), as proposed by Stewart et al. (2006). Using this decision strategy, the decision-maker can determine which option is the best, for example, by simply counting how many times each option was better than other options on each dimension (in the context of salient comparison items from memory). Suppose, for example, that the key choice is between computer A, with 20-in screen and 200-Gb hard disk; and computer B, with 25-in screen and 100-Gb hard disk. Comparison with a sample of other computers with 120-, 140-, 160-, and 180-Gb hard disks, but 15-in screens will tend to amplify the perceived relative importance of the difference in disk size—because computers A and B are at opposite ends of the ranking for hard disk size, but quite close in ranking on screen size. So computer A will tend to be preferred to computer B. Conversely, sampling computers with 21-, 22-, 23-, and 24-in screens, all with 50-Gb hard disks, will amplify the perceived difference in screen size, rather than hard disk size, and so computer B will tend to be preferred to computer A, thus leading to a preference reversal. And, in particular, this type of pattern—in which the impact of comparison on choice is *local* with respect to the contextually available comparison items—cannot be accounted for by value-based theories of choice. This conclusion follows, irrespective of whether value is interpreted in psychological, neural, or, as in classical economics, purely instrumental terms.

More generally, to the extent that people cannot assign the attributes of an item a stable value (but are rather influenced by comparison with attributes of other contextually available items), then *tradeoffs* between different attributes will be highly unstable. Indeed, from the present perspective, local comparisons are basic—and such comparisons are, in the first instance, based on comparisons along specific dimensions. Thus, there is no straightforward way of comparing between (and in particular trading off between) different dimensions—we do not appear, after all, to be able meaningfully to ask an experimental participant whether a light is brighter than a sound is loud. On the other hand, we can say that a light is bright *relative to other lights in the scene*; and that a sound is quiet *relative to other sounds we can currently hear*. So we might conclude, in one context, that the light is more "salient;" but such a judgment would be reversed, by appropriately switching the comparison lights and sounds.

In trying to decide between items with multiple attributes, the decision maker may often be in just the same state as our hapless psychophysics participant. Comparing screen sizes and hard disk capacities is no more meaningful than comparing brightnesses and sounds. Ranking along each dimension provides one mechanism by which people may, as we have suggested above, make such comparisons; but other decision rules are possible—for example, people might choose the item that "wins" on the most important dimension (e.g., screen size) and ignore all other dimensions entirely (e.g., Brandstätter et al., 2006; Gigerenzer and Goldstein, 1996); or they may rule out items that do not meet a threshold on each dimension (e.g., Tversky, 1972).

The psychological approach outlined here assumes also that sampling from memory is extremely limited, and also stochastic, which implies that people's judgments concerning magnitudes will be strongly influenced by the particular items that they happen to sample (see Stewart et al., 2006, for a precise specification of this sampling model and some simulation results). In this account, comparison items may be drawn from long-term memory of recent events, but also from magnitudes that have been presented in the current decision context. Hence, people's assessments of payoffs, probabilities, and intervals of time will vary capriciously, and may be highly malleable, rather than corresponding to a stable ordering, as in normative economic theory. Indeed, the effects of sequential and simultaneous context, discussed in the next section, confirm this prediction.

If choice depends on context, then a crucial issue is to describe typical contexts in which choices are made, e.g., by considering statistical distributions of relevant "economic" magnitudes encountered by the decision maker. The hope is that properties of these distributions may help explain typical patterns of decision-making behavior. In particular, Stewart et al. (2006) are able to account for incremental wealth having diminishing incremental utility (i.e., risk aversion); losses looming larger than gains; sub-hyperbolic temporal discounting, with a dependency of magnitude and nature of the outcome; and overestimation of small probabilities and underestimation of large probabilities. Roughly, this type of account works as follows. If small amounts of monetary gain are encountered more often than large amounts, then changing a prize from $5 and $10 may improve its rank position substantially (the latter seems a much better prize); but changing between $1000 and $1005 will be indiscernible—both will have the same rank position in almost all samples. This observation can be used to explain the apparent decreasing marginal utility of money. Probabilities, by contrast, are most commonly encountered in discourse close to 0 and 1; hence the ends of the probability scale are "artificially expanded" when considered in terms of ranks, yielding the inverted S-shaped weighting function of prospect theory (Kahneman and Tverksy, 1979).

In addition, decision-by-sampling can be extended to make the assumption that the attribute values of an option are simply averaged to reach an overall evaluation of an item. If the value of an item on each of its attributes is sensitive to context, this implies that the tradeoff between attributes will not be stable. Suppose, for example, that item A is superior on dimension x, and item B is superior on dimension y. If many alternative items in the decision context (whether given in the experiment, or sampled from memory) have values on dimension x that are intermediate between A and B, then this difference on dimension x will be perceived as large (i.e., in terms of rank position in this sample); and if there are few or no items with values on y between those of A and B, then the difference on dimension y will be perceived as small. This might be expected to lead to a preference for A over B. But, if the sample has the opposite pattern with respect to the two dimensions, the reverse would be expected: B would be preferred to A. Thus, the instability of the representation of individual dimensions leads to the prediction of systematic preference reversals—which are, of course, not compatible with the existence of a stable utility scale, whether ordinal or cardinal.

In summary, our major claim is that when people judge the attributes of choice options (like utilities, payoffs, and probabilities), they are not able to represent the absolute magnitudes of these attributes; instead, they represent magnitudes using *local comparisons*—in relation to whether they are larger or smaller than other magnitudes sampled from the environment or from memory. This implies that the difference between two items in relation to any dimensions will be highly context-sensitive—depending on the number of intervening values for other items in the sample, as we have seen. Additional evidence for this claim comes from behavioral research on the effects of context on decision making, and also from recent research in neuroscience, which we consider in the next sections.

4.3 Comparison and value I: behavioral data

Existing models of choice, including expected utility theory or prospect theory (Kahneman and Tversky, 1979), assume that the utility of a risky prospect or strategy is determined by the utility of the outcomes of the prospect or game, and transforms of the probabilities of each outcome. Decisions are assumed to be based on these utilities, embodying a value-based theory of choice. Such theories are typically based on the underlying assumption that only an option's own attributes are relevant in determining its perceived value—and that the only relevance of other choices is via their overall values.

There is recent evidence, however, that the attributes of the previously or currently seen risky prospects and games influence the evaluation of the attributes of the current prospect (or game), which suggests that prospects are not considered independently of previously cases (Stewart et al., 2003; Vlaev and Chater, 2006; Vlaev et al., 2007). In particular, Stewart et al. (2003) have argued for the existence of what they call *prospect relativity*: that the perceived value of a risky prospect (e.g., "*p* chance of *x*") is relative to other prospects with which it is presented. In particular, Stewart et al. studied peoples' perception of utilities in individual decision-making tasks in gambling situations. The initial expectation, based on the psychophysical studies described above, is that the option set (i.e., the context) will affect peoples' choices because there is no fixed internal scale according to which people make their judgments of the values of certain options. The results demonstrated a powerful context effect in judging the value of different risky prospects. The set of non-options offered as potential certainty equivalents for simple prospects was shown to have a large effect on the certainty equivalents selected. For example, suppose we are asked to judge the certain amount of money equivalent to the value of a 50% chance of winning £200. If people have options of £40, £50, £60, and £70, the most popular choice is £60 and then second choice is £50. When people have options of £90, £100, £110, £120, the most popular choice is £100, and then second choice is £110. So, the set of alternatives affects the modal choice of the optimal balance of risk and return almost by a factor of 2.

This effect was replicated, despite monetary incentives designed to encourage participants to deliver accurate and truthful certainty equivalents. In another experiment, the set from which a simple prospect was selected was also shown to have a large effect on the prospect that was chosen. Vlaev et al. (2007) further illustrated prospect relativity, by demonstrating relativity of human preferences in financial decision making under risk. This study investigated how the range and the rank of the options offered as saving amounts and levels of investment risk influence people's decisions about these variables. In the range manipulation, participants were presented with either a full range of choice options or a limited subset, while in the rank manipulation they were presented with a (positively or negatively) skewed set of feasible options. The results showed that choices of saving rates and investment risk are affected by the position of each option in the range and the rank of presented options, which suggests that such judgments and choices are relative.

Similar context effects were also found in a sequential setting during interactive decision making when people play many one-shot Prisoner's Dilemma games with appropriate anonymity (Vlaev and Chater, 2006), thus providing a new type of anomaly for orthodox game theory. In particular, participants were asked on each round of the game to predict the likelihood that their co-player will cooperate, and then to make a decision as to whether to cooperate or defect. The results demonstrated that the average cooperation rate and the mean predicted cooperation of the co-player in each game strongly depended on the cooperativeness of the preceding games (defined by the cooperation index proposed by Rapoport and Chammah, 1965). Thus, the perceived cooperativeness of a game did not depend only on the absolute value of its cooperation index, because people cooperated more and expected more cooperation in a game with higher rank position (in terms of its cooperation index) relative to the other games in the sequence. These results present a challenge to game-theoretic models that assume that the attributes of each game in a sequence are valued independently from the other games that are played.

A recent experiment suggests that people do not have stable representations of utility, even for immediate subjective experiences, such as pain. Vlaev et al. (2009) show that valuation is highly contextual, in that the price people pay for relief of pain is remarkably susceptible to the momentary contingencies of the market. In an auction-based market experiment, subjects received a single electrical shock and were then asked to decide how much they were willing to pay, from an initial monetary endowment for that trial (40 pence or 80 pence), to avoid fifteen further shocks. Participants made higher price offers for medium-pain relief, which they experienced in a sequence of low-pain trials, compared to when the same pain was experienced among high-pain trials. That is, individuals were willing to pay more to avoid the same pain when that pain was relatively more painful, rather than relatively less painful, compared to recent trials. Furthermore, the price people are willing to pay for pain relief was strongly determined by "money-in-the-pocket" (i.e., the amount they were allowed to "bid" on that particularly trial), rather than overall wealth. This suggests that the subjective value people attribute to non-market products, here relief of suffering, is remarkably malleable. The estimated consumer demand curves for pain relief exhibited the relativistic patterns described above. However, whereas the demand to avoid the medium pain was substantially affected by whether the other pain was higher or lower, the high and low pains were less affected by the context pairing, consistent with the idea that participants pay attention mainly to the rank order of pains (and not to absolute pain level). More recently, similar effects have been demonstrated where people gain money or suffer mild electric shocks, in a perceptuo-motor task (Kurniawan et al., 2010).

A number of other experiments have also investigated the effect of the context, i.e., the set of available options, on decision making in a way analogous to the effects we have described in a psychophysical context. These contextual effects provide further evidence against an internal value scale that mediates judgment and choice. For example, the set of options available as potential certainty equivalents has been shown to affect the choice of certainty equivalent for risky prospects (gambles). In making a certainty equivalent judgment, participants suggest, or select from, a set of options, the amount of money for certain that is worth the same to them as a single chance to play the prospect. Birnbaum (1992) demonstrated that skewing the distribution of options offered as certainty equivalents for simple prospects, whilst holding the maximum and minimum constant, influenced the selection of a certainty equivalent. When the options were positively skewed (i.e., most values were small) prospects were under-valued, compared to when the options were negatively skewed (i.e., most values were large).

Benartzi and Thaler (2001) have found evidence of another effect of the choice set by studying how people allocate their retirement funds across various investment vehicles. In particular, they find evidence for a diversification bias, which they call the $1/n$ heuristic. The idea is that when an employee is offered n funds to choose from in her retirement plan, she divides the money approximately evenly among the funds offered. Use of this heuristic, or others only slightly more sophisticated, implies that the asset allocation an investor chooses will depend strongly on the array of funds offered in the retirement plan. Thus, in a plan that offered one stock fund and one bond fund, the average allocation would be 50% stocks, but if another stock fund were added, the allocation to stocks would jump to two thirds. Read and Loewenstein (1995) also reported that people tend to diversify equally between the set of available options. Finally, the notion of (constant) risk aversion has come under criticism from behavioral economics. According to Rabin (2000), a consumer who, from any initial wealth level, turns down gambles where she loses $100 or gains $110, each with 50% probability, will turn down 50–50 bets of losing $1000 or gaining any credible sum of money. The point is that the constant determining relative risk aversion in the first small-stakes gamble, applied to gambles with larger stakes, leads to absurd predictions. The bottom line is that we cannot infer risk aversion from one gamble and expect it to scale up to larger gambles. One solution to the problem observed by Rabin is that proposed by prospect theory (Kahneman and Tversky, 1979), where outcomes are considered relative to a reference point (usually the status quo), rather than to consider only the final wealth.

Simonson and Tversky (1992) also reported strong context effects but their evidence was that there is a general preference for the central options in each choice set, which they explained with what they called the compromise effect. For example, when participants had to choose between $6 or a famous brand pen, the introduction of a pen from a lesser known brand name increased the proportion of participants selecting the famous brand pen, and reduced the proportion selecting the $6. A plausible account for this type of data is the notion of tradeoff contrast, where participants, who are assumed to have little knowledge about the tradeoff between two properties, i.e., they do not have a clear idea what is the exact utility of each option, deduce what the average tradeoff is, from the current or earlier choice sets. These data may reflect a more general tendency to prefer central options when choosing amongst set of options (also called extremeness aversion), which might also be due to the relativistic way people derive the utilities of the choice options. Similar trends were observed when people chose between products on a supermarket shelf (Christenfeld, 1995). These results back up the earlier suggestion that preferences between different types of good may be unstable.

Simonson and Tversky (1992) also provide several cases where preceding material significantly influences current judgments in decision making. For example, when choosing between pairs of computers that vary in price and amount of memory, the tradeoff between the two attributes in the previous choice affects the current choice. This result shows that, by varying the preceding products, the preference can be reversed. Such an effect of the preceding material is similar to the sequential context effects found in the psychophysical studies of perceptual judgment reported in the previous section.

Furthermore, Tversky and Simonson (1993) proposed the *componential-context model* as a comparison-based model of context-dependent preference devised to provide an account of tradeoff contrast and extremeness aversion (Simonson and Tversky, 1992). According to the model, each attribute has a subjective value depending on its magnitude and the value of an option is a weighted sum of its attribute values. The background context is assumed to be the previous choice set, which modifies the weighting of each attribute (dimension) according to the tradeoff between the attributes in that set. Thus, after the weighting of each attribute has been modified, the value of an option in the current set is then modified by the relative value of the option averaged over *pair-wise comparisons* with the other options in the choice set (i.e., the choice between options is made again in relative terms).

In summary, these findings on the role of context in decision making, which are reviewed here, present a challenge to standard rational choice theory and game theory as descriptive models. But they also challenge descriptive theories of decision making under uncertainty, including rank-dependent utility theory (Quiggin, 1982, 1993), configural weight models (Birnbaum, et al., 1999), and prospect and cumulative prospect theories (Kahneman and Tversky, 1979; Tversky and Kahneman, 1992), which all assign a risky prospect with a value or utility that depends only on the attributes of that prospect. In addition, the results by Vlaev and Chater (2006) present a challenge to the descriptive adequacy of standard game theory, which assumes that games in a sequence are considered independently (e.g., Fudenberg and Tirole, 1991). Therefore, the comparative theory of choice presented here departs fundamentally from previous work in this field, by modeling the highly flexible and contextually variable way in which people represent magnitudes (like sums of money, probabilities, time intervals, cooperativeness, etc.), rather than assuming that these magnitudes can be represented on absolute internal (cardinal) psychological scales. Our conjecture is that the results from the studies presented here suggest that people use context in order to derive the attractiveness of a risky prospect or a strategy. Thus, if absolute judgments are impossible, then the only reliable judgment that can be made is that one option is just better/worse than the other (without being able to say by how much). Next we discuss evidence from neuroscience, which suggests that similar processes take place at the level of neural responses.

4.4 **Comparison and value II: neuroscientific data**

The behavioral results discussed so far do not necessarily imply that the brain does not have stable representations of utility, but they do suggest that it cannot readily translate such representations into choices. However, there is also evidence that such relativistic effects may exist at a biological level. For example, although the neurophysiological basis of aversive (pain) valuation is complex (Dayan and Seymour, 2008), there is evidence that relativistic effects similar to the ones observed by Vlaev et al. (2009) may indeed exist at an underlying biological level. Neurophysiological recordings in both monkeys and humans have shown evidence of relative reward coding in neural substrates (for instance, via dopamine projections to the striatum and the orbitofrontal cortex) strongly implicated in simple choice behavior (Tremblay and Schultz, 1999; Nieuwenhuis et al., 2005; Tobler, Fiorillo, and Schultz, 2005), suggesting that value relativity may exist at a more fundamental level in the brain.

The proponents of the existence of a common currency of value, on the other side, argue that neural signals in certain areas of the brain reflect tradeoffs between value signals coming from different brain areas (e.g., Knutson et al., 2007, have shown that when an explicit tradeoff is made between a stated price and an every-day good, there appear to be separate representations of the value of the item to be gained in nucleus accumbens, and the financial loss in insula cortex). Plassmann et al. (2007) report evidence that the brain integrates and compares such gain and loss information in terms of common value currency—subjects' willingness to pay for goods correlates with orbitofrontal cortical activity.

However, the brain area (i.e., the medial orbitofrontal cortex) involved in such willingness-to-pay broadly co-localizes with that involved in the establishment of context-related judgments, which implies that such currency tradeoffs might equally well proceed via some (relativistic) comparative mechanisms instead of value-based one. Thus, Tremblay and Schultz (1999) report evidence for relative coding in the orbitofrontal neurons of monkeys when presented with varying juice rewards, which were presented in pairs within each block of trials; such coding appears to be highly local, i.e., dependent on the local context of alternative options. The recorded neuronal activity depended on whether or not the juice was the more preferred one in that block, rather than its absolute value—the neurons did not fire if the alternative juice was more preferable. Elliott et al. (2008) report an analogous fMRI study with humans, which found similar results in the medial orbitofrontal cortex—a brain with a well-understood role in basic value coding. Hosokawa et al. (2007) found similar effects with aversive outcomes: if a neutral outcome is presented alongside an electric shock, orbitofrontal neurons respond to the neutral outcome precisely as they do to juice reward presented alongside the neutral outcome. That is, in both studies, stimuli activate orbitofrontal neurons when they are comparatively better than the alternatives.

The evidence presented so far demonstrates that neurons record how much better an outcome is in the context of others, which is clearly useful for adaptation, and such relative encoding is analogous to the prediction error—the learning signal responsible for updating values as a consequence of trial-and-error experience (Sutton and Barto, 1998). Schultz et al. (1997) demonstrate that dopamine projections from the midbrain to the striatum carry this signal.

Theories of relative judgment also imply that values should scale to match the relevant range of magnitudes in the decision context. Tobler et al. (2005) found that dopamine neurons in monkeys exhibit this property. When the monkeys were presented with cues that predicted two equally likely amounts of fruit juice, the dopamine neurons coded the relative value of the outcomes, with larger juice volumes eliciting phasic activations and smaller volumes causing deactivations, independent of absolute juice quantity (the animals had to learn to predict varying quantities of fruit juice). Critically, however, the difference between the activity associated with the higher and lower magnitudes were essentially constant, despite the fact that the juice volume ranges were substantially different. This result suggests that the neuronal sensitivity adapts to the range of magnitudes expected. Seymour and McClure (2008) argue that the fact such scaling (matching the relevant range of magnitudes) may occur in some form of another is not surprising, and that it would be remarkable if neurons accurately encoded on the same scale the value of all goods—from the cheapest ones like chocolate bar to the most expensive ones such as a new house. If they do indeed adapt, then comparisons across scales might be hazardous. Seymour and McClure point out that the evidence suggests that the benefit of adaptive scaling outweighs the costs from neuronal inability to integrate across transactions in separate contexts in an individual's daily life. But an alternative viewpoint that such scales are never constructed—instead, neural activity represents the transient results of comparison to the specific set of items which form the local perceptual or cognitive context.

In summary, this evidence suggests that there is no stable neural common currency that is used to independently value stimuli across contexts. And even in a specific context, it may be that the brain can find, at best, the ordinal position of goods in a range of options. Thus, object or price anchors can establish the boundaries and sensitivity (or gain) of a value scale, determining whether a given transaction will appear relatively good or bad. Therefore, so far, we suggest, there is no convincing evidence that absolute values are coded in the brain.

4.5 Implications

If the value-based account of human choice were correct, the consequences could potentially be astonishingly far-reaching. Suppose that it were possible, from behavioral or neuroscientific data, to determine the underlying value of arbitrarily different options on a single scale of value. Then, it would be possible directly to determine which options people will choose, when given arbitrary options; and, moreover, where people fail to make such choices, perhaps due to one or other of the innumerable contextual forces operative in human judgment and decision making, it might nonetheless be possible to advise people concerning what options they should choose, to act in their own interests. Thus a cognitive or neural theory of valuation would provide a powerful descriptive, and potentially, prescriptive, tool at the level of individual behavior. One could imagine that, by uncovering a scale of value, it would be possible to help people tradeoff apparently incommensurable goods, such as present pleasures vs. future ill-health; or tradeoff the effort involved in pro-social or pro-environment behaviors, against the immediate personal "cost." According to the value-based approach, people assign values to all manner of different goods; the task of the psychologist, neuroscientist, or economist, may be merely to infer these values, and predict and/or advise according.

The implications might be more far-reaching still. Perhaps it would be possible to use such valuations as a yard-stick for public policy. If a "neural signal" for value were relatively stable within individuals, and, crucially, also across individuals, then it would be possible to imagine directly measuring the neural correlates of human well-being. A natural aim of public policy would then, of course, be to maximize the expected level of such well-being. One could imagine a science-fiction future in which each person might be fitted with a "hedonometer," streaming back data concerning their well-being, or perhaps their valuation of particular types of experience, event, or outcome; and public policy might be shaped appropriately. The utilitarian approach to ethics and politics could finally be put on a scientific basis.

Such optimistic suggestions are, we suspect, not so far from the long-term aims of many researchers at the intersection of psychology, economics, and the neurosciences. This idea has a long history going back to Bentham's (1789/1970) utilitarianism. However, the assumption that people do not have internal scales for value potentially undermines Bentham's notion of utility.

As we noted above, mainstream economics has moved away from assuming the existence of internal utility scales. For example, the standard "revealed preference" interpretation of utility in economics (Samuelson, 1937) takes utilities to be revealed by observable choices without further specification about the psychological nature of these utilities; and Savage (1954) generalized this assumption to utilities and probabilities by showing that preferences over gambles could be used to "reveal" utility and probability information simultaneously. Thus, from the revealed preference perspective, the utility and probability scales are derived from choice preferences, rather than from assumptions about psychological scales.

4.5.1 Implication for economics

The conceptual framework presented here has interesting similarities with respect to this traditional view in economics. In both the revealed preference perspective and the decision-by-sampling approach proposed by Stewart et al. (2006), people are assumed to have access only to their own binary preferences (or more generally, to binary comparisons between magnitudes). Therefore, to the extent that people have a broader grasp of their own, more global, values (probabilities, etc.), this must be inferred from sampling their own past choices and other memories, thus revealing their preferences. So, for a given person to gain any "global" insight into how much pleasure is gained from consuming a specific product, this person has to sample from her memory for some related, comparable events where she consumed that product or comparable products. If the consumption episode in question is preferred to these events sampled from memory, this "reveals" to the person that this was a good experience; if it is preferred to some past episodes, but dispreferred to as many, this reveals to the same person that the experience was moderate, and so on. Thus, to the extent that people have any global grasp of their views concerning their perspective on how valuable (or, similarly, how probable) some event is, they must "reveal" this, by sampling from their own binary preferences, just as the economist attempts to reconstruct utility and probability values from the entire set of a person's binary preferences.

However, if both choices and utility judgments are radically influenced by contextual factors, and hence subject to systematic reversals of preference, how can we develop measurement tools to establish what people "really" want? How much do they really value aspects of their own future, environmental or health outcomes? Indeed, only to the extent that it is possible to find ways of avoiding large contextual influence can we be confident that the question of what people really want is even well-defined. According to the "constructive" preference viewpoint (Slovic, 1995; Tversky et al., 1988), the picture is bleak—people are assumed to construct their judgments on-line, rather than having access to any stable preferences. If this conclusion is correct, the implications for normative theories of decision making are disturbing, whether in political philosophy, the valuation of non-market goods (such as environmental and health goods), or, indeed, in the foundations of micro-economics.

An immediate acceptance to constructive preferences may, however, be too swift. The psychophysical case is illustrative. Using binary choices, as noted above, people can reliably discriminate about 100 loudnesses (for a single type of stimulus, e.g., tones). Thus, following Fechner (1966) and Thurstone (1959), we can construct a loudness scale from a careful selection of binary options, which is vastly more precise than a scale about which people can make direct judgments. This loudness scale will reliably predict which pairs of tones will be judged to be louder (and, indeed, even the precision of discrimination can be enhanced, if people make multiple judgments on each pair of tones). And the predictions about binary judgments, and hence the Fechnerian scale derived from them, are themselves not context dependent (or are at least marginally so). So, we have the somewhat paradoxical result that, although people cannot locate items on a psychophysical scale, they can provide binary judgments from which such a scale can be derived (or revealed). So it is at least conceivable that people's binary judgments might be used to construct a scale measuring their values or utility, which is much more stable than any judgments that they could provide directly. That is, it might be possible to "knit together" people's local judgments into a global theory of preference, even though people are unable to do this "from the inside." The results of any such scaling procedure would inevitably clash with the highly labile and context-driven choices that people actually make, given a fixed set of options. How clashes between the theoretically-derived prescription (perhaps that, given my global wants, I should prefer salad to cake) would be resolved with actual choices (that I choose cake not salad) is not clear.

4.5.2 Health economics

Explicit judgments concerning pain, and other subjective health-state experiences, are typically expressed in complex social and economic contexts. This is the case, firstly, when consumers (including patients) are forced to make abstract comparisons between experienced or imagined primary affective health states and other non-health-related goods, such as money. Furthermore, a particular difficulty in trading off such different quantities to inform our purchasing behavior is generated by the fact that health products are naturally inhibitory, in that one pays to avoid a certain aversive symptom, rather than to receive a positive good. Note also that the products of health purchase embody the positively valenced property of relief, because states that are associated with termination of aversive events acquire rewarding valence (Seymour et al., 2005). Lack of valuation scales would require increasing experience in order to mitigate this tradeoff problem, but experience cannot easily do so for products that buy relief for never-experienced symptoms, a central "commodity" in modern preventative healthcare markets.

Explicit valuation judgments are also required when economists and policy makers quantify adverse clinical states, to inform decisions regarding pricing strategy, investment in research, and cost-effectiveness of treatments. Pain, in particular, is a major public health issue, not least given the fact that approximately 20% of the general population suffer from clinically significant pain (Eriksen et al., 2003; Macfarlane, Jones, and McBeth, 2005). Importantly, pain rarely occurs in isolation, and is usually being experienced in the general symptomatic and temporal context of an illness. The comparative theory of choice outlined here (and the lack of intrinsic human value representations) would require new methods of health-state valuations, because of the susceptibility to relativistic judgment biases shaped by context, which is likely to have substantial economic consequences. Future research should explore methods for obtaining stable valuations for various clinical symptoms as such methods play a very important role in healthcare policy and markets.

4.6 **Conclusions**

Theories of decision making, in neuroscience, psychology, and economics, divide fundamentally on the role of utility. The strongest position, which we call *neuro-utility*, is that utility is computed by the brain, and that this computed utility drives choice. The intermediate position, which we call *behavioral-utility*, is that utility is not computed by the brain; but people, and non-human animals, may behave as if their choices are driven by utility, and hence that utility is useful as a prediction device for future behavior. The final position, *utility-scepticism*, is that utility plays neither of these roles. What makes utility normatively appealing in the first two positions is exactly what makes it psychologically unappealing—its ability to bridge across domains. However, the evidence here implies that utility is unstable, even within the same domain, which implies that it will be even more malleable across domains. For these reasons, we tentatively defend the third position, which avoids the concept of underlying utility altogether, and instead looks at preferences as derived from the fundamental process of local comparison.

References

Barlow, H. B. (1991). Possible principles underlying the transformation of sensory messages. In **W. A. Rosenblith** (ed.) *Sensory communication* (pp. 217–34). Cambridge, MA: MIT Press.

Benartzi, S. and Thaler, R. (2001). Naive diversification strategies in defined contribution saving plans. *American Economic Review*, **91**, 79–98.

Bentham, J. (1970). *An introduction to the principles of morals and legislation* (**J. H. Burns and H. L. A. Hart,** eds). London: The Athlone Press. (Original work published in 1789.)

Birnbaum, M. H. (1992). Violations of monotonicity and contextual effects in choice-based certainty equivalents. *Psychological Science*, **3**, 310–4.

Birnbaum, M. H., Patton, J. N., and Lott, M. K. (1999). Evidence against rank-dependent utility theories: Tests of cumulative independence, interval independence, stochastic dominance, and transitivity. *Organizational Behavior and Human Decision Processes*, **77**, 44–83.

Brandstätter, E., Gigerenzer, G., and Hertwig, R. (2006). The priority heuristic: Making choices without tradeoffs. *Psychological Review*, **113**, 409–32.

Brown, G.D.A., Neath, I., and Chater, N. (2007). A temporal ratio model of memory. *Psychological Review*, **114**, 539–76.

Camerer, C., Loewenstein, G., and Prelec, D. (2005). Neuroeconomics: how neuroscience can inform economics. *Journal of Economic Literature*, **XLIII**, 9–64.

Christenfeld, N. (1995). Choices from identical options. *Psychological Science*, **6**, 50–55.

Cooter, R. and Rappoport, P. (1984). Were the ordinalists wrong about welfare economics? *Journal of Economic Literature*, **22**, 507–30.

Dayan, P. and Seymour, B. (2008). Value and actions in aversion. In: P. W. Glimcher, C. F. Camerer, E. Fehr, and R. A. Poldrack (eds) *Neuroeconomics: Decision making and the brain*. London, UK: Elsevier.

Elliott, R., Agnew, Z., and Deakin, J. F. (2008). Medial orbitofrontal cortex codes relative rather than absolute value of financial rewards in humans. *European Journal of Neuroscience*, **27**, 2213–2218.

Eriksen, J., Jensen, M. K., Sjogren, P., Ekholm, O., and Rasmussen, N. K. (2003). Epidemiology of chronic non-malignant pain in Denmark. *Pain*, 106, 221–28.

Fechner, G. T. (1966). *Elements of psychophysics* (H. E. Adler, Trans.). New York: Holt, Rinehart, and Winston. (Original work published 1860).

Fudenberg, D. and Tirole J. (1991). *Game theory*. Cambridge, MA: MIT Press.

Garner, W. R. (1962). *Uncertainty and structure and psychological concepts*. New York: Wiley.

Gigerenzer, G. and Goldstein, D (1996). Reasoning the fast and frugal way: models of bounded rationality. *Psychological Review*, 103, 650–69.

Hosokawa, T., Kato, K., Inoue, M., and Mikami, A. (2007). Neurons in the macaque orbitofrontal cortex code relative preference of both rewarding and aversive outcomes. *Neuroscience Research*, 57, 434–45.

Kahneman, D. and Tversky, A. (1979). Prospect theory: an analysis of decision under risk. *Econometrica*, 47, 263–91.

Knutson, B., Rick, S., Wimmer, G., Prelec, D., and Loewenstein, G. (2007). Neural predictors of purchases. *Neuron*, 53, 147–56.

Kurniawan, I.T., Seymour, B., Vlaev, I., Trommershäuser, J., Dolan, R. J., and Chater, N. (2010). Pain relativity in motor control. *Psychological Science*, 21, 840–7.

Laming, D. R. J. (1984). The relativity of "absolute" judgments. *British Journal of Mathematical and Statistical Psychology*, 37, 152–83.

Laming, D. R. J. (1997). *The measurement of sensation*. London: Oxford University Press.

Loomes, G. and Sugden, R. (1982). Regret theory: an alternative theory of rational choice under uncertainty. *Economic Journal*, 92, 805–24.

Macfarlane, G. J., Jones, G. T., and McBeth, J. (2005). Epidemiology of pain. In S. B. McMahon and M. Koltzenburg (eds.) *Wall and Melzack's textbook of pain*, 5th edn (pp. 1199–214). Philadelphia: Elsevier.

Miller, G. A. (1956). The magical number seven, plus or minus two: some limits on our capacity for information processing. *Psychological Review*, 63, 81–97.

Nieuwenhuis, S., Heslenfeld, D. J., von Geusau, N. J., Mars, R. B., Holroyd, C. B., and Yeung, N. (2005). Activity in human reward-sensitive brain areas is strongly context dependent. *Neuroimage*, 25, 1302–1309.

Padoa-Schioppa, C. and Assad, J. A. (2008). The representation of economic value in the orbitofrontal cortex is invariant for changes of menu. *Nature Neuroscience*, 11, 95–102.

Plassmann, H., O'Doherty, J., and Rangel A. (2007). Orbitofrontal cortex encodes willingness to pay in everyday economic transactions. *Journal of Neuroscience*, 27, 9984–88.

Quiggin, J. (1982). A theory of anticipated utility. *Journal of Economic Behavior and Organisation*, 3, 323–43.

Quiggin, J. (1993). *Generalized expected utility theory: the rank-dependent model*. Boston: Kluwer Academic.

Rabin, M. (2000). Diminishing marginal utility of wealth cannot explain risk aversion. In D. Kahneman and A. Tversky (eds) *Choices, values, and frames* (pp. 202–208). New York: Cambridge University Press.

Rapoport, A. and Chammah, A. (1965). *Prisoner's dilemma: a study in conflict and cooperation*. Ann Arbor: University of Michigan Press.

Read, D. and Loewenstein, G. (1995). Diversification bias: explaining the discrepancy in variety seeking between combined and separated choices. *Journal of Experimental Psychology: Applied*, 1, 34–49.

Samuelson, P. (1937). A note on the measurement of utility. *Review of Economic Studies*, 4, 155–61.

Savage, L. J. (1954). *The foundations of statistics*. New York: Wiley.

Schultz, W., Dayan, P., and Montague, P. R. (1997). A neural substrate of prediction and reward. *Science*, 275, 1593–99.

Seymour, B. and McClure, S. (2008). Anchors, scales and the relative coding of value in the brain. *Current Opinion in Neurobiology*, **18**, 173–78.

Seymour, B., O'Doherty, J. P., Koltzenburg, M., Wiech, K., Frackowiak, R., Friston, K., and Dolan, R. (2005). Opponent appetitive-aversive neural processes underlie predictive learning of pain relief. *Nature Neuroscience*, **8**, 1234–40.

Shiffrin, R. M. and Nosofsky, R. M. (1994). Seven plus or minus two: a commentary on capacity limitations. *Psychological Review*, **101**, 357–61.

Simonson, I. and Tversky, A. (1992). Choice in context: tradeoff contrast and extremeness aversion. *Journal of Marketing Research*, **29**, 281–95.

Slovic, P. (1995). The construction of preferences. *American Psychologist*, **50**, 364–71.

Stevens, S. S. (1957). On the psychophysical law. *Psychological Review*, **64**, 153–81.

Stewart, N., Brown, G. D. A., and Chater, N. (2005). Absolute identification by relative judgment. *Psychological Review*, **112**, 881–911.

Stewart, N., Chater, N., Stott, H. P., and Reimers, S. (2003). Prospect relativity: how choice options influence decision under risk. *Journal of Experimental Psychology: General*, **132**, 23–46.

Stewart, N., Chater, N., and Brown, G. D. A. (2006). Decision by sampling. *Cognitive Psychology*, **53**, 1–26.

Sutton, R. S. and Barto, A. G. (1998). *Reinforcement learning: an introduction*. MIT Press.

Thurstone, L. L. (1959). *The measurement of values*. Chicago: University of Chicago Press.

Tobler, P. N., Fiorillo, C. D., and Schultz, W. (2005). Adaptive coding of reward value by dopamine neurons. *Science*, **307**, 1642–45.

Tremblay, L. and Schultz, W. (1999). Relative reward preference in primate orbitofrontal cortex. *Nature*, **398**, 704–708.

Tverksy, A. (1972). Elimination by aspects: atheory of choice. *Psychological Review*, **79**, 281–99.

Tversky, A. and Kahneman, D. (1992). Advances in prospect theory: cumulative representation of uncertainty. *Journal of Risk and Uncertainty*, **5**, 204–217.

Tversky, A. and Simonson, I. (1993). Context-dependent preferences. *Management Science*, **39**, 1179–89.

Tversky, A., Sattah, S., and Slovic, P. (1988). Contingent weighting in judgment and choice. *Psychological Review*, **95**, 371–84.

Vlaev, I. and Chater, N. (2006). Game relativity: how context influences strategic decision making. *Journal of Experimental Psychology: Learning, Memory, and Cognition*, **32**, 131–49.

Vlaev, I., Chater, N., and Stewart, N. (2007). Financial prospect relativity: context effects in financial decision making under risk. *Journal of Behavioral Decision making*, **20**, 273–304.

Vlaev, I., Seymour, B., Dolan, R., and Chater, N. (2009). The price of pain and the value of suffering. *Psychological Science*, **20**, 309–17.

Wallach, H. (1948). Brightness constancy and the nature of achromatic colors. *Journal of Experimental Psychology*, **38**, 310–24.

Chapter 5

Do intransitive choices reflect genuinely context-dependent preferences?

Tobias Kalenscher and Cyriel M.A. Pennartz

Abstract

A multitude of theories on decision making suppose that individuals choose between different prospects by placing a value, or utility, on these prospects and selecting whichever prospect has the highest value. If decisions were at all times value-based, then choices should always be transitive. Transitivity holds that, if prospect A is preferred over prospect B, and B is preferred over C, A should also be preferred over C. Despite its intuitive appeal, individuals often show striking violations of transitivity. Intransitive decisions could be the consequence of asymmetrically distributed errors made during the implementation of transitively organized values because individuals may be more likely to erroneously choose against their true preference when the discrimination between the prospects' values is difficult compared to situations where the prospect with the highest value is clearly and easily detectable. Alternatively, intransitive choices may reflect genuinely context-dependent preferences because individuals may compare the options' multiple attributes separately, not in an integrated fashion. In this study, we replicate intransitive choices in a risky decision-making task, and present a novel analysis that argues against the noisy implementation of transitive value account. We maintain that choices reflect truly intransitive and context-dependent preferences and discuss several possible explanations why individuals make decisions in such a way.

5.1 Introduction

Let's assume you want to eat dessert, and you are pondering whether to eat two apples or one cup of *mousse au chocolat*. How do you decide between such qualitatively different commodities? Many, if not the majority, of theories on decision making assume that individuals solve such decision problems by assigning a subjective value ("*utility*") to the available choice options. The value of an option is a function of the option's attributes (e.g., identity and quantity in the example above), personal preference, waiting time, and other factors. Encoding choice options in terms of subjective value allows different commodities to be represented on a common scale, and therefore ranked, and otherwise incommensurable outcomes can be compared (cf. Shizgal, 1997; Montague and Berns, 2002). The greater the difference between the assigned values, the more likely it is that a decision maker chooses the option with the higher value. We refer to theories making this assumption as "simple scalability" or "value-based decision models" (Navarick and Fantino, 1975; Rangel et al., 2008).

Value-based decision models explicitly assert that observable choices reflect a hierarchically ordered, internally represented ranking of subjective values. Therefore, even though values are not visible or directly measurable, they can be inferred from overt choice relations (Samuelson, 1937; von Neumann and Morgenstern, 1944; Friedman and Savage, 1952; Afriat, 1967; Varian, 1982). However, such inference is only possible if choices are transitive (Afriat, 1967; Varian, 1982). Transitivity holds that, if commodity A is preferred over B, and B is preferred over C, then A should also be preferred over C. More precisely, three levels of intransitive preferences can be defined. Where $P(X, Y)$ indicates the probability of choices for X over Y, and $P(A, B) \geq 0.5$ and $P(B, C) \geq 0.5$, choice satisfies:

- weak stochastic transitivity if $P(A, C) \geq 0.5$;
- moderate transitivity if $P(A, C) \geq \text{minimum}[P(A, B), P(A, C)]$;
- strong transitivity if $P(A, C) \geq \text{maximum}[P(A, B), P(A, C)]$.

If any of these levels of transitivity is not satisfied, a correspondence between choice relations and value relations cannot be straightforwardly assumed, and conclusions about internal value rankings may not be possible without making further assumptions.

Despite its intuitive nature, human and non-human individuals often show striking violations of transitivity (Tversky, 1969; Lindman and Lyons, 1978; Budescu and Weiss, 1987; Loomes et al., 1991; Shafir, 1994; Roelofsma and Read, 2000; Waite, 2001; Shafir et al., 2002; Bateson et al., 2003). It is presently unclear why intransitive choices occur. A stochastic specification of simple scalability posits that the core theory is true, i.e., the choice-underlying values are fixed and uniquely hierarchically ordered, but they are noisily implemented, so that subjects occasionally choose against their true preference (Sopher and Gigliotti, 1993; Hey, 1995; Loomes and Sugden, 1998; Birnbaum and Gutierrez, 2007; Birnbaum and Schmidt, 2009). The degree of noise, i.e., the likelihood of choosing against the true preference, may not be identical for all decision problems, but may depend on the difference between the alternatives' subjective values. If the difference in values is high, the alternatives are easy to discriminate, and subjects are likely to detect and choose the alternative yielding the highest value. However, if the subjective values are very similar, the options are difficult to discriminate, and individuals may be more prone to choose against their true preference. In the following, we will refer to this theory as the *noisy implementation of value account*.

Another class of theories states that subjects do not make decisions by assessing the alternative values independently, but they compare and integrate the difference in the alternatives' attributes separately (Tversky, 1969; Lindman and Lyons, 1978; Russo and Dosher, 1983; Roelofsma and Read, 2000; Brandstätter et al., 2006). For example, a subject choosing between risky positive prospects may first compare the difference in probabilities between the prospects, then the difference in gain magnitudes, and then weigh and integrate the differences in an attribute-wise fashion. According to a mathematical formalization of this idea (Tversky, 1969), prospect X would be preferred over Y if:

$$\sum_{i=1}^{n} \Phi_i [u_i(X_i) - u_i(Y_i)] \geq 0 \qquad (5.1)$$

where n is the number of attributes (two attributes in the case of risky choice between positive gains: gain magnitude and probability), $[u_i(X_i) - u_i(Y_i)]$ is the difference in utilities of attribute i between alternatives X and Y, and Φ_i is the weighting function that determines the impact of the difference in utility of attribute i on the overall decision. For example, a risky prospect X would be preferred over Y if:

$$\Phi_{Probability}[u(X_{Probability}) - u(Y_{Probability})] + \Phi_{Gain}[u(X_{Gain}) - u(Y_{Gain})] \geq 0 \qquad (5.2)$$

that is, when the difference in probabilities between gambles X and Y has a higher influence on the decision than the difference in gains. Depending on the shape of the weighting functions and the actual differences in gains and probabilities, a decision may be more strongly determined by gains than probabilities in one situation, but more by probabilities than gains in another situation (see below for explanation). Inconsistent choices would be the consequence. In the following, we will refer to the theory outlined in eqn. 5.1 as the *additive-difference model*.

The two theories make different predictions. If the *noisy implementation of value account* was true, then decisions between prospects with similar subjective values should be more difficult and more error prone than decisions between prospects with clearly different values (Hey, 1995). Hence, reactions times as a measure of choice difficulty should negatively correlate with the difference in values. Furthermore, with diminishing discriminability[1] between the prospects' subjective values, participants should be increasingly indifferent between the prospects (this prediction is more extensively discussed below). Thus, when discriminability is minimal, the choice distribution should not significantly deviate from indifference.

If the *additive-difference model* was true, then intransitive choices should not be the consequence of erroneous implementations of preferences, but follow systematic patterns. Specifically, the theory predicts that individuals systematically prefer safe prospects when the difference in the alternatives' attributes is big because their decision should be more strongly influenced by probabilities than by gains; but when the difference in the

---

[1] We do not refer to perceptual discrimination, but to the ability to tell the values of the choice alternatives apart. The better the discriminability, the easier it is to detect the alternative with the highest value.

attributes is small, they should systematically prefer risky prospects because gains should matter more to them than probabilities (Tversky, 1969; Brandstätter et al., 2007).

We tested 27 subjects in a risky choice task in which they made pairwise choices between prospects that differed in probability and gain magnitude: 18 out of 27 subjects showed several instances of intransitive choice. An analysis of the choices and reaction times provided little evidence for the *noisy implementation of value account,* suggesting that intransitive choices did not merely result from noisily implemented hierarchical preferences. Conversely, our analysis did support the *additive-difference model,* according to which intransitive choices were the consequence of local, context-dependent shifts in the importance of gains and probabilities for the decision.

5.2 Methods

5.2.1 Participants

Altogether, 27 participants (16 female, age 18–28, mean age 22.8), recruited from the University of Amsterdam, participated in this experiment. All participants were right-handed with no history of neurological problems. They were paid between €25 and €30 for participation, depending on whether they won or not. Participants gave their informed consent and the study met all criteria for approval of the Academic Medical Center Medical Ethical Committee. The behavioral data presented here were collected as part of a neuroimaging experiment that has been published elsewhere (Kalenscher et al., 2010).

5.2.2 Experimental design and task

Subjects were making choices between risky gambles. In short, each gamble offered a different gain magnitude (range $400 to $500) with a different probability (range 0.41 to 0.29) (Fig. 5.1A and 1B). On every trial, two out of a total of five gambles were presented, and subjects indicated which of the two gambles they would prefer to play. Within a presented gamble pair, one gamble had always a higher gain magnitude (the risky gamble, G_{risky}), and the other had a higher winning probability (the safe gamble, G_{safe}). To avoid an accumulated wealth effect, the gambles were not resolved during testing, and subjects were instructed that only one of the chosen gambles would be selected, played, and payed out (in case of a win) at the end of the experiment.

Prior to testing, participants were informed that they would be reimbursed with €25 for their participation, but that they could add up to €5 to this sum, depending on whether they win in this game or not. They were instructed that they were playing for dummy dollars, and the final gain in Euro would be determined by dividing the won sum of dummy dollars by 100. No losses were possible, and in case of a no-win, nothing would be added to the initial imbursement of €25. Subjects were further instructed that they would not receive feedback about the success or failure of their chosen gamble, but that, at the end of the experiment, one trial would be selected at random by the computer, and only the chosen gamble in this randomly selected trial would be played and paid out (in case of a win).

A

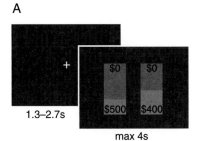

1.3–2.7s

max 4s

B

	Probability	Gain	Expected value
Gamble A	0.29	$500	145
Gamble B	0.32	$475	152
Gamble C	0.35	$450	158
Gamble D	0.38	$425	161
Gamble E	0.41	$400	164

Fig. 5.1 (A) Task design. Each trial began with an inter-trial interval (ITI) of variable duration, followed by the presentation of a pair of gambles. Each bar represents one gamble, which contained information about the potential monetary gain to be won by selecting it (numbers at the bottom of the bars) and the probability of winning this money, as specified by the expanse covered by a light gray area at the bottom of each bar (in the actual task the colors indicating winning and non-winning were green and red respectively). The $0 at the top of the bars indicated that subjects would receive no money in case they didn't win. Money was in dummy-dollars that could be exchanged against Euros at a rate of 1/100 in case of a win. Subjects had a maximum of 4 s to indicate which of the two gambles they would prefer to play. The gambles were not resolved during task performance, and subjects were instructed that one of the trials would be selected at random at the end of the experiment, and the selected gamble in this trial would be played. (B) Gambles used in the experiment. There were five different gambles that were presented in all ten possible pairwise combinations in a randomized fashion. The winning probability increased from gamble A to E in steps of 0.03, and the gain magnitude decreased from A to E in steps of $25, so that a gamble with a high gain had a low probability and vice versa. The expected value (product of gain and probability) was not identical across gambles but increased from gamble A to E in conjunction with the increase in probability. In each trial, two gambles were presented one of which always had a lower winning probability but a higher potential gain (the risky gamble, G_{risky}), and the other had a higher probability with a lower potential gain (the safe gamble, G_{safe}). Note that the differences are relative, and a given gamble that has a relatively low probability in one gamble pair may have a relatively high probability in another pair. The relative difference in gain and probability between gambles was quantified as *gamble-distance* (see text for details). Note that we also included control-trials in which either probability, but not gain, or only gain, but not probability was varied (not shown here, see methods section for details).

Participants were presented with 440 trials, divided into five blocks of 80 trials, and one block of 40 trials. Blocks were separated by a break of approximately one minute duration. The trials comprised 200 experimental trials and 240 control trials. Each trial began with an inter-trial interval (ITI) of variable duration (mean length 1.72 s, range 1.3–2.7 s), as indicated by a white fixation cross on the screen, and then the presentation of two gambles. In every trial, subjects had 4 s time to indicate which of the two gambles they would prefer to play. The difference between the actual response time and 4 s was added to the ITI, failure to respond within 4 s resulted in a missed trial. After indicating the response, the chosen gamble was enlarged for 500 ms to indicate that the response was registered by the computer. The entire experiment took approximaely 45 min.

In each experimental trial, two out of five different gambles were presented (Fig. 5.1A and B). All ten possible binary combinations of these five gambles were presented 20 times each. The degree by which the gains and probabilities of the two presented gambles differed varied between gamble pairs and was characterized by the variable *gamble-distance* (see below).

Furthermore, we included control trials in which gambles were presented that differed only in probability, but not in gain (probability-controls), or only in gain, but not in probability (gain-controls). Probability- and gain-control trials had the purpose of ensuring that subjects could perceptually discriminate between small differences in probability or gain, and to exclude subjects that made entirely random decisions. They were not further analyzed. None of the subjects was eventually excluded for making random decisions, since all subjects, without any exception, always selected the more valuable control gamble (i.e., the richer of the two gambles with equal probability, or the more certain one of the two gambles with equal gain magnitude).

Control trials were intermixed with experimental trials. The sequence of presentation of all trials was randomized between subjects, and the side of gamble presentation was randomized within each subject across all trial repetitions.

In the current version of the task, gain magnitudes were presented as numbers, and probabilities as bar-graphs. In preceding piloting sessions, we tested different presentation formats. For example, gain- and probability-information were both presented as numbers (probabilities were either presented as floating points, percentages or fractions), or probabilities were displayed as pie-charts. Intransitive preferences were found with all presentation formats and always in about an identical fraction of subjects (between 1/2 to 2/3 of all subjects tested in a given presentation format showed the effect), indicating that the effect seemed to be independent of the way the problem was presented.

After the experiment, the basic assumption of value-based decision making and the implications for transitivity were explained to our subjects. They did not seem to be aware of having made intransitive choices because, when asked, without exception, all subjects reported that they had made decisions by assigning values to each gamble, and claimed that their choices would be transitive. When confronted with the intransitivity of their choice pattern, they responded with astonishment. When further asked about the rules they applied to make their decisions, all intransitive subjects testified that they used a rule that was reminiscent of the predictions of the *additive-difference model* (Tversky, 1969). That is, they reported that they would generally prefer the gamble with the higher probability, and neglect gains, but that they opted for the gamble with the higher gain when the difference in probabilities was minute. Transitive subjects reported having either maximized reward amount (three participants) or probability (six participants). None of the transitive subjects stated having made decisions based on expected-value estimates.

5.2.3 Detection of intransitive preferences

The terminology of strong, moderate, and weak stochastic transitivity (see above) is somewhat misleading, as weak stochastic transitivity is the most conservative definition, and actually represents the most compelling form of transitivity (not every preference chain that violates moderate or strong transitivity also violates weak transitivity, but every violation of weak transitivity also violates moderate or strong transitivity). Therefore, here, we focus on violations of weak transitivity.

We used graph theory to detect intransitive cycles in our subjects' choices (Choi et al., 2007). In short, we tested they hypothesis that, if gamble X is (directly or indirectly) preferred to gamble Z, then Z is not strictly preferred to X (Varian, 1982). This was probed by representing choices between gambles graphically and testing for acyclicity: preferred gambles were connected to non-preferred gambles by an arrow pointing in the direction of the unpreferred gamble. Indifferent gamble-pairs were connected by two arrows pointing in both directions. We deemed a gamble as preferred over another gamble if the preferred gamble was chosen in more than 50% of the presentations of that pair. Indifference was assumed when both gambles in a pair were chosen with equal frequency (50%).[2]

Transitivity requires that such directed graphs representing choices are acyclical. If there are one or more loops in the graph, we can conclude that the subject had one or more occurrences of intransitive choices. For example, if a subject prefers gamble A over B, and B over C, but C over A, then the arrows will point from A→B→C and back from C→A. Hence, the existence of such a loop implies intransitivity. Real choice data often contain at least one violation of transitivity. It is, therefore, important to quantify the extent of intransitivity. We used a quantity that was inspired by Afriat's (1972) critical cost-efficiency index. Our quantity measures, for each subject, the smallest possible amount by which all choices must be adjusted in order to remove all violations of transitivity. A value of 0 means that a subject is perfectly transitive (no choice must be adjusted), a value of 1 means that a subject is perfectly intransitive (the maximum number of choices must be adjusted). We classified subjects as intransitive if they scored higher than 0.3 on our measure. See Kalenscher et al., (2010) for more details on detection of intransitive preferences.

5.2.4 Distance between gambles

Intransitive preferences imply that the frequency of choices of a given gamble is variable and depends on local context, i.e., which other gamble it is paired with. To characterize the effect of context, we examined choice as a function of *distance* between gambles. Distance is a quantity that measures how different two gambles are: the greater the difference in gain

---

[2] We opted for this very strict indifference criterion because more relaxed definitions would bias our selection against the *noisy implementation of value account*. Assume, for example, that an individual has a very slight preference for option A over B, a strong preference for B over C, and a likewise strong preference for A over C. The *noisy implementation of value account* predicts that this individual may choose B more often than A (against his true preference) because the values of A and B are difficult to discriminate, and choices are thus more error-prone. If we opted for a relaxed indifference criterion, we may classify the choice between A and B as indifferent, and, because A and B both equally dominate C, we would categorize this gamble set as transitive. Hence, we would artificially remove gamble combinations from the intransitive data set that contain near-indifferent statements. Because near-indifferent statements are one of the predictions of the *noisy implementation of value account,* we would bias our dataset against this account by removing data that meet the predictions.

and probability between the gambles, the greater the distance. Distance is correlated with discriminability: because the values of two gambles are easier to tell apart when their attributes are greatly different, discriminability increases with increasing distance.

We used the minimum step-size of changes in probability (0.03) and gain magnitude ($25) to measure the distance between G_{risky} and G_{safe} (cf. Fig. 5.1B). Adjacent gambles, i.e., gambles that are one step apart along the probability and gain scale (e.g., gamble pairs AB, or BC, etc.), are classified as distance 1. Gambles that are two steps apart are classified as distance 2 (e.g., gamble pairs AC or BD). The attributes in gamble pair AE are maximally different and this pair is, therefore, assigned the highest distance. In total, gamble pairs could be classified into four distances.

5.2.5 A few notes on the additive-difference model

Figure 5.2 illustrates hypothetical weighting functions according to which probabilities and gains have a differential, context-dependent importance for the decision. This is because of the different sigmoidal shapes of the weighting functions for probabilities ($\Phi_{Probabilities}$, black line) and gains (Φ_{Gains}, gray line): Φ_{Gains} is higher than $\Phi_{Probabilities}$ when the difference in gains and probabilities is minute, e.g., at a small distance between the gambles (left gamble pair). However, when the difference in both attributes increases (greater distance, right gamble pair), the sign of the difference in the weights reverse and $\Phi_{Probabilities}$ grows

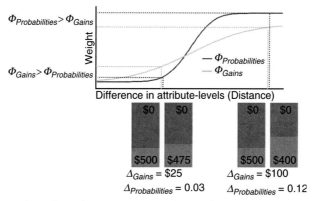

Fig. 5.2 Hypothetical weighting-functions in the additive-difference model. The x-axis depicts the difference in gains or probabilities, respectively, and the y-axis the decision weight of the difference in attributes. Because of the different sigmoidal shapes of the weighting functions for probabilities ($\Phi_{Probabilities}$, black line) and gains (Φ_{Gains}, gray line), subjects reverse their choice pattern: Φ_{Gains} is higher than $\Phi_{Probabilities}$ when the difference in gains and probabilities is minute, i.e., at a small distance between the gambles (left gamble pair). However, when the difference in both attributes increases (greater distance, right gamble pair), the weights reverse and $\Phi_{Probabilities}$ is larger than Φ_{Gains}. As a consequence, at distance 1, decisions should be more strongly influenced by gains than by probabilities, and individuals should have a higher propensity to choose the gamble with the higher gain (G_{risky}). Conversely, at higher distances, decisions should be more strongly influenced by probabilities than by gains, and individuals should be more likely to choose the gamble with the higher probability (G_{safe}).

larger than Φ_{Gains}. As a consequence, at distance 1, decisions should be more strongly influenced by gains than by probabilities, and individuals should have a higher propensity to choose the gamble with the higher gain (G_{risky}). Conversely, at higher distances, decisions should be more strongly influenced by probabilities than by gains, and individuals should be more likely to choose the gamble with the higher probability (G_{safe}).

How can this model explain intransitive preferences? Take the adjacent gamble pair AB: because the gambles' attributes are very similar, the theory predicts choices of the gamble with the higher gain (gamble A). The same rationale applies to the adjacent gamble pair BC (choice of gamble B). However, when the choice is between gambles A and C, the difference between both attributes is relatively large, and subjects should therefore prefer the gamble with the higher probability (gamble C). Hence, although A should be preferred over B, and B should be preferred over C, A should not be preferred over C.

5.2.6 A few notes on the noisy implementation of value account

We assumed that, if participants made decisions based on independently assessed subjective values, then each gamble's subjective value should be either a function of the gamble's probability (probability-maximizing subjects), gain magnitude (reward-maximizing subjects), or expected value or expected utility (subjects maximizing the product of probability and gain magnitude, or a subjective representation thereof). Independent of what the actual basis of gamble evaluation was, the discriminability between gambles should always be minimal at gamble-distance 1, because the difference in gains, probabilities, and expected values was smallest. Discriminability increased with increasing gamble distance, i.e., increasing difference in gains, probabilities, and expected values.

The *noisy implementation of value account* states that, when the discriminability between the gambles is minimal (distance 1), choices should approach equal distribution for the following reasons: it is possible that the subject is truly indifferent between the gambles, in which case choice distribution should be equal. Alternatively, if the subject is *not* indifferent, it has been hypothesized that, if people made no errors, a decision maker would always choose the preferred option on every trial (Birnbaum and Gutierrez, 2007; Birnbaum and Schmidt, 2009). It is further assumed that the error rate e is independent and $e < \frac{1}{2}$ (Birnbaum and Gutierrez, 2007; Birnbaum and Schmidt, 2009). An error rate of $e < \frac{1}{2}$ implies that participants make decisions against their true preference in less than 50% of the times. Or, in other words, with an error rate approaching its asymptote of 0.5, the choice distribution for binary decisions (such as the present task) should approach indifference (50:50 distribution), but should not exceed indifference in favor of the unpreferred option.

One can easily see that this strict model fails to explain the intransitive choices reported above, because an error rate $e < \frac{1}{2}$ implies that a participant would always decide more often in accordance with his true preference than against his true preference. Hence, according to this model, choice distributions in our repeated measures design (remember that every gamble pair presentation was repeated 20 times) should yield reasonably accurate estimates of our participants' true preferences for each pair. If it was true that the more frequently chosen gamble in a given pair was generally also the "truly" preferred gamble, how could this error model reconcile the striking intransitive choices (reported below) with the core theory of hierarchically ordered, transitive preferences? For example, how could the model account for the decisions made by subject 22, who selected gamble A over gamble B in 100% of the times when gamble A was paired with B, and opted for B over C in 80% of times of BC presentations, but when the choice was between A and C, chose A only in 5% of cases (see Section 5.3)?

In order to reconcile the assumption of transitively ordered preferences with our participants' actual choices, an error model would need to consider the possibility that the actually unpreferred option is occasionally chosen *more* often than in 50% of gamble pair presentations. Therefore, we relax the assumptions made above. A more lenient assumption states that also *error-free* choice distributions are stochastic[3], and that the ratio of choices of one option over another should match the ratio of the options' subjective values (Herrnstein, 1961, 1970). This implies that the more equal the options' subjective values, the more likely a subject will be to choose both options equally often. Yet, subjects *do* make errors. Hence, in trials with minimal discriminability, *error-free* choices should be equally distributed between the options, but the error rate may skew this equal choice distribution towards the actually unpreferred option, thus allowing for selections of the unpreferred gamble in more than 50% of the times. Assuming that errors are independent and symmetrically distributed, choices against true preference can thus occur on an individual level (and can therefore explain intransitivity), but should range around indifference on the inter-subject level. Hence, we tested the prediction that, at gamble-distance 1, choices were roughly equally distributed between the two gambles.

5.2.7 Analysis

To test whether intransitive choices were merely caused by a higher number of errors in low discriminability trials (*noisy implemention of value account*), we tested whether choices differed significantly from indifference (50%) in trials with lowest discriminability, i.e., at distance 1, where the difference in probability and gain was minimal, using parametric one-sample t-tests and non-parametric binomial tests. Furthermore, we assessed whether the reaction times were correlated with discriminability between gambles, i.e., distance, using analysis of variance (ANOVA) for repeated measures. Also, we assessed whether the frequency of G_{risky} and G_{safe} choices systematically depended on distance, as predicted by the *additive-difference model*, using an ANOVA for repeated measures.

5.3 Results

5.3.1 Intransitive choices

Our measure based on directed graph theory found intransitive choices in 18 out of 27 subjects, i.e., 18 subjects had a score higher than 0.3 on our intransitivity index. Nine subjects made consistently transitive choices, or scored lower than 0.3. All further

---

[3] An error-free but stochastic choice distribution may arise, for instance, through a tendency to occasionally deliberately sample the unpreferred option to remain fully informed.

analyses are based on the intransitive subjects, unless indicated otherwise. Subject 22 showed a typical chain of intransitive choices. She preferred gamble A over gamble B in 100% of the times when gamble A was paired with B, and she preferred B over C in 80% of times of BC presentations, but when the choice was between A and C, A was only chosen in 5% of cases even though A should be clearly preferred over C according to transitivity. This pattern goes on: while gamble B was preferred over C (B was chosen in 80% of the cases) and C was preferred over D (90%), B was not preferred over D (11%); likewise, although C was preferred over D (90%) and D was preferred over E (85%), C was not preferred over E (25%).

Figure 5.3A–D shows the averaged choices across all identified intransitive gamble sets and subjects (choices of gamble X over Y, where X and Y represent the two gambles in a given gamble pair). Because not all subjects showed intransitive choices in the same gamble combinations, statistics were calculated across different sets of gambles. Here, gamble number 1 is a placeholder that represents the first gamble in any given intransitive gamble set (according to the order of gambles in Fig. 5.1B, e.g., gamble A in gamble set ABC, or C in gamble set CDE), and gamble numbers 2–5 represent the second, third, fourth, and fifth gambles, respectively (e.g., B and C in gamble set ABC, or BCDE in gamble set ABCDE). Horizontal lines represent the mean percentage of choices of one gamble over another, boxes encompass the standard error of the means (SEM), and whiskers indicate 2∗SEM. Figure 5.3A shows that, even though subjects preferred gamble 1 over 2, and gamble 2 over 3, they did not prefer 1 over 3. Figure 5.3B shows that subjects preferred gamble 1>2>3>4, but not 1>4, and Fig. 5.3C shows the same rationale for all five gambles. Figure 5.3D shows intransitive gamble sets with indifference between two gambles (see paragraph above on the detection of intransitive gamble sets with indifference). This panel shows that, even though subjects were indifferent between one pair of gambles (named gamble 1 and 2 in Fig. 3D), choice proportions of both indifferent gambles with another gamble were clearly different. Again, intransitive choices with one or more indifferent statements occurred in different gamble sets across subjects. For the purpose of this figure, we classified the indifferent gamble pair as "1 vs 2," the dominating gamble pair as "1 vs 3," and the dominated pair as "2 vs 3." This classification is somewhat arbitrary and should therefore be interpreted with caution, but it is useful to illustrate that indifference between two gambles does not predict the same choice relation with other gambles.

We tested whether the choice patterns were significantly inhomogeneous across gamble pair presentations (cf. Fig. 5.3). For example, in Fig. 5.3A, we tested whether gamble pairs "1 vs 2," "2 vs 3" and "1 vs 3" had an effect on choices of gambles "1 over 2," "2 over 3" or "1 over 3." An ANOVA for repeated measures revealed a significant effect of gamble pair on choice for triplet gamble sets (Fig. 5.3A, $F_{(2,106)} = 112.69$, $P<10^{-27}$), quadruples (Fig. 5.3B, $F_{(3,159)} = 120.74$, $P<10^{-41}$), and quintuples (Fig. 5.3C, $F_{(4,44)} = 81.4$, $P<10^{-20}$). Furthermore, within-subject contrasts showed that the frequency of choices of X over Y in outlier gamble pairs in figure panels Fig. 5.3A–C (e.g., gamble pair 1 vs 3 in Fig. 5.3A) were significantly different from all other gamble pairs (all $F>46$, all $P<10^{-5}$). This result is not very surprising, given that the data entering the statistic were pre-selected

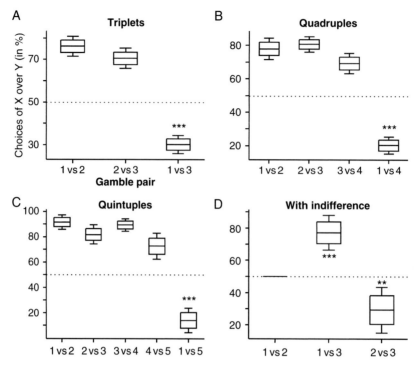

Fig. 5.3 Intransitive choices in gamble-triplets (A), -quadruples (B), -quintuples (C), and gamble sets involving indifference statements (D). Horizontal lines represent the mean percentage of choices of gamble X over Y, where X and Y refer to the two gambles in the gamble pair specified on the x-axis. Boxes encompass the standard error of the means (SEM), and whiskers indicated 2*SEM. Numbers on the x-axis are placeholders for gambles, e.g., 1 vs 2 in panel (A) refers to the first and second gambles in a given gamble set, e.g., gambles A and B in gamble set ABC, or gambles C and D in gamble set CDE. (A) Triplets refer to all intransitive gamble sets across three gambles (e.g., gamble sets ABC, ABD, BDE, etc., where A>B, B>C, but A<C, etc.); (B) quadruples refer to all gamble sets involving four gambles (e.g., ABCD, ACDE, etc.);and (C) quintuples refer to the gamble set involving five gambles (ABCDE). (D) Intransitive gamble sets with indifference refer to situations where a subject was indifferent between two gambles (e.g., between gambles A and B), but the choice relation between these two gambles with a third gamble was not identical. See text for further details. ** $P<0.01$. *** $P<10^{-5}$

to be intransitive. However, even when including all data in the analysis, i.e., also including transitive gamble sets, there was a significant effect of pair on choice (all $F>55.45$, all $P<10^{-20}$), and the same outliers as in figure panels Fig. 5.3A–C also differed significantly from the rest of the gamble pairs (all $F>38.74$, all $P<10^{-6}$). The analysis of the intransitive gamble sets containing indifference statements (Fig. 5.3D) yielded similar results: there was a significant effect of gamble pair on choice ($F(2,28) = 27.04$, $P<10^{-7}$), and choices at both non-indifferent gamble pairs deviated significantly from indifference (all $F>8.4$, all $P<0.01$). This analysis confirms that choices were clearly intransitive.

5.3.2 Choices at distance 1

The *noisy implementation of value account* states that choices should be nearly equally distributed when the discriminability between the gambles is minimal, and any choice distributions against true preference should be due to errors in choice. However, an analysis of choices at distance 1 (minimum discriminability between the gambles) revealed that the subjects' preferences clearly deviated from indifference. Intransitive subjects had a general preference for the risky gamble G_{risky} at distance 1 (choices of G_{risky} in 76.9% ±4.2; Fig. 5.4A). A one-sample t-test revealed that choices of G_{risky} were significantly different from 50% ($t(17) = 6.41$, $P<10^{-6}$). This was confirmed by a non-parametrical binomial test ($P = 0$). Thus, it is unlikely that choices of G_{risky} merely reflected an error component.

5.3.3 Reaction times

The *noisy implemention of value account* furthermore predicts that choices should be most difficult when discriminability is minimal, and that task difficulty should decrease with discriminability (Hey, 1995). However, the analysis of our intransitive participants' reaction times as a proxy for choice difficulty (Hey, 1995) showed that they were not longest at distance 1, but rather followed an inverted U-shaped curve as a function of distance (Fig. 5.4B). An ANOVA for repeated measures revealed that reaction times were significantly modulated by distance ($F(3, 1056) = 23.55$, $P<10^{-15}$), and that they were significantly shorter at distance 1 than at distance 2 ($F(1,355) = 42.68$, $P<10^{-10}$) and distance 3 ($F(1,355) = 55,68$, $P<10^{-13}$). Hence, reaction times did not correlate with the degree of discriminability, but, on the contrary, they seemed to be shortest in trials with low discriminability.

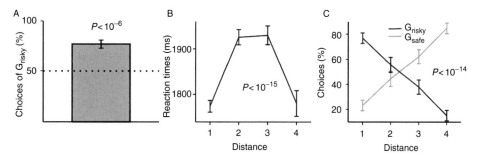

Fig. 5.4 Behavioral results. Panel (A) shows the percentage of choices of the risky gamble at distance 1. The risky gamble yields a relatively higher gain magnitude with a relatively lower probability compared to the safe gamble. Subjects' preference for the risky gamble was significantly different from indifference (50%). (B) Reaction times (in milliseconds) as a function of distance. Contrary to the prediction of the *noisy implementation of value account*, reaction times did not decrease linearly with gamble-distance, and hence discriminability, but seemed to follow an inverted U-shape function. (C) Proportion of choices in percent of the risky gamble (black line) and safe gamble (gray line) as a function of distance (means±SEM), *** $P<10^{-6}$.

5.3.4 **Choices as a function of distance**

The *additive-difference model* predicts that, when the attributes between the gambles are quite similar, differences in gains have a higher impact on the decision than differences in probabilities, but probabilities are more important than gains when the gambles' attributes are clearly different. Consequently, subjects should prefer G_{risky} over G_{safe} at small distances, but this preference should reverse with higher distances. Figure 5.4C shows the average choices of G_{risky} (black line, ±SEM) and G_{safe} (gray line, ±SEM) as a function of distance. Consistent with the predictions of the *additive-difference model*, subjects prefer G_{risky} at distance 1 (see also Fig. 5.4A), but choices of G_{risky} linearly decrease with distance, and choices of G_{safe} linearly increase with distance. An ANOVA for repeated measures confirmed that choices of G_{risky} and G_{safe} were significantly distance-dependent ($F(3,51) = 44.09$, $P<10^{-14}$). Tests of the within-subject contrasts showed that choices of G_{risky} and G_{safe} varied linearly with distance ($F(1,17) = 89.05$, $P<10^{-8}$). This analysis suggests that it is unlikely that variations in choice reflected a stochastic component, but that choices followed the systematic pattern suggested by the *additive-difference model*.

5.4 **Discussion**

We addressed whether intransitive choices reflected genuinely intransitive, context-dependent preferences, or whether they were simply the consequence of noisily implemented transitive preferences. Individuals made decisions between probabilistic prospects that differed in probability and gain. In every trial, one gamble had a higher winning probability (the safe gamble), and the other gamble offered a higher gain magnitude (the risky gamble). We found that about two-thirds of our participants made intransitive choices.

Rational choice theories predict that the bigger the difference in values between two options, the more likely an individual is to choose the option with the higher value. Hence, according to the *noisy implementation of value account*, the degree of error would depend on the discriminability between options. Adopting a lenient assumption that choices are stochastic, even in the absence of errors (see above for discussion), individuals should be nearly indifferent when both options are only poorly discriminable, and choices should reflect indifference plus an error term. The same rationale holds when assuming that subjects are truly indifferent between gambles. Moreover, decisions should be most difficult when discriminability is minimal because they would entail a higher degree of uncertainty and conflict.

However, our analysis fails to support this idea. The examination of intransitive gamble sets (Fig. 5.3) shows that preferences were strong and rarely ranged around indifference. It is important to note that indifference in one gamble pair cannot necessarily be taken as evidence for the *noisy implementation of value account* if there is no indifference between other gamble pairs (see Fig. 5.3D). For example, if preferences were transitive, indifference between gambles A and B would imply that the preference between A and C should be equal to preference between B and C. Take a case where a subject is indifferent between

A and B, and prefers A over C, but does not prefer B over C. The *noisy implementation of value account* predicts that the subject should be indifferent between gamble pairs AC and BC, too. However, Fig. 5.3D shows that choices often clearly deviated from indifference.

Moreover, at distance 1 (minimal discriminability), subjects had a clear and significant preference for the gamble yielding the higher gain magnitude. It is, hence, unlikely that deviations from indifference were merely due to errors in choice. In support of this conclusion, reaction times at distance 1 were lower than at distances 2 and 3, and less variable than at distance 4, speaking against the hypothesis that decisions at distance 1 were more difficult than decisions in trials with higher discriminability.

It is possible that objective discriminability, i.e., the objective difference in gains, magnitudes and expected values, was not equivalent to the subjective difference in values; for example, because of a non-linear integration of gain and probability. Hence, the discriminability of the gambles at distance 1 may be objectively minimal, but the difference in subjective values may be not. If this was the case, one would not expect near-indifference at distance 1, but at other distances. And indeed, our participants' choices ranged around indifference at distance 2 (Fig. 5.4C). Apart from the fact that it is difficult to explain why subjective values should be indiscriminable at distance 2, but not at distance 1, we consider it unlikely that minimal discriminability and hence higher error rates at distance 2 produced intransitive choices because one would *not* expect intransitive choices in gambles sets excluding distance 2 pairs, such as intransitive quadruples and quintuples (Fig. 5.3B–C). In addition, theories of subjective utility, such as expected utility theory (von Neumann and Morgenstern, 1944), posit that subjective values do not considerably differ from a linear value function for small cashflows, such as the reward amounts used in the present study. Hence, if subjective cashflow values approximated objective values, it follows that the difference in subjective values was smaller (and hence less discriminable) at distance 1 than distance 2, but not the other way around.

Furthermore, intransitive subjects showed a clear and significant context-dependent shift in choice. When the difference in both attributes was small (distance 1), gains were given priority over probabilities, and, out of the two gambles, subjects preferred the one yielding a higher gain magnitude, but lower winning probability. However, with increasing difference between gain *and* probability (increasing distance), the priorities reversed, and subjects eventually preferred the safe gamble with the higher probability, but lower gain (Fig. 5.4C). This suggests that the subjects' choices followed a systematic and predictable pattern, which is consistent with the predictions of the *additive-difference model* of choice (Tversky, 1969). According to this model, decisions are not based on hierarchically ordered fixed values, but are the consequence of comparing and integrating the options' attributes, such as probability and gain, independently (cf. Brandstätter et al., 2006). Hence, we conclude that choices in this task reflected genuinely intransitive preferences, and not merely noisy implementations of uniquely ranked, hierarchically organized independent values.

Other authors came to a different conclusion. For example, Birnbaum and Gutierrez (2007) or Birnbaum and Schmidt (2009) conducted internet-based experiments with gambles, similar to the ones used here, and concluded that the evidence from their experiments was not sufficient to reject value-based, transitive decision models. Why did we find intransitive choices in the present task, whereas other authors did not? There are numerous differences in the experimental procedures that may explain the diverging results. For example, Birnbaum's studies were mainly internet-based, whereas our subjects performed the task inside a functional magnetic resonance imaging (fMRI) scanner. Making intransitive choices is effortful because participants consistently need to consider all gamble dimensions, and flexibly adjust the priority placed on them. Hence, participants probably need to be dedicated, committed, and motivated to show intransitive choices. It is possible that participants' commitment and dedication is generally lower when performing an internet-based task, which can be completed on the run between other activities, than when volunteering for an fMRI study, which is highly time-consuming and requires a high base motivation. Moreover, unlike tasks used by other authors, subjects in the present experiment had to make their decision within a 4-s reaction time window, following the onset of gamble presentation. This time restriction may have influenced the selection of a decision rule in favor of fast attribute-based heuristics. Most importantly, however, we think that the main reason for the difference between ours and Birnbaum's findings (2007, 2009) lies in the number of trial repetitions: whereas in the present task, each gamble-pair combination was presented 20 times, Birnbaum presented each pair only twice. Birnbaum used the number of preference reversals within these two repetitions to estimate error rates for each gamble pair (a preference reversal occurred if, in AB choices, a participant selected gamble A once and gamble B once). However, such a low number of trial repetitions does not allow for accurate estimation of error rates for each participant individually. Hence, because a higher number of trial repetitions affords a more accurate assessment, we argue that our task permits a much better inference which gamble in a given pair was the "truly" preferred one. Finally, the analytical approach in our study was different to Birnbaum and colleagues. We classified subjects as transitive or intransitive based on formal criteria (see above) and then asked whether the intransitive decisions can be better explained by the *noisy implementation of value account* or the *additive-difference model*. Conversely, Birnbaum and colleagues (2007, 2009) calculated the probability that their subjects' observable choice sequences were more likely to be consistent with intransitive or transitive preference chains, based on an underlying error model, and asked how many choice patterns could be classified as intransitive with sufficient certainty. However, again, it is possible that the task design, the experimental procedures, and the model assumptions underlying certainty estimation may have biased the analysis towards underestimating the number of intransitive instances. In conclusion, we argue that the intransitive choices observed in the present experiment were real and can be best explained by the *additive-difference model*. Future research needs to identify the circumstances under which (and the underlying reasons why) participants have a tendency to make transitive or intransitive decisions.

Only about one-third of our participants made consistent, transitive choices. Of these, six participants consistently preferred the gamble with the higher probability (G_{safe}), and rarely chose the gamble yielding higher gain magnitudes (G_{risky}), and three participants consistently preferred G_{risky} over G_{safe}. We can infer with reasonable certainty that subjects preferring G_{risky} over G_{safe} maximized reward amount at the expense of outcome certainty. However, because expected value was correlated with probability, our design does not allow unequivocal conclusions whether participants preferring G_{safe} over G_{risky} maximized probability (at the expense of outcome magnitude), or made decisions based on expected value. Yet, the informal interviews following task completion suggested that those participants primarily focused on maximizing probability, and did not compute or consider expected values. Is the fact that some subjects make consistent choices a challenge for our rejection of the *noisy implementation of value account*? We think not for the following reasons. First, it is not surprising that there is individual variability in how people make decisions. Such variability can be simply modeled with the *additive-difference model* by fitting the weighting functions $\Phi_{Probabilities}$ and Φ_{Gains} to the individual preference pattern, e.g., $\Phi_{Probabilities} \gg \Phi_{Gains}$ at all attribute levels for strong preference for certainty, and $\Phi_{Gains} \gg \Phi_{Probabilities}$ at all attribute levels for strong preference for reward magnitude. Furthermore, as mentioned, making intransitive choices requires flexibility in weighing gains and probabilities, and thus necessitates a high degree of dedication and cognitive effort. The post-hoc interviews suggested that, compared to the intransitive participants, many transitive participants made less effort in completing the task. For example, several participants reported having made up their mind to generally prefer G_{safe} after only a few trials, and then automatically went on selecting G_{safe} without further consideration. Hence, it is possible that transitive participants would have showed intransitive choices, too, had they completed the task more assiduously. Future research needs to determine whether transitive choices can be attributed to cognitive inflexibility and/or inertia. The remainder of the discussion will focus on the intransitive participants' choices.

Why do the priorities given to gains and probabilities shift as a function of the overall difference in the gambles' attributes in our intransitive participants? Several explanations are conceivable. It is well established that the probability weighting function is not well defined for small probabilities (Kahneman and Tversky, 1979), and, therefore, the weight attached to small *differences* in probabilities may be just as poorly defined. Hence, subjects may cognitively treat very similar probabilities as equal, and base their choice on the remaining discriminator–gain magnitude. When the difference in probabilities increases, the likelihood that they are also *interpreted* as different increases, too, and their importance for the decision consequently grows proportionally. This theory makes the implicit assumption that the "default" preference is the safe gamble with the higher probability, and that higher gains are only preferred when the probabilities are perceived as being equal. This assumption is not unreasonable given that most subjects are risk-averse and have a natural bias towards low-variance outcomes (van Neumann and Morgenstern, 1948; Friedman and Savage, 1949, 1952; Kahneman and Tversky, 1979; Kacelnik and Bateson, 1996). If this assumption was true, then manipulation of risk attitude (Kahneman and Tversky, 1984; Knoch et al., 2006) should reverse the "default" preference: a strongly risk-seeking subject should by default place higher priorities on gains than on probabilities, even at large distances. However, this theory cannot explain why small differences in probabilities are cognitively neglected, whereas small differences in gains are not. This could be due simply to the selection of parameters in the present study. That is, had we opted for smaller absolute gains in our experimental design, subjects may potentially have neglected small differences in gains as well.

A different theory to account for the order in which gains and probabilities are considered states that the different cognitive treatment of the gambles' attributes could be related to the way the brain treats stimulus magnitudes. Chater and Brown (1999) argued that the structures of many aspects in the environment are invariant over change of scale. For example, the visual perception of brightness, colors, and contrasts can be virtually unaffected, although luminance may vary by a factor of 10,000 between sunlight and shade. Hence, perception seems to be more sensitive to the ratio between stimulus magnitudes rather than absolute magnitudes. Chater and Brown (1999) maintained that scale invariance is a universal information processing principle that may apply not only to perception, but general cognition and representation of non-physical parameters, too. If scale invariance applies to the processing of gains and probabilities, it is conceivable that their weighting functions follow similar transformation rules that produce scale invariance in other domains, such as visual or time perception. One such transformation is a power function of the following form (Chater and Brown, 1999):

$$\Phi_i = -a_i(X_i/Y_i)^{b_i} \tag{5.3}$$

where a_i and b_i are attribute-specific parameters that determine the scaling and the steepness of the ratio of X_i over Y_i, X_i and Y_i are the quantitative values of the attribute i of the two gambles, and Φ_i is the weight, of attribute i.

Because probabilities are on a bounded scale (they range between 0 and 1), but gains are unbounded quantities (they range between 0 and ∞), the measurement scales of the two attributes are not identical. It is, therefore, reasonable to assume that the parameters a and b in eqn. 5.3 are different for gains than for probabilities. If this is the case, then the power functions for gains and probabilities will cross, which would correspond to the shift in priority given to gains and probabilities. This variant of the *additive-different model* provides an alternative to the hypothetical weighting function illustrated in Fig. 5.2 (see above), and has the advantage that it does not make assumptions about a "default" preference as in the small-difference model explained above. Risk attitudes, priorities given to gains and probabilities, and shifts thereof, would be the consequence of the differential shapes of the attributes' power functions. Future research is needed to determine whether this model holds for intransitive choice.

Neither theory can explain why subjects did not base their decisions on independently calculated subjective values, but decided on the basis of a comparison of the gambles' attributes. It is possible that we artificially biased subjects to this end by using different stimulus classes to present gains and probabilities: whereas probabilities were presented graphically, gains were presented as numbers. However, previous studies using text-only versions of risky (Russo and Dosher, 1988) or intertemporal (Roelofsma and Read, 2000) choice problems have also shown that subjects make systematic risky intransitive choices, even though all information was given within the same stimulus class. In line with this, pilot studies in our lab have shown that the intransitive effect occurs independently of the way the current task is presented and in always about the same fraction of subjects: we consistently found intransitive choices in approximately 1/2 to 2/3 of our subjects, when probabilities *and* gains were presented as numbers (probabilities were presented either as floating numbers, fractions or percentages), or when probabilities were presented as pie charts. Hence, in line with previous findings (Russo and Dosher, 1983; Roelofsma and Read, 2000), we conclude that subjects robustly and consistently made attribute-based decisions that are not attributable to the particular presentation format.

Besides biasing subjects, it is also possible that individuals make attribute-wise comparisons because they are less effortful than first computing the integrated values, and then comparing those values (cf. Russo and Dosher, 1983). When compared independently, attributes can be readily evaluated within their proper scale and there is no need to perform a costly transformation into a common currency, which, however, is required when making value-based decisions. For example, it is easy to detect which of two probabilities is higher, but it is more difficult, costly, and error-prone to integrate gain and probability into a common currency because these attributes are differently scaled and thus not directly comparable. Hence, the processing strategy (e.g., attribute-wise versus value-based[4] comparisons) affects choice accuracy. In the present task, attribute-wise decision rules produce different and irrational choices compared to what would be expected from a decision maker using value-based decision rules, but it is easy to construct examples in which both rules produce identical results. In such examples, the decision rule that is less error-prone would more reliably prescribe the correct, i.e., most optimal choice, and should therefore be preferred. Take the following example (Russo and Dosher, 1983): subjects are instructed to rate which of two scholarship applicants deserve to be awarded a grant. Applicant A has an annual family income of $7920, has a high school performance (GPA) of 3.51 and an academic potential (SAT) of 1440. Applicant B has an annual family income of $7920, too, but has a lower high school performance (GPA) of 3.43 and a lower academic potential (SAT) of 1260. Attribute-wise comparisons reveal right away that applicant A is superior to B in two out of three attributes (GPA and SAT). Hence, applicant A should be preferred over B with very little chance of choosing the wrong candidate. A value-based decision rule would imply that the utilities of income, GPA, and SAT will be estimated and then integrated for each applicant separately (e.g., through multiplication), and the integrated utility then compared across applicants. Even though the value-based heuristic should, on average, recommend applicant A, too, computational outcomes are more inconsistent and error-prone because of the variability in utility estimation, and the high computational demand.

---

[4] Note that most value-based models do not make claims about the underlying choice mechanisms and heuristics. However, here, we use the term "value-based heuristic" in the sense that some computation must take place that integrates the attributes of one alternative into a common currency. Thus, unlike many models, here we do refer to a specific integrating mechanism.

A value-based decision maker will hence be more likely to choose the wrong candidate (applicant B may be preferred over A, although A is better qualified) than an attribute-wise decision maker.

In summary, attribute-wise decision rules recommend non-optimal choices in some special cases, like the present task, but they seem to perform better than value-based heuristics in other situations, like the scholarship example above. It is possible that most decision problems in the real world are structured in such a way that the benefits of attribute-wise heuristics outweigh their drawbacks. Therefore, decision rules that rely on attribute-wise comparisons may have evolved because they provided an evolutionary advantage for fitness maximization, despite of their apparent non-optimality in special cases (cf. Houston, 1997, 2007). Hence, maybe intransitive choices are not so irrational after all.

A consequence of this thought implies that the cognitive processes associated with attribute-wise option evaluations should have neural substrates that should be identifiable with standard neuroimaging methods. For example, in the present task, the desirability of any given gamble was not independent, but was local and depended on which other gamble was present at the time of choice. Such choice-set-dependent desirabilities should be represented in brain areas previously shown to encode goal values and decision parameters, such as ventromedial (Hare et al., 2008, 2009) or lateral prefrontal cortex (McClure et al., 2004; Kalenscher and Pennartz, 2008; Kim et al., 2008). Moreover, the prominent shift in priority placed on gain magnitudes and probabilities during the decision (cf. Fig. 5.4C)—the presumed cause of intransitive choices—should also have a neural substrate. Specifically, we hypothesize that brain structures previously associated with choices of larger, but riskier (Huettel et al., 2006; Smith et al., 2009) or larger, but delayed rewards (Tanaka et al., 2004; Wittmann et al., 2007), such as insular cortex, represent the priority given to gains over probabilities. Conversely, we predict that brain regions that have been shown to play a role in incorporating individual risk attitude into reward preference (McCoy and Platt, 2005), such as posterior cingulate cortex, represent the priority given to probabilities over gains. We have recently presented evidence supporting our hypothesis elsewhere (Kalenscher et al., 2010).

Acknowledgments

TK is supported by grants from the Nederlandse Organisatie voor Wetenschappelijk Onderzoek (NWO-VENI 016.081.144) and SenterNovem (BSIK-03053).

References

Afriat, S.N. (1967). The construction of utility functions from expenditure data. *International Economic Review*, **8**: 67–77.

Afriat, S.N. (1972). Efficiency estimation of production functions. *International Economic Review*, **13**: 568–98.

Bateson, M., and Kacelnik, A. (1998). Risk-sensitive foraging: decision making in variable environments. In: *Cognitive ecology* (Dukas R, ed), pp 297–341. Chicago, Illinois: University of Chicago Press.

Bateson, M., Healy, S.D. and Hurly, T.A. (2003). Context-dependent foraging decisions in rufous hummingbirds. *Proceedings of the Royal Society of London. Series B, Biological Sciences*, **270**: 1271–76.

Birnbaum, M.H., and Gutierrez, R.J. (2007). Testing for intransitivity of preferences predicted by a lexicographic semi-order. *Organizational Behavior and Human Decision Processes*, **104**: 96–112.

Birnbaum, M.H., and Schmidt, U. (2009). Testing transitivity in choice under risk. *Theory and Decision*, **69**: 599–614.

Brandstätter, E., Gigerenzer, G., and Hertwig, R. (2006). The priority heuristic: making choices without trade-offs. *Psychological Review*, **113**: 409–32.

Budescu, D.V., and Weiss, W. (1987). Reflection of transitive and intransitive preferences: a test of prospect theory. *Organizational Behavior and Human Decision Processes*, **39**: 184–202.

Chater, N., and Brown, G.D. (1999). Scale-invariance as a unifying psychological principle. *Cognition*, **69**: B17–24.

Choi, S., Fisman, R., Gale, D., and Kariv, S. (2007) Consistency and heterogeneity of individual behavior under uncertainty. *American Economic Review*, **97**: 1921–38.

Friedman, M., and Savage, L.J. (1948) The utility analysis of choices involving risk. *The Journal of Political Economy*, **56**: 279–304.

Friedman, M., Savage, L.J. (1952) The expected-utility hypothesis and the measurability of utility. *The Journal of Political Economy*, **60**: 463–74.

Hare, T.A., O'Doherty, J., Camerer, C.F., Schultz, W., and Rangel, A. (2008) Dissociating the role of the orbitofrontal cortex and the striatum in the computation of goal values and prediction errors. *Journal of Neuroscience*, **28**: 5623–30.

Hare, T.A., Camerer C.F., and Rangel, A. (2009). Self-control in decision making involves modulation of the vmPFC valuation system. *Science*, **324**: 646–48.

Herrnstein, R.J, (1961), Relative and absolute strength of response as a function of frequency of reinforcement. *Journal of the Experimental Analysis of behavior*, **4**: 267–72.

Herrnstein, R.J. (1970). On the law of effect. Journal of the Experimental Analysis of Behavior **2**: 243–66.

Hey, J.D. (1995). Experimental investigations of errors in decision making under risk. *European Economic Review*, 39 **3-4**: 633–40.

Houston, A.I. (1997). Natural selection and context-dependent values. *Proceedings of the Royal Society of London. Series B, Biological Sciences*, **264**: 1539–41.

Houston, A.I., McNamara, J.M., and Steer, M.D. (2007). Violations of transitivity under fitness maximization. *Biology Letters*, **3**: 365–67.

Huettel, S.A., Stowe, C.J., Gordon, E.M., Warner, B.T., and Platt, M.L. (2006). Neural signatures of economic preferences for risk and ambiguity. *Neuron*, **49**: 765–75.

Kacelnik, A., and Bateson, M. (1996). Risky theories the effects of variance on foraging decisions. *American Zoologist*, **36**: 402–34.

Kahneman, D., and Tversky, A. (1979). Prospect theory: an analysis of decision under risk. *Econometrica*, **47**: 263–91.

Kahneman, D., and Tversky, A. (1984). Choices, values, and frames. *American Psychologist*, **39**: 341–50.

Kalenscher, T., and Pennartz, C.M. (2008). Is a bird in the hand worth two in the future? The neuroeconomics of intertemporal decision making. *Progress in Neurobiology*, **84**: 284–315.

Kalenscher, T., Daselaar, S.M., Huijbers, W., Tobler, PN., and Pennartz, C.M.A. (2010) Neural signatures of intransitive preferences. *Frontiers in Human Neuroscience*, **4**: 1–14.

Kim, S., Hwang, J., and Lee, D. (2008). Prefrontal coding of temporally discounted values during intertemporal choice. *Neuron*, **59**: 161–72.

Knoch, D., Gianotti, L.R., Pascual-Leone, A., Treyer, V, Regard, M., Hohmann, M., and Brugger, P. (2006). Disruption of right prefrontal cortex by low-frequency repetitive transcranial magnetic stimulation induces risk-taking behavior. *Journal of Neuroscience*, **26**: 6469–72.

Lindman, H.R., and Lyons, J. (1978). Stimulus complexity and choice inconcistency among gambles. *Organizational Behavior and Human Performance,* **21**: 146–59.

Loomes, G., and Sugden, R. (1998). Testing different stochastic specifications of risky choice. *Economica,* **65**: 581–98.

Loomes, G., Starmer, C., and Sugden, R. (1991). Observing violations of transitivity by experimental methods. *Econometrica,* **59**: 425–39.

McClure, S.M., Laibson, D.I., Loewenstein, G., and Cohen, J.D. (2004). Separate neural systems value immediate and delayed monetary rewards. *Science,* **306**: 503–507.

McCoy, A.N., and Platt, M.L. (2005). Risk-sensitive neurons in macaque posterior cingulate cortex. *Nature Neuroscience,* **8**: 1220–27.

Montague, P.R., and Berns, G.S. (2002). Neural economics and the biological substrates of valuation. *Neuron,* **36**: 265–84.

Navarick, D.J., and Fantino, E. (1975). Stochastic transitivity and the unidimensional control of choice. *Learning and Motivation,* **6**: 179–201.

Rangel, A., Camerer, C., and Montague, P.R. (2008). A framework for studying the neurobiology of value-based decision making. *Nature Reviews Neuroscience,* **9**: 545–56.

Roelofsma, P.H.M.P. and Read, D. (2000). Intransitive intertemporal choice. *Journal of Behavioural Decision Making,* **13**: 161–77.

Russo, J.E., and Dosher, B.A. (1988). Strategies for multiattribute binary choice. *Journal of Experimental Psychology, Learning, Memory and Cognition,* **9**: 676–96.

Samuelson, P.A. (1937). A note on measurement of utility. *The Review of Economic Studies,* **4**: 155–61.

Shafir, S. (1994). Intransitivity of preferences in honey bees: support for "comparative" evaluation of foraging options. *Animal Behavior,* **48**: 55–67.

Shafir, S., Waite, T.A., and Smith, B.H. (2002). Context-dependent violations of rational choice in honeybees (*Apis mellifera*) and gray jays (*Perisoreus canadensis*). *Behavioral Ecology and Sociobiology,* **51**: 180–87.

Shizgal, P. (1997). Neural basis of utility estimation. *Current Opinion in Neurobiology,* **7**: 198–208.

Smith, B.W., Mitchell, D.G., Hardin, M.G., Jazbec, S., Fridberg, D., Blair, R.J., and Ernst, M. (2009). Neural substrates of reward magnitude, probability, and risk during a wheel of fortune decision making task. *Neuroimage,* **44**: 600–609.

Sopher, B., and Gigliotti, G. (1993). Intransitive cycles: rational choice or random error? An answer based on estimation of error rates with experimental data. *Theory and Decision,* **35**: 311–36.

Tanaka, S.C., Doya, K., Okada, G., Ueda, K., Okamoto, Y., and Yamawaki, S. (2004). Prediction of immediate and future rewards differentially recruits cortico-basal ganglia loops. *Nature Neuroscience,* **7**: 887–93.

Tversky, A. (1969). Intransitivity of preferences. *Psychological Review,* **76**: 31–48.

Varian, H.R. (1982). The nonparametric approach to demand analysis. Econometrica **50**: 945–73.

von Neumann, J., and Morgenstern, O. (1944). *Theory of games and economic behavior.* Princeton, NJ: University Press.

Waite, T.A. (2001). Intransitive preferences in hoarding gray jays (Perisoreus canadensis). *Behavioral Ecology and Sociobiology,* **50**: 116–21.

Wittmann, M., Leland, D.S., and Paulus, M.P. (2007). Time and decision making: differential contribution of the posterior insular cortex and the striatum during a delay discounting task. *Experimental Brain Research,* **179**: 643–53.

Section II

Neural systems of decision making

Chapter 6

On the difficulties of integrating evidence from fMRI and electrophysiology in cognitive neuroscience

(Tutorial Review)

Benjamin Y. Hayden and Michael L. Platt

Abstract

Functional magnetic resonance imaging (fMRI) and single unit physiology are two of the most widely-used methods in cognitive neuroscience and neuroeconomics. Despite the fact that practitioners of both methods share a common goal–understanding the mechanisms underlying behavior and cognition–their efforts are rarely directly linked. Here we consider some of the reasons for apparent discrepancies between findings of fMRI and electrophysiological studies. We examine these problems through the lens of two case studies—decision making under uncertainty and fictive learning— derived from our own research program. Despite this narrow focus, these arguments are likely to extend to other areas of study. We find that major differences in the neural events measured by the two methods, the behavioral techniques employed with animal and human subjects, and the intellectual history and unique culture of each discipline, contribute to difficulties in providing a wholly synthetic account of the mechanisms underlying cognition and decision making. These observations endorse more collaborative efforts conducting parallel research using analogous, if not identical, behavioral techniques using both brain imaging and single unit physiology.

6.1 Introduction

Neuroimaging in general, and fMRI in particular, have revolutionized cognitive neuro-science (Huettel et al., 2008; Logothetis and Wandell, 2004; Ogawa et al., 1990) and use of these techniques now permeates diverse fields, including psychology, neuroscience, and economics, and has begun to influence sociology, law, philosophy, anthropology, and other related fields. The popularity of neuroimaging springs both from its wide availability (e.g., nearly every major hospital in the US and Europe has an MRI machine) and its ability to provide noninvasive access to covert mental events in conscious, behaving human subjects.

Prima facie, single-unit physiology and functional neuroimaging should be highly complementary techniques. Scientists who use the two methods are generally interested in the exact same problems and aim to provide a material answer to important questions in psychology, cognitive science, and philosophy (e.g., Greene et al., 2001), as well as economics (Camerer, 2008), political science (Amodio et al., 2007), sociology (Amodio et al., 2004; Harris and Fiske, 2006), and other fields. The need for communication between practitioners of these diverse methods is further motivated by the insight they can provide on debilitating diseases, including addiction, depression, autism, and other pathologies. Despite common interests and goals, however, there is a surprising disconnect between

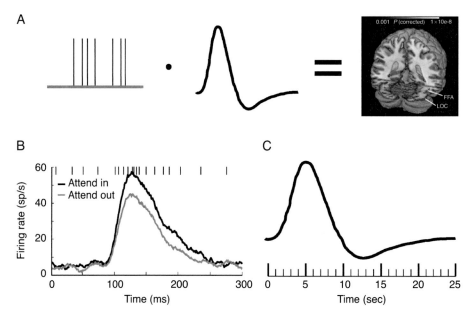

Fig. 6.1 (A) Schematic of the inferred relationship between spiking activity and bold activity. BOLD activation (right) reflects a convolution of individual action potentials (left) with an idealized hemodynamic response function (center). (B) Single-unit physiology studies typically plot peristimulus time histograms, reflecting averaged responses of single units across multiple trials. These are then compared in different conditions, such as two attention conditions in the example data drawn from area V4. Single-unit responses typically last a few hundred milliseconds, and are characterized by a low baseline firing rate, a rapid transient response, followed by a longer lasting sustained response. This entire response typically lasts around 250–500 ms. (C) The idealized hemodynamic responses function is characterized by a very small initial dip, a large and relatively brisk enhancement, and a long, slow suppression, followed by a return to baseline. The entire process typically lasts about 15 s.

Reprinted from Hayden et al. (2008a) Posterior cingulate cortex mediates outcome-contingent allocation of behavior. Neuron, with permission from Elsevier.

the data and interpretations issuing from imaging and neurophysiological studies (see, for example, Huk et al., 2001; Nir et al., 2007; Sirotin and Das, 2009; Yoshor et al., 2007).

The signal measured by fMRI depends on the relaxation times in the spin of hydrogen atoms that have been aligned by a large magnetic field (Huettel et al., 2008). The quantity most often measured by fMRI is known as the blood-oxygen-level-dependent change (BOLD). Specifically, fMRI measures changes in relaxation times due to changes in levels of deoxyhemoglobin in small units of brain volume referred to as voxels. Each voxel is typically about 3–4 mm on a side. An implicit assumption in many people's minds is that the BOLD response is the outcome of a convolution between acute spiking activity and a canonical hemodynamic impulse response function (Fig. 6.1A) (Huettel et al., 2008; Logothetis and Wandell, 2004). Thus fMRI studies typically assume that BOLD activity reflects underlying neural events, and these events are inferred through a simple process of deconvolution.

Although developed much earlier than fMRI, single-unit physiology (which measures single-unit activity, SUA) remains a core method in cognitive neuroscience. The term "single unit" refers to the single neuron whose spiking responses are recorded by an electrode placed near to, but outside of, the cell membrane. The techniques necessary to record extracellular potentials from awake, behaving monkeys were developed by Ed Evarts (Evarts, 1966) at the NIH in the late 1960s, and had their antecedents in earlier research by Penfield, and in the anesthetized recordings made in the labs of Kuffler and others (Barlow et al., 1957; Penfield and Jasper, 1954). Originally used to study motor control (Evarts, 1968), sensory perception (Goldberg and Wurtz, 1972a; Mays and Sparks, 1980; Mountcastle et al., 1975), memory (Funahashi et al., 1989; Fuster and Alexander, 1971; Kubota and Niki, 1971), and attention (Goldberg and Wurtz, 1972b), processes studied by single-unit physiology quickly grew to include executive control (Hanes and Schall, 1996; Niki and Watanabe, 1979), face recognition (Gross et al., 1979), sensory (Shadlen and Newsome, 1996), and economic decision making (Platt and Glimcher, 1999), among other cognitive processes. Other closely related techniques include local field potential (LFP) recording and multi-unit recording (MUA). In contrast to fMRI, these methods typically employ animal subjects (with some exceptions, see below), and thus require behavioral training, surgical support, and reliance on simple tasks. Single-unit physiology can be performed on awake, behaving monkeys, rats, mice, birds, and ferrets, among other animals.

Thus, BOLD and SUA measure distinct aspects of neural processing, in much the same way that different prismatic lenses image separate parts of the spectrum of visible light. Single-unit physiology measures spiking activity—predominantly generated by the cell bodies of large pyramidal neurons—and thus emphasizes outputs of local processing. Although less certain, BOLD appears to reflect a blend of high-frequency synchronized spiking, synaptic potentials in dendrites, and membrane oscillations—processes that reflect inputs, local computations, and outputs, albeit indirectly. We note that, at the present time, none of these physiological processes has privileged status in explaining the mechanisms underlying cognition.

Given these differences in measurement focus, it is difficult to draw a straight line connecting single-unit and fMRI studies, even when they address the same questions. In the following sections, we discuss this problem in a detailed fashion by examining two case studies of single-unit physiological experiments designed to tackle neuroeconomic questions that have also been explored with brain imaging. In addition to discussing the specific results of these studies, we also dwell on the thorny issues raised by these same physiological results for interpreting comparable BOLD data. Despite many fundamental differences between the two methods, we remain optimistic that additional work, both empirical and sociological, can help bridge these gaps and lead to greater understanding of the neural basis of cognition.

6.1.1 Case study 1: spiking activity and decision making under uncertainty

Decision making under uncertainty is an economic problem that has received scrutiny from both physiologists (Barraclough et al., 2004; Fiorillo et al., 2003; Hayden et al., 2008a; McCoy and Platt, 2005) and neuroimagers (Daw et al., 2006; Hsu et al., 2005; Kuhnen and Knutson, 2005; Weber and Huettel, 2008), as well as from economists (Samuelson, 1963; Von Neumann and Morgenstern, 1944), psychologists (Heilbronner et al., 2008; Kacelnik and Bateson, 1996) and theorists (Yu and Dayan, 2005).

Several recent neuroimaging studies in human subjects reported distinct foci of activation associated with risk and uncertainty, and making decisions in volatile environments, including posterior and anterior cingulate cortices, dorsal and ventral striatum, obritofrontal cortex, and lateral prefrontal cortex (for reviews, see: Platt and Huettel, 2008; Rushworth and Behrens, 2008). To understand these processes at the neuronal level, we first probed the spiking activity of single neurons in monkeys making simple decisions between probabilistic and deterministic fluid rewards (Fig. 6.2a; Hayden and Platt, 2007, 2009a; Hayden et al., 2008a, 2008b). On each trial, monkeys chose between two options of equal expected value (typically 200 microliters of an immediate fruit juice reward), but differing in the variability, and thus economic risk, of the potential outcomes. The variance in reward payout of the risky option was adjusted randomly every 50 trials, while the safe option was fixed at an intermediate value. Monkeys preferred the risky option in this task, and preference increased with increasing variance in reward. Moreover, local patterns of choice strongly depended on the recent history of rewards and choices (Hayden et al. 2008a).

To understand the neuronal mechanisms underlying this behavior, we began by recording spiking activity of neurons in the posterior cingulate cortex (CGp). CGp is a large brain region located in a belt around the corpus collosum, lying posterior to the central sulcus and likely to be homologous to the human posterior cingulate cortex (Hayden and Platt, 2009b; Vincent et al., 2007; Vogt et al., 1992, 1993). CGp is strongly and reciprocally interconnected with the anterior cingulate cortex, medial temporal lobe, and hippocampus, as well the parietal lobe, and is therefore well-positioned to integrate information about action, reward, and risk and guide choice (Hayden et al., 2008a).

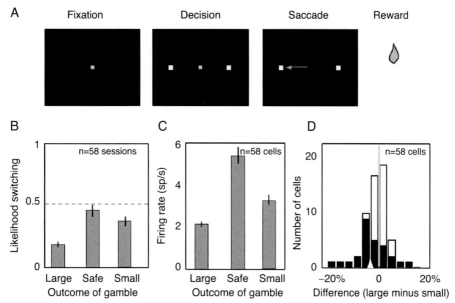

Fig. 6.2 Neuronal spiking and risky decision making. (A) Schematic of task used to study risky behavior in monkey (McCoy and Platt, 2005; Hayden et al., 2008a). First, small fixation square appears centrally. Once fixation is acquired and maintained for one second, two eccentric targets appear to the left and right of the central fixation square. Central square is then extinguished, signaling that a saccade to one of the targets is required. Following saccade, reward is given. (B) Likelihood that monkey will switch from risky to safe target or vice verse from one trial to the next depends on the outcome of the trial. Switching likelihood is greater following smaller than expected outcomes than following large outcomes. Likelihood is about even following safe choices. (C) Plot of average firing rate of all CGp neurons in population following large and small outcomes of gambles, as well as following safe choices. Firing rates of all neurons during a 500 ms epoch after saccades is closely aligned with the likelihood of switching. (D) Plot of the distribution of firing rate changes associated with large and small outcomes of gambles. The distribution of response properties within CGp is highly heterogeneous (panels B–D based on Hayden et al., 2008a). Black regions indicate neurons with significant modulations (p<0.05); white regions indicate neurons with non-significant modulations.

(A) Reprinted by permission from Macmillan Publishers Ltd: *Nature Neuroscience*, 8(9), 1220–7. A.N. McCoy and M.L. Platt, Risk-sensitive neurons in macaque posterior cingulate cortex, Copyright 2005. (B–D) Reprinted from *Neuron*, 60(1), B.Y. Hayden, A.C. Nair, A.N. McCoy, and M.L. Platt, Posterior Cingulate Cortex Mediates Outcome-Contingent Allocation of Behaviour, Copyright 2008, with permission from Elsevier.

We found that tonic firing rates of single CGp neurons systematically varied with the variance in reward associated with the risky option (McCoy and Platt, 2005). Spiking activity also predicted whether the risky option would be subsequently chosen (McCoy and Platt, 2005). We also found that firing rates changed following reward delivery, signaling the size of the reward obtained from a risky option and predicting subsequent changes in choice behavior (Hayden and Platt, 2009b). When rewards are deterministic,

CGp neurons encode reward value monotically (McCoy et al., 2003), but when rewards are uncertain CGp neurons signal reward size with respect to the best obtainable reward, i.e., ditonically (Hayden and Platt, 2009b). This pattern of spiking also predicted the likelihood that the animal would adjust his behavior (Fig. 6.2B–D), suggesting that CGp contributes to risky decision making by signaling the need to change behavioral strategies (see also Pearson et al., 2009). These results clearly and unequivocally implicate CGp in the representation of variables that contribute to risky decision making.

It remains unclear whether neuroimaging studies would replicate these results. Most importantly, we observed consistent heterogeneity of modulation in spiking activity across the population of studied neurons. Approximately half the neurons in our sample showed elevated spiking activity following larger than expected rewards, and about half showed significantly decreased spiking following such outcomes. Although we did detect a statistically significant preponderance of neurons with larger firing-rate changes to smaller outcomes, the bias was not overwhelming, and a substantial minority of neurons showed stronger spiking activity for better-than-expected outcomes. This heterogeneity may reflect the existence of two fundamentally distinct classes of neuronal spiking responses, with two different outputs that happen to be intercalated. Alternatively, these two types of neurons may converge on a single output structure, where they are gated in a non-linear competition (Gold and Shadlen, 2002; Lee et al., 1999; Salzman and Newsome, 1994). Heterogeneity in neuronal spiking responses appears to be quite common in cortical areas in particular (see Table 6.1 for a partial list of examples).

Unlike single-unit spiking, BOLD measures aggregate neuronal processing in a given brain region and is thus blind to anything other than the mass action effects within a given voxel. Consequently, the BOLD signal fails to capture diversity in the functional properties of different categories of neurons in a given voxel—at least given current spatial sensitivity. To our knowledge, very little empirical work has investigated how the BOLD signal varies with the activity of heterogeneous populations of neurons with excitation and suppression of spiking. It thus remains unclear how BOLD signal in CGp would vary in this task. In the worst case, the BOLD signal would not distinguish between enhanced and suppressed spiking, leading to false negative results. Alternatively, the BOLD signal may reflect slight variations in the balance between excitation and suppression.

Another closely related problem is that many neurophysiological studies report the presence of neurons with significant effects—even if the percentages are a small proportion of all neurons in the area. In this case, it is possible that BOLD activation would be too weak to reach significance. In general, we know very little about the mapping between the proportion of neurons activated in a study and the expected BOLD signal.

Thus, it is not hard to imagine situations in which BOLD signals would diverge quite strongly from the observed physiological responses. Collectively, these caveats demonstrate the potential problems of intercalated neuronal spiking properties for brain-imaging studies. Indeed, BOLD activation is typically not reported in posterior cingulate cortex in studies of risky decision making in human subjects (Huettel et al., 2006; Kuhnen and Knutson, 2005; Tom et al., 2007). Lack of BOLD signal in posterior cingulate cortex

Table 6.1 Examples of intercalated functional effects among neurons

Area	Effect	Comment	Reference
LIP	Gaze following	Positive responses to gaze cue vs negative responses to gaze cue	Shepherd et al. (2009)
ACC	Conflict	Turns out to be direction selection	Nakamura et al. (2005)
CGp	Reward outcomes	Positive responses to outcomes vs negative responses to outcomes	Hayden et al. (2008a)
CGp	Reward tuning	Positive tuning for reward vs negative tuning for reward	McCoy et al. (2003)
Area 46	Direction tuning	Tuning for different directions in working memory	Funahashi et al. (1989)
striatum	Reward tuning	Positive and negative reward encoding (TANs medium spiny neurons)	Aosaki et al. (1995)
LIP	Numerosity tuning	Positive and negative tuning for numerosity	Roitman et al. (2007)
OFC	Decision variables	Various variables related to reward and decision making	Kennerley et al. (2009)
LIP	Saccade tuning	Neurons and anti-neurons	Shadlen and Newsome (1996)
ACC	Reward tuning	Positive and negative responses	Matsumoto et al. (2007)
ACC	Reward variable tuning	Recent history vs RPEs	Seo and Lee (2007)
Hippocampus	Learning-related changes	Positive vs negative learning related	Wirth et al. (2003)
ACC	Task stage	Explore vs exploit	Procyk et al. (2000)
ACC	Task stage	Each of four task events	Shidara and Richmond (2002)
OFC	Value encoding	Chosen value vs offer value vs taste	Padoa-Schioppa and Assad (2006)
striatum	Action value	Left vs right	Samejima et al. (2005)
amygdala	State encoding	Positive vs negative	Belova et al. (2008)
entorhinal	Match encoding	Match enhancement vs match suppression	Suzuki et al. (1997)
OFC	Operant phase	Specific phases	Kravitz and Peoples (2008)
ACC/DLPFC	Reward variable	S-R, reward-error, timing	Niki and Watanabe (1979)
LPFC	Reward context	Reward value independent of category and reward value within context	Pan et al. (2008)
Hippocampus	Outcome encoding	Positive and negative responses to rewards	Wirth et al. (2009)

during risky decision making may reflect the highly heterogeneous and intercalated functional response properties in CGp. The converse problem is just as vexing. If we had BOLD signal from CGp or any other brain region, it would be nearly impossible to infer the underlying neuronal spiking events in the absence of corresponding single-unit data.

These results point to another problem raised by our findings. We showed that CGp neurons multiplex information about multiple variables related to risky decision making, including reward variance, whether a risky option will be chosen, and the reward outcome of the previous two or three trials. This type of multiplexing is quite common in neuronal spiking patterns but is often overlooked in neuroimaging studies, which typically rely on analytical subtraction of two conditions to generate a signal. This technique leads to a preponderance of studies reporting that a brain region mediates a single cognitive process. In the extreme case, this can lead to neurorealism, the reification of a hypothesized theoretical variable based on a neural correlate (Racine et al., 2005).

6.1.2 Case study 2: neural representation of fictive outcomes

People routinely recognize and respond to information about outcomes that would have occurred had they chosen differently (Byrne, 2002; Camille et al., 2004; Chiu et al., 2008; Epstude and Roese, 2008; Lohrenz et al., 2007; Roese, 1997; Ursu and Carter, 2005). Such outcomes are known as fictive or counterfactual outcomes. The ability to understand such outcomes may be a precursor to the emotion of regret and is a hallmark of higher cognitive functions (Camille et al., 2004; Coricelli et al., 2005; Coricelli et al., 2007; Hofstadter, 1979; Ursu and Carter, 2005).

Two recent neuroimaging studies have examined the neural bases of fictive learning and reasoning (Chiu et al., 2008; Lohrenz et al., 2007). In one study, people played a stock market simulation game in which they found out what outcomes they could have obtained had they chosen differently (Lohrenz et al., 2007). The authors found BOLD activation in the ventral caudate nucleus of the striatum that reflected fictive outcomes. Moreover, they found that the size of these activations predicted the size of subsequent adjustments in behavior. A subsequent study reported that, although fictive information activates these same areas in the brains of smokers, the observed activations did not predict behavior (Chiu et al., 2008).

To complement these studies, we measured neuronal spiking in anterior cingulate cortex (ACC) while monkeys responded to fictive reward outcomes (Hayden et al., 2009a). To do this, we developed a novel task that provided information about rewards associated with options that could have been chosen (Fig. 6.3a). On each trial of our eight-point gambling task, monkeys chose one of eight identical-looking targets arrayed in a circle. Through training, the monkeys learned that seven of these targets provided a small and fixed reward (low-value, or LV target), while the other one provided a variable, but usually larger, reward (high-value, or HV target). The location of the HV target changed in a stochastically predictable manner from trial to trial by remaining in the same position with a 60% probability and moving one position clockwise with a 40% probability. Following choices, the outcome associated with each of the eight targets was revealed by a change in their color. Thus, when monkeys chose one of the small, safe options—which they did on about 50% of trials—they learned the size of the reward they would have obtained had they chosen the HV target. We called this "could-have-been" reward the fictive outcome (Hayden et al., 2009a).

Monkeys successfully chose the HV target on about 45% of trials, which is about 75% of the accuracy of an ideal observer. Critically, the likelihood that a monkey would successfully choose the HV target on a trial depended strongly on the fictive outcome on the previous trial (Fig. 6.3B). Thus, monkeys recognize and respond to fictive outcomes in a way that is very similar to the way people do. We next recorded spiking activity of single neurons in the anterior cingulate cortex while monkeys performed this task. The ACC is a brain region that contributes to several cognitive processes, including representing uncertainty (Behrens et al., 2007; Rushworth and Behrens, 2008), representing effort costs (Rudebeck et al., 2006a), social decision making (Hadland et al., 2003; Rudebeck, 2006b) and, most relevant for our study, representing reward outcomes and signaling subsequent adjustments in behavior (Amiez et al., 2006; Holroyd and Coles, 2002; Matsumoto et al., 2007).

We found that ACC neurons fire a clear phasic burst of action potentials following saccades to targets in this task, and that the size of this burst is a roughly linear function of the amount of reward expected on trials when the monkeys chose the HV target (Fig. 6.3C). Importantly, firing rate was also a roughly linear function of the amount of fictive reward signaled on trials when the monkeys choose the LV target (Fig. 6.3D). Spiking activity was generally higher for larger outcomes—a positive monotonic encoding—and this trend was observed for both experienced and fictive outcomes. A plurality of individual neurons exhibited significant correlations between firing rate and both types of outcomes. These results demonstrate that ACC neurons signal both experienced and fictive outcomes, and do so using a similar coding scheme, in their spiking activity.

One the one hand, these results appear to be more straightforwardly amenable to comparison with neuroimaging data than our results studying the neuronal spiking correlates of risk in CGp, since there was a low degree of heterogeneity of neuronal tuning for fictive rewards. However, given a BOLD signal, without knowledge of the underlying single-unit responses, one would not know whether separate populations of intercalated neurons encoded fictive and experienced rewards or whether a single population encoded both types of rewards. Thus, as in the other case study, the possibility that there might be neurons with distinct functional properties potentially clouds the interpretation of any neuroimaging study.

We also observed that individual neurons fired more weakly overall to fictive outcomes than to experienced outcomes. This asymmetry can potentially pose another challenge for understanding the relationship between BOLD and SUA. If we assume, for simplicity, that BOLD activation is a roughly linear function of neuronal spiking activity (see below), then activation will be stronger for experienced than for fictive outcomes. In voxels that are homologous to the ones we recorded, different BOLD changes would be observed, but in more distant voxels, BOLD activity may just barely cross the threshold for significance for experienced outcomes, but may fall just below it for fictive outcomes. Consequently, there will be voxels that appear to encode experienced outcomes but not fictive outcomes. Consequently, it may appear that these two outcomes have distinct spatial activation patterns, and thus are mediated by distinct neuronal processes.

In fact, the two neuroimaging studies that have studied fictive learning and reasoning found results that only partially overlapped ours. Specifically, Lohrenz and colleagues found no activation in ACC associated with fictive outcomes. The lack of effects observed

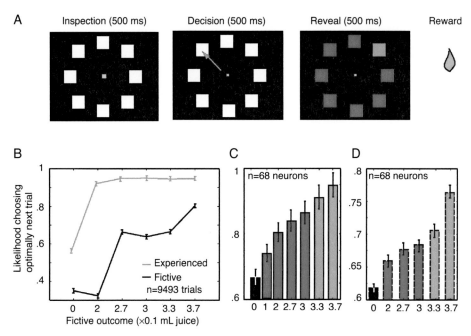

Fig. 6.3 Fictive learning and spiking activity. (A) Schematic of task used to study fictive learning in monkeys. Monkeys are presented with an array of eight identical targets arrayed in a circle and a small, yellow, fixation square in the center. On acquisition of fixation, the square shrinks, and fixation is maintained for 500 ms. Following this, square disappears, and monkey saccades to one of the targets. Immediately following choice, information about the reward that would have been obtained for each of the eight targets is revealed by a change in color of each target. Following another half second, reward corresponding to chosen target is provided. Monkey is attempting to choose variable high-value target (here, green square) and not the seven low-value targets. (B) Likelihood of correctly choosing the high-value variable target on a trial following choice of LV targets depends on the fictive outcome on previous trial (black line). Following HV choices, likelihood is affected by whether HV target provided zero reward or other reward (gray line). (C) and (D) Firing rates of ACC neurons following choices depends on both experienced (C) and fictive (D) outcomes (panels A–D, Hayden et al., 2009a). Monkeys understood the values of the targets by their colors. Colors in these panels indicate reward category experienced by monkey: black (zero reward), red (low-value reward), green (medium rewards) and orange (high-value rewards).

From *Science*, B.Y. Hayden, J.M. Pearson, and M.L. Platt, Fictive Reward Signals in the Anterior Cingulate Cortex, Copyright 2009. Reprinted with permission from AAAS.

in ACC, where we observed changes in neuronal spiking rate, may reflect any of the reasons expressed above, including fundamental differences between the information measured by single unit activity and BOLD, as well as task differences, species differences in neural processing as well as species differences in strategy. The study by Chiu and colleagues similarly found no main effect of fictive outcomes in ACC. However, BOLD activity in this region was positively correlated with the interaction between cigarette craving and fictive outcomes. Together, these results present a mixed picture of consistency between BOLD and single-unit data.

6.2 Model selection and the nature of animal and human behavior

Aside from differences in the way brain events are measured, single-unit physiology and functional neuroimaging generally employ different model organisms that differ in many fundamental ways. The differences in these organisms strongly constrain the behavioral tools that can be used in these methods, thereby strongly influencing the type of information gathered. Thus, these distinctions lead directly to important differences between fMRI and single-unit studies in cognitive neuroscience and neuroeconomics. Consider decision making in the face of risk. Humans are generally regarded as risk-averse (Holt and Laury, 2002; Rabin and Thaler, 2001; Samuelson, 1977; Tom et al., 2007; Von Neumann and Morgenstern, 1944), while animals are often risk-seeking (Hayden and Platt, 2007; Hayden et al., 2008a, 2008b; McCoy and Platt, 2005).

In a typical experiment, humans are offered a single choice between a certain reward and a gamble associated with a larger and a smaller reward (or losses; see, e.g., Hayden and Platt, 2009c; Huettel et al., 2006; Kuhnen and Knutson, 2005). Animals cannot spontaneously understand explicit verbal or symbolic offers, and so must be trained to associate outcomes with prior events and choices over multiple, repeated trials. Learning from experience demands the use of specialized neural machinery for forming associations that differs from the mechanisms used to glean information from explicit instructions. Explicit cuing of task parameters has behavioral consequences as well; in the domain of risk, even in humans, trial repetition tends to promote risk-seeking (Hertwig et al., 2004; Lopes, 1981, 1996; Wedell and Boeckenholt, 1994; Barron and Erev, 2003), and is thus not favored in many economic studies. More importantly, this difference suggests that behavior for one-shot and repeated gambles—whether in humans or animals—may reflect distinct cognitive processes.

Our own work suggests that the way experiments are conducted with animal and human subjects has profound effects on behavior, and thus colors our interpretation of the underlying neurobiology. For these reasons, we advocate using behavioral methods that are closely analogous, if not identical, in comparative studies using fMRI in humans and single-unit physiology in animals. For example, if one is faced with multiple gambles with a positive expected value (amount multiplied by probability of reward), one has the opportunity to make up for stochastic losses. In other words, as the gamble repeats, the law of large numbers ensures that the possibility of bad luck is reduced and the average

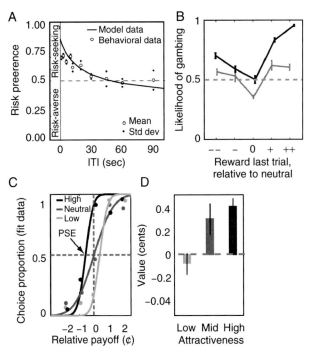

Fig. 6.4 Results of recent studies from our lab aimed at bridging the gap between behavioral methods used in physiological studies and neuroimaging studies. (A) Monkeys' preference for a risky option gradually approaches neutrality as the delay between trials increases from a few seconds to 90 s (after Hayden and Platt, 2007). (B) Humans' preference for risky options (gray line) depends strongly on recent outcomes when they choose between different juice options in a task designed to mimic conditions used in monkey studies. These results qualitatively match those found in monkey studies (black line) (after Hayden and Platt, 2009). (C) Humans' ability to discriminate tone duration is influenced by the attractiveness of the photo they will see if they choose one of the images. From the bias in the discrimination function, we extract the point of subjective equivalence (PSE), which in turn approximates the subjective value of the opportunity to view the image. (D) Human males have a significant positive PSE for photos of high- and mid-level attractiveness females, suggesting that these stimuli can be used as primary rewards in neuroimaging experiments (panels C–D after Hayden et al, 2007).

(A) Reprinted from *Current Biology*, 17(1) B.Y. Hayden and M.L. Platt, Temporal Discounting Predicts Risk Sensitivity in Rhesus Macaques, Copyright 2007, with permission from Elsevier. (C–D) Reprinted from Proceedings of the Royal Society B: *Biological Sciences*, 274 (1619): 1751. Hayden, B.Y., Parikh, P.L., Deaner, R.O., and Platt, M.L., Economic principles motivating social attention in humans, Copyright 2007. Reprinted with permission from the Royal Society.

payoff regresses toward expectation (Lopes, 1981). Indeed, many people switch their risk preferences when faced with multiple repeats of a single gamble (Hertwig et al., 2004; Lopes, 1981, 1996; Samuelson, 1963; Wedell and Boeckenholt, 1994).

For comparison, we studied this problem in rhesus monkeys—the favored animal model in single-unit studies in cognitive neuroscience and neuroeconomics (Hayden and Platt, 2007). Specifically, we examined the influence of delays between sequential choices on risk preferences in rhesus monkeys. We found that increasing the normally short inter-trial interval from 1 s to 45 s reduced risk-seeking (Fig. 6.4A). The precise pattern of decrease in risk-seeking was well-explained by a model that specifically assumes that the monkey makes prospective judgments over the next several trials, amortizing any potential loss from the present choice by the increasing probability of a potential gain in the long run (Rachlin et al., 1988). Increasing delays reduces this amortization, and thus induces more frequent choices of the guaranteed option (Hayden and Platt, 2007). These results are consistent with the idea that one-shot gambles and repeated gambles recruit different cognitive processes, including prospective thinking and interval timing (Hayden and Platt, 2007).

Risk is not the only domain in which task repetition may influence behavior and the cognitive processes that support it. For example, when human subjects are asked to decide on which candy bar they will receive for the next several weeks, they are more variety-seeking than they are when they decide each week which candy bar to take (Simonson, 1990). Trial repetition also impacts behavior in complex choice tasks, where behavior reflects low-level biases, such as alternation and perseveration (Lau and Glimcher, 2005), as well as local estimates of reward rate (Corrado et al., 2005; Hayden et al., 2008a; Lau and Glimcher, 2008). Trial repetition can influence choice and normative strategy in game theoretic contexts as well. For example, Nash equilibrium strategy can switch from defection to tit-for-tat when moving from a single-shot to an iterated Prisoner's Dilemma problem (Axelrod, 1984). Behavior is influenced by the outcomes of recent trials in both simple discrimination tasks (Law and Gold, 2009) and in more complex executive control tasks (Emeric et al., 2007), and some functions may be improved by practice (Muraven et al., 1999). These and other effects of trial repetition indicate the importance of care in comparing experiments in which the amount of repetition can vary—especially when comparing fMRI results with humans to physiological studies with animals.

There is another potentially important difference between experiments structured around sequences of trials and those structured around one-time decisions. In one-time decisions, subjects do not have experience with previous trials, whereas in trial sequences, they may. In primate studies, where primary rewards are used exclusively, subjects inevitably have information about outcomes of previous trials. In many studies of risky choice in humans, even with sequences of gambles, the gambles are not resolved until the end of the session. It is generally assumed, in most animal experiments, that the task is well-learned and thus that behavior does not reflect the history of recent rewards and choices. This assumption does not generally hold, however (Corrado et al., 2005; Hayden et al., 2008a; Lau and Glimcher, 2008; Sugrue et al., 2004). For example, we found that choices made by monkeys in a simple gambling task strongly reflect reward outcomes of the most recent trials (Hayden et al., 2008a, 2009a). These patterns are consistent with simple reinforcement learning models, suggesting that learning continues, even after a task is well practiced. Such behavioral adjustment is strong enough that it occurs even for fictive outcomes—rewards that have been observed, but not directly experienced (Hayden et al., 2009a). In both cases, outcomes were found to contribute to neuronal spiking as well, thus underscoring the importance of repetition frequency and learning in neurophysiological studies with animals.

Yet another difference is that animals typically work for primary rewards that they consume immediately, such as food or drink (but see Seo and Lee, 2009). The use of primary rewards as motivators may strongly influence decisions (McClure et al., 2007). Moreover, since motivation must be maintained across multiple trials, animals are typically given very small rewards on each trial. It is generally assumed that satiety does not occur in most human studies—particularly those involving monetary rewards—and that diminishing marginal utility for goods does not apply to the small rewards typically used in the lab. In any case, small non-hypothetical rewards promote risk-seeking in humans, possibly because they engage different cognitive processes than those engaged by hypothetical or extremely large rewards (Barron and Erev, 2003).

To address these issues, we investigated the importance of task design in risky decision making. We examined choices made by undergraduates in a gambling task that was as close as possible to the one we use with monkeys (Hayden and Platt, 2008). Specifically, thirsty participants sat in an anechoic chamber with a juice tube in their mouth, saw the same computer display that monkeys do, and received squirts of Gatorade of variable volumes as rewards. The rules were only explained in a minimal way, so that participants would have to learn the task structure and probabilistic nature of rewards by experience. We found that, under these conditions, risk aversion disappeared, and choices depended strongly on recent reward outcomes—just like the behavior of monkeys in the same situation (Fig. 6.4B, Hayden and Platt, 2008; Hayden et al.,2008a; McCoy and Platt, 2005).

In summary, the specific experimental paradigms used to study risk-sensitive decision making in animals clearly deviate from the standard questionnaire approach used in behavioral economics. However, this does not mean that either one of these approaches is inferior or unrealistic. Indeed, real-life economic choices come in many forms, and any complete theory of the psychology and neuroscience of decision making must account for all of them. More generally, laboratory measures of psychological processes should demonstrate their generality to real-life situations.

6.3 Establishing behavioral homologies

The above discussion highlights the critical importance of simple, straightforward behavioral studies designed to determine how behavior, and its underlying neural mechanisms, vary across different experimental task domains. Within the realm of risk, an important series of studies has looked at how decisions are influenced by learning through experience (Barron and Erev, 2003; Erev and Barron, 2005; Hertwig et al., 2004; Klos et al., 2005; Stewart et al., 2006). Furthermore, the application of reinforcement learning theory to the study of decision making in uncertain environments has made it possible to take advantage of local reinforcement dynamics in studying risky decisions (Corrado et al., 2005; Dorris and Glimcher, 2004; Lau and Glimcher, 2005, 2007, 2008; Sugrue et al., 2004). Finally, it is critical to obtain input from experts in both qualitative and quantitative aspects of animal behavior, as they can provide a useful assessment of the applicability of economic models and tests to animal behavior (Bateson and Kacelnik, 1997; Kacelnik and Bateson, 1996; Stephens and Anderson, 2001; Stephens and Krebs, 1986; Stephens and McLinn, 2003).

One possible way to aid communication between physiologists and neuroimagers is to examine the behavior of humans making decisions about primary rewards—the currency of choice in animal studies. It is, in practice, very difficult to provide primary rewards to humans while they are in an MRI machine—although a few recent studies have either done so or come close (McClure et al., 2007; O'Doherty et al., 2002; Plassmann et al., 2007). One potentially valuable tool in this regard is the use of photographs, especially pictures of other people, which have been demonstrated to have reward value for individual subjects (Aharon et al., 2001; Hayden et al., 2007; O'Doherty et al., 2003). For example, we recently showed that the decisions men make about viewing photographs of females are consistent with economic theory in three ways (Fig. 6.4C, D; Hayden et al., 2007). First, opportunities to view photographs are discounted with time; second, they substitute for monetary rewards; third, they reinforce work (see also Aharon et al., 2001). In fact, such photos activate the same reward circuitry as other types of rewards like food and money (Aharon et al., 2001; O'Doherty et al., 2003). Photographic rewards are experimentally appealing, as they do not diminish in value with satiety; do not require movements that introduce artifacts, such as swallowing; cannot be saved (thus promoting discounting); and are not messy and sticky, as many food rewards are.

A second solution is to train non-human animals to perform tasks that are more similar to those used in studies with humans. We have begun preliminary studies using explicit symbolic stimuli that do not require complicated reward-learning—similar to using symbolic task instructions with human subjects (Hayden et al., 2010) see also So and Stuphorn, 2010. These preliminary studies demonstrate that it is possible, in theory, for monkeys, at least, to use explicit cues about the probability, timing, and size of rewards. Using novel tasks to enhance comparability between studies with humans and animals is advisable for a range of economic problems, such as delay discounting, economic exchange (Deaner et al., 2005; Klein et al., 2008), and strategic interactions.

Perhaps most importantly, all these behavioral approaches should inspire the use of neurometric measures to infer whether different decision problems are mediated by the same neural substrates (Britten et al., 1996; Glimcher, 2003; Kable and Glimcher, 2007; Klein et al., 2008). If, for example, risky decisions based on experiential learning engage brain regions distinct from those engaged by risky decisions based on verbal instructions, this will have important implications for related studies such as those designed to examine whether preferences for risk and time are mediated by the same underlying brain mechanisms.

6.4 Conclusion: a call for parallel studies using fMRI and single-unit recording in neuroeconomics and cognitive neuroscience

fMRI and single-unit activity, and other measures of brain function, are useful to cognitive neuroscience and neuroeconomics only to the extent that they can provide insight into the mechanisms underlying behavior. We have argued that the information offered by these measures is substantially different, and that understanding the nature of these differences is critical for developing a synthetic understanding of brain function.

These differences are manifest in two case studies from our own laboratory. We showed that monkeys' risk preferences diverge strikingly from those of humans, and that these differences may reflect the specifics of task design, rather than fundamental species' differences in behavior and cognition. Moreover, although CGp neurons in tracks several relevant variables, functionally distinct subpopulations that carry multiple forms of information can frustrate attempts to link CGp neuronal activity like BOLD. Consequently, the corresponding BOLD signal remains difficult to predict, and, conversely, it seems unlikely that these neuronal response patterns could be inferred based on fMRI data alone. We also showed that spiking of single ACC neurons tracks both experienced and fictive outcomes, and do so in a monotonic fashion. The critical finding of this study—that single neurons rather than overlapping populations—track both experienced and fictive outcomes in their spike rates, would be invisible to fMRI analysis, as would the precise time-course of these signals—at least given current imaging techniques. Moreover, the weaker, but still significant effects of fictive outcomes relative to experienced outcomes, could potentially lead to the conclusion that subregions within the ACC are specialized for experienced and fictive outcomes.

Based on these case studies, we argue that a deeper comprehension of brain function demands a fuller understanding of the discontinuities between behavioral methods used by physiologists and neuroimagers. Nonetheless, we contend that the single, largest problem is the fundamental uncertainty in the nature of the hemodynamic response. Beginning with Cajal, a large body of foundational literature has supported the centrality of synaptic transmission and single-neuron activity for computation in the brain (Barlow, 1972; Bullock, 1959). However, despite nearly 20 years of progress, the biophysical processes underlying the BOLD signal are less well-understood than those associated with neuronal spiking. Yet clear biases in neuronal selection and recording, the difficulty of recording from multiple areas simultaneously, and the limitations of an animal model, warrant caution in the abstemious focus on single-unit recording as the ultimate arbiter of neuroscientific understanding. Clearly, progress is being made; however, until a much more sophisticated understanding is obtained, we must resist the urge to rush to strong conclusions based on fMRI or single-unit data alone.

An often ignored, yet critical, set of differences between fMRI studies and single-unit studies comes in the form of experimental design. Indeed, two otherwise analogous experiments designed to isolate a cognitive variable of interest may have entirely different implementations in a single-unit study in an animal and an imaging experiment using human participants. Such differences can have direct ramifications on how these cognitive processes are recruited, and this difference can in turn influence neural data acquired. We therefore heartily endorse studies designed to directly examine the influence of the specifics of task design on both behavior and brain function.

Given these considerations, methodological convergence will demand an understanding of neural processing at multiple levels—ideally in animals and humans performing precisely the same tasks. The emergence of sophisticated data collection hardware, increasing access to intracranial recordings in humans (albeit in rare and restricted circumstances), and rich new analytical methods, will facilitate this process. A fundamental goal of such studies should be to continue to delineate the relationships between SUA, LFPs, and BOLD in various cognitive states and processes. Coupling functions between these measures will most likely depend on location within the brain, as well as various cognitive and non-cognitive factors. It will be equally important to more fully understand the suite of biophysical processes that contribute to spiking, including dendritic computation, signal summation, neuromodulation, local inhibition, and so on. In these endeavors, the use of fMRI and single-unit physiology on the same monkeys, while they perform the same tasks, will be an invaluable tool—a method that is much easier and more practical than recordings in humans. This coordination of methods will permit perfect control for species, for specific subject, for idiosyncrasies in task design, and cognitive variability. Finally, it is paramount to perform single-unit physiology studies on humans when the rare opportunity arises, so as to reduce the potentially confounding effects of species' differences in brain function and task demands. If all these measures can be successfully combined, their separate domains of information are likely to be quite beneficial for neuroscience, since averaging multiple independent sources of information generally reduces entropy (Shannon and Weaver, 1963).

References

Ackermann, R. F., Finch, D. M., Babb, T. L., and Engel, J., Jr. (1984). Increased glucose metabolism during long-duration recurrent inhibition of hippocampal pyramidal cells. *J Neurosci*, 4(1), 251–64.

Aharon, I., Etcoff, N., Ariely, D., Chabris, C. F., O'Connor, E., and Breiter, H. C. (2001). Beautiful faces have variable reward value: fMRI and behavioral evidence. *Neuron*, 32(3), 537–51.

Amiez, C., Joseph, J. P., and Procyk, E. (2006). Reward encoding in the monkey anterior cingulate cortex. *Cereb Cortex*, 16(7), 1040–55.

Amodio, D. M., Harmon-Jones, E., Devine, P. G., Curtin, J. J., Hartley, S. L., and Covert, A. E. (2004). Neural signals for the detection of unintentional race bias. *Psychol Sci*, 15(2), 88–93.

Amodio, D. M., Jost, J. T., Master, S. L., and Yee, C. M. (2007). Neurocognitive correlates of liberalism and conservatism. *Nat Neurosci*, 10(10), 1246–47.

Aosaki, T., Kimura, M., and Graybiel, A. M. (1995). Temporal and spatial characteristics of tonically active neurons of the primate's striatum. *J Neurophysiol*, 73(3), 1234–52.

Aston-Jones, G., and Cohen, J. D. (2005). An integrative theory of locus coeruleus-norepinephrine function: adaptive gain and optimal performance. *Annu Rev Neurosci*, 28, 403–50.

Attwell, D. and Iadecola, C. (2002). The neural basis of functional brain imaging signals. *Trends Neurosci*, 25(12), 621–25.

Axelrod, R. (1984). *The evolution of cooperation*. New York: Basic Books.

Barash, S. (2003). Paradoxical activities: insight into the relationship of parietal and prefrontal cortices. *Trends Neurosci*, 26(11), 582–89.

Barlow, H. B. (1972). Single units and sensation: a neuron doctrine for perceptual psychology. *Perception*, 1(4), 371–94.

Barlow, H. B., Fitzhugh, R., and Kuffler, S. W. (1957). Change of organization in the receptive fields of the cat's retina during dark adaptation. *J Physiol*, 137(3), 338–54.

Barraclough, D. J., Conroy, M. L., and Lee, D. (2004). Prefrontal cortex and decision making in a mixed-strategy game. *Nat Neurosci*, 7(4), 404–410.

Barron, G. and Erev, I. (2003). Small feedback-based decisions and their limited correspondence to description-based decisions. *J Behav Decis making,* **16**, 215–33.

Bartels, A., Logothetis, N. K., and Moutoussis, K. (2008). fMRI and its interpretations: an illustration on directional selectivity in area V5/MT. *Trends Neurosci,* **31**(9), 444–53.

Bateson, M. and Kacelnik, A. (1997). Starlings' preferences for predictable and unpredictable delays to food. *Anim Behav,* **53**(6), 1129–42.

Behrens, T. E., Berg, H. J., Jbabdi, S., Rushworth, M. F., and Woolrich, M. W. (2007). Probabilistic diffusion tractography with multiple fibre orientations: what can we gain? *Neuroimage,* **34**(1), 144–55.

Belova, M. A., Paton, J. J., and Salzman, C. D. (2008). Moment-to-moment tracking of state value in the amygdala. *J Neurosci,* **28**(40), 10023–30.

Bisley, J. W. and Goldberg, M. E. (2006). Neural correlates of attention and distractibility in the lateral intraparietal area. *J Neurophysiol,* **95**(3), 1696–1717.

Bisley, J. W., Krishna, B. S., and Goldberg, M. E. (2004). A rapid and precise on-response in posterior parietal cortex. *J Neurosci,* **24**(8), 1833–38.

Blake, R. and Logothetis, N. K. (2002). Visual competition. *Nat Rev Neurosci,* **3**(1), 13–21.

Botvinick, M. M., Braver, T. S., Barch, D. M., Carter, C. S., and Cohen, J. D. (2001). Conflict monitoring and cognitive control. *Psychol Rev,* **108**(3), 624–52.

Boynton, G. M., Engel, S. A., Glover, G. H., and Heeger, D. J. (1996). Linear systems analysis of functional magnetic resonance imaging in human V1. *J Neurosci,* **16**(13), 4207–21.

Brefczynski, J. A. and DeYoe, E. A. (1999). A physiological correlate of the "spotlight" of visual attention. *Nat Neurosci,* **2**(4), 370–74.

Brinker, G., Bock, C., Busch, E., Krep, H., Hossmann, K. A., and Hoehn-Berlage, M. (1999). Simultaneous recording of evoked potentials and T2*-weighted MR images during somatosensory stimulation of rat. *Magn Reson Med,* **41**(3), 469–73.

Britten, K. H., Shadlen, M. N., Newsome, W. T., and Movshon, J. A. (1992). The analysis of visual motion: a comparison of neuronal and psychophysical performance. *J Neurosci,* **12**(12), 4745–65.

Britten, K. H., Shadlen, M. N., Newsome, W. T., and Movshon, J. A. (1993). Responses of neurons in macaque MT to stochastic motion signals. *Vis Neurosci,* **10**(6), 1157–69.

Britten, K. H., Newsome, W. T., Shadlen, M. N., Celebrini, S., and Movshon, J. A. (1996). A relationship between behavioral choice and the visual responses of neurons in macaque MT. *Vis Neurosci,* **13**(1), 87–100.

Bullock, T. H. (1959). Neuron doctrine and electrophysiology. *Science,* **129**(3355), 371–94.

Buzsaki, G. and Draguhn, A. (2004). Neuronal oscillations in cortical networks. *Science,* **304**(5679), 1926–29.

Byrne, R. M. (2002). Mental models and counterfactual thoughts about what might have been. *Trends Cogn Sci,* **6**(10), 426–31.

Camerer, C. F. (2008). Neuroeconomics: opening the gray box. *Neuron,* **60**(3), 416–419.

Camille, N., Coricelli, G., Sallet, J., Pradat-Diehl, P., Duhamel, J. R., and Sirigu, A. (2004). The involvement of the orbitofrontal cortex in the experience of regret. *Science,* **304**(5674), 1167–70.

Canolty, R. T., Edwards, E., Dalal, S. S., Soltani, M., Nagarajan, S. S., Kirsch, H. E. et al. (2006). High gamma power is phase-locked to theta oscillations in human neocortex. *Science,* **313**(5793), 1626–28.

Chiu, P. H., Lohrenz, T. M., and Montague, P. R. (2008). Smokers' brains compute, but ignore, a fictive error signal in a sequential investment task. *Nat Neurosci,* **11**(4), 514–20.

Coricelli, G., Critchley, H. D., Joffily, M., O'Doherty, J. P., Sirigu, A., and Dolan, R. J. (2005). Regret and its avoidance: a neuroimaging study of choice behavior. *Nat Neurosci,* **8**(9), 1255–62.

Coricelli, G., Dolan, R. J., and Sirigu, A. (2007). Brain, emotion and decision making: the paradigmatic example of regret. *Trends Cogn Sci,* **11**(6), 258–65.

Corrado, G. S., Sugrue, L. P., Seung, H. S., and Newsome, W. T. (2005). Linear-nonlinear-Poisson models of primate choice dynamics. *J Exp Anal Behav,* **84**(3), 581–617.

Daw, N. D., O'Doherty, J. P., Dayan, P., Seymour, B., and Dolan, R. J. (2006). Cortical substrates for exploratory decisions in humans. *Nature,* **441**(7095), 876–79.

Deaner, R. O., Khera, A. V., and Platt, M. L. (2005). Monkeys pay per view: adaptive valuation of social images by rhesus macaques. *Curr Biol,* **15**(6), 543–48.

Desimone, R. and Schein, S. J. (1987). Visual properties of neurons in area V4 of the macaque: sensitivity to stimulus form. *J Neurophysiol,* **57**(3), 835–68.

Devor, A., Hillman, E. M., Tian, P., Waeber, C., Teng, I. C., Ruvinskaya, L. et al. (2008). Stimulus-induced changes in blood flow and 2-deoxyglucose uptake dissociate in ipsilateral somatosensory cortex. *J Neurosci,* **28**(53), 14347–57.

Donoghue, J. P., Sanes, J. N., Hatsopoulos, N. G., and Gaal, G. (1998). Neural discharge and local field potential oscillations in primate motor cortex during voluntary movements. *J Neurophysiol,* **79**(1), 159–73.

Dorris, M. C. and Glimcher, P. W. (2004). Activity in posterior parietal cortex is correlated with the relative subjective desirability of action. *Neuron,* **44**(2), 365–78.

Emeric, E. E., Brown, J. W., Boucher, L., Carpenter, R. H., Hanes, D. P., Harris, R. et al. (2007). Influence of history on saccade countermanding performance in humans and macaque monkeys. *Vision Res,* **47**(1), 35–49.

Engel, A. K., Fries, P., and Singer, W. (2001). Dynamic predictions: Oscillations and synchrony in top-down processing. *Nat Rev Neurosci,* **2**(10), 704–16.

Epstude, K. and Roese, N. J. (2008). The functional theory of counterfactual thinking. *Pers Soc Psychol Rev,* **12**(2), 168–92.

Erev, I. and Barron, G. (2005). On adaptation, maximization, and reinforcement learning among cognitive strategies. *Psychol Rev,* **112**(4), 912–31.

Evarts, E. V. (1968). Relation of pyramidal tract activity to force exerted during voluntary movement. *J Neurophysiol,* **31**(1), 14–27.

Evarts, E. V. (1966). Methods for recording activity of individual neurons in moving animals. In *Methods in medical research*. Rushmer, R.F., (ed), pp. 241–50. Chicago: Year Book Medical Publishers.

Fan, J., Byrne, J., Worden, M. S., Guise, K. G., McCandliss, B. D., Fossella, J. et al. (2007). The relation of brain oscillations to attentional networks. *J Neurosci,* **27**(23), 6197–6206.

Fiorillo, C. D., Tobler, P. N., and Schultz, W. (2003). Discrete coding of reward probability and uncertainty by dopamine neurons. *Science,* **299**(5614), 1898–1902.

Floresco, S. B., West, A. R., Ash, B., Moore, H., and Grace, A. A. (2003). Afferent modulation of dopamine neuron firing differentially regulates tonic and phasic dopamine transmission. *Nat Neurosci,* **6**(9), 968–73.

Ford, K. A., Gati, J. S., Menon, R. S., and Everling, S. (2009). BOLD fMRI activation for anti-saccades in nonhuman primates. *Neuroimage,* **45**(2), 470–76.

Fox, M. D. and Raichle, M. E. (2007). Spontaneous fluctuations in brain activity observed with functional brain imaging. *Nat Rev Neurosci,* **8**, 700–11.

Fox, S. E., Wolfson, S., and Ranck, J. B., Jr. (1986). Hippocampal theta rhythm and the firing of neurons in walking and urethane anesthetized rats. *Exp Brain Res,* **62**(3), 495–508.

Funahashi, S., Bruce, C. J., and Goldman-Rakic, P. S. (1989). Mnemonic coding of visual space in the monkey's dorsolateral prefrontal cortex. *J Neurophysiol,* **61**(2), 331–49.

Fuster, J. M. and Alexander, G. E. (1971). Neuron activity related to short-term memory. *Science,* **173**(997), 652–54.

Gandhi, S. P., Heeger, D. J., and Boynton, G. M. (1999). Spatial attention affects brain activity in human primary visual cortex. *Proc Natl Acad Sci USA,* **96**(6), 3314–19.

Gattass, R., Sousa, A. P., and Gross, C. G. (1988). Visuotopic organization and extent of V3 and V4 of the macaque. *J Neurosci*, **8**(6), 1831–45.

Glimcher, P. W. (2003). *Decisions, uncertainty, and the brain: the science of neuroeconomics*. Cambridge, MA: The MIT Press.

Glover, G. H. (1999). Deconvolution of impulse response in event-related BOLD fMRI. *Neuroimage*, **9**(4), 416–29.

Gold, J. I. and Shadlen, M. N. (2002). Banburismus and the brain: decoding the relationship between sensory stimuli, decisions, and reward. *Neuron*, **36**(2), 299–308.

Goldberg, M. E. and Wurtz, R. H. (1972a). Activity of superior colliculus in behaving monkey. I. Visual receptive fields of single neurons. *J Neurophysiol*, **35**(4), 542–59.

Goldberg, M. E. and Wurtz, R. H. (1972b). Activity of superior colliculus in behaving monkey. II. Effect of attention on neuronal responses. *J Neurophysiol*, **35**(4), 560–74.

Greene, J. D., Sommerville, R. B., Nystrom, L. E., Darley, J. M., and Cohen, J. D. (2001). An fMRI investigation of emotional engagement in moral judgment. *Science*, **293**(5537), 2105–2108.

Gross, C. G., Bender, D. B., and Gerstein, G. L. (1979). Activity of inferior temporal neurons in behaving monkeys. *Neuropsychologia*, **17**(2), 215–29.

Gusnard, D. A. and Raichle, M. E. (2001). Searching for a baseline: functional imaging and the resting human brain. *Nat Rev Neurosci*, **2**(10), 685–94.

Hadland, K. A., Rushworth, M. F., Gaffan, D., and Passingham, R. E. (2003). The effect of cingulate lesions on social behavior and emotion. *Neuropsychologia*, **41**(8), 919–31.

Haenny, P. E., Maunsell, J. H., and Schiller, P. H. (1988). State dependent activity in monkey visual cortex. II. Retinal and extraretinal factors in V4. *Exp Brain Res*, **69**(2), 245–59.

Hanes, D. P. and Schall, J. D. (1996). Neural control of voluntary movement initiation. *Science*, **274**(5286), 427–30.

Harris, L. T. and Fiske, S. T. (2006). Dehumanizing the lowest of the low: neuroimaging responses to extreme out-groups. *Psychol Sci*, **17**(10), 847–53.

Hayden, B. Y. and Platt, M. L. (2007). Temporal discounting predicts risk sensitivity in rhesus macaques. *Curr Biol*, **17**(1), 49–53.

Hayden, B. Y. and Platt, M. L. (2009a). Gambling for Gatorade: risk-sensitive decision making for fluid rewards in humans. *Anim Cogn*, **12**(1), 201–7.

Hayden, B. Y. and Platt, M. L. (2009b). Cingulate cortex. In *Encyclopedia of neuroscience* (Vol. 2). L. R. Squire (ed.), pp. 887–92. Oxford: Academic Press.

Hayden, B. Y. and Platt, M. L. (2009c). The mean, the median, and the St. Petersburg Paradox. *Judgment and Decision making*, **4**, 256–73.

Hayden, B. Y., Parikh, P. C., Deaner, R. O., and Platt, M. L. (2007). Economic principles motivating social attention in humans. *Proc Biol Sci*, **274**(1619), 1751–56.

Hayden, B. Y., Nair, A. C., McCoy, A. N., and Platt, M. L. (2008a). Posterior cingulate cortex mediates outcome-contingent allocation of behavior. *Neuron*, **60**(1), 19–25.

Hayden, B. Y., Heilbronner, S. R., Nair, A. C., and Platt, M. L. (2008b). Cognitive influences on risk-seeking by rhesus macaques. *Judgment and Decision making*, **3**(5), 389–95.

Hayden, B. Y., Pearson, J. M., and Platt, M. L. (2009a). Fictive reward signals in the anterior cingulate cortex. *Science*, **324**(5929), 948–50.

Hayden, B. Y., Smith, D. V., and Platt, M. L. (2009b). Electrophysiological correlates of default-mode processing in macaque posterior cingulate cortex. *Proc Natl Acad Sci USA*, **106**(14), 5948–53.

Hayden, B. Y., Heilbronner, S. R., and Platt, M. L. (2010). Ambiguity aversion in rhesus macques. *Front Neurosci*, **4**, 166.

Heilbronner, S. R., Rosati, A. G., Stevens, J. R., Hare, B., and Hauser, M. D. (2008). A fruit in the hand or two in the bush? Divergent risk preferences in chimpanzees and bonobos. *Biol Lett,* **4**(3), 246–49.

Hertwig, R., Barron, G., Weber, E. U., and Erev, I. (2004). Decisions from experience and the effect of rare events in risky choice. *Psychol Sci,* **15**(8), 534–39.

Hofstadter, D. R. (1979). *Gödel, Escher, Bach.* New York: Basic Books.

Holroyd, C. B. and Coles, M. G. (2002). The neural basis of human error processing: reinforcement learning, dopamine, and the error-related negativity. *Psychol Rev,* **109**(4), 679–709.

Holt, C. A. and Laury, S. K. (2002). Risk aversion and incentive effects. *Am Econ Rev,* **92**(5), 1644–55.

Hsu, M., Bhatt, M., Adolphs, R., Tranel, D., and Camerer, C. F. (2005). Neural systems responding to degrees of uncertainty in human decision making. *Science,* **310**(5754), 1680–83.

Huettel, S. A., Song, A. W., and McCarthy, G. (2008). *Functional magnetic resonance imaging, 2nd edn.* New York, NY: Sinauer Associates, Inc.

Huettel, S. A., Stowe, C. J., Gordon, E. M., Warner, B. T., and Platt, M. L. (2006). Neural signatures of economic preferences for risk and ambiguity. *Neuron,* **49**(5), 765–75.

Huk, A. C., Ress, D., and Heeger, D. J. (2001). Neuronal basis of the motion aftereffect reconsidered. *Neuron,* **32**(1), 161–72.

Hyder, F., Rothman, D. L., and Shulman, R. G. (2002). Total neuroenergetics support localized brain activity: implications for the interpretation of fMRI. *Proc Natl Acad Sci USA,* **99**(16), 10771–76.

Jacobs, J., Kahana, M. J., Ekstrom, A. D., and Fried, I. (2007). Brain oscillations control timing of single-neuron activity in humans. *J Neurosci,* **27**(14), 3839–44.

Jokisch, D. and Jensen, O. (2007). Modulation of gamma and alpha activity during a working memory task engaging the dorsal or ventral stream. *J Neurosci,* **27**(12), 3244–51.

Kable, J. W. and Glimcher, P. W. (2007). The neural correlates of subjective value during intertemporal choice. *Nat Neurosci,* **10**(12), 1625–33.

Kacelnik, A. and Bateson, M. (1996). Risky theories the effects of variance on foraging decisions. *Am Zool,* **36**, 402–34.

Kastner, S. and Ungerleider, L. G. (2000). Mechanisms of visual attention in the human cortex. *Annu Rev Neurosci,* **23**, 315–41.

Kayser, C., Kim, M., Ugurbil, K., Kim, D. S., and Konig, P. (2004). A comparison of hemodynamic and neural responses in cat visual cortex using complex stimuli. *Cereb Cortex,* **14**(8), 881–91.

Kennerley, S. W., Dahmubed, A. F., Lara, A. H., and Wallis, J. D. (2009). Neurons in the frontal lobe encode the value of multiple decision variables. *J Cogn Neurosci,* **21**(6), 1162–78.

Keshavan, M. S., Reynolds, C. F., 3rd, Miewald, M. J., Montrose, D. M., Sweeney, J. A., Vasko, R. C., Jr. et al. (1998). Delta sleep deficits in schizophrenia: evidence from automated analyses of sleep data. *Arch Gen Psychiatry,* **55**(5), 443–48.

Klein, J. T., Deaner, R. O., and Platt, M. L. (2008). Neural correlates of social target value in macaque parietal cortex. *Curr Biol,* **18**(6), 419–24.

Klos, A., Weber, E. U., and Weber, M. (2005). Investment decisions and time horizon: risk perception and risk behavior in repeated gambles. *Manage Sci,* **51**, 1777–90.

Kravitz, A. V. and Peoples, L. L. (2008). Background firing rates of orbitofrontal neurons reflect specific characteristics of operant sessions and modulate phasic responses to reward-associated cues and behavior. *J Neurosci,* **28**(4), 1009–18.

Kriegeskorte, N., Mur, M., Ruff, D. A., Kiani, R., Bodurka, J., Esteky, H. et al. (2008). Matching categorical object representations in inferior temporal cortex of man and monkey. *Neuron,* **60**(6), 1126–41.

Kubota, K. and Niki, H. (1971). Prefrontal cortical unit activity and delayed alternation performance in monkeys. *J Neurophysiol,* **34**(3), 337–47.

Kuhnen, C. M. and Knutson, B. (2005). The neural basis of financial risk taking. *Neuron,* **47**(5), 763–70.

Lakatos, P., Chen, C. M., O'Connell, M. N., Mills, A., and Schroeder, C. E. (2007). Neuronal oscillations and multisensory interaction in primary auditory cortex. *Neuron,* **53**(2), 279–92.

Lau, B. and Glimcher, P. W. (2005). Dynamic response-by-response models of matching behavior in rhesus monkeys. *J Exp Anal Behav,* **84**(3), 555–79.

Lau, B. and Glimcher, P. W. (2007). Action and outcome encoding in the primate caudate nucleus. *J Neurosci,* **27**(52), 14502–14514.

Lau, B. and Glimcher, P. W. (2008). Value representations in the primate striatum during matching behavior. *Neuron,* **58**(3), 451–63.

Law, C. T. and Gold, J. I. (2009). Reinforcement learning can account for associative and perceptual learning on a visual-decision task. *Nat Neurosci,* **12**(5), 655–63.

Lee, D. K., Itti, L., Koch, C., and Braun, J. (1999). Attention activates winner-take-all competition among visual filters. *Nat Neurosci,* **2**(4), 375–81.

Lee, H., Simpson, G. V., Logothetis, N. K., and Rainer, G. (2005). Phase locking of single neuron activity to theta oscillations during working memory in monkey extrastriate visual cortex. *Neuron,* **45**(1), 147–56.

Leopold, D. A., Murayama, Y., and Logothetis, N. K. (2003). Very slow activity fluctuations in monkey visual cortex: implications for functional brain imaging. *Cereb Cortex,* **13**(4), 422–33.

Libet, B., Gleason, C. A., Wright, E. W., and Pearl, D. K. (1983). Time of conscious intention to act in relation to onset of cerebral activity (readiness-potential). The unconscious initiation of a freely voluntary act. *Brain,* **106** (Pt 3), 623–42.

Logothetis, N. K. (2008). What we can do and what we cannot do with fMRI. *Nature,* **453**(7197), 869–78.

Logothetis, N. K. and Wandell, B. A. (2004). Interpreting the BOLD signal. *Annu Rev Physiol,* **66**, 735–69.

Logothetis, N. K., Pauls, J., Augath, M., Trinath, T., and Oeltermann, A. (2001). Neurophysiological investigation of the basis of the fMRI signal. *Nature,* **412**(6843), 150–57.

Lohrenz, T., McCabe, K., Camerer, C. F., and Montague, P. R. (2007). Neural signature of fictive learning signals in a sequential investment task. *Proc Natl Acad Sci USA,* **104**(22), 9493–98.

Lopes, L. L. (1981). Decision making in the short run. *J Exp Psychol Learn,* **7**(5), 377–85.

Lopes, L. L. (1996). When time is of the essence: averaging, aspiration, and the short run. *Organ Behav Hum Dec,* **65**(3), 179–89.

Luck, S. J., Chelazzi, L., Hillyard, S. A., and Desimone, R. (1997). Neural mechanisms of spatial selective attention in areas V1, V2, and V4 of macaque visual cortex. *J Neurophysiol,* **77**(1), 24–42.

MacKay, W. A. and Mendonca, A. J. (1995). Field potential oscillatory bursts in parietal cortex before and during reach. *Brain Res,* **704**(2), 167–74.

Maier, A., Wilke, M., Aura, C., Zhu, C., Ye, F. Q., and Leopold, D. A. (2008). Divergence of fMRI and neural signals in V1 during perceptual suppression in the awake monkey. *Nat Neurosci,* **11**(10), 1193–1200.

Mangia, S., Giove, F., Tkac, I., Logothetis, N. K., Henry, P. G., Olman, C. A. et al. (2009). Metabolic and hemodynamic events after changes in neuronal activity: current hypotheses, theoretical predictions and in vivo NMR experimental findings. *J Cereb Blood Flow Metab,* **29**(3), 441–63.

Mathiesen, C., Caesar, K., Akgoren, N., and Lauritzen, M. (1998). Modification of activity-dependent increases of cerebral blood flow by excitatory synaptic activity and spikes in rat cerebellar cortex. *J Physiol,* **512** (Pt 2), 555–66.

Mathiesen, C., Caesar, K., and Lauritzen, M. (2000). Temporal coupling between neuronal activity and blood flow in rat cerebellar cortex as indicated by field potential analysis. *J Physiol,* **523** Pt 1, 235–46.

Matsumoto, M., Matsumoto, K., Abe, H., and Tanaka, K. (2007). Medial prefrontal cell activity signaling prediction errors of action values. *Nat Neurosci,* **10**(5), 647–56.

Mays, L. E. and Sparks, D. L. (1980). Dissociation of visual and saccade-related responses in superior colliculus neurons. *J Neurophysiol,* **43**(1), 207–32.

McClure, S. M., Ericson, K. M., Laibson, D. I., Loewenstein, G., and Cohen, J. D. (2007). Time discounting for primary rewards. *J Neurosci,* **27**(21), 5796–5804.

McCoy, A. N. and Platt, M. L. (2005). Risk-sensitive neurons in macaque posterior cingulate cortex. *Nat Neurosci,* **8**(9), 1220–27.

McCoy, A. N., Crowley, J. C., Haghighian, G., Dean, H. L., and Platt, M. L. (2003). Saccade reward signals in posterior cingulate cortex. *Neuron,* **40**(5), 1031–40.

Miller, E. K. and Desimone, R. (1994). Parallel neuronal mechanisms for short-term memory. *Science,* **263**(5146), 520–22.

Miller, E. K. and Wilson, M. A. (2008). All my circuits: using multiple electrodes to understand functioning neural networks. *Neuron,* **60**(3), 483–88.

Montemurro, M. A., Rasch, M. J., Murayama, Y., Logothetis, N. K., and Panzeri, S. (2008). Phase-of-firing coding of natural visual stimuli in primary visual cortex. *Curr Biol,* **18**(5), 375–80.

Moore, C. I. and Cao, R. (2008). The hemo-neural hypothesis: on the role of blood flow in information processing. *J Neurophysiol,* **99**(5), 2035–47.

Moran, J. and Desimone, R. (1985). Selective attention gates visual processing in the extrastriate cortex. *Science,* **229**(4715), 782–84.

Mountcastle, V. B., Lynch, J. C., Georgopoulos, A., Sakata, H., and Acuna, C. (1975). Posterior parietal association cortex of the monkey: command functions for operations within extrapersonal space. *J Neurophysiol,* **38**(4), 871–908.

Mukamel, R., Gelbard, H., Arieli, A., Hasson, U., Fried, I., and Malach, R. (2005). Coupling between neuronal firing, field potentials, and fMRI in human auditory cortex. *Science,* **309**(5736), 951–54.

Muraven, M., Baumeister, R. F., and Tice, D. M. (1999). Longitudinal improvement of self-regulation through practice: building self-control strength through repeated exercise. *J Soc Psychol,* **139**(4), 446–57.

Muthukumaraswamy, S. D. and Singh, K. D. (2008). Spatiotemporal frequency tuning of BOLD and gamma band MEG responses compared in primary visual cortex. *Neuroimage,* **40**(4), 1552–60.

Nakamura, K., Roesch, M. R., and Olson, C. R. (2005). Neuronal activity in macaque SEF and ACC during performance of tasks involving conflict. *J Neurophysiol,* **93**(2), 884–908.

Nasrallah, F. A., Griffin, J. L., Balcar, V. J., and Rae, C. (2007). Understanding your inhibitions: modulation of brain cortical metabolism by GABA(B) receptors. *J Cereb Blood Flow Metab,* **27**(8), 1510–20.

Newsome, W. T., Britten, K. H., Salzman, C. D., and Movshon, J. A. (1990). Neuronal mechanisms of motion perception. *Cold Spring Harb Symp Quant Biol,* **55**, 697–705.

Niessing, J., Ebisch, B., Schmidt, K. E., Niessing, M., Singer, W., and Galuske, R. A. (2005). Hemodynamic signals correlate tightly with synchronized gamma oscillations. *Science,* **309**(5736), 948–51.

Niki, H. and Watanabe, M. (1979). Prefrontal and cingulate unit activity during timing behavior in the monkey. *Brain Res,* **171**(2), 213–24.

Nir, Y., Fisch, L., Mukamel, R., Gelbard-Sagiv, H., Arieli, A., Fried, I. et al. (2007). Coupling between neuronal firing rate, gamma LFP, and BOLD fMRI is related to interneuronal correlations. *Curr Biol,* **17**(15), 1275–85.

Nudo, R. J. and Masterton, R. B. (1986). Stimulation-induced [14C]2-deoxyglucose labeling of synaptic activity in the central auditory system. *J Comp Neurol,* **245**(4), 553–65.

O'Doherty, J. P., Deichmann, R., Critchley, H. D., and Dolan, R. J. (2002). Neural responses during anticipation of a primary taste reward. *Neuron*, **33**(5), 815–26.

O'Doherty, J., Winston, J., Critchley, H., Perrett, D., Burt, D. M., and Dolan, R. J. (2003). Beauty in a smile: the role of medial orbitofrontal cortex in facial attractiveness. *Neuropsychologia*, **41**(2), 147–55.

O'Keefe, J. and Recce, M. L. (1993). Phase relationship between hippocampal place units and the EEG theta rhythm. *Hippocampus*, **3**(3), 317–30.

Ogawa, S., Lee, T. M., Kay, A. R., and Tank, D. W. (1990). Brain magnetic resonance imaging with contrast dependent on blood oxygenation. *Proc Natl Acad Sci USA*, **87**(24), 9868–72.

Ogawa, S., Lee, T. M., Stepnoski, R., Chen, W., Zhu, X. H., and Ugurbil, K. (2000). An approach to probe some neural systems interaction by functional MRI at neural time scale down to milliseconds. *Proc Natl Acad Sci USA*, **97**(20), 11026–31.

Padoa-Schioppa, C. and Assad, J. A. (2006). Neurons in the orbitofrontal cortex encode economic value. *Nature*, **441**(7090), 223–26.

Padoa-Schioppa, C. and Assad, J. A. (2008). The representation of economic value in the orbitofrontal cortex is invariant for changes of menu. *Nat Neurosci*, **11**(1), 95–102.

Pan, X., Sawa, K., Tsuda, I., Tsukada, M., and Sakagami, M. (2008). Reward prediction based on stimulus categorization in primate lateral prefrontal cortex. *Nat Neurosci*, **11**(6), 703–712.

Parker, A. J. and Newsome, W. T. (1998). Sense and the single neuron: probing the physiology of perception. *Annu Rev Neurosci*, **21**, 227–77.

Pearson, J. M., Hayden, B. Y., and Platt, M. L. (2009). Neurons in posterior cingulate cortex signal exploratory decisions in a dynamic multi-option choice task. *Curr Biol*, **19**(18), 1–6.

Penfield, W. and Jasper, H. (1954). *Epilepsy and the functional anatomy of the human brain*. Boston: Little, Brown.

Pesaran, B., Nelson, M. J., and Andersen, R. A. (2008). Free choice activates a decision circuit between frontal and parietal cortex. *Nature*, **453**(7193), 406–409.

Pesaran, B., Pezaris, J. S., Sahani, M., Mitra, P. P., and Andersen, R. A. (2002). Temporal structure in neuronal activity during working memory in macaque parietal cortex. *Nat Neurosci*, **5**(8), 805–811.

Plassmann, H., O'Doherty, J., and Rangel, A. (2007). Orbitofrontal cortex encodes willingness to pay in everyday economic transactions. *J Neurosci*, **27**(37), 9984–88.

Platt, M. L. and Glimcher, P. W. (1999). Neural correlates of decision variables in parietal cortex. *Nature*, **400**(6741), 233–38.

Platt, M. L. and Huettel, S. A. (2008). Risky business: the neuroeconomics of decision making under uncertainty. *Nat Neurosci*, **11**(4), 398–403.

Poldrack, R. A. (2006). Can cognitive processes be inferred from neuroimaging data? *Trends Cog Sci*, **10**, 59–63.

Procyk, E., Tanaka, Y. L., and Joseph, J. P. (2000). Anterior cingulate activity during routine and non-routine sequential behaviors in macaques. *Nat Neurosci*, **3**(5), 502–508.

Rabin, M. and Thaler, R. H. (2001). Risk aversion. *J Econ Perspect*, **15**(1), 219–32.

Rachlin, H. (2000). *The science of self-control*. Cambridge, MA: Harvard University Press.

Racine, E., Bar-Ilan, O., and Illes, J. (2005). fMRI in the public eye. *Nat Rev Neurosci*, **6**(2), 159–64.

Raichle, M. E. (2006). The brain's dark energy. *Science*, **314**(5803), 1249–50.

Raichle, M. E. and Mintun, M. A. (2006). Brain work and brain imaging. *Annu Rev Neurosci*, **29**, 449–76.

Raichle, M. E., MacLeod, A. M., Snyder, A. Z., Powers, W. J., Gusnard, D. A., and Shulman, G. L. (2001). A default mode of brain function. *Proc Natl Acad Sci USA*, **98**(2), 676–82.

Rauch, A., Rainer, G., and Logothetis, N. K. (2008). The effect of a serotonin-induced dissociation between spiking and perisynaptic activity on BOLD functional MRI. *Proc Natl Acad Sci USA,* **105**(18), 6759–64.

Redgrave, P. and Gurney, K. (2006). The short-latency dopamine signal: a role in discovering novel actions? *Nat Rev Neurosci,* **7**(12), 967–75.

Rees, G., Friston, K., and Koch, C. (2000). A direct quantitative relationship between the functional properties of human and macaque V5. *Nat Neurosci,* **3**(7), 716–23.

Riehle, A., Grun, S., Diesmann, M., and Aertsen, A. (1997). Spike synchronization and rate modulation differentially involved in motor cortical function. *Science,* **278**(5345), 1950–3.

Robson, M. D., Dorosz, J. L., and Gore, J. C. (1998). Measurements of the temporal fMRI response of the human auditory cortex to trains of tones. *Neuroimage,* **7**(3), 185–98.

Roese, N. J. (1997). Counterfactual Thinking. *Psychol Bull,* **121**(1), 133–48.

Roitman, J. D., Brannon, E. M., and Platt, M. L. (2007). Monotonic coding of numerosity in macaque lateral intraparietal area. *PLoS Biol,* **5**(8), e208.

Romo, R., Hernandez, A., Zainos, A., Brody, C. D., and Lemus, L. (2000). Sensing without touching: psychophysical performance based on cortical microstimulation. *Neuron,* **26**(1), 273–78.

Rudebeck, P. H., Walton, M. E., Smyth, A. N., Bannerman, D. M., and Rushworth, M. F. (2006a). Separate neural pathways process different decision costs. *Nat Neurosci,* **9**(9), 1161–68.

Rudebeck, P. H., Buckley, M. J., Walton, M. E., and Rushworth, M. F. (2006b). A role for the macaque anterior cingulate gyrus in social valuation. *Science,* **313**(5791), 1310–12.

Rushworth, M. F. and Behrens, T. E. (2008). Choice, uncertainty and value in prefrontal and cingulate cortex. *Nat Neurosci,* **11**(4), 389–97.

Rushworth, M. F., Kennerley, S. W., and Walton, M. E. (2005). Cognitive neuroscience: resolving conflict in and over the medial frontal cortex. *Curr Biol,* **15**(2), R54–56.

Salzman, C. D. and Newsome, W. T. (1994). Neural mechanisms for forming a perceptual decision. *Science,* **264**(5156), 231–37.

Samejima, K., Ueda, Y., Doya, K., and Kimura, M. (2005). Representation of action-specific reward values in the striatum. *Science,* **310**(5752), 1337–40.

Samuelson, P. A. (1963). Risk and uncertainty: a fallacy of large numbers. *Scientia,* **98**, 108–113.

Samuelson, P. A. (1977). St. Petersburg paradoxes: defanged, dissected, and historically described. *Journal of Economic Literature,* **15**(1), 24–55.

Sanes, J. N. and Donoghue, J. P. (1993). Oscillations in local field potentials of the primate motor cortex during voluntary movement. *Proc Natl Acad Sci USA,* **90**(10), 4470–74.

Schall, J. D., Stuphorn, V., and Brown, J. W. (2002). Monitoring and control of action by the frontal lobes. *Neuron,* **36**(2), 309–22.

Schein, S. J. and Desimone, R. (1990). Spectral properties of V4 neurons in the macaque. *J Neurosci,* **10**(10), 3369–89.

Schmolesky, M. T., Wang, Y., Hanes, D. P., Thompson, K. G., Leutgeb, S., Schall, J. D. et al. (1998). Signal timing across the macaque visual system. *J Neurophysiol,* **79**(6), 3272–78.

Schridde, U., Khubchandani, M., Motelow, J. E., Sanganahalli, B. G., Hyder, F., and Blumenfeld, H. (2008). Negative BOLD with large increases in neuronal activity. *Cereb Cortex,* **18**(8), 1814–27.

Seo, H. and Lee, D. (2007). Temporal filtering of reward signals in the dorsal anterior cingulate cortex during a mixed-strategy game. *J Neurosci,* **27**(31), 8366–77.

Seo, H. and Lee, D. (2009). Behavioral and neural changes after gains and losses of conditioned reinforcers. *J Neurosci,* **29**(11), 3627–41.

Shadlen, M. N. and Newsome, W. T. (1994). Noise, neural codes and cortical organization. *Curr Opin Neurobiol,* **4**(4), 569–79.

Shadlen, M. N. and Newsome, W. T. (1996). Motion perception: seeing and deciding. *Proc Natl Acad Sci USA,* **93**(2), 628–33.

Shannon, C. E. and Weaver, W. (1963). *The mathematical theory of communication.* Urbana and Chicago: University of Illinois Press.

Shepherd, S. V., Klein, J. T., Deaner, R. O., and Platt, M. L. (2009). Mirroring of attention by neurons in macaque parietal cortex. *Proc Natl Acad Sci USA,* **106**(23), 9489–94.

Shidara, M., and Richmond, B. J. (2002). Anterior cingulate: single neuronal signals related to degree of reward expectancy. *Science,* **296**(5573), 1709–1711.

Shmuel, A. and Leopold, D. A. (2008). Neuronal correlates of spontaneous fluctuations in fMRI signals in monkey visual cortex: implications for functional connectivity at rest. *Hum Brain Mapp,* **29**(7), 751–61.

Shmuel, A., Augath, M., Oeltermann, A., and Logothetis, N. K. (2006). Negative functional MRI response correlates with decreases in neuronal activity in monkey visual area V1. *Nat Neurosci,* **9**(4), 569–77.

Silberberg, A., Murray, P., Christensen, J., and Asano, T. (1988). Choice in the repeated-gambles experiment. *J Exp Anal Behav,* **50**(2), 187–95.

Simonson, I. (1990). The effect of purchase quantity and timing on variety seeking behavior. *J Marketing Res,* **32**, 150–62.

Sirotin, Y. B. and Das, A. (2009). Anticipatory haemodynamic signals in sensory cortex not predicted by local neuronal activity. *Nature,* **457**(7228), 475–79.

Smith, A. J., Blumenfeld, H., Behar, K. L., Rothman, D. L., Shulman, R. G., and Hyder, F. (2002). Cerebral energetics and spiking frequency: the neurophysiological basis of fMRI. *Proc Natl Acad Sci USA,* **99**(16), 10765–70.

So, N. and Stuphorn, V. (2010). Supplementary eye field encodes option and action value for Saccades with variable reward, *J Neurophysiol* [E-pub].

Stefanovic, B., Warnking, J. M., and Pike, G. B. (2004). Hemodynamic and metabolic responses to neuronal inhibition. *Neuroimage,* **22**(2), 771–78.

Stephens, D. W. and Anderson, D. (2001). The adaptive value of preference for immediacy: when shortsighted rules have farsighted consequences. *Behav Ecol,* **12**(3), 330–39.

Stephens, D. W. and Krebs, J. R. (1986). *Foraging theory.* Princeton, NJ: Princeton University Press.

Stephens, D. W. and McLinn, C. M. (2003). Choice and context: testing a simple short-term choice rule. *Anim Behav,* **66**(1), 59–70.

Stewart, N., Chater, N., and Brown, G. D. (2006). Decision by sampling. *Cogn Psychol,* **53**(1), 1–26.

Stone, J. (1973). Sampling properties of microelectrodes assessed in the cat's retina. *J Neurophysiol,* **36**(6), 1071–79.

Sugrue, L. P., Corrado, G. S., and Newsome, W. T. (2004). Matching behavior and the representation of value in the parietal cortex. *Science,* **304**(5678), 1782–87.

Sugrue, L. P., Corrado, G. S., and Newsome, W. T. (2005). Choosing the greater of two goods: neural currencies for valuation and decision making. *Nat Rev Neurosci,* **6**(5), 363–75.

Suzuki, W. A., Miller, E. K., and Desimone, R. (1997). Object and place memory in the macaque entorhinal cortex. *J Neurophysiol,* **78**(2), 1062–81.

Thorpe, S., Delorme, A., and Van Rullen, R. (2001). Spike-based strategies for rapid processing. *Neural Networks,* **14**, 715–25.

Tolias, A. S., Smirnakis, S. M., Augath, M. A., Trinath, T., and Logothetis, N. K. (2001). Motion processing in the macaque: revisited with functional magnetic resonance imaging. *J Neurosci,* **21**(21), 8594–8601.

Tom, S. M., Fox, C. R., Trepel, C., and Poldrack, R. A. (2007). The neural basis of loss aversion in decision making under risk. *Science,* **315**(5811), 515–518.

Tong, F., and Engel, S. A. (2001). Interocular rivalry revealed in the human cortical blind-spot representation. *Nature*, **411**(6834), 195–99.

Towe, A. L. and Harding, G. W. (1970). Extracellular microelectrode sampling bias. *Exp Neurol*, **29**(2), 366–81.

Tsao, D. Y., Freiwald, W. A., Tootell, R. B., and Livingstone, M. S. (2006). A cortical region consisting entirely of face-selective cells. *Science*, **311**(5761), 670–4.

Turken, A. U., Vuilleumier, P., Mathalon, D. H., Swick, D., and Ford, J. M. (2003). Are impairments of action monitoring and executive control true dissociative dysfunctions in patients with schizophrenia? *Am J Psychiatry*, **160**(10), 1881–3.

Ursu, S., and Carter, C. S. (2005). Outcome representations, counterfactual comparisons and the human orbitofrontal cortex: implications for neuroimaging studies of decision making. *Brain Res Cogn Brain Res*, **23**(1), 51–60.

Van Rullen, R. and Thorpe, S. J. (2002). Surfing a spike wave down the ventral stream. *Vision Res*, **42**(23), 2593–2615.

Van Rullen, R., Gautrais, J., Delorme, A., and Thorpe, S. (1998). Face processing using one spike per neurone. *Biosystems*, **48**(1-3), 229–39.

van Veen, V., Cohen, J. D., Botvinick, M. M., Stenger, V. A., and Carter, C. S. (2001). Anterior cingulate cortex, conflict monitoring, and levels of processing. *Neuroimage*, **14**(6), 1302–8.

Vincent, J. L., Snyder, A. Z., Fox, M. D., Shannon, B. J., Andrews, J. R., Raichle, M. E. et al. (2006). Coherent spontaneous activity identifies a hippocampal-parietal memory network. *J Neurophysiol*, **96**(6), 3517–31.

Vincent, J. L., Patel, G. H., Fox, M. D., Snyder, A. Z., Baker, J. T., Van Essen, D. C. et al. (2007). Intrinsic functional architecture in the anaesthetized monkey brain. *Nature*, **447**(7140), 83–U84.

Viswanathan, A. and Freeman, R. D. (2007). Neurometabolic coupling in cerebral cortex reflects synaptic more than spiking activity. *Nat Neurosci*, **10**(10), 1308–12.

Vogt, B. A. and Gabriel, M. (1993). *Neurobiology of cingulate cortex and limbic thalamus*. Boston: Birkhauser.

Vogt, B. A., Finch, D. M., and Olson, C. R. (1992). Functional heterogeneity in cingulate cortex: the anterior executive and posterior evaluative regions. *Cereb Cortex*, **2**(6), 435–43.

Von Neumann, J. V. and Morgenstern, O. (1944). *Theory of games and economic behavior*. Princeton, NJ: Princeton University Press.

von Stein, A., Chiang, C., and Konig, P. (2000). Top-down processing mediated by interareal synchronization. *Proc Natl Acad Sci USA*, **97**(26), 14748–53.

Waldvogel, D., van Gelderen, P., Muellbacher, W., Ziemann, U., Immisch, I., and Hallett, M. (2000). The relative metabolic demand of inhibition and excitation. *Nature*, **406**(6799), 995–8.

Wandell, B. A. (1999). Computational neuroimaging of human visual cortex. *Annu Rev Neurosci*, **22**, 145–73.

Weber, B. J. and Huettel, S. A. (2008). The neural substrates of probabilistic and intertemporal decision making. *Brain Res*, **1234**, 104–115.

Wedell, D. H. and Boeckenholt, U. (1994). Contemplating single vs multiple encounters of a risky prospect. *Am J Psychol*, **107**(4), 499–518.

Wirth, S., Avsar, E., Chiu, C. C., Sharma, V., Smith, A. C., Brown, E. et al. (2009). Trial outcome and associative learning signals in the monkey hippocampus. *Neuron*, **61**(6), 930–40.

Wirth, S., Yanike, M., Frank, L. M., Smith, A. C., Brown, E. N., and Suzuki, W. A. (2003). Single neurons in the monkey hippocampus and learning of new associations. *Science*, **300**(5625), 1578–81.

Yoshor, D., Ghose, G. M., Bosking, W. H., Sun, P., and Maunsell, J. H. (2007). Spatial attention does not strongly modulate neuronal responses in early human visual cortex. *J Neurosci*, **27**(48), 13205–13209.

Yu, A. J., and Dayan, P. (2005). Uncertainty, neuromodulation, and attention. *Neuron*, **46**(4), 681–92.

Chapter 7

Neuroeconomics of risky decisions: from variables to strategies

Vinod Venkatraman, John W. Payne, and Scott A. Huettel

Abstract

We make a variety of decisions throughout our lives. Some decisions involve outcomes whose values can be readily compared, especially when those outcomes are simple, immediate, and familiar. Other decisions involve imperfect knowledge about their potential consequences: Should I accept the job offer I have now or wait for a possible better offer in the future? Should I put my retirement money into volatile stocks or into predictable money market funds? Understanding the choice process when consequences are uncertain—often called the study of decision making under risk—remains a key goal of behavioral economics, cognitive psychology, and now neuroscience. An ongoing challenge, however, lies in the substantial individual differences in how people approach risky decisions. Using a novel choice paradigm, we demonstrate that people vary in whether they adopt compensatory rules (i.e., tradeoffs between decision variables) or non-compensatory rules (i.e., a simplification of the choice problem) in economic decision making. Then, using functional magnetic resonance imaging (fMRI), we show that distinct neural mechanisms support variability in choices and variability in strategic preferences. Specifically, compensatory choices were associated with activation in anterior insula and ventromedial prefrontal cortex, while non-compensatory choices were associated with increased activation in dorsolateral prefrontal cortex and posterior parietal cortex. The dorsomedial prefrontal cortex shaped decision making at a strategic level, through its functional connectivity with these regions. We argue for the importance of individual-difference analyses as a key direction through which neuroscience can influence models of choice behavior.

The science of decision making has a remarkably rich history that reaches from the early insights of Pascal and Bernoulli (Bernoulli, 1738), through axiomatic formalizations of rational choice under risk by von Neumann and Morgenstern (von Neumann and Morgenstern, 1944) and Savage (Savage, 1954), to recent explorations of seemingly "irrational" biases in choice by Kahneman, Tversky, and many others (Kahneman and Tversky, 1979; Loewenstein, Weber, Hsee, and Welch, 2001; Slovic and Lichtenstein, 1968; Tversky and Kahneman, 1974, 1981). Throughout most of this history, there has been a focus on abstracting the risky decision problem into small sets of decision variables that combine into simple compensatory functions. The decision variables of most historical interest have included aspects of option value (e.g., magnitude, valence), the probability of option delivery (e.g., risk, ambiguity), and the delay until outcomes are resolved (e.g., immediate vs. distal rewards). In the late-twentieth century, contextual factors, such as the regret one experiences when another option would have had a better outcome than the one chosen (Zeelenberg, 1999; Zeelenberg and Pieters, 2004) or whether the outcomes of a gamble are framed as gains or losses (Tversky and Kahneman, 1981), rose to the fore in response to robust violations of existing models of choice. Traditionally, decision scientists posit that the observed choice reflects tradeoffs between two or more of these variables (Slovic and Lichtenstein, 1968; Tversky and Fox, 1995; Tversky and Kahneman, 1992). Further, it has often been assumed that every individual can be represented by the same compensatory model, with individual differences in choice reflecting differences in model parameters (Birnbaum, 2008). Yet, there exists broad evidence that people adaptively draw upon multiple models for choice, some compensatory and some non-compensatory, depending on context, individual preferences and task structure (Gigerenzer and Goldstein, 1996; Payne et al., 1988, 1992).

7.1 Neural correlates of decision variables

Studies using the techniques of neuroscience to understand decision making—often described as the emerging discipline of neuroeconomics (Glimcher and Rustichini, 2004)—have heretofore adopted a similar focus on identifying decision variables within a general compensatory model framework. In particular, the vast majority of neuroeconomic studies target a particular decision variable (e.g., temporal delay), incorporate that variable into a model function (e.g., hyperbolic discounting), manipulate the level of that variable across a range of stimuli (e.g., monetary gambles), and then identify aspects of brain function that track changes in that variable (Platt and Huettel, 2008). Using this approach, researchers have identified potential neural underpinnings of nearly all of the core variables present in standard descriptive economic models, including value of monetary rewards (Knutson et al., 2003; Yacubian et al., 2007) and other rewards (Aharon et al., 2001; Berns et al., 2001), risk (Huettel, 2006; Preuschoff et al., 2006), ambiguity (Hsu et al., 2005; Huettel et al., 2006), probability weighting (Berns et al., 2008; Hsu et al., 2009), and temporal delay (Kable and Glimcher, 2007; McClure et al., 2004). Moreover, recent studies have identified effects of complex variables implied by particular frameworks for decision making, such as framing strength (De Martino et al., 2006), regret

(Camille et al., 2004; Coricelli et al., 2005) and other fictive signals (Chiu et al., 2008; Hayden et al., 2009; Lohrenz et al., 2007), and even unexpected changes in risk over time (Preuschoff et al., 2008).

The focus of neuroeconomics on decision variables plays into the strengths of neuroscience methods. Functional magnetic resonance imaging (fMRI), in particular, provides robust information about metabolic changes that pervade a particular brain region for a period of several seconds (Logothetis, 2008; Logothetis et al., 2001). To the degree that a decision variable influences computations within a region, and thus alters local metabolism, fMRI can be very useful for mapping its neural correlates. Conversely, by assuming that choice reflects the interactions of particular variables within a well-defined function, neuroscience researchers can ignore other complexities of the decision environment, from variability in how a given individual approaches choices over time, to potential differences among individuals in their choice behavior. Excluding these latter factors simplifies analyses, ameliorating the weakness of neuroscience methods in dealing with complex sets of predictors that could combine in an unexpected manner.

Yet, despite many real advances, an emphasis on compensatory interactions between variables has some clear limitations. For example, it leads to the intuitive, but often misleading, interpretation that brain systems interact competitively to generate choices. Most common is the canonical rational-affective distinction, also referred to as "Hot vs. Cold" or "System 1 vs. System 2" (Bernheim and Rangel, 2004; Greene et al., 2001; Kahneman, 2003; McClure et al., 2004; Sanfey et al., 2003). And, even when other models have been proposed (Kable and Glimcher, 2007), they still assume that individual differences reflect the relative strength of a parameter within a decision function. To the extent that individuals' choices reflect fundamentally different valuation or comparison functions—not merely differences in parameter values—then the underlying mechanisms would be invisible to standard neuroeconomic analyses. In short, a focus on tradeoffs between decision variables risks missing the very ways people represent and process decision problems, or their decision *strategies*.[1]

In the following sections, we describe strategies used by many individuals to solve complex risky decision problems, show how those strategies relate to the predictions of canonical decision models (i.e., those common in neuroeconomic research),[2] and outline an approach to elucidating individual differences in use of those strategies using neuroscience. We are hopeful that understanding *variability* in strategic preferences will

---

[1] We note that the term "strategy" has different meanings in different contexts. Within game theory it refers to a particular choice option available to one player (Camerer, 2003a), whereas within cognitive psychology it refers to the manner in which people seek out and use information in the pursuit of some goal (Cope and Murphy, 1981). We adopt this term based on the latter connotation, but we note that similar concepts are implied by terms like "decision modes" or "heuristics."

[2] Cumulative prospect theory is the most frequently cited model for decision making under risk. However, it is important to note that even in the original description of that model (Tversky and Kahneman, 1992), its authors clearly acknowledge that multiple decision strategies contribute to risky choices—"when faced with a complex problem, people employ a variety of heuristic procedures in order to simplify the representation and the evaluation of prospects" (p. 317).

facilitate construction of models that are both parsimonious and biologically plausible (Clithero et al., 2008; Glimcher and Rustichini, 2004), the cardinal goals of neuroeconomics.

7.2 Strategic influences on choice: the probability-maximizing heuristic

Most studies of risky choice behavior have used very simple gambles for reasons of experimental control and simplicity. Typical decision scenarios juxtapose two gambles of the form ($x, p; 0, 1–p) where one receives $x with probability p or $0 with probability 1–p. The utility of such a simple gamble is modeled, for obvious reasons, using a function that combines the probability and utility of each outcome and sums the weighted outcome values over all the possible outcomes. Such models suffice even when using mixed gambles, typically one non-zero gain and one non-zero loss outcome ($x>0, p; $y<0, 1–p). Yet, as argued by Lopes among others, more complex gambles with multiple gain and loss outcomes are needed to simulate real-world choice scenarios (Lopes, 1995; Lopes and Oden, 1999). Most notably, complex mixed gambles with more than two outcomes allow researchers to identify simplifying strategies (heuristics) that may guide more complex risky choice behavior.

One potentially valuable, and computationally tractable, strategy for simplifying a complex gamble is to make decisions based on the overall probability of winning. This strategy was explored by Payne, who created a novel incentive-compatible decision-making task in which subjects added money to (i.e., improved) specific options within complex gambles (Payne, 2005). In this task, subjects viewed a five-outcome gamble $G = (x_1, p_1; x_2, p_2; x_3, p_3; x_4, p_4; x_5, p_5)$, where p_i indicates the probability of monetary outcome x_i. The outcomes are rank-ordered $x_1>x_2>x_3>x_4>x_5$, where at least two outcomes are strict gains ($x_1>x_2>\$0$) and two are strict losses ($x_5<x_4<\$0$). The value of the middle, referent outcome (x_3) varies across trials, but is typically $0 or slightly negative (Fig. 7.1A).

Subjects then chose between different ways of improving this gamble (Fig. 7.1B). Adding money to the extreme positive outcome, x_1, would be a *gain-maximizing* (G_{max}) choice, whereas adding money to the extreme negative outcome, x_5, would be a *loss-minimizing* (L_{min}) choice. As discussed more extensively below, the gambles were constructed so that these two sorts of choices have the greatest effect on the overall subjective value of the gamble, as calculated using well-known descriptive models of choice like cumulative prospect theory along with standard parameter values (Tversky and Kahneman, 1992). Thus, we hereafter describe them collectively as *value-maximizing* choices. Conversely, adding money to the middle outcome, x3, increases the overall probability of winning or decreases the overall probability of losing. We refer to such choices as *probability-maximizing* (P_{max}). Note that in the terminology of Payne (2005), the bias toward options that minimize the probability of losing compared to winning, was called the "Probability-of-Winning Heuristic."

Responses from more than 500 subjects demonstrated that choices in this task systematically violated the predictions of models like expected utility theory (EU) and

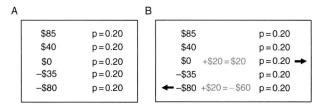

Fig. 7.1 Experimental stimuli and paradigm. (A) Subjects initially viewed a multi-attribute mixed gamble consisting of five different outcomes, each associated with a probability of occurrence. The outcomes were rank-ordered and typically consisted of two gains, two losses and a central reference outcome. (B) Subjects had to choose between two options for improving the gamble, highlighted in red. Here, the addition of $20 to the central, reference outcome would maximize the overall probability of winning (P_{max} choice), whereas the addition of $20 to the extreme loss would reflect a loss-minimizing (L_{min}) choice. In other trials, subjects could have a chance to add money to the extreme gain outcome ($85), reflecting a gain-maximizing (G_{max}) choice. For the fMRI experiment, subjects had 6 s to make their choice after which two arrows identified the buttons corresponding to the two options. Subjects indicated their choice by pressing the corresponding button as soon as possible.

cumulative prospect theory (CPT), such that subjects sacrificed considerable expected value in favor of maximizing the overall probability of winning compared to losing (Payne, 2005). Most subjects (over two-thirds) preferred to add money to the central reference outcome (x_3) that improved the overall probability of winning (or not losing) for the gamble. These results provided strong evidence that many, but not all, individuals incorporate information about the overall probabilities of positive and negative outcomes into their decision making, consistent with both older (Lopes and Oden, 1999) and recent frameworks that include aspiration levels in utility calculations (Diecidue and van de Ven, 2008). Coding an outcome or attribute as good or bad relative to an aspiration level has often been seen as one important form of cognitive simplification. Simon uses such an aspiration level concept in the "satisficing" strategy for decision making (Simon, 1957). That is, a satisficing person is hypothesized to select the first option that meets minimum aspiration levels on all the relevant attributes. Alba and Marmorstein suggest that people may choose alternatives based simply upon the counts of the good or bad features that the alternatives possess (Alba and Marmorstein, 1987). Similarly, the probability-maximizing choices in our task improve the overall probability of winning relative to a neutral aspiration level.

7.3 **Individual differences in the probability-maximizing strategy**

In follow-up experiments, hereafter drawn from Venkatraman and colleagues (Venkatraman et al., 2009), we modified the above decision-making paradigm to explore, in greater detail, individual differences in the bias toward maximizing the probability of winning compared to losing (i.e., a probability-maximizing strategy). To match the procedure of Payne (2005), subjects (N = 71) chose among two of the above ways to improve five-outcome mixed gambles, but those gambles were not resolved and subject compensation was unrelated to their decisions. Across a set of conditions, we modified the payoff structure of the gambles in ways theorized to bias subjects toward or against use of a probability-maximizing strategy (Fig. 7.2A).

A first test was designed to replicate the basic phenomenon from Payne (2005), while also demonstrating that subjects' choices are still sensitive to expected value. When subjects chose between gain-maximizing and probability-maximizing choices, each associated with similar improvements in the expected value of the gamble, they selected the probability-maximizing option approximately two-thirds of the time (Fig. 7.2B). (Similar effects were observed when subjects chose between loss-minimizing and probability-maximizing options.) But, when the probability-maximizing choice was associated with reduced expected value (i.e., if only $10 could be added to the middle option, compared to $15 to the extreme), the bias toward probability maximizing was reduced but still present (58% of all choices). This bias towards probability-maximizing choices is

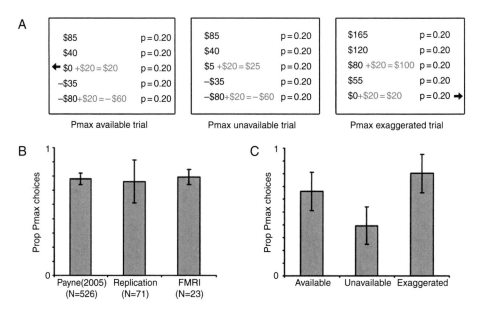

Fig. 7.2 Subjects prefer choices that increase the overall probability of winning. (A) In a behavioral experiment (N = 71), we manipulated the gamble attributes across multiple conditions. In the P_{max}-unavailable trials, none of the options would result in a change in the overall probability of winning. In the P_{max}-exaggerated trial, the gambles were modulated such that the P_{max} choice now reflects moving from an uncertain gain to a certain gain gamble. (B) Subjects show a significant bias towards P_{max} choices across three independent experiments. (C) More importantly, the preference for the P_{max} choices can be reversed or accentuated by experimental manipulations. When none of the options changed the overall probability, subjects now preferred value-maximizing choices. Similarly, when provided with an option to eliminate the possibility of losing, P_{max} choices (indicated with arrows) increased dramatically. Note that the P_{max}-unavailable condition did not have any choice that changed the overall probability, and the value in the plot represents the proportion of choices of the central outcome in these gambles.

consistent with a recent dual-criterion model for risky choice (Diecidue and van de Ven, 2008), in which an overall probability criterion can be traded off against other decision variables. Moreover, subjects were significantly faster for probability-maximizing choices compared to either sort of value-maximizing choice, consistent with a less effortful strategy (Shah and Oppenheimer, 2008). Finally, and most critically, we found that there was tremendous variability in subjects' relative preference for different strategies, such that some subjects nearly exclusively adopted a probability-maximizing strategy, while others nearly exclusively adopted a value-maximizing strategy.

A second condition included decision problems identical in format to those from Payne (2005), save for one small change: the middle option (x_3) was subtly modified such that the subject's decision could not change its valence (e.g., on some trials, it started at $5, so adding money might increase it to $20). Note that this change is miniscule compared to the gamble's overall range, which was typically greater than $150. Under these task conditions, subjects now only chose the middle option on 39% of trials (Fig. 7.2C), a highly significant decrease from the first condition. These results confirm that many subjects who do preferentially adopt a probability-maximizing strategy when such choices are available in the decision problem, will readily switch to a value-maximizing strategy otherwise.

Our third condition included problems that would exaggerate the probability-maximizing strategy. Based on earlier behavioral studies (Payne et al., 1980, 1981), we hypothesized that people will be particularly attracted to changes in overall probabilities that involve moving from an uncertain gain to a certain gain or from a certain loss to an uncertain loss. We selected gambles used in the first condition above, and then translated all values by adding the magnitude of the largest loss (i.e., the worst outcome became $0) or subtracting the magnitude of the largest gain (i.e., the best outcome became $0). When faced with such gambles, subjects indeed showed a significantly increased tendency to choose the option that altered the overall probability of winning (e.g., 82% for gambles that improved the overall probability of winning from 0.8 to 1; Fig. 7.2C). Thus, the use of the overall probability of winning strategy (heuristic) has been shown to be used by many (but not all) subjects, and to be sensitive in its use to the specific task factors.

To identify potential individual trait correlates of this strategic variability, we collected psychometric data that included tendency toward satisficing (Schwartz et al., 2002) and emotional sadness (Fordyce, 1988). Across our subject sample, increased maximizing trait responses predicted a decreased bias toward probability-maximizing choices. In other words, satisficers preferred the probability-maximizing choices more than maximizers, consistent with these choices representing a simplifying strategy. Similarly, an increase in the sadness trait measure also predicted a decreased bias towards probability maximizing. Sadness has also been typically associated with reduced certainty, increased elaboration, and reduced heuristic processing (Bodenhausen et al., 1994; Schwarz et al., 1991).

In summary, we show a consistent strong bias towards probability-maximizing choices. Within subjects, we demonstrate that this bias is indeed related to the overall probability of winning and that it can be attenuated or exaggerated by subtle manipulations in decision context. Across subjects, we show that differences in decision strategies can be explained by individual variability in trait measures like satisficing. Taken together, these strategy-trait relationships suggest that the robust individual differences in these risky choice paradigms (and, presumably, other settings) may reflect measurable cognitive or affective differences across individuals. We return to this idea further in our discussion of the fMRI experiment below.

7.4 Evaluations of consistency with economic models

Given the overall bias towards the probability-maximizing strategy in the previous experiments, we next sought to explicitly evaluate whether choices associated with this response strategy were consistent with traditional economic models such as expected utility (EU) maximization and cumulative prospect theory (CPT). For this test, we used behavior from 72 trials of the task described above, collected during an fMRI study with 23 subjects (neural data will be discussed in a subsequent section). The fMRI experiment used an incentive-compatible payment method, such that subjects were provided an initial unknown but fixed endowment and were later paid for a subset of their improved gambles, selected randomly. (See Venkatraman et al., 2009, for complete experimental details.)

Our model comparisons used both standard and free parameters for the EU and CPT models. Note that we did not include original prospect theory (OPT), since it was meant for simple two-outcome gambles. All gambles used in this study were of the form $G = \{x_1,p_1; x_2,p_2; x_3,p_3; x_4,p_4; x_5,p_5\}$. The expected utility (EU) of each gamble is given by:

$$EU = \sum_{i=1}^{5} u(x_i)p_i, \quad \text{where } u(x_i) = \begin{cases} x_i^{\beta}, & x_i \geq 0 \\ -|x_i|^{1+(1-\beta)}, & x_i < 0 \end{cases}.$$

The cumulative prospect theory (CPT) predictions were obtained using:

$$CPT = \sum_{i=1}^{5} v(x_i)c(i) \quad \text{where } v(x_i) = \begin{cases} x_i^{\beta}, & x_i \geq 0 \\ -\lambda|x_i|^{\beta}, & x_i < 0 \end{cases},$$

$$c(i) = \begin{cases} w^+(p_i), & i=1 \\ w^+\left(\sum_{j=1}^{i} p_j\right) - w^+\left(\sum_{j=1}^{i-1} p_j\right), & i=2,..,k \ (gains) \\ w^-\left(\sum_{j=i}^{5} p_j\right) - w^-\left(\sum_{j=i+1}^{5} p_j\right), & i=k+1,..,4 \ (losses) \\ w^-(p_i), & i=5 \end{cases},$$

$$w^+(p) = \frac{p^{\gamma^+}}{[p^{\gamma^+} + (1-p)^{\gamma^+}]^{1/\gamma^+}} \quad \text{and} \quad w^-(p) = \frac{p^{\gamma^-}}{[p^{\gamma^-} + (1-p)^{\gamma^-}]^{1/\gamma^-}}.$$

For the first level of model comparisons, we determined the model predictions for each of 72 trials in which expected value was approximately matched between possible choices. We first tested models using parameters drawn from the prior literature. Our EU model used a concave utility function with $\beta = 0.88$. For the CPT model, we used parameter values of $\gamma^+ = 0.61$, $\gamma^- = 0.69$ and $\lambda = 2.25$ (Tversky and Kahneman, 1992; Tversky and Wakker, 1995). Despite these standard parameters, neither model was a good predictor of subjects' aggregate choices. As one example, consider a trial on which a subject chooses whether to add a fixed amount of money either to a large negative outcome (e.g., –$75) or to a middle outcome of $0, each of which is equally likely to occur. Both EU and CPT models predict that subjects should always add the money to the large negative outcome (i.e., minimizing the worst loss). However, subjects showed an opposite effect, adding money to the middle outcome 68% of the time (i.e., typically making a probability-maximizing choice). This and other observations indicated that subjects' behavior in these experiments was inconsistent with standard model predictions.

To account for potential individual differences in model parameter values, we performed a robustness check using a split-sample analysis. We used one half of the choices of each subject to estimate model parameters: for EU, β; and for CPT, β and γ, keeping λ fixed at 2.25. We also simplified the equation for CPT in our estimation by assuming $\gamma^+ = \gamma^-$. We then assessed the performance of the EU and CPT models by estimating the reliability of the fitted model in predicting the other half of that subject's data. We found that parameters estimated from one half of the sample showed poor reliability in predicting choices in the complementary sample (EU: Cronbach $\alpha = 0.37$; CPT: $\alpha = 0.39$). However, the proportion of probability-maximizing choices was much more reliable across the two samples ($\alpha = 0.78$), indicating that subjects remained highly consistent in their strategy preference across the experiment.

We stress that these results should not be interpreted to imply that the probability-maximizing strategy provides a new, better, and general model of risky choice behavior. On the contrary, this particular simplifying strategy only applies to a subset of decision problems—those that involve comparisons between similar gambles that differ in their overall probability of winning—and cannot be used for choice problems that involve only gains or only losses, or that involve constant probability of winning. In such cases, people may use other heuristic strategies such as the priority heuristic advocated by Gigerenzer and colleagues (Brandstätter et al., 2006) that focuses more on the outcomes of the gambles. We do suggest that, under certain contexts, most individuals adopt heuristic decision strategies not encapsulated in standard models (but see Birnbaum, 2008). Clarifying the neural mechanisms that support such strategies will be the focus of the remainder of this chapter.

7.5 Neural substrates for the strategic control of behavior

Prior research in cognitive neuroscience provides candidate brain regions that may contribute to sorts of the computations necessary for strategic control. As a broad beginning, nearly all models of neural control posit an important role for regions within the prefrontal cortex (Miller and Cohen, 2001), which in turn is argued to shape processing in other cortical and subcortical brain regions. Substantial evidence in support of this perspective comes from studies of patients with lesions to prefrontal cortex, who exhibit impairments in changing behavior based on current task context (Bechara et al., 2000). Importantly, this inflexibility is not always economically irrational or even maladaptive. For example, Shiv and colleagues demonstrated that patients with PFC damage did better than individuals with intact prefrontal cortex on a gambling game; examination of the specific pattern of choices revealed that the patients were less likely to shift away from high expected-value but risky options following negative feedback (Shiv et al., 2005). That is, the patients exhibited less of a risk-aversion bias than neurologically normal individuals. Note that patients with similar damage would show considerably worse performance than control individuals in decision scenarios where increased risk is associated with reduced expected value.

Moreover, new conceptions of prefrontal function have argued that specific subregions of PFC may be critical for contextual control. A commonly held framework, one advanced in different guises by different theorists, suggests that lateral prefrontal cortex contains a topographic organization along its posterior to anterior axis (Koechlin et al., 2000; Koechlin et al., 2003). More posterior regions, those immediately adjacent to premotor cortex, are associated with setting up general rules for behavior. Conversely, more anterior regions support the instantiation of rules for behavior based on the current context. Findings from functional neuroimaging studies argue for further divisions within anterior prefrontal cortex, such that regions around the frontal pole support relational integration, or the combination of disparate information into a single judgment (Christoff et al., 2001). An open, but critical, question is how the computational capacities of these distinct regions differentially contribute to decisions under different contexts.

In recent years, there has been substantial interest in the dorsomedial prefrontal cortex (dmPFC)—also called the anterior cingulate cortex (ACC)—as playing a key role in assessing and/or shaping behavior based on context (Hadland et al., 2003; Kennerley et al., 2006; Rushworth et al., 2004). Several independently arising lines of evidence have contributed to the interest in dmPFC. First, electrophysiological studies, in both human and non-human primates, have identified neuronal signatures of a very rapid response to events that signal a change in the current task demands (Nieuwenhuis et al., 2004). These have included, but are not limited to, external feedback about errors (Holroyd and Coles, 2002; Miltner et al., 1997; Ruchsow et al., 2002), self-recognition that an action was likely to be an error (Gehring and Fencsik, 2001), and even the quality of monetary outcomes (Gehring and Willoughby, 2002). For example, a recent study from our group found that the scalp-recorded ERP signal over fronto-central cortex to a monetary outcome, as obtained in a probabilistic guessing task, depended on the valence and magnitude of that outcome, as well as the history of outcomes over preceding trials (Goyer et al., 2008).

Second, a large corpus of functional neuroimaging research has shown that dmPFC activation is evoked by task contexts that involve conflict, particularly between competing response tendencies. Many such studies have used variants of the Stroop paradigm

(MacLeod, 1992), which requires individuals to inhibit a fast, prepotent response (e.g., color word reading) and instead engage in a slower, less common process (e.g., naming an ink color). Under such task conditions, a very large number of studies have reported activation in dmPFC (Bush et al., 1998; Derrfuss et al., 2005), as reviewed by Bush and colleagues (Bush et al., 2000). (Note, however, that a simple contrast of response conflict versus non-conflict conditions also evokes activation in many other regions, reflecting that other processes are brought online, as well.) Subsequent work has greatly refined the description of this dmPFC activation, such that current theories of dmPFC function emphasize its role in coordinating activation in other regions (Beckmann et al., 2009; Cohen et al., 2005; Meriau et al., 2006). For example, a seminal study by Kerns and colleagues demonstrated that the magnitude of activation change in dmPFC on one trial predicted the subsequent change in lateral PFC activation on the next trial, suggesting that dmPFC may engage executive control regions based on task demands (Kerns et al., 2004).

Third, recent work has implicated dmPFC in the detection of environmental volatility, or the degree to which the current task context is static or variable over time. In an elegant set of studies, Rushworth and colleagues have shown that volatility in the mappings of responses to outcomes is associated with increased dmPFC activity, even when controlling for variability in responses, outcomes, learning rates, and other factors (Behrens et al., 2007). Moreover, these authors have suggested the possibility of a spatial topography within dmPFC such that distinct subregions support volatility associated with social and non-social contexts, and that those subregions have distinct functional connectivity to regions in ventral PFC (Rudebeck et al., 2008; Rushworth et al., 2007). Collectively, these studies point to dmPFC as a likely candidate for implementing the strategic control of behavior.

7.6 Functional neuroimaging of strategic control

Our fMRI experiment sought to dissociate the neural mechanisms that underlie choices from those that shape strategic preferences in risky decision making (Venkatraman et al., 2009). Subjects completed a series of choices using the basic paradigm described in the previous experiments. In each trial, subjects chose between a probability-maximizing simplifying option and a value-maximizing compensatory option (which could be gain-maximizing in some trials and loss-minimizing in others). Subjects made these choices without feedback, so that their decisions would not be shaped by outcome learning. We characterized our subjects' strategic preferences according to their relative proportion of simplifying (P_{max}) versus compensatory (G_{max} or L_{min}) choices. Such a definition creates a continuum with a high value indicating an individual who prefers a simplifying strategy and a low value indicating an individual who prefers a compensatory strategy. Like in the previous experiments, there was substantial variability across individuals in their strategic preferences.

Our first analyses identified regions whose activation during the decision phase of the task, but before responses were indicated, predicted the type of choice made on a given trial (Fig. 7.3). Somewhat counterintuitively, increased activation in nominally emotional

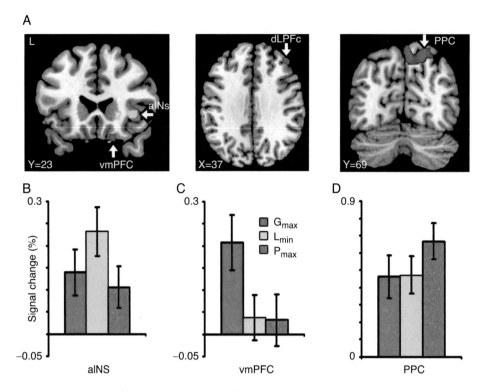

Fig. 7.3 Distinct sets of brain regions predict choices. (A) Increased activation in the right anterior insula (peak MNI space coordinates: x = 38, y = 28, z = 0) and in the ventromedial prefrontal cortex (x = 16, y = 21, z = −23) predicted L_{min} and G_{max} choices, respectively, while increased activation in the lateral prefrontal cortex (x = 44, y = 44, z = 27) and posterior parietal cortex (x = 20, y = −76, z = 57) predicted P_{max} choices. Activation maps show active clusters that surpassed a threshold of z>2.3 with cluster-based Gaussian random field correction. (B–D) Percent signal change in these three regions to each type of choice. On this and subsequent figures, error bars represent ±1 standard error of the mean for each column.

regions predicted that a subject would make choices consistent with economic models: activation in anterior insula (aINS) predicted loss-minimizing choices, whereas activation in vmPFC predicted gain-maximizing choices. Conversely, activation in the nominally cognitive regions of dorsolateral prefrontal cortex (dlPFC) and posterior parietal cortex (PPC) predicted probability-maximizing choices (i.e., simplifying). These results are inconsistent with the canonical neural dual-systems model for decision making, namely that economic rationality results from the activation of cognitive brain systems and that the opposing activation of emotional brain systems drives people toward simplifying and heuristic choices. Instead, these data support an interpretation in terms of the specific consequences of choices in this task: anterior insula activation reflects aversion to potential negative consequences (Kuhnen and Knutson, 2005), whereas vmPFC activation reflects the magnitude of the greatest gain (Bechara et al., 2000). We emphasize, based on these results and those highlighted in the previous section, that economic

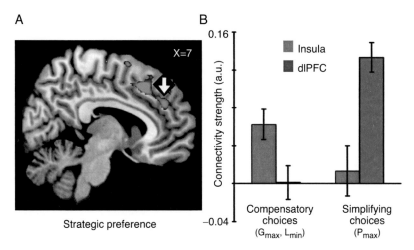

Fig. 7.4 Dorsomedial prefrontal cortex predicts strategy use during decision making. (A) Activation in dorsomedial prefrontal cortex (dmPFC, x = 10, y = 22, z = 45; indicated with arrow) tracked strategic preferences, such that the difference in activation between probability-maximizing (i.e., simplifying) and value-maximizing (i.e., compensatory) choices was significantly correlated with variability in strategic preference across individuals. (B) Additionally, we also found that this region exhibited differential functional connectivity with choice-related regions: there was increased connectivity with dlPFC (and PPC) for probability-maximizing choices and increased connectivity with aINS (and amygdala) for value-maximizing choices.

rationality reflects an idealized model of behavior, not the output of a specific brain region. Regions within prefrontal cortex, for example, may shape behavior in a manner consistent with—or contrary to—a particular economic model, depending on task and context.

Furthermore, activation in a third region, dorsomedial PFC (dmPFC), predicted strategic preferences across subjects (Fig. 7.4A). Specifically, activation in this region increased when subjects made choices that were inconsistent with their preferred strategy (i.e., greater activation when people with a preference for probability-maximizing choices made value-maximizing choices, and vice versa). (Note that activation was minimal, regardless of choice, in those individuals who found the two strategies similarly preferable, consistent with a strategy-conflict explanation but inconsistent with a response-conflict explanation.) We also found differential functional connectivity of this region to dlPFC and anterior insula (Fig. 7.4B), two regions that predicted different types of choices. These findings support the interpretation that control signals from dmPFC modulate the activation of choice-related brain regions, with the strength and directionality of this influence dependent on an individual's preferred strategy.

Finally, we found that individual differences in strategic preferences were also correlated with neural sensitivity to reward outcomes. At the end of the experiment, we resolved a subset of the gambles for real rewards, during which we measured the neural response to anticipation of reward, to gain outcomes, and to loss outcomes. Across subjects, a neurometric measure of reward sensitivity, namely the difference between responses to

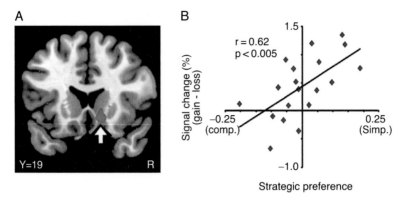

Fig. 7.5 Ventral striatal sensitivity to rewards predicts strategic bias. At the end of the experiment, some gambles were resolved to monetary gains or losses. (A) Activation in the ventral striatum (x = 14, y = 16, z = −10) increased to realized gains but decreased to realized losses. (B) Notably, the difference in activation to gains and losses in this region correlated with variability in strategic preferences across subjects, with subjects who were most likely to prefer the probability-maximizing strategy exhibiting the greatest neural sensitivity to rewards.

gain outcomes and loss outcomes in the ventral striatum, was positively correlated with bias toward a probability-maximizing strategy (Fig. 7.5). Finally, we also found that the neurometric measure of differential reward sensitivity to gain versus loss outcomes in the ventral striatum was negatively correlated with the trait measure of maximizing (r = −0.69), indicating that satisficers were more sensitive than maximizers to the reward consequences of their decisions. While these results by itself provides no information about the direction of causation, we can speculate that increased neural sensitivity to reward outcomes may underlie preferences for decision strategies that seek to maximize the probabilities of winning over losing.

7.7 Implications for future research

Neuroeconomic research will, for the foreseeable future, continue to be focused on identifying neural mechanisms that underlie decision variables and the operators that process those variables. We do not disagree with this focus—simply put, many factors that contribute to even simple decisions deserve elucidation. However, we predict that identifying the factors that shape how people differentially represent decision problems, both across contexts and across individuals, will become an increasingly critical topic.

An increased focus on strategic variability would have several salutary consequences. First, it would provide an avenue by which neuroscience data could be extended to modeling in economics (and other social sciences). A common criticism of neuroeconomics, at least among economic theorists, is that neuroscience data is simply irrelevant for core models in economics. Where such theories cannot be derived from first principles, it is argued, they can be identified based on expressed behavior without recourse to internal neural mechanisms. This criticism, which we have labeled the "behavioral sufficiency" argument, can be countered on several grounds (Clithero et al., 2008). Most relevant for the current topic, economic models of behavior are disconnected from the substantial psychological and neuroscientific literature on individual differences. Because of this disconnect, a model may well describe behavior of young adults making decisions in a relaxed setting, but nevertheless have little predictive validity when applied to older adults making decisions under time pressure. To the extent that neuroscience can illuminate the mechanisms underlying individual choice biases and strategic preferences, it may become critical for creating robust and flexible models of real-world decision behavior.

Second, there will be substantial value in moving descriptions of decision mechanisms—within neuroeconomics, cognitive psychology, behavioral economics, and even the lay public—away from the oft-claimed interaction between competing decision systems. Clearly, based on the many studies cited at the outset of this chapter, there has been substantial progress in mapping specific decision variables to specific brain regions. Yet, considering decisions to reflect the simple interactions between sets of these regions would be, much like hydraulic theories of personality, an unnecessary and misleading oversimplification. No one region, nor any set of regions, can be unambiguously claimed to implement a rational decision-making process. Instead, specific brain regions contribute to particular computations, which may or may not be consistent with models for rational behavior. Some such regions may even exert context-dependent influences, like that shown for dmPFC in the final experiment, making it impossible to categorize them within a two-systems framework (Frank et al., 2009).

Third, an important direction for neuroeconomics will be to strengthen its connections to the broader cognitive neuroscience literature. For example, our results are consistent with the growing consensus that dmPFC reflects a mechanism for identifying and responding adaptively to changes in the context for behavior. The postulated computations for dmPFC, which involve broad cognitive control functions like alerting (Gehring and Willoughby, 2002) or monitoring (Carter et al., 1998) changes in the external (or internal) milieu, may reflect specific physiological constraints in the implementation of adaptive behavior. Notably, complex aspects of behavior, like full consideration of decision problems, require a wide range of processes of executive control. By adopting simplifying rules for behavior, and only changing those rules when environmental conditions change, the brain can operate with a much-reduced metabolic demand. We contend that dmPFC plays such a role in complex decision making: it signals changes in how a decision problem is represented, and thus shapes computational processing elsewhere in the brain based on the current decision strategy. We note that such strategic considerations are unlikely to limited to abstract economic decisions; they are also likely to be critical for interpersonal interactions in social contexts (Camerer, 2003b). Initial converging evidence from primate lesion studies and functional neuroimaging data indicate a dissociation between contributions of the anterior cingulate sulcus and the anterior cingulate gyrus to non-social and social behavior, respectively (Behrens et al., 2008, 2009). Future studies need to extend these findings to the role of trust and reputation in influencing decision strategies (King-Casas et al., 2005).

Fourth, and finally, given a potentially large repertoire of strategies, how could individuals determine which one to employ in a particular situation? Cognitive models of strategy selection often argue that strategy selection occurs through a simple cost/benefit analysis (Payne et al., 1988). In other words, an adaptive decision maker often evaluates costs (effort and computational resources) and benefits (outcomes, potential regret, ease of justification) before selecting and applying a strategy. Like other aspects of decision making, strategic preferences can vary both as a function of the decision context (like complexity of the problem and timing constraints) and the decision maker. However, it is unclear how the trade off works at a computational level (Busemeyer and Townsend, 1993). Alternatively, strategy selection may represent a learned response that is based on past experiences with different strategies (Rieskamp and Hoffrage, 2008; Rieskamp and Otto, 2006), such that the decision maker merely chooses the most efficient strategy for each situation based on prior experience (e.g., reward history, consistent with Fig. 7.5). Neuroscience may help answer the metacognitive question of how people decide how to decide.

References

Aharon, I., Etcoff, N., Ariely, D., Chabris, C. F., O'Connor, E., and Breiter, H. C. (2001). Beautiful faces have variable reward value: fMRI and behavioral evidence. *Neuron, 32*(3), 537–51.

Alba, J. W. and Marmorstein, H. (1987). The effects of frequency knowledge on consumer decision-making. *The Journal of Consumer Research, 14*(1), 14–25.

Bechara, A., Tranel, D., and Damasio, H. (2000). Characterization of the decision-making deficit of patients with ventromedial prefrontal cortex lesions. *Brain, 123*(Pt 11), 2189–2202.

Beckmann, M., Johansen-Berg, H., and Rushworth, M. F. S. (2009). Connectivity-based parcellation of human cingulate cortex and its relation to functional specialization. *Journal of Neuroscience, 29*(4), 1175–90.

Behrens, T. E., Woolrich, M. W., Walton, M. E., and Rushworth, M. F. (2007). Learning the value of information in an uncertain world. *Nature Neuroscience, 10*(9), 1214–21.

Behrens, T. E., Hunt, L. T., Woolrich, M. W., and Rushworth, M. F. (2008). Associative learning of social value. *Nature, 456*(7219), 245–49.

Behrens, T. E., Hunt, L. T., and Rushworth, M. F. (2009). The computation of social behavior. *Science, 324*(5931), 1160–64.

Bernheim, B. D. and Rangel, A. (2004). Addiction and cue-triggered decision processes. *American Economic Review, 94*(5), 1558–90.

Bernoulli, D. (1738). Specimen theoriae novae de mensura sortis. *Commentarii Academiae Scientarum Imperialis Petropolitanae, 5*, 175–92.

Berns, G. S., McClure, S. M., Pagnoni, G., and Montague, P. R. (2001). Predictability modulates human brain response to reward. *Journal of Neuroscience, 21*(8), 2793–98.

Berns, G. S., Capra, C. M., Chappelow, J., Moore, S., and Noussair, C. (2008). Nonlinear neurobiological probability weighting functions for aversive outcomes. *Neuroimage, 39*(4), 2047–57.

Birnbaum, M. H. (2008). New paradoxes of risky decision-making. *Psychological Review, 115*(2), 463–501.

Bodenhausen, G. V., Sheppard, L. A., and Kramer, G. P. (1994). Negative affect and social judgment the differential impact of anger and sadness. *European Journal of Social Psychology, 24*(1), 45–62.

Brandstätter, E., Gigerenzer, G., and Hertwig, R. (2006). The priority heuristic: making choices without trade-offs. *Psychological Review, 113*(2), 409–32.

Busemeyer, J. R. and Townsend, J. T. (1993). Decision field-theory - a dynamic cognitive approach to decision-making in an uncertain environment. *Psychological Review, 100*(3), 432–59.

Bush, G., Luu, P., and Posner, M. I. (2000). Cognitive and emotional influences in anterior cingulate cortex. *Trends in Cognitive Science*, **4**(6), 215–22.

Bush, G., Whalen, P. J., Rosen, B. R., Jenike, M. A., McInerney, S. C., and Rauch, S. L. (1998). The counting Stroop: an interference task specialized for functional neuroimaging validation study with functional MRI. *Human Brain Mapping*, **6**(4), 270–82.

Camerer, C. F. (2003a). Behavioral studies of strategic thinking in games. *Trends in Cognitive Science*, **7**(5), 225–31.

Camerer, C. (2003b). *Behavioral game theory: experiments in strategic interaction*. Princeton, NJ.: Princeton University Press.

Camille, N., Coricelli, G., Sallet, J., Pradat-Diehl, P., Duhamel, J.R., and Sirigu, A. (2004). The involvement of the orbitofrontal cortex in the experience of regret. *Science*, **304**(5674), 167–70.

Carter, C. S., Braver, T. S., Barch, D. M., Botvinick, M. M., Noll, D., and Cohen, J. D. (1998). Anterior cingulate cortex, error detection, and the online monitoring of performance. *Science.*, **280**(5364), 747–49.

Chiu P. H., Lohrenz T. M., and Montague P. R. (2008). Smokers' brains compute, but ignore, a fictive error signal in a sequential investment task. *Nature Neuroscience*, **11**(4), 514–20.

Christoff, K., Prabhakaran, V., Dorfman, J., Zhao, Z., Kroger, J. K., Holyoak, K. J. et al. (2001). Rostrolateral prefrontal cortex involvement in relational integration during reasoning. *Neuroimage*, **14**(5), 1136–49.

Clithero, J. A., Tankersley, D., and Huettel, S. A. (2008). Foundations of neuroeconomics: from philosophy to practice. *Plos Biology*, **6**(11), 2348–53.

Cohen, M. X., Heller, A. S., and Ranganath, C. (2005). Functional connectivity with anterior cingulate and orbitofrontal cortices during decision-making. *Cognitive Brain Research*, **23**(1), 61–70.

Cope, D. E. and Murphy, A. J. (1981). The value of strategies in problem-solving. *Journal of Psychology*, **107**(1), 11–16.

Coricelli G., Critchley H. D., Joffily M., O'Doherty J. P., Sirigu A., and Dolan R. J. (2005). Regret and its avoidance: a neuroimaging study of choice behavior. *Nature Neuroscience*, **8**(9), 1255–62.

De Martino, B., Kumaran, D., Seymour, B., and Dolan, R. J. (2006). Frames, biases, and rational decision-making in the human brain. *Science*, **313**(5787), 684–87.

Derrfuss, J., Brass, M., Neumann, J., and von Cramon, D. Y. (2005). Involvement of the inferior frontal junction in cognitive control: meta-analyses of switching and Stroop studies. *Human Brain Mapping*, **25**(1), 22–34.

Diecidue, E. and van de Ven, J. (2008). Aspiration level, probability of success and failure, and expected utility. *International Economic Review*, **49**(2), 683–700.

Fordyce, M. W. (1988). A review of research on the happiness measures - a 60 second index of happiness and mental-health. *Social Indicators Research*, **20**(4), 355–81.

Frank, M. J., Cohen, M. X., and Sanfey, A. G. (2009). Multiple systems in decision-making: a neurocomputational perspective. *Current Directions in Psychological Sciences*, **18**(2), 73–77.

Gehring, W. J. and Fencsik, D. E. (2001). Functions of the medial frontal cortex in the processing of conflict and errors. *Journal of Neuroscience*, **21**(23), 9430–37.

Gehring, W. J. and Willoughby, A. R. (2002). The medial frontal cortex and the rapid processing of monetary gains and losses. *Science*, **295**(5563), 2279–82.

Gigerenzer, G. and Goldstein, D.G. (1996). Reasoning the fast and frugal way: Models of bounded rationality. *Psychological Review*, **103**, 650–69.

Glimcher, P. W. and Rustichini, A. (2004). Neuroeconomics: the consilience of brain and decision. *Science*, **306**(5695), 447–52.

Goyer, J. P., Woldorff, M. G., and Huettel, S. A. (2008). Rapid electrophysiological brain responses are influenced by both valence and magnitude of monetary rewards. *Journal of Cognitive Neuroscience*, **20**(11), 2058–69.

Greene, J. D., Sommerville, R. B., Nystrom, L. E., Darley, J. M., and Cohen, J. D. (2001). An fMRI investigation of emotional engagement in moral judgment. *Science,* **293**(5537), 2105–08.

Hadland, K. A., Rushworth, M. F. S., Gaffan, D., and Passingham, R. E. (2003). The effect of cingulate lesions on social behavior and emotion. *Neuropsychologia,* **41**(8), 919–31.

Hayden B.Y., Pearson J.M., Platt M.L. (2009). Fictive reward signals in the anterior cingulate cortex. *Science,* **324**(5929), 948–50.

Holroyd, C. B., and Coles, M. G. (2002). The neural basis of human error processing: reinforcement learning, dopamine, and the error-related negativity. *Psychological Review,* **109**(4), 679–709.

Hsu, M., Bhatt, M., Adolphs, R., Tranel, D., and Camerer, C. F. (2005). Neural systems responding to degrees of uncertainty in human decision-making. *Science,* **310**(5754), 1680–3.

Hsu, M., Krajbich, I., Zhao, C., and Camerer, C. F. (2009). Neural response to reward anticipation under risk is nonlinear in probabilities. *Journal of Neuroscience,* **29**(7), 2231–7.

Huettel, S. A. (2006). Behavioral, but not reward, risk modulates activation of prefrontal, parietal, and insular cortices. *Cognitive, Affective, and Behavioral Neuroscience,* **6**(2), 141–51.

Huettel, S. A., Stowe, C. J., Gordon, E. M., Warner, B. T., and Platt, M. L. (2006). Neural signatures of economic preferences for risk and ambiguity. *Neuron,* **49**(5), 765–75.

Kable, J. W., and Glimcher, P. W. (2007). The neural correlates of subjective value during intertemporal choice. *Nature Neuroscience,* **10**(12), 1625–33.

Kahneman, D. (2003). Maps of bounded rationality: Psychology for behavioral economics. *American Economic Review,* **93**(5), 1449–75.

Kahneman, D. and Tversky, A. (1979). Prospect theory: An analysis of decision under risk. *Econometrica,* **47**(2), 263–91.

Kennerley, S. W., Walton, M. E., Behrens, T. E., Buckley, M. J., and Rushworth, M. F. (2006). Optimal decision-making and the anterior cingulate cortex. *Nature Neuroscience,* **9**(7), 940–47.

Kerns, J. G., Cohen, J. D., MacDonald, A. W., 3rd, Cho, R. Y., Stenger, V. A., and Carter, C. S. (2004). Anterior cingulate conflict monitoring and adjustments in control. *Science,* **303**(5660), 1023–26.

King-Casas, B., Tomlin, D., Anen, C., Camerer, C. F., Quartz, S. R., and Montague, P. R. (2005). Getting to know you: reputation and trust in a two-person economic exchange. *Science,* **308**(5718), 78–83.

Knutson, B., Fong, G. W., Bennett, S. M., Adams, C. M., and Hommer, D. (2003). A region of mesial prefrontal cortex tracks monetarily rewarding outcomes: characterization with rapid event-related fMRI. *NeuroImage,* **18**(2), 263–72.

Koechlin, E., Corrado, G., Pietrini, P., and Grafman, J. (2000). Dissociating the role of the medial and lateral anterior prefrontal cortex in human planning. *Proceedings of National Academy of Science USA,* **97**(13), 7651–56.

Koechlin, E., Ody, C., and Kouneiher, F. (2003). The architecture of cognitive control in the human prefrontal cortex. *Science,* **302**(5648), 1181–5.

Kuhnen, C. M. and Knutson, B. (2005). The neural basis of financial risk taking. *Neuron,* **47**(5), 763–70.

Loewenstein, G. F., Weber, E. U., Hsee, C. K., and Welch, N. (2001). Risk as feelings. *Psychological Bullet,* **127**(2), 267–86.

Logothetis, N.K. (2008). What we can do and what we cannot do with fMRI. *Nature,* **453**(7197), 869–878.

Logothetis, N.K., Pauls, J., Augath, M., Trinath, T., and Oeltermann, A. (2001). Neurophysiological investigation of the basis of the fMRI signal. *Nature,* **412**(6843), 150–7.

Lohrenz T, McCabe K, Camerer C.F., and Montague, P.R. (2007). Neural signature of fictive learning signals in a sequential investment task. *Proceedings of National Academy of Science USA,* **104**(22), 9493–8.

Lopes, L. L. (1995). Algebra and process in the modeling of risky choice. In J. R. Busemeyer, R. Hastie, and D. L. Medin (Eds.), *Decision-making from a cognitive perspective.* San Diego: Academic Press.

Lopes, L. L. and Oden, G. C. (1999). The role of aspiration level in risky choice: a comparison of cumulative prospect theory and sp/a theory. *Journal of Mathematical Psychology,* **43**(2), 286–313.

MacLeod, C. M. (1992). The Stroop task: The "gold standard" of attentional measures. *Journal of Experimental Psychology: General,* **121**(1), 12–14.

McClure, S. M., Laibson, D. I., Loewenstein, G., and Cohen, J. D. (2004). Separate neural systems value immediate and delayed monetary rewards. *Science,* **306**(5695), 503–507.

Meriau, K., Wartenburger, I., Kazzer, P., Prehn, K., Lammers, C. H., van der Meer, E. et al. (2006). A neural network reflecting individual differences in cognitive processing of emotions during perceptual decision-making. *Neuroimage,* **33**(3), 1016–27.

Miller, E. K. and Cohen, J. D. (2001). An integrative theory of prefrontal cortex function. *Annual Review of Neuroscience,* **24**, 167–202.

Miltner, W. H. R., Braun, C. H., and Coles, M. G. H. (1997). Event-related brain potentials following incorrect feedback in a time-estimation task: evidence for a "generic" neural system for error-detection. *Journal of Cognitive Neuroscience,* **9**, 788–98.

Nieuwenhuis, S., Holroyd, C. B., Mol, N., and Coles, M. G. (2004). Reinforcement-related brain potentials from medial frontal cortex: origins and functional significance. *Neuroscience Biobehavioral Reviews,* **28**(4), 441–48.

Payne, J. W. (2005). It is whether you win or lose: The importance of the overall probabilities of winning or losing in risky choice. *Journal of Risk and Uncertainty,* **30**(1), 5–19.

Payne, J. W., Laughhunn, D. J., and Crum, R. (1980). Translation of gambles and aspiration level effects in risky choice behavior. *Management Science,* **26**(10), 1039–60.

Payne, J. W., Laughhunn, D. J., and Crum, R. (1981). Further tests of aspiration level effects in risky choice behavior. *Management Science,* **27**(8), 953–58.

Payne, J. W., Bettman, J. R., and Johnson, E. J. (1988). Adaptive strategy selection in decision-making. *Journal of Experimental Psychology-Learning Memory and Cognition,* **14**(3), 534–52.

Platt, M. L., and Huettel, S. A. (2008). Risky business: the neuroeconomics of decision-making under uncertainty. *Nat Neurosci,* **11**(4), 398–403.

Preuschoff, K., Bossaerts, P., and Quartz, S. R. (2006). Neural differentiation of expected reward and risk in human subcortical structures. *Neuron,* **51**(3), 381–90.

Preuschoff, K., Quartz, S. R., and Bossaerts, P. (2008). Human insula activation reflects risk prediction errors as well as risk. *Journal of Neuroscience,* **28**(11), 2745–52.

Rieskamp, J. and Hoffrage, U. (2008). Inferences under time pressure: how opportunity costs affect strategy selection. *Acta Psychologica,* **127**(2), 258–76.

Rieskamp, J. and Otto, P. E. (2006). SSL: a theory of how people learn to select strategies. *Journal of Experimental Psychology-General,* **135**(2), 207–36.

Ruchsow, M., Grothe, J., Spitzer, M., and Kiefer, M. (2002). Human anterior cingulate cortex is activated by negative feedback: evidence from event-related potentials in a guessing task. *Neuroscience Letters,* **325**(3), 203–206.

Rudebeck, P. H., Bannerman, D. M., and Rushworth, M. F. S. (2008). The contribution of distinct subregions of the ventromedial frontal cortex to emotion, social behavior, and decision-making. *Cognitive Affective and Behavioral Neuroscience,* **8**(4), 485–97.

Rushworth, M. F. S., Behrens, T. E. J., Rudebeck, P. H., and Walton, M. E. (2007). Contrasting roles for cingulate and orbitofrontal cortex in decisions and social behavior. *Trends in Cognitive Sciences,* **11**(4), 168–76.

Rushworth, M. F. S., Walton, M. E., Kennerley, S. W., and Bannerman, D. M. (2004). Action sets and decisions in the medial frontal cortex. *Trends in Cognitive Sciences,* **8**(9), 410–417.

Sanfey, A. G., Rilling, J. K., Aronson, J. A., Nystrom, L. E., and Cohen, J. D. (2003). The neural basis of economic decision-making in the Ultimatum Game. *Science.,* **300**(5626), 1755–58.

Savage, L. J. (1954). *Foundations of statistics*. New York: Wiley.

Schwarz, N., Bless, H., and Bohner, G. (1991). Mood and persuasion affective states influence the processing of persuasive communications. *Advances in Experimental Social Psychology*, 24, 161–99.

Schwartz, B., Ward, A., Monterosso, J., Lyubomirsky, S., White, K., and Lehman, D. R. (2002). Maximizing versus satisficing: happiness is a matter of choice. *Journal of Personality and Social Psychology*, 83(5), 1178–97.

Shah, A. K. and Oppenheimer, D. M. (2008). Heuristics made easy: an effort-reduction framework. *Psychological Bulletin*, 134(2), 207–22.

Shiv, B., Loewenstein, G., and Bechara, A. (2005). The dark side of emotion in decision-making: when individuals with decreased emotional reactions make more advantageous decisions. *Cognitive Brain Research*, 23(1), 85–92.

Simon, H. A. (1957). *Models of man: social and rational*. New York: Wiley.

Slovic, P. and Lichtenstein, S. (1968). The relative importance of probabilities and payoffs in risk-taking. *Journal of Experimental Psychology Monograph Supplement*, 72, 1–18.

Tversky, A. and Fox, C. R. (1995). Weighing risk and uncertainty. *Psychological Review*, 102(2), 269–83.

Tversky, A. and Kahneman, D. (1974). Judgment under uncertainty: heuristics and biases. *Science*, 185, 1124–31.

Tversky, A. and Kahneman, D. (1981). The framing of decisions and the psychology of choice. *Science*, 211(4481), 453–58.

Tversky, A. and Kahneman, D. (1992). Advances in prospect theory: cumulative representation of uncertainty. *Journal of Risk and Uncertainty*, 5, 297–323.

Tversky, A. and Wakker, P. (1995). Risk attitudes and decision weights. *Econometrica*, 63(6), 1255–80.

Venkatraman, V., Payne, J. W., Bettman, J. R., Luce, M. F., and Huettel, S. A. (2009). Separate neural mechanisms underlie choice and strategic preference in risky decision-making. *Neuron*, 62(4), 593–602.

von Neumann, J. and Morgenstern, O. (1944). *Theory of games and economic behavior*. Princeton, NJ: Princeton University Press.

Yacubian, J., Sommer, T., Schroeder, K., Glascher, J., Braus, D. F., and Buchel, C. (2007). Subregions of the ventral striatum show preferential coding of reward magnitude and probability. *Neuroimage*, 38(3), 557–63.

Zeelenberg, M. (1999). Anticipated regret, expected feedback and behavioral decision-making. *Journal of Behavioral Decision-making*, 12(93–106).

Zeelenberg, M. and Pieters, R. (2004). Consequences of regret aversion in real life: The case of the Dutch postcode lottery. *Organizational Behavior and Human Decision Processes*, 93(2), 155–68.

Chapter 8

Multiple neural circuits in value-based decision making

Manami Yamamoto, Xiaochuan Pan,
Kensaku Nomoto, and Masamichi Sakagami

Abstract

Valuation is an essential process and function in decision making. The variety and organization of such valuation systems characterize the decision making of animals. To understand the nature of the distinct neural systems used in such valuation, we performed monkey single-unit recording experiments together with a human fMRI experiment using (1) a perceptual discrimination task with asymmetric reward, and (2) a reward inference task. The results suggest that both the primate and human brain have, at least, two distinct valuation systems: one in the nigro-striatal circuit (here, referred to as the "stimulus-based valuation system") and the other in the prefrontal cortex (PFC) circuit (here, referred to as the "knowledge-based valuation system"). We believe that the nigro-striatal circuit calculates values based on the empirical and probabilistic relation between an event and its outcome. The PFC circuit, on the other hand, generates values by further extension of directly-experienced association through categorical processes and rules, thereby enabling animals to predict the outcome of an inexperienced event.

8.1 **Introduction**

The brain is an organ able to select an appropriate behavior in an ever-changing environment. Smaller brains are thought to generate behavior corresponding to a specific environmental stimulus in a one-to-one fashion. This type of action may be called a reflex or involuntary action. Although a smaller brain would effectively work as a "relay machine," a larger brain seems able to select more appropriate behaviors among available choices, depending on the context of the stimulus environment. Such processes of selection may be loosely termed "thought" or "decision making." Recent studies in neuroscience have begun to reveal brain mechanisms used in decision making, taking into account knowledge from other fields, such as economics (Glimcher, 2009) and philosophy (Levy, 2007). Some of these new findings are challenging long-established beliefs.

Decision making does not involve a single process, as previously believed. For example, Rangel et al. (2008) suggested that value-based decision making is composed of five processes: (1) state representation, (2) valuation, (3) action selection, (4) outcome evaluation, and (5) learning. Among these, the valuation process is critical in decision making because the evolution of the animal brain has developed multiple valuation systems (e.g., conditioned, goal-directed, as well as others), and the divergence of decision making mainly depends on the variation of said valuation systems. In this chapter, we will see some evidence bearing on the diverse contributions of cortical and subcortical neural circuits in both the non-human and human primate brain, and also discuss the nature of the decision-making function.

8.2 The dual nature of valuation, and two neural circuits

When we select a behavior from several options, the brain may calculate values, or so-called "utilities," of the consequent behavioral outcomes in order to compare the cost and benefit of the consequences of those behaviors in a single dimension (Glimcher et al., 2003). These values may depend on the environmental context. For example, when we go to a grocery store to buy ingredients for dinner, we collect vegetables, meat, and spices necessary for a planned dish (let's say a steak). While shopping, we activate a plan, or an internal model related to our goal, which is for making the dish. According to the plan, each ingredient would have a particular value. However, it is possible that something more interesting, such as the sight of fresh tuna, may change the dinner plan. We may have considered tuna-sushi as a candidate for tonight's dinner and rejected it due to a lower value, but the newly acquired value, activated automatically by the actual image of tuna, could exceed the planned value of the steak. Why does the fresh tuna suddenly receive such a high value for dinner, even though the plan was to buy steak?

It seems that we have at least two distinct systems, which work independently to calculate such values. One serves to calculate values based on knowledge organized by planning and reasoning, while the other automatically calculates values independent of plan or context. In other words, both an automatic system and a more rational system appear to interact in making a choice.

Several lines of psychological studies have provided evidence for dual forms of valuation. For example, Johansson et al. (2005) performed an experiment where they asked subjects to choose the most attractive person from two photos. After the subject chose one, the experimenter laid the photos face down. Then, the experimenter showed the one that had been chosen by the subject and asked why he or she had chosen it. Once in a few trials, the experimenter showed the photo that had not been chosen by the subject and asked why he or she had "chosen" it. We might think that the subject should not be able to explain why he or she had "chosen" it because he or she had actually not done so. However, in many such trials, the subject actually gave a reason why he or she had "chosen" the photo that in fact had not been chosen, as if the subject was unaware that the photo shown was not his or her choice. These results suggest that subjects not only calculate a value for choice by preference, but that explicit reasoning is not necessarily made based on value, thus suggesting that valuation by reasoning may exist in parallel with valuation by more automatic processes.

As pertains to psychological findings, Shimojo and colleagues have investigated human brain activity using functional magnetic resonance imaging (fMRI), while a subject performed a preference task (Kim et al., 2007). In this experiment, two photos were serially presented to a subject two or more times until he or she was finally able to decide which photo was more preferable. The brain activity was analyzed during the presentation of the photo for which the subject had ultimately shown a preference. The researchers found that different brain areas had been activated, in accordance with the first and final presentations of the photo. They found that the nucleus accumbens (NAC) in the basal ganglia, (which receives strong projections from dopamine neurons), had been strongly activated when the ultimately preferable photo was presented the first time, and that this activity disappeared on final presentation of the photo. At that moment, the medial orbitofrontal cortex (mOFC) was activated instead of the NAC. Kim et al. (2007) interpreted that the activity in the NAC was related to an initial rapid and automatic choice, and that the activity in the mOFC reflected the explicit process of reasoning with referring to the output of NAC.

Several lines of clinical studies have also suggested the disparate contributions of cortical and subcortical circuits possibly involved in the valuation process. Lhermitte et al. (1986) reported behavioral deficits in PFC-lesioned patients. They indicated that many PFC patients could not suppress the mimicking of others (in imitation behavior), and to utilize tools presented in front of them, which were not immediately necessary (for so-called utilization behavior). As an example, when a patient was invited to a doctor's house, as soon as he found the bedroom, he would get into the bed with his clothes off. This would not be strange if it were his own bedroom. However, in the context of his being invited to someone else's house, his behavior of getting into the bed with his clothes off would have been expected to be suppressed. Nevertheless, PFC patients can maintain habitual decision making, apparently based on the statistical probabilities of their experiences, yet they seem to have problems controlling other types of decision making that depend on environment. In relation to such problems in context-dependent decision making, PFC patients also showed poor performance on the Stroop test, the Wisconsin Card Sorting Test, and the Iowa Gambling Test (Bechara et al., 1996; Lauwereyns et al., 2001; Luria., 1980; Perret., 1974; Sakagami et al., 2001, 2006).

In the following sections, we will see some experimental evidence of dissociation between the cortical valuation system (in particular, the PFC), and the subcortical (nigrostriatal) valuation system, using: (1) the perceptual discrimination task with asymmetric reward, and (2) the reward inference task.

8.3 Reward prediction under stimulus ambiguity

When an ambiguous stimulus is used as a reward-indicative cue, an animal may predict reward by at least two distinct ways. One way is for the animal to probabilistically predict reward on the basis of stimulus–outcome (or stimulus–response–outcome), i.e., association through classical conditioning. In this system (stimulus-based), the value of a predicted reward depends on the physical salience of a stimulus, as well as the probability of stimulus–outcome pairing in the training history. Another way is for the animal to predict reward based on a mental representation of a stimulus. In this system (knowledge-based), a cue activates representations, or knowledge, of stimulus and associated outcome. In the ambiguous stimulus situation, the dependence on mental representation in the decision making is expected to increase in inverse proportion to the salience of a target stimulus.

To test this hypothesis, that separate neural mechanisms underlie these processes, we recorded brain activity during the performance of a random dot motion discrimination task using an asymmetric reward schedule (Fig. 8.1) in both human fMRI and monkey neurophysiology experiments (Nomoto et al., 2007, 2010; Yamamoto et al., 2007). The subject was presented with random dot motion, which has been used in studies on motion perception (Parker and Newsome, 1998), and required to report its motion direction (rightward or leftward). In a given block, while one direction of motion stimuli was associated with more valuable reward (in terms of quality or quantity), the other direction was associated with less valuable reward. To manipulate discrimination difficulty, several levels of coherence were used. Although small details of the task were adapted to work well with different species, the task structure was basically the same. Whereas the stimulus-based valuation system shows reward prediction based on the motion stimulus itself, the knowledge-based valuation system shows reward prediction based on the subject's reported perceptual discrimination. Dissociation between these two systems is discernable in error trials.

In the human fMRI experiment, we were able to show that the caudate nucleus and the medial prefrontal cortex (MPFC) are involved in distinct reward predictions. Whereas the caudate activity shows stimulus-based reward prediction, the MPFC activity is consistent with the knowledge-based reward prediction. The activity in the caudate nucleus predicted reward based on the sensory input of cues (direction and coherence of the motion stimuli), irrespective of the subjects' perceptual decision on the motion direction (Fig. 8.2A). In contrast, the MPFC seemed to use the output of perceptual decision to

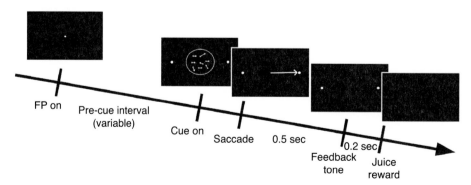

Fig. 8.1 Time course of random-dot motion discrimination task.

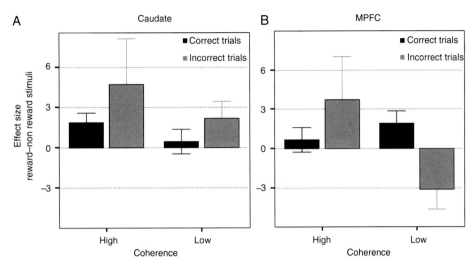

Fig. 8.2 fMRI signal on reward prediction in random-dot discrimination task. (A) Caudate nucleus shows greater reward-predicting activity for high-coherence stimuli than for low-coherence stimuli, depending upon the direction of the stimulus input. (B) Medial prefrontal cortex (MPFC) shows a reversal of direction of the reward-predicting activity in the low-coherence stimuli with significant interaction between stimulus (high/low) and trial types (correct/incorrect). Error bar shows 1 SEM.

predict reward, especially in the low-coherence trials, where the sensory input of the cue stimuli was limited (Fig. 8.2B). These results suggest that the striatum generates a stimulus-driven reward value based on the probabilistic relation between stimulus input and reward, whereas the MPFC incorporates the output of the stimulus processes (i.e., the percept), to compensate for weak sensory-dependent prediction by the striatum.

The monkey neurophysiology experiment complements this idea with the finding that midbrain dopamine neurons, which provide abundant projections to the striatum (Haber, 2003), show reward-predictive activity based on the stimulus-based system. In agreement with previous findings (Schultz, 1998), dopamine neurons responded to reward-indicative cues (i.e., direction of motion stimuli). Importantly, dopamine responses in the small-reward error trials are similar to those in the small-reward correct trials (as shown in Fig. 8.3), even if perceptual decisions were in the opposite direction, suggesting that dopaminergic responses were not consistent with reward prediction associated with behavioral reports. Rather, dopaminergic responses reflected reward prediction associated with actual motion stimuli. These results suggest that dopaminergic activity reflects external stimulus-based reward prediction, irrespective of the monkey's report. Accordingly, dopaminergic neurons may influence the stimulus-based striatal activity through dopaminergic projections to the striatum.

Our results demonstrate that two distinct systems are differently involved in reward prediction under stimulus ambiguity. The caudate activity reflected reward prediction based on the physical properties of external stimuli in a probabilistic manner. This

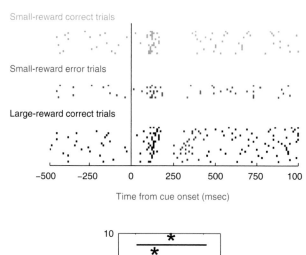

Fig. 8.3 Stimulus-dependent prediction error of a dopamine neuron. Raster plots (the top panel) and firing rates (the bottom panel) of this neuron are shown. Gray levels indicate trial types: small-reward correct trials (light gray), small-reward error trials (dark gray), and large-reward correct trials (black). Horizontal axis indicates time from cue onset. Vertical line indicates time of cue onset.

is consistent with previous studies (Tobler et al., 2007). Moreover, we found that dopamine-reward-predictive activity was also based on the motion stimulus itself, but not on behavioral report. Given that the striatum receives massive dopaminergic inputs (Haber, 2003), these subcortical structures collaboratively provide reward prediction on the basis of the external stimulus-based system. Unlike this subcortical circuit, the MPFC activity was correlated with perceptual judgment on motion direction. We observed this feature only for the lower coherence level. This suggests that knowledge-based reward prediction by the MPFC is particularly effective when the external stimulus is weak, or stimulus input is limited. In the context of perceptual decision making, a previous study has shown that the MPFC holds predictive codes for perceptual categorization (Summerfield et al., 2006). Thus, our results suggest that the MPFC activity supplements limited stimulus information with reward prediction based on perceptual judgment. This would entail that the coding of the MPFC is consistent with a knowledge-based system.

8.4 Reward prediction for different time scales

Our previous study showed another example of multiple neural circuits for valuation: whereas the prefrontal activity incorporated reward prediction over subsequent trials, the caudate activity only reflected reward prediction based on the current trial (Kobayashi et al., 2007). We show the activities of the lateral prefrontal cortex (LPFC) and the caudate of the monkey performing a reward-biased visually-guided saccade task (Fig. 8.4).

In a given block, whereas the cue in one position was assigned to be the rewarded target (i.e., the reward condition), the cue in the other position was not rewarded, even if the monkey made correct responses (i.e., the no-reward condition). Since error trials were followed by a trial with the same condition, the monkeys should make a correct response even in the no-reward condition in order to escape the no-reward condition.

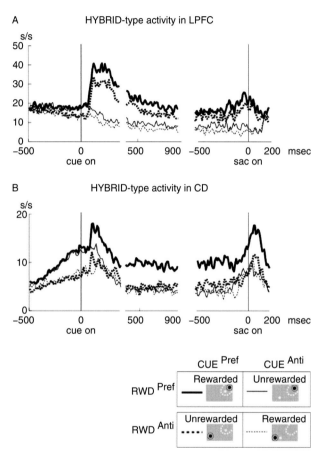

Fig. 8.4 Population histograms of integration-type neurons in the lateral prefrontal cortex (LPFC) (A) and in the caudate nucleus (CD) (B). The cue was presented either in the preferred direction (CUE[Pref], white circle inside the white dashed line in the inset; thick line in the histograms) or anti-preferred direction (CUE[Anti]; white circle out of the white dashed line in inset; thin line in the histograms). Immediate reward was associated either with the preferred direction (RWD[Pref], bull's eye mark inside the white dashed line in the inset; solid line in the histograms) or non-preferred direction (RWD[Anti], bull's eye mark out of the white dashed line; dashed line in the histograms). Immediate reward was available in the CUE[Pref]–RWD[Pref] condition and the CUE[Anti]–RWD[Anti]-conditions, whereas immediate reward was not available in the CUE[Pref]–RWD[Anti] condition and the CUE[Anti]–RWD[Pref] conditions. The left vertical line indicates the time of cue onset and the right vertical line indicates the time of saccade onset.

With kind permission from Springer Science and Business Media: *Experimental Brain Research*, Functional diffference between macaque prefrontal cortex and caudate nucleus during eye movements with and without reward, 176(2), 2006, Shunsuke Kobayashi.

Highly trained monkeys showed as high correct performance rates in the no-reward condition as monkeys in the reward condition, probably because, through extensive training, the monkeys may have acquired knowledge of the task structure, indicating that they would obtain rewards within the next few trials.

We recorded the LPFC and the caudate activities during this task. In general, while the LPFC neurons had spatial selectivity of cue position (Fig. 8.4A), the caudate neurons responded to the reward-associated cue position if the position corresponded to neurons' receptive field (Fig. 8.4B). In the no-reward condition, whereas the LPFC neurons maintained spatial selectivity, although the activity was modulated by the reward condition (Fig. 8.4A), the caudate neurons lost spatial selectivity (Fig. 8.4B). These results suggest that the caudate neurons were more affected by the immediate reward expectation, but the LPFC neurons were not. This might reflect a difference as to how far the neurons code for the future reward. Since the LPFC neurons remained active even in the no-reward condition, their responses might have been driven by the afore-mentioned knowledge-based system posited to expect reward in the near future. In contrast, as the caudate neurons lost selectivity in the no-reward condition, their activity was consistent with the stimulus-based valuation system.

8.5 **Reward inference by prefrontal and striatal neurons**

In the previous sections, we presented evidence for two distinct valuation systems: a stimulus-based valuation system operating within a nigro-striatal circuit, and a knowledge-based valuation system by a PFC circuit. While reward prediction in the stimulus-based system depends on stimulus–reward association learned through direct experience (e.g., conditioning), the one in the knowledge-based system is not limited by the range of direct experience. Organized representations in the knowledge network enable us to predict an outcome from a series of actions, which can be called the goal-directed value (Rangel et al., 2008). Animals with developed prefrontal cortices, such as human and non-human primates, are able to infer the outcomes of future events, even without the prior experience of events (Liberman and Trope, 2008). To understand how the PFC integrates independently acquired knowledge so as to infer the outcome of future events, we recorded neural activity from the LPFC of monkeys performing a sequential paired association task with an asymmetric reward schedule (Pan et al, 2008). In this task, the monkeys first learned two stimulus–stimulus association sequences (here denoted: A1→B1→C1 and A2→B2→C2, where A1, B1, C1, A2, B2, and C2 were six different visual stimuli), in sequential paired association trials (SPATs) (Fig. 8.5). After having mastered the task, the monkeys were taught the asymmetric reward schedule using reward instruction trials, in which one stimulus (C1 or C2) was paired with a large reward (0.4 ml of water) and another stimulus (C2 or C1) with a small reward (0.1 ml of water). Reward instruction trials were followed by SPATs in one block. In the SPATs, the amount of reward at the end of correct trials was also asymmetric: if C1 had been paired with the large reward, and C2 with the smaller, in the reward instruction trials, the sequence A1→B1→C1 would lead to the larger reward, while the sequence

A2→B2→C2 would lead to the smaller reward, and vice versa. Our question was whether the monkeys would transfer the reward information associated with C1 and C2 to the first visual stimuli, A1 and A2, in the SPATs. Stimuli A1 and A2 were not directly paired with the different amount of reward, but if the monkeys could generate the stimulus–reward relation (C with reward amount), and stimulus–stimulus (A→B→C) associations, we could expect them to predict reward amount at the time of the first stimulus presentation of A1 or A2 in a SPAT, just after reward instruction with C1 and C2. Our results showed that the monkeys and LPFC neurons discriminated the large reward condition from the small reward condition from the first SPATs (Pan et al, 2008). In particular, we found that a group of LPFC neurons predicted reward information specific to a group of relevant visual stimuli that required the same behavioral response (e.g., the A1-group including A1, B1, and C1, and the A2-group including A2, B2, and C2) (Fig. 8.6). These neurons responded to each stimulus from the preferred group in the preferred reward condition (large or small), and showed no response to the stimuli from the non-preferred group, irrespective of the reward condition. Thus, these neurons (category-reward neurons) likely coded both the category information of visual stimuli (either the A1 or A2 groups), and reward information (either large or small), simultaneously. The monkeys might group the relevant stimuli according to intended behavior requiring the same matching response, together as a functional category through extensive training with the paired association task. When the monkeys learned that C1 (or C2) was paired with a large reward, category-reward neurons combined the stimulus–reward relation and the category information to relay the reward information to other category members, which would allow the monkeys to predict reward on the basis of A1 (or A2) just after the reward instruction of C1 or C2.

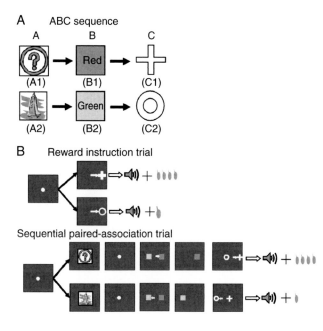

A ABC sequence

A   B   C

(A1)   Red (B1) → (C1)

(A2)   Green (B2) → (C2)

B Reward instruction trial

Sequential paired-association trial

Fig. 8.5 Scheme of sequential paired association task. (A) Two associative sequences (ABC sequence) learned by monkeys. The monkeys also learned two other sequences: BCA and CAB sequences. (B) Asymmetric stimulus–reward contingency in one block.

Reprinted by permission from Macmillan Publishers Ltd: *Nature Neuroscience*, Reward prediction based on stimulus categorization in primate lateral prefrontal cortex, 11(6), pp.703–12, X.Pan, K.Sawa, I.Tsuda, M.Tsukada, and M.Sakagami, Copyright 2008.

In the present experiment, we used such stimulus–reward reversal repeatedly; i.e., in one block, the A1 group was associated with a large reward and the A2 group with a small reward, and in the other, the A1 group was associated with a small reward and the A2 group with a large reward. One possibility is that monkeys used conditional discrimination to predict reward, rather than categorical inference, because the monkeys had repeatedly experienced the stimulus–reward association. Thus, the follow-up question was whether the monkeys and PFC neurons could carry out similar reward prediction with newly introduced category members. To answer this question, we introduced new category members for the A1 and A2 groups. Monkeys were trained to learn associations between new visual stimuli and B1 or B2 (e.g., for a new pair of stimuli (N1 and N2),

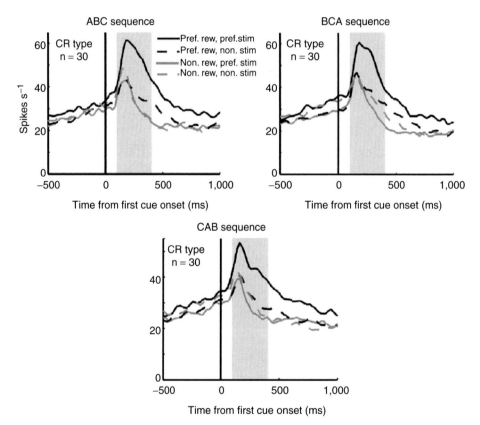

Fig. 8.6 Population histograms of category-reward (CR) neurons in three sequences (ABC, BCA and CAB). All trials were sorted into four conditions: preferred stimulus and preferred reward condition (solid black curve), non-preferred stimulus and preferred reward condition (dashed black curve), preferred stimulus and non-preferred reward condition (solid gray curve), and non-preferred stimulus and non-preferred reward condition (dashed gray curve). The gray areas indicate the first cue period used for analysis of neuronal activity.

Reprinted by permission from Macmillan Publishers Ltd: *Nature Neuroscience*, Reward prediction based on stimulus categorization in primate lateral prefrontal cortex, 11(6), pp.703–12, X.Pan, K.Sawa, I.Tsuda, M.Tsukada, and M.Sakagami, Copyright 2008.

N1→B1 and N2→B2). During the learning of the new associations, the monkeys received a constant, medium-sized reward, neither large nor small, for all new stimuli in correctly performed trials. In so doing, the monkeys were able to learn to categorize new stimuli, through common stimuli B1 and B2, into the current A1 and A2 groups. Behaviorally, we found that the correct rate of the first choice (selection of B on the basis of the first cue), for new stimuli on their first presentation, was significantly higher in large reward trials than in small ones, demonstrating that the monkeys could predict the size of the reward by the new stimulus in the first reward inference trial. Category-reward neurons showed similar response patterns to both the old and new stimuli, and predicted the reward information from the first presentation of new stimuli in the first SPATs after reward instructions C1 and C2. These results suggest that LPFC neurons could transfer reward information to new members on the basis of category membership, and may reflect a neural basis for the posited category-based reward inference.

Our results are consistent with the predictions from the model-based process proposed by Daw et al. (2005), which stands on higher order computations that allow simulations to predict outcomes using internal models. Daw et al (2005) also suggest that the striatum codes for stimulus–outcome relations through direct experiences, as a result of a model-free process, which is different from the prefrontal model-based process. To investigate this difference, we simultaneously recorded neural activity from the LPFC and striatum of the third monkey in the reward-instructed sequential paired association task with the first cues of old stimuli (A1 and A2). This third monkey was unable to perform the task well with new stimuli; however, we found that many striatal neurons showed reward-predictive activity to the first cue stimuli (A1 and A2), and that the activity was independent of the visual properties of the stimuli (as in the reward neurons studied in Pan and Sakagami, 2008)—a finding that is consistent with those of previous studies (Hollerman et al, 1998; Kawagoe et al, 1998; Samejima et al, 2005). However, careful analysis revealed that the reward neurons in the striatum showed different response patterns when compared to those in the LPFC (Fig. 8.7). After reward instruction with C1 and C2, the striatal neurons showed no differential activity between the large and small reward conditions in the first SPAT. In other words, these neurons were unable to predict the reward based on the first cue stimuli in the first trials, but could do so from the second SPATs. The results suggest that the striatal neurons, unlike the LPFC neurons, cannot transfer reward information associated with C1 and C2 to the first cues, A1 and A2, in the SPATs without direct experience. Therefore, there may be different mechanisms in the LPFC and striatum for reward prediction. Thus, we propose that the LPFC represents the category of a relevant stimulus as knowledge or an internal model, and predicts reward for the stimulus based on its category membership without requiring the direct experience of stimulus-reward associations. Furthermore, the striatum appears to predict reward for stimuli after directly experiencing each stimulus-reward relation.

In the fMRI experiment using random-dot motion discrimination, knowledge-based valuation-related activity was found in the MPFC, whereas in the LPFC, we found category-reward neurons. Although several lines of studies have indicated close functional and anatomical relations among sub-areas within the PFC (Hare et al., 2009; Rushworth and

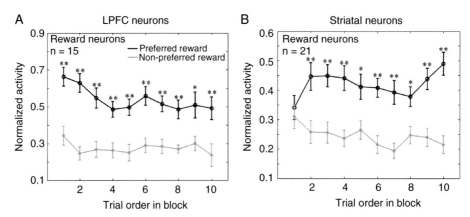

Fig. 8.7 Activity of simultaneously recorded neurons from LPFC and striatum. (A) Population-averaged activity of 15 LPFC neurons in first cue period as a function of SPAT order in blocks. (B) Population-averaged activity of 21 striatal neurons. Activities were sorted into two conditions: preferred reward condition (black curves) and non-preferred reward condition (gray curves). Statistical significance was checked by two tailed t-test (* $p<0.05$, ** $p<0.01$). Error bars: SEM.

Behrens, 2008), additional evidence is needed to support the hypothesis that functional cooperation among sub-areas of PFC may underlie knowledge-based valuation.

8.6 **Summary and implication**

Valuation is a key function in decision making. Variety and organization of valuation systems appear to be essential to decision making. In this chapter, we have suggested, by showing experimental data from our laboratory, that the primate brain has at least two distinct valuation systems that cooperate in one situation but compete in another. One of these systems is a part of the nigro-striatal circuit (which we refer to as the stimulus-based valuation system); and the other, a part of the PFC circuit (which we refer to as the knowledge-based valuation system). The nigro-striatal circuit appears to calculate values based on the empirical and probabilistic relation between an event and the ensuing reward or punishment. On the other hand, the PFC circuit appears to generate reward values in a more elaborate process that applies categorical information and rules to previously experienced association in order to make reward predictions, and thereby enabling an animal to predict the outcome of an inexperienced event. Although some groups have proposed ideas on how the brain integrates values from different valuation systems (Behrens et al., 2009; Hare et al., 2009), not much is known about the relationship between these systems. However, the evolution of the brain may provide hints. The basal ganglia are evolutionarily older than the cerebral cortex, particularly the PFC. From rodents to primates, mammals share homologous structures in the basal ganglia, but the PFC is highly developed in the primate brain, and particularly so in that of humans. From this structural viewpoint, we could say that the stimulus-based valuation system is common to the mammalian brain, while the knowledge-based valuation system differs among species. Differences in the knowledge-based system may also account for differences in intelligence.

In the course of evolution, the brain has preserved some older structures. For example, primates and humans have several neural circuits related to eye movement; some controlled by older brain regions and others by newer ones. When these compete, higher brain circuits often suppress lower ones, as in the competition between fixation (controlled by the cortex) and the vestibulo-ocular reflex (controlled by the brain stem). We can interpret the imitation behavior and the utilization behavior of prefrontal patients as examples of a deficit in this suppression (Sakagami and Pan, 2007; Sakagami et al., 2001, 2006). The valuation system in the nigro-striatal circuit plays a critical role in habitual and conditioned responses, such as the triggering of hand extension to reach out for a cup when thirsty. This system collects the information on the outcome value based on statistical evidence and the information is used for generating a behavioral decision. Ignoring more contextual cues in such decision making, reaching for a cup and drinking its contents would be the most common behavior when one is thirsty. However, the knowledge-based system activates representations regarding context (e.g., the position of a wine glass in relation to one and others, the social relations among the other people, etc.), and generates predictions using knowledge of the consequences— and thereby we raise our glasses in unison. Our findings suggest that the PFC neural network builds links among the representations in a goal-directed manner, as explained above, and generates an internal model based on current circumstances to make a prediction. If the predicted outcome is one of punishment, the PFC neural network has to suppress more automatic commands resulting from habit or conditioning. PFC patients have been observed to falter in their suppression of more automated processes that do not take social values into account. However, we do not know much about the functional relationships between different systems yet. Of course, further investigation will be necessary to better elucidate the neural mechanisms of valuation and decision making. In particular, an important next step would be to clarify the involvement and interaction of emotion in the valuation process.

Acknowledgments

Our research was supported by the 21st Century Center of Excellence (COE) program (Integrative Human Science Program, Tamagawa University) and the global COE program (Origins of the Social Mind, Tamagawa University) from the Japan Society for Promotion of Science (JSPS), and Grants-in-Aid for Scientific Research on Priority areas from the Ministry of Education, Culture, Sports, Science and Technology, Japan.

References

Bechara, A., Tranel, D., Damasio, H., and Damasio, A. R. (1996). Failure to respond autonomically to anticipated future outcomes following damage to prefrontal cortex. *Cereb Cortex,* **6**(2), 215–25.

Behrens, T. E., Hunt, L. T., and Rushworth, M. F. (2009). The computation of social behavior. *Science,* 324(5931), 1160–64.

Daw, N. D., Niv, Y., and Dayan, P. (2005). Uncertainty-based competition between prefrontal and dorsolateral striatal systems for behavioral control. *Nat Neurosci,* **8**(12), 1704–1711.

Glimcher, P. W. (2003). The neurobiology of visual-saccadic decision-making. *Annu Rev Neurosci,* **26**, 133–79.

Glimcher, P. W., Camerer, C., Poldrack, R. A., and Fehr, E. (2009). Neuroeconomics: Decision-making and the Brain. London: Academic Press.

Haber, S. N. (2003). The primate basal ganglia: parallel and integrative networks. *J Chem Neuroanat,* **26**(4), 317–30.

Hare, T. A., Camerer, C. F., and Rangel, A. (2009). Self-control in decision-making involves modulation of the vMPFC valuation system. *Science,* **324**(5927), 646–48.

Hollerman, J. R., Tremblay, L., and Schultz, W. (1998). Influence of reward expectation on behavior-related neuronal activity in primate striatum. *J Neurophysiol,* **80**(2), 947–63.

Johansson, P., Hall, L., Sikstrom, S., and Olsson, A. (2005). Failure to detect mismatches between intention and outcome in a simple decision task. *Science,* **310**(5745), 116–19.

Kawagoe, R., Takikawa, Y., and Hikosaka, O. (1998). Expectation of reward modulates cognitive signals in the basal ganglia. *Nat Neurosci,* **1**(5), 411–16.

Kim, H., Adolphs, R., O'Doherty, J. P., and Shimojo, S. (2007). Temporal isolation of neural processes underlying face preference decisions. *Proc Natl Acad Sci USA,* **104**(46), 18253–58.

Kobayashi, S., Kawagoe, R., Takikawa, Y., Koizumi, M., Sakagami, M., and Hikosaka, O. (2007). Functional differences between macaque prefrontal cortex and caudate nucleus during eye movements with and without reward. *Exp Brain Res,* **176**(2), 341–55.

Lauwereyns, J., Sakagami, M., Tsutsui, K., Kobayashi, S., Koizumi, M., and Hikosaka, O. (2001). Responses to task-irrelevant visual features by primate prefrontal neurons. *J Neurophysiol,* **86**(4), 2001–10.

Levy, N. (2007). *Neuroethics: challenges for the 21st century.* New York: Cambridge University Press.

Lhermitte, F., Pillon, B., and Serdaru, M. (1986). Human autonomy and the frontal lobes. Part I: Imitation and utilization behavior: a neuropsychological study of 75 patients. *Ann Neurol,* **19**(4), 326–34.

Liberman, N. and Trope, Y. (2008). The psychology of transcending the here and now. *Science,* **322**(5905), 1201–5.

Luria, A. R. (1980). *Higher cortical functions in man.* New York: Basic Books, Inc.

Nomoto, K., Watanabe, T., and Sakagami, M. (2007) Dopamine responses to complex reward-predicting stimuli. *Soc. Neurosci. Abstr.* 749.5.

Nomoto, K., Schultz, W., Wanatabe, T., and Sakagami, M. (2010). Temporally extended dopamine responses to perceptually demanding reward-predictive stimuli. *J Neurosci,* **30**(32), 10692–702.

Pan, X. and Sakagami, M. (2008) Dissociable roles of lateral prefrontal cortex and striatum for reward prediction. *Japanese Soc. Neurosci. Abstr.* 3.16.

Pan, X., Sawa, K., Tsuda, I., Tsukada, M., and Sakagami, M. (2008). Reward prediction based on stimulus categorization in primate lateral prefrontal cortex. *Nat Neurosci,* **11**(6), 703–12.

Parker, A. J. and Newsome, W. T. (1998). Sense and the single neuron: probing the physiology of perception. *Annu Rev Neurosci,* **21**, 227–77.

Perret, E. (1974). The left frontal lobe of man and the suppression of habitual responses in verbal categorical behaviour. *Neuropsychologia,* **12**(3), 323–30.

Rangel, A., Camerer, C., and Montague, P. R. (2008). A framework for studying the neurobiology of value-based decision-making. *Nat Rev Neurosci,* **9**(7), 545–56.

Rushworth, M. F. and Behrens, T. E. (2008). Choice, uncertainty and value in prefrontal and cingulate cortex. *Nat Neurosci,* **11**(4), 389–97.

Sakagami, M. and Pan, X. (2007). Functional role of the ventrolateral prefrontal cortex in decision-making. *Curr Opin Neurobiol*, **17**(2), 228–33.

Sakagami, M., Tsutsui, K., Lauwereyns, J., Koizumi, M., Kobayashi, S., and Hikosaka, O. (2001). A code for behavioral inhibition on the basis of color, but not motion, in ventrolateral prefrontal cortex of macaque monkey. *J Neurosci*, **21**(13), 4801–8.

Sakagami, M., Pan, X., and Uttl, B. (2006). Behavioral inhibition and prefrontal cortex in decision-making. *Neural Netw*, **19**(8), 1255–65.

Samejima, K., Ueda, Y., Doya, K., and Kimura, M. (2005). Representation of action-specific reward values in the striatum. *Science*, **310**(5752), 1337–40.

Schultz, W., Dayan, P., and Montague, P. R. (1997). A neural substrate of prediction and reward. *Science*, **275**(5306), 1593–99.

Summerfield, C., Egner, T., Mangels, J., and Hirsch, J. (2006). Mistaking a house for a face: neural correlates of misperception in healthy humans. *Cereb Cortex*, **16**(4), 500–8.

Tobler, P. N., O'Doherty, J. P., Dolan, R. J., and Schultz, W. (2007). Reward value coding distinct from risk attitude-related uncertainty coding in human reward systems. *J Neurophysiol*, **97**(2), 1621–32.

Yamamoto, M., Okuda, J., Samejima, K., and Sakagami, M. (2007) Differential reward prediction on salient and uncertain perception as revealed by random dot motion stimuli and fMRI. *Soc Neurosci Abstr* 311.12.

Chapter 9

Model-based analysis of decision variables

Kenji Doya, Makoto Ito, and Kazuyuki Samejima

Abstract

When determining the neural correlates of decision making, a major difficulty is the non-stationarity of the brain's response. The evaluation of the same action should vary over time depending on the subject's choice and reward history. The speed at which such subjective evaluations changes should differ among subjects, or even in the same subject in different sessions. A recently emerging paradigm for coping with this difficulty is to estimate the time course of the internal variables of a mathematical model of decision making from each subject's sequence of stimuli, actions, and obtained rewards in each experimental session, and use that as a marker for detecting the neurons or brain regions implicated. This chapter reviews mathematical models describing the adaptive process of decision making, computational methods for estimating the model variables from observed data, and examples of applications of such model-based analysis to behavioral tests, neural recording, and functional brain imaging.

9.1 **Introduction**

What makes the study of decision making difficult and interesting is its voluntary and subjective nature. The evaluation of action candidates keeps changing depending on past actions, the resulting outcomes, and the subject's own needs. In the studies of information coding in the brain, the most successful way has been to correlate the neural signals, such as single-neuron firing and MRI signals, with sensory stimuli and motor outputs (Fig. 9.1). The classic examples are identification of stimulus tuning of visual cortical neurons (Hubel, 1959) and direction tuning of motor cortical neurons (Georgopoulos et al., 1986; Kakei et al., 1999). By sufficient pre-training of sensory-motor mapping, it is possible to assess the neural correlates of subjective interpretation of ambiguous sensory stimuli (Newsome et al., 1989) and visuo-spatial targets of motor output (Kakei et al., 1999). However, in trying to find the neural correlates of highly adaptive cognitive processes like decision making, a major difficulty is the non-stationarity of the brain's response.

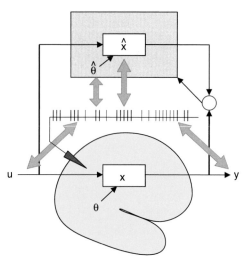

Fig. 9.1 The paradigm of learning model-based analysis of neural signal. Search for neural correlates of sensory perception and motor action can be done by seeking correlation with the sensory stimulus u and motor output y. To search for the neural correlates of the brain's internal variable x or the parameters that affect the dynamics θ, we assume a dynamic of model of adaptation, estimate its internal variables and parameters, and seek any correlation with then in the neural signal.

For example, the evaluation of the same action should vary over time, depending on the subject's choice and reward history and the speed at which such subjective evaluations change should differ among subjects, or even in the same subject in different sessions. How can we keep track of such a moving target in the subject's brain and find any signal that represents it?

This is exactly the motivation behind the recent trend of using mathematical models of the brain's adaptive process for the analysis of behaviors, neural recording, and functional brain imaging data (Daw and Doya, 2006; Corrado and Doya, 2007). The main idea is to estimate the time course of the internal variables of a mathematical model of decision making from each subject's sequence of stimuli, actions, and rewards in each experimental session and use that as the fingerprint for detecting the responsible neurons or brain regions.

Below we will overview the mathematical models that describe the adaptive process of decision making, the computational methods for estimating the model variables from observed data, and the examples of application of such model-based analysis to behavioral tests, neural recording, and function brain imaging.

9.2 Modeling frameworks

In capturing the process of decision making, the framework of the Markov decision process (Sutton and Barto, 1998) is the simplest and most widely applicable. In this framework, a subject observes the state s of the world, selects an action a, and receives a reward r, and the world state changes to s'. The subject aims to find a mapping from each state to an action, called a policy, that maximizes the expected amount of forthcoming rewards. In an animal experiment, the state may be notified by a light in a box, the action can be a lever press, and the reward would be a food pellet. In human economic decisions, the state would be the subject's needs and budget, the action is a purchase of a good, and the reward is the benefit enjoyed minus the price paid. Below we overview representative models that describe how a subject changes its action policy depending on its past experience.

9.2.1 Markov models

One way of modeling a subject's choice sequence is to consider it as an output of a higher order Markov model (Ito and Doya, 2009). In general, the subject's action $a(t)$ at time t can depend on the sequence of all the past states, actions, and rewards $\{s(1), a(1), r(1), s(2), a(2), r(2),\ldots, s(t{-}1), a(t{-}1), r(t{-}1)\}$. However, as the memory of a subject should not be infinite, it is reasonable to assume that the choice $a(t)$ depends mostly on recent states, actions, and rewards. Suppose there are m possible actions $\{1,\ldots,m\}$ and n possible states $\{1,\ldots,n\}$, we can store how many times each action a was taken at state s, $N(a,s)$, in a table and estimate the action choice probability[1] as:

$$P(a|s) = N(a, s)/\Sigma_{i=1}^{m} N(i, s). \tag{9.1}$$

This is the simplest Markov model that takes into account only the present state. We can consider an augmented model that takes into account the action and the reward the subject experienced previously at the same state:

$$P(a|s, a_1, r_1) = N(a, s, a_1, r_1)/\Sigma_{i=1}^{m} N(i, s, a_1, r_1), \tag{9.2}$$

where $N(a, s, a', r)$ is the number of choice a at state s after a previous choice a_1 resulted in a reward r_1 at the same state. This is the first order Markov model. By taking into account even more previous experiences at the state, $P(a|s, a_1, r_1, a_2, r_2)$, $P(a|s, a_1, r_1, a_2, r_2, a_3, r_3),\ldots$ higher order Markov models can capture arbitrary rule of choice probability change. However, an obvious problem is that the counting table becomes huge as we increase the number of past experiences considered, and there is a possibility of overfitting with a limited number of data.

9.2.2 Reinforcement learning models

While the Markov model is a purely descriptive model of choice sequence, the reinforcement learning model is a normative model that has been proven to derive a policy that maximizes the acquired reward (Sutton and Barto, 1998; Doya, 2007). The criterion of reinforcement learning is the expected cumulative future rewards:

$$R = E[r(t) + \gamma\, r(t{+}1) + \gamma^2\, r(t{+}2) +\ldots], \tag{9.3}$$

where $E[]$ represents the average over experience given by a certain policy. The parameter γ is called the *temporal discount factor*. If $\gamma{=}0$, only the immediate reward $r(t)$ is considered. As γ is increased closer to one, further future rewards are taken into account.

---

[1] N is often incremented by one for a better estimate under small samples.

Among a number of algorithms of reinforcement learning, so-called "Q-learning" is the most popular one. The main machinery in Q-learning is called the *action value function Q(s,a)*, which is an estimate of the cumulative future rewards after taking action *a* at state *s*. Given an accurate action value function, the optimal action policy is to take an action *a* that gives the largest value of $Q(s,a)$ at each state *s*. However, when the action value is not completely learned, it is better to take some exploratory actions. A common way, inspired by statistical physics, is to consider the action value as a negative energy and take an action in proportion to the exponential of the action value:

$$P(a \mid s) = \exp[\beta Q(s,a)] / \sum_{i=1}^{m} \exp[\beta Q(s,i)]. \tag{9.4}$$

Here, the denominator is to normalize the action selection probability so that it sums up to one. This is called the *softmax* or *Boltzmann* action selection and the gain parameter β is called the *inverse temperature*. If $\beta = 0$, since $\exp[0] = 1$, all actions are taken randomly with probability $1/m$, corresponding to a very high temperature. As the coefficient β is increased, any small difference in the action value is magnified and the action with the largest expected reward is taken with probability close to one. This is a greedy or exploitative action selection. For the simplest case of two actions, the softmax function reduces to a sigmoid function of the difference of two action values:

$$P(a_1|s) = 1/(1 + \exp[-\beta (Q(s,a_1) - Q(s,a_2))])$$

and the inverse temperature β determines the slope of the sigmoid function.

After an action is taken and a reward (positive, negative, or zero) is received, the action value is updated according to the inconsistency of the action values of consecutive states. In Q-learning, the inconsistency is given by:

$$\delta(t) = r(t) + \gamma \max_{a'} Q(s(t+1),a') - Q(s(t),a(t)), \tag{9.5}$$

which is the difference between the reward prediction before action, $Q(s(t),a(t))$, and the sum of the reward acquired, $r(t)$, and the maximal reward further expected, $\max_{a'} Q(s(t+1),a')$ after the action. This called the *temporal difference (TD) error*. The action value for the chosen action is then updated by the *delta rule*:

$$Q(s(t),a(t)) := Q(s(t),a(t)) + \alpha \, \delta(t), \tag{9.6}$$

where α is the *learning rate* parameter.

The action values are usually stored in a n-by-m matrix Q and the components of the matrix is updated by the learning eqns (9.5) and (9.6). The Q-learning algorithm has three major parameters: the learning rate α, the inverse temperature β, and the temporal discount factor γ. These are often called *meta-parameters* because they specify how the regular parameters, the components of the matrix Q, change by learning (Doya, 2002).

There are several variants of action value-based reinforcement learning models. For action selection, ϵ-*greedy* is another popular way of exploration, in which a random action is selected at probability ϵ and otherwise the action with the highest action value is selected. Another action selection method is the *matching law*:

$$P(a|s) = Q(s, a)/\Sigma_{i=1}^{m} Q(s, i), \qquad (9.7)$$

in which each action is selected in proportion to the expected amount of reward (Sugrue et al., 2004). This is overly exploratory in the Markovian setting, but is optimal in a harvesting problem, in which a reward persists with an action until harvested.

The update of action values by (9.6) is usually applied only to the selected action and the action values for actions not chosen stay fixed. A variant is to introduce forgetting of action values that were not chosen (Barraclough et al., 2004; Ito and Doya, 2009).

9.3 Estimation methods

Given a dynamic model of decision making and behavioral data of individual subjects, how can we estimate the time course of its variables, such as the action value function, the TD errors, and the parameters of learning (as summarized in Table 9.1)? Below are basic strategies for doing such model fitting to the data. After model fitting, an essential process before utilizing them for analysis is validation of the model and comparison of alternative models.

9.3.1 A priori choice

In some studies, the time course of the variables of a learning model is estimated by a priori assumptions on the learning parameters. For example, in a seminal fMRI study that revealed the TD-error related activity in the ventral striatum and the orbitofrontal cortex (O'Doherty et al., 2003), the authors took a fixed set of parameters common to all subjects (e.g., learning rate $\alpha = 0.2$). This arbitrary choice was justified by verifying that the result was robust under different choices of the parameter.

In another imaging experiment that revealed the ventro-dorsal segregation within the striatum in terms of the time scale of reward prediction (Tanaka et al., 2004), the authors set six different levels of the temporal discount factor γ and computed the time course of the value function and the TD error, and used them as the regressors for the BOLD signals. They assumed an optimal scheduling of learning rate (α decays hyperbolically).

9.3.2 Maximum likelihood estimation

A standard way of fitting the model parameters to observed data is the maximum likelihood estimation. Given a series of state, action and reward until t-th trial $y(1:t) = \{s(1),$

Table 9.1 Major variables and parameters in reinforcement learning models

Symbol	Name	Meaning
$Q(s,a)$	action value function	predicted reward by taking action a at state s
δ	temporal difference error	inconsistency in reward prediction
α	learning rate	rate of update of memory by new experience
β	inverse temperature	sensitivity of choice to predicted reward
γ	temporal discount factor	exponential weight to future rewards

$a(1)$, $r(1)$,…,$s(t)$, $a(t)$, $r(t)$}, we can compute the time course of the action values {$Q(1)$,…,$Q(t)$} by the learning eqns (9.5) and (9.6) for a set of parameters $\theta = (\alpha, \beta, \gamma)$. The initial action values are often set as zero, meaning no expectation, but they can also be tuned as a part of the parameters. For a given new state $s(t+1)$, we can predict the action selection probability $P(a|s(t+1); y(1:t), \theta)$ for each action candidate from $Q(t)$, β, and the action selection rule (9.4). Given the actual choice by the subject $a(t+1)$, the fitness of the model with the parameter setting is measured by $P(a(t+1)|s(t+1); y(1:t), \theta)$, which is called the *likelihood* when considered as the function of the parameter θ. For a series of T actions, the average log likelihood:

$$L(\theta) = 1/T \sum_{t=1}^{T} \log P(a(t)|s(t); y(1:t-1), \theta) \qquad (9.8)$$

is the standard measure of the fitness of the parameter θ to the subject's choice data. For a given model, the set of parameters θ that gives the maximum of the average log likelihood, or the maximum likelihood estimate (MLE), can be found by scanning the parameter space with a certain mesh grid, or using function maximization algorithms like gradient ascent or genetic algorithms.

9.3.3 Dynamic Bayesian filters

One assumption in the maximum likelihood method above is that the parameters are fixed during the experimental session, which may or may not be true. If not, how can we keep track of the moving parameters? This is a problem encountered in target tracking, such as following the trajectory of an aircraft despite noisy radar signals. The most popular solution is the dynamic Bayesian filters (Bishop, 2006).

In the Bayesian framework, we assume a certain model of how the hidden variable x evolves, $P(x'|x)$, and how the observation depends on the hidden variables, $P(y|x)$, and estimate the probability distribution of $x(t)$ given the observable variables $y(1:t) =$ {$y(1)$,…,$y(t)$} in an iterative way:

Prediction of $x(t+1)$ from $x(t)$:

$$P(x(t+1)|y(1:t)) \propto \int P(x(t+1)|x(t)) \, P(x(t)|y(1:t)) \, dx(t). \qquad (9.9)$$

Correction of $x(t+1)$ with a new observation $y(t+1)$:

$$P(x(t+1)|y(1:t+1)) \propto P(y(t+1)|x(t+1)) \, P(x(t+1)|y(1:t)). \qquad (9.10)$$

The first equation predicts the probability distribution of the hidden variables given our assumption about how they change. The second equation takes the result of prediction as the prior distribution and trims it down in reference to the likelihood given a new observation $y(t+1)$, which produces a new posterior distribution of the hidden variable $x(t+1)$ given the past observations $y(1:t+1)$.

In the decision-making model, the hidden variables are the action values and the parameters, $x = (Q, \alpha, \beta, \gamma)$, and the observable variables are the state, action, and reward, $y = (s, a, r)$ (Fig. 9.2). The learning eqns. (9.5) and (9.6) define the transition of the action values Q. For the parameters (α, β, γ), we can assume a Gaussian random walk model that allows

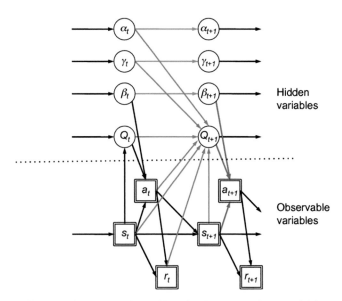

Fig. 9.2 Bayesian inference of the internal variables of a decision-making model (Samejima et al., 2004). The prior probability of the hidden variables is given by the learning rule (red arrows) and a random walk model (orange arrows). They are used for prediction of the next action (green arrows). The actual action by the subject gives the likelihood of the hidden variables (green arrows backward). The combination of the prior probability and the likelihood by the Bayes' rule gives a new posterior probability of the internal variables.

gradual shift in the parameters with a small variance parameter. The likelihood of these variables for a given action is defined by the action choice eqn. (9.4). In general, the combined dynamics of the action values and the parameters are nonlinear and non-Gaussian. Thus Samejima et al. (2004) proposed the application of *particle filtering* (Doucet et al., 2001), which keeps track of the posterior distribution using a large population of sample points. Figure 9.3 shows an example of particle filtering for estimating the time course of the action values and the parameters in a binary choice task (Ito and Doya, 2009).

Daw et al. (2006) took a hybrid approach of using dynamic Bayesian filtering for the action values and the maximal likelihood estimate for the parameters. In this case, the dynamics of the action values given the parameters and the subject's data become linear, so that the use of the Kalman filter is possible. The main difference from the basic maximum likelihood method is to keep track of not only the action value, or mean reward, but also the variance of the reward, and use the variance to adjust the update of the action value.

9.3.4 Model validation and comparison

An important step, after estimating the variables of interest of a model, is to test if the model reasonably captures the process of decision making and to compare it with other possible models, to pick the best one. An obvious first step is to check if the average likelihood is better than the chance level or that for a heuristic strategy, such as simple repetitive actions or the *win–stay–lose–switch*.

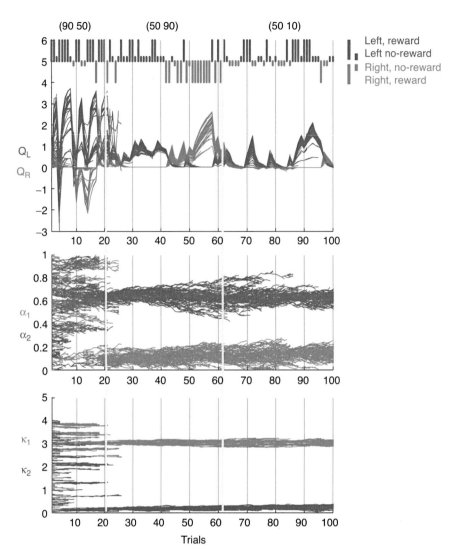

Fig. 9.3 Estimation of the time course of action values and parameters by particle filtering (Ito and Doya, 2009). There were 5000 particles, or imaginary subjects, initialized with the action values set as zero and the parameters uniformly distributed. Only 100 of them are plotted here for clarity. The particles move according to the learning rule and the random walk model and predict the action choice probability. Depending on the fitness with the real subject's choice, the particles are duplicated or discarded, so that the population of the particles keep track of the posterior distribution of the action values and the parameters. This model had two learning rates (α_1 for chosen action, α_2 for forgetting) and two parameters (κ_1 for reinforcement by a food pellet, κ_2 for aversion by no reward) in place of β.

When there are multiple models with the same level of complexity, the model with the highest maximum likelihood best captures the subject's behaviors. When we compare models of different complexities, we need to consider the risk of overfitting: a model with many parameters can replicate a particular set of data well, but does not generalize to new data. A convenient way of giving a penalty to complex models is *Akaike's* Information Criterion (AIC):

AIC $\propto$ – average log likelihood + number of parameters/number of data.

The validity of AIC is based on a number of assumptions, so it has to be used with care. In Bayesian inference, the normalizing denominator of the posterior probability, called the marginal likelihood or *evidence*, can be used as the criterion for model selection, although its exact computation is usually quite costly (Bishop, 2006).

A more general method for comparison of models is *cross validation*. When there are sufficient data, they are divided into two sets of comparable sizes, one for parameter setting, or training, and another for testing. The average log likelihood for the data not used for parameter setting is a reliable measure of predictive capability of the model. When the number of data is limited, so-called leave-one-out cross validation can be used.

9.4 Application to decision mechanisms

Here we review classic and recent (as of 2009) studies that utilized a model-based behavioral analysis paradigm for detecting the change in decision parameters, analysis of single-neuron activities, and analysis of fMRI signals.

9.4.1 Behavioral analysis

What makes decision making difficult is a number of tradeoffs. Should we stick to what we learned or should we forget it and adapt quickly to a new situation? Should we focus on what's happening immediately or consider what will come out in a long run? A virtue of reinforcement learning models is that these tradeoffs are resolved by the parameters, such as the learning rate α and the temporal discount factor γ. Estimation of these parameters can be an effective way of quantifying the change of decision strategies with the environmental setting and the subject's own needs.

9.4.1.1 Temporal discounting

Tanaka et al. (2006) devised a four-state Markov decision task and tested whether subjects' RL model parameters change with the change of the predictability of the environmental dynamics. By comparing two settings of the Markov process, "regular" condition with deterministic transition and "random" condition with totally random state transition, they found that the estimates of the temporal discount factor γ were significantly higher in the regular condition. This suggests that the subjects can tune their temporal focus of reward evaluation depending on the environment. Furthermore, Schweighofer et al. (2008) tested whether the decision parameters can be affected by the serotonergic system using acute tryptophan depletion and loading paradigm. They found that under the tryptophan depletion condition, where the synthesis of central serotonin is expected to be lower, the estimated discount factor was lower than in the control condition (Fig. 9.4). This is consistent with the hypothesis that the serotonergic system regulates temporal discounting (Doya, 2002).

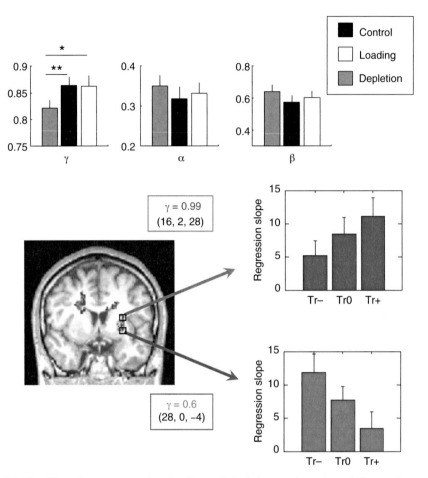

Fig. 9.4 The effect of acute tryptophan loading and depletion on the temporal discounting parameter and the brain activity correlated with the value function. By maximum likelihood estimation from the subjects' choice sequence in a dynamic inter-temporal choice task, a decrease in the temporal discount factor γ was detected under tryptophan depletion condition, in which the subjects' serotonergic function should have been reduced (Schweighofer et al., 2008). Using the value functions computed with different levels of the discount factor ($\gamma = 0.6$ and 0.99) as the regressors, activity loci were found in ventral and dorsal parts of the striatum. The activities correlated with the steeply discounted valuation in the ventral striatum and the very slowly discounted valuation in the dorsal striatum, were differentially affected by tryptophan loading and depletion (Tanaka et al., 2007).

9.4.1.2 Exploration

Luksys et al. (2009) studied how mice genotypes, phenotypes, stress, motivation, and noradrenergic drugs affect decision parameters. By fitting a reinforcement learning model to the mice performance in a nose poking task, they estimated the change of the parameters α, β, and γ during the courses of training. While stress during training made the mice more exploitative with a higher β, stress before training made the mice more explorative with a lower β. Pharmacological reduction of the noradrenergic level made the mice less impulsive with a higher γ and more explorative with a lower β. specifically in the anxious DBA/2 strain. Increase in the noradrenergic level made the mice more impulsive with a lower γ. The result showed that the anxious genotype, stress, and increased noradrenergic transmission cause more impulsive and exploitative behaviors.

9.4.1.3 Learning rate

Behrens et al. (2007) tested whether the volatility of the environment affects the subjects' learning rates. Bayesian estimation of the parameter revealed that the learning rate α was larger in the environment where the expected rewards for two choice cues change rapidly over time. Frank et al. (2009) applied the model-based estimation framework for behavioral analysis of different genetic groups. They found that subjects with DARPP-32 T/T genotype, which facilitates the D1-type dopamine receptor system in the striatum, have higher learning rates for reward gains, while subjects with DRD2 T/T genotype, which facilitates D2 receptor system in the striatum, have higher learning rates for reward losses. Subjects with COMT met genotype, which facilitates dopamine functions in the prefrontal cortex, have higher rates of uncertainty-based exploration.

9.4.2 Neural recording

Trial-by-trial estimation of the decision variables has turned out to be a quite effective tool for characterizing the neural firing recorded in decision-making tasks.

9.4.2.1 Action value

Samejima et al. (2005) trained monkeys to perform a choice task with different reward probabilities for left and right lever turns. They estimated the time course of action values by the Bayesian inference framework (Samejima et al., 2004) and showed that the monkeys' choices were well predicted by a Q-learning model. Through trial-by-trial regression analysis of neural firing before action initiation, they showed that more than one-third of the neurons in the striatum was selective to an action value.

Sugrue et al. (2004) used a reward harvesting task and showed that the monkeys' saccadic choice performance was well predicted by a local matching law, in which action choice probabilities are proportional to the action values. They found that the parietal cortical neurons changed their firing depending on the estimated action values. Other studies also found neural firing correlated with action values in the dorsal striatum (Lau and Glimcher, 2007, 2008), the parietal cortex (Seo et al., 2009), and the prefrontal cortex (Kim et al., 2008). The nucleus accumbens of rodents has been suggested to play an important role in reward-oriented behaviors based on lesion studies. However, model-based analysis of neuron recording data showed that remarkably few neurons in the nucleus accumbens encode action values (Kim et al., 2007; Ito and Doya, 2009).

9.4.2.2 TD error

Dopamine neurons have been shown to encode the TD error (Schultz et al., 1997). However, Nakahara et al. (2004) analyzed the dopamine neuron activity during a reward-biased saccade task based on a reinforcement learning model and found a subtle inconsistency with the standard TD learning model. By incorporating the fact that the reward was given only once in each four-trial block in that task, the dopamine neuron firing was better modeled, suggesting that the monkey's brain could capture the hidden dynamic structure of the task. In a delayed saccade task in which the most rewarding timing of saccade was varied, Bayer et al. (2007) analyzed the dopamine neuron firing by multiple regression with rewards in previous trials. As a result, they found nearly exponential weighting on previous rewards, which is consistent with the update of the value function by the delta rule (9.6).

9.4.3 Functional brain imaging

9.4.3.1 Temporal discounting

In a series of fMRI studies on the regulation of temporal discount factor, Tanaka and colleagues (Tanaka et al., 2004, 2006, 2007) showed a functional dissociation within the striatum; the ventral part of the striatum is involved in prediction of immediate rewards (small γ) and the dorsal part of the striatum is involved in prediction of long-term rewards (large γ). Using the tryptophan depletion and loading method, they further showed that the ventral activity correlated with short-term reward prediction is facilitated under lower serotonin function and that the dorsal activity correlated with long-term reward prediction is facilitated under higher serotonin function (Fig. 9.4). Such a differential regulation of short- and long-term reward prediction could be a mechanism of regulation of the temporal discount factor by serotonin (Doya, 2002).

In inter-temporal choice tasks using imagined rewards (e.g., $20 now vs $21 tomorrow), one group of researchers found correlates of immediate reward choices with the ventral striatum and delay-independent choices in the prefrontal cortex (McClure et al., 2004). Another group reported that the activity of the ventral striatum and the medial prefrontal cortex is correlated with the subjectively discounted value, despite the wide subject-wise discrepancy of the rate of discounting (Kable and Glimcher, 2007).

9.4.3.2 Exploration

Daw et al. (2006) analyzed the brain substrate for exploratory behaviors in a four-armed banded task. By comparing three different models of exploration, they found a model with Boltzmann selection explained the subjects' data best. They then found that the activity of the medial prefrontal cortex is correlated with the choice probability of the action, meaning confident, exploitive actions. On the other hand, activities in the frontopolar cortex were correlated with exploratory trials in which an action with the second highest or lower action value was chosen.

In a related study with a binary choice task, (Hampton et al., 2006) showed that the subject's performance was better fit by a predictive model-based strategy, rather than by a simple reinforcement learning strategy. They found that medial PFC activity was higher in switch trials following one unrewarded trial, which is a feature of model-based decision making. The authors also found in the "inspector game" that the subjects' behaviors are best fit by an extended RL model called influential model, and that the expected value signal estimated by the model is correlated with the activation of the medial prefrontal cortex (Hampton et al., 2008).

9.4.3.3 Learning rate

In an aforementioned experiment on volatility (Behrens et al., 2007), the activity related to the environmental volatility and corresponding increase in the learning rate was correlated with the activity of the anterior cingulate cortex.

9.5 Future directions

As we reviewed above, the use of reinforcement learning models for characterization of individual behavioral data and analysis of neural recording and fMRI data has become increasingly popular over the last five years. There are a number of issues to be resolved to make the framework a reliable standard tool in neuroscience. First is the choice of the learning models and estimation methods. Researchers so far picked arbitrary combinations of the learning models and estimation methods, which makes the comparison of results from different groups difficult. The second is more systematic use of model validation and selection methods. One way for promoting standard procedures is to package them in a software tool. The brain-imaging community has benefitted profoundly with a standard tool like SPM (http://www.fil.ion.ucl.ac.uk/spm/), which did not only make the complex preprocessing and statistical testing procedures accessible to a wide range of researchers, but also helped standardize the analysis procedures.

References

Barraclough, D, J., Conroy, M,L., and Lee, D. (2004). Prefrontal cortex and decision making in a mixed-strategy game. *Nat Neurosci*, 7:404–10.

Bayer, H.M., Lau, B., and Glimcher, P.W. (2007). Statistics of midbrain dopamine neuron spike trains in the awake primate. *J Neurophysiol*, 98:1428–39.

Behrens, T.E., Woolrich, M.W., Walton, M.E., and Rushworth, M.F. (2007). Learning the value of information in an uncertain world. *Nat Neurosci*, 10:1214–21.

Bishop, C.M. (2006). *Pattern recognition and machine learning*. New York: Springer.

Corrado, G., and Doya, K. (2007). Understanding neural coding through the model-based analysis of decision making. *J Neurosci*, 27:8178–80.

Daw, N.D., and Doya, K. (2006). The computational neurobiology of learning and reward. *Curr Opin Neurobiol*, 16:199–204.

Daw, N.D., O'Doherty, J.P., Dayan. P., Seymour, B., and Dolan, R.J. (2006). Cortical substrates for exploratory decisions in humans. *Nature*, 441:876–79.

Doucet, A., Freitas, N.d., Gordon, N. (2001). *Sequential Monte Carlo methods in practice*. New York: Springer.

Doya, K. (2002). Metalearning and neuromodulation. *Neural Netw,* 15:495–506.

Doya, K. (2007). Reinforcement learning: computational theory and biological mechanisms. *HFSP Journal,* 1:30–40.

Frank, M.J., Doll, B.B., Oas-Terpstra, J., and Moreno, F. (2009). Prefrontal and striatal dopaminergic genes predict individual differences in exploration and exploitation. *Nat Neurosci,* 8:1062–8.

Georgopoulos, A.P., Schwartz, A.B., and Kettner, R.E. (1986). Neuronal population coding of movement direction. *Science,* 233:1416–9.

Hampton, A.N., Bossaerts, P., and O'Doherty, J.P. (2006). The role of the ventromedial prefrontal cortex in abstract state-based inference during decision making in humans. *J Neurosci,* 26:8360–67.

Hampton, A.N., Bossaerts, P., and O'Doherty, J.P. (2008). Neural correlates of mentalizing-related computations during strategic interactions in humans. *Proc Natl Acad Sci USA,* 105:6741–46.

Hubel, D.H., and Wiesel, T. N. (1959). Receptive fields of single neurones in the cat's striate cortex. *J Physiol,* 148:574–91.

Ito, M., and Doya, K. (2009). Validation of decision making models and analysis of decision variables in the rat basal ganglia. *J Neurosci,* 29:9861–74.

Kable, J.W., and Glimcher, P.W. (2007). The neural correlates of subjective value during intertemporal choice. *Nat Neurosci,* 10:1625–33.

Kakei, S., Hoffman, D.S., and Strick, P.L. (1999). Muscle and movement representations in the primary motor cortex. *Science,* 285:2136–39.

Kim, Y.B., Huh, N., Lee, H., Baeg, E.H., Lee, D., and Jung, M.W. (2007). Encoding of action history in the rat ventral striatum. *J Neurophysiol,* 98:3548–56.

Kim, S., Hwang, J., and Lee, D. (2008). Prefrontal coding of temporally discounted values during intertemporal choice. *Neuron,* 59:161–72.

Lau, B., and Glimcher, P.W. (2007). Action and outcome encoding in the primate caudate nucleus. *J Neurosci,* 27:14502–14.

Lau, B., Glimcher, P.W. (2008). Value representations in the primate striatum during matching behavior. *Neuron,* 58:451–63.

Luksys, G., Gerstner, W., and Sandi, C. (2009). Stress, genotype and norepinephrine in the prediction of mouse behavior using reinforcement learning. *Nat Neurosci,* 12:1180–6.

McClure, S.M., Laibson, D.I., Loewenstein, G., and Cohen, J.D. (2004). Separate neural systems value immediate and delayed monetary rewards. *Science,* 306:503–7.

Nakahara, H., Itoh, H., Kawagoe, R., Takikawa, Y., and Hikosaka, O. (2004). Dopamine neurons can represent context-dependent prediction error. *Neuron,* 41:269–80.

Newsome, W.T., Britten, K.H., and Movshon, J.A. (1989). Neuronal correlates of a perceptual decision. *Nature,* 341:52–4.

O'Doherty, J.P., Dayan, P., Friston, K., Critchley, H., and olan, R.J. (2003). Temporal difference models and reward-related learning in the human brain. *Neuron,* 38:329–37.

Samejima, K., Doya, K., Ueda, Y., and Kimura, M. (2004). *Advances in neural processing systems 16.* Cambridge, Massachusetts, London, England: The MIT Press.

Samejima, K., Ueda, Y., Doya, K., and Kimura, M. (2005). Representation of action-specific reward values in the striatum. *Science,* 310:1337–40.

Schultz, W., Dayan, P., and Montague, P.R. (1997). A neural substrate of prediction and reward. *Science,* 275:1593–99.

Schweighofer, N., Bertin, M., Shishida, K., Okamoto, Y., Tanaka, S.C., Yamawaki, S., and Doya, K. (2008). Low-serotonin levels increase delayed reward discounting in humans. *J Neurosci,* 28:4528–32.

Seo, H., Barraclough, D.J., and Lee, D. (2009). Lateral intraparietal cortex and reinforcement learning during a mixed-strategy game. *J Neurosci,* 29:7278–89.

Sugrue, L.P., Corrado, G.S., and Newsome, W.T. (2004). Matching behavior and the representation of value in the parietal cortex. *Science,* **304**:1782–87.

Sutton, R.S., Barto, A.G. (1998). *Reinforcement learning.* Cambridge, MA: MIT Press.

Tanaka, S.C., Doya, K., Okada, G., Ueda, K., Okamoto, Y., and Yamawaki, S. (2004). Prediction of immediate and future rewards differentially recruits cortico-basal ganglia loops. *Nat Neurosci,* **7**:887–93.

Tanaka, S.C., Samejima, K., Okada, G., Ueda, K., Okamoto, Y., Yamawaki, S., and Doya, K. (2006). Brain mechanism of reward prediction under predictable and unpredictable environmental dynamics. *Neural Netw,* **19**:1233–41.

Tanaka, S.C., Schweighofer, N., Asahi, S., Shishida, K., Okamoto, Y., Yamawaki, S., and Doya, K. (2007). Serotonin differentially regulates short- and long-term prediction of rewards in the ventral and dorsal striatum. *PLoS ONE,* **2**:e1333.

Chapter 10

Reversal learning in fronto-striatal circuits: a functional, autonomic, and neurochemical analysis

H.F. Clarke and A.C. Roberts

Abstract

The orbitofrontal cortex (OFC) is intimately associated with the processes underlying behavioral flexibility that allow us to successfully interact with our ever-changing environment. Dysfunction within the OFC and its associated circuitry, including the striatum and amygdala, is an important feature of many psychiatric disorders in which behavioral inflexibility is a prominent symptom. The discrimination reversal learning task is a commonly used test of behavioral flexibility, and impaired performance on this test is not only associated with damage to the OFC in rats, monkeys, and humans, but has also been described in patients suffering from a variety of neuropsychiatric disorders, including schizophrenia and psychopathy. In addition, reversal learning-related hypofunction within the OFC may act as a vulnerability marker for obsessive-compulsive disorder. This chapter discusses the role of the OFC in reversal learning from an anatomical, motivational, and neurochemical perspective. The effect of OFC lesions on discrimination reversal learning in monkeys and rats is reviewed, along with the anatomical and psychological issues arising from these studies. Evidence is provided that supports a role for the OFC in adapting the autonomic, as well as the behavioral, responses in reversal learning, with consideration of the relevance of these results to the emotional uncoupling reported in a number of psychiatric disorders. The monoaminergic modulation of the OFC, and, in particular, the dissociable roles of dopamine and serotonin in behavioral flexibility, are discussed in the context of their relationship to current psychiatric treatments. Finally, the roles of the striatum and amygdala are evaluated in the light of recent findings highlighting the role of serotonin and dopamine in modulating the effectiveness of prefrontal top-down control of these structures.

10.1 **Introduction**

Dysfunction within the orbitofrontal cortex (OFC) and related circuitry, including the striatum and amygdala, has been implicated in a number of neuropsychiatric disorders including depression, schizophrenia, and a variety of anxiety disorders, including obsessive-compulsive disorder (OCD; Saxena and Rauch, 2000; Drevets, 2007; Milad and Rauch, 2007; Chamberlain et al., 2008; Floresco et al., 2008). This dysfunction is thought to contribute to both the negative symptoms seen in depression, schizophrenia, and anxiety, and the compulsive responding of OCD patients. Current treatments for these affective and compulsive symptoms are drugs that primarily target the monoaminergic nuclei, a group of chemically specific neurons residing in the brainstem that provide widespread monoaminergic innervation of OFC circuitry (Ichikawa and Meltzer, 1999; Saxena et al., 1999; Meltzer et al., 2003; Cowen, 2008). Not only is this circuitry innervated by the monoamines, but reciprocal pathways enable this circuitry to modulate the monoaminergic activity in turn (Porrino and Goldman-Rakic, 1982; Sesack et al., 1989; Holets, 1990; Gaykema et al., 1991; Mesulam and Geula, 1992; Azmitia and Whitaker-Azmitia, 1995; Zaborszky et al., 1997; Jodo et al., 1998; Celada et al., 2001). Thus, an understanding of the interaction between the monoamines and these structures is of particular relevance to our understanding of the overall functioning of the circuit and the underlying causes and treatment of the psychiatric disorders mentioned above.

In addition to monoaminergic regulation, activity in this OFC-striatal-amygdala circuitry is also affected by peripheral states of arousal, mood, and emotion via reciprocal connections with regions involved in the monitoring of our internal state, including the hypothalamus (Ongur and Price, 2000; Barbas, 2007) and insular cortex (Craig, 2002). Thus, along with its connections with other sensory processing regions, the OFC is in a position to integrate peripheral awareness of the animal's internal state with cognitive knowledge of the motivational and emotional meaning of stimuli in the outside world, enabling animals to respond appropriately to motivationally salient stimuli. It has been proposed that mismatches between these signals may contribute to the aberrant behavior and negative symptoms of disorders such as anxiety, schizophrenia, and autism (Pantelis et al., 1999; Bachevalier and Loveland, 2006; Paulus and Stein, 2006).

Whilst damage to the OFC has been reported to disrupt complex decision making, it can also disrupt behavior in remarkably simple situations. Thus, lesions of the OFC in rats have been shown to disrupt the acquisition, but not expression, of a food-approach response in Pavlovian conditioning (Chudasama and Robbins, 2003). Another relatively simple behavior, that of re-directing responding from one stimulus to another, based upon a change in reward contingencies (discrimination reversal learning) has been shown to be impaired in rats (Schoenbaum et al., 2002; Chudasama and Robbins, 2003), monkeys (Jones and Mishkin, 1972; Dias et al., 1996; Izquierdo et al., 2003), and humans (Rolls et al., 1994; Fellows and Farah, 2003; Hornak et al., 2004) alike, following damage to the OFC. Such reversal learning deficits are also apparent in schizophrenics (Pantelis et al., 1999), cocaine addicts (Ersche et al., 2008), and children and adults with psychopathic traits (Blair et al., 2001; Budhani and Blair, 2005). Moreover, reversal learning related hypofunction has been reported in OCD patients and healthy first-degree relatives, which may act as a vulnerability marker or endophenotype for OCD (Menzies et al., 2007; Chamberlain et al., 2008). Given the relevance of OFC-dependent reversal learning to our understanding of a variety of neuropsychiatric conditions, this paper will consider reversal learning from a functional, autonomic, and neurochemical perspective.

10.2 Discrimination reversal learning and the OFC

In a typical reversal learning task, animals are initially presented with two stimuli, one of which is always associated with reward, the other, never associated with reward. Usually, the animal has to respond to the reward-associated stimulus in order to gain access to the reward (instrumental version). Once the animal has learnt the discrimination and is responding primarily to the rewarded stimulus, the contingencies are reversed and the previously unrewarded stimulus is now rewarded and vice versa. The OFC-induced deficit is seen at the reversal stage of the task. There have been a number of hypotheses as to the nature of the underlying deficit responsible for the OFC lesion-induced reversal impairment. For example, there is accumulating evidence for a role of the OFC in predicting specific outcomes based on their relationship with discrete environmental cues. Electrophysiological studies in primates and rats have identified outcome-related neural activity in the OFC (Thorpe et al., 1983; Schoenbaum et al., 1998; Tremblay and Schultz, 2000). In addition, lesions of the OFC abolish the sensitivity of conditioned approach behavior to both outcome devaluation (Gallagher et al., 1999; Pickens et al., 2003; Pickens et al., 2005) and stimulus–outcome contingency degradation in rats (Ostlund and Balleine, 2007), and similarly disrupt the ability of rhesus monkeys to alter their selection of specific objects as a consequence of reinforcer devaluation (Izquierdo et al., 2004). Thus, it has been suggested that a loss of outcome prediction may underlie disrupted reversal learning, as old, associative encoding in other brain regions would be slow to be updated when actual outcomes no longer match expectations (Schoenbaum et al., 2007). Whilst plausible, it should be noted that a recent study investigating the effects of localized lesions within rhesus monkey OFC, restricted to areas 11 and 13 (Fig. 10.1a), has shown that insensitivity to reinforcer devaluation can occur in the absence of deficits in discrimination reversal (Kazama and Bachevalier, 2009). Thus, if behavioral insensitivity to reward devaluation reflects the role of the OFC in acquiring and maintaining predictions of outcome value, then this function may not play an essential role in reversal learning. This single dissociation highlights the fact that the OFC is made up of a number of cytoarchitectonically distinct regions in rats, monkeys, and humans (Carmichael and Price, 1994; Petrides and Pandya, 1994; Preuss, 1995; Ongur and Price, 2000) that may also be functionally dissociable. Moreover, homology between subregions of rat and monkey OFC have yet to be identified (see Uylings et al., 2003). Whilst, to date, only a handful of studies have directly compared the effects of lesions to distinct regions within the OFC, those that have, report differential effects. Thus, medial and lateral OFC lesions in rats augment and attenuate, respectively, cocaine-primed reinstatement of responding

Evaluation of the OFC on reversal learning:
variations in lesion location in rhesus monkeys and rats

(a) Rhesus monkey studies

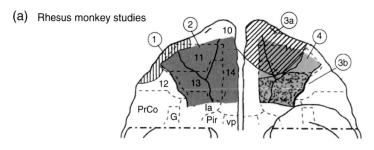

(b) Rat studies

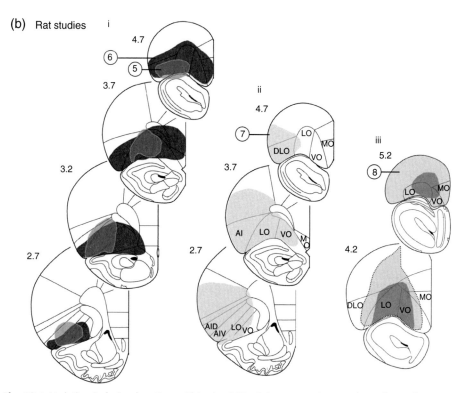

Fig. 10.1 Variation in lesion location within the OFC of rhesus monkeys and rats in studies investigating the role of the OFC in reversal learning. For illustrative purposes, lesions are depicted on one side of the brain only. In rhesus monkeys (a), lesions targeting area 12 (1) and areas 11/13/14 (2) disrupt reversal learning, whereas lesions that include areas 10/11 (3a), 13/Ia (3b) and 11/13 (4) are without effect. Cytoarchitectonic fields are as described by Carmichael and Price (1994). In rats (b), reversal learning is impaired by lesions restricted to (i) the lateral orbital (LO) region with partial damage to ventral orbital (VO), dorsolateral orbital (DLO) and agranular insula (AI) (5), as well as more extensive lesions of the LO, VO, medial orbital (MO), and AI (6). In addition, large lesions (ii) focusing on lateral regions including DLO, AI, dorsal AI (AID), and ventral AI (AIV) with partial damage to LO and VO also disrupt reversal learning (7). Finally, (iii) lesions focusing on LO and VO and partial damage to MO, DLO, and adjacent dorsal

Fig. 10.1 (*Contd*). regions of prefrontal cortex disrupt reversal learning (8). The region consistently damaged in all these studies is LO, although there is sparing of its most anterior extent in study 5 and 7. Prefrontal parcellation is as described by Paxinos and Watson (1997). (Note that area VLO is not shown on this particular parcellation. VLO includes the lateral part of VO and the medial part of LO.) Lesions have been re-drawn based on illustrations from their source studies. They vary as to whether they depict the largest lesion, a representative lesion or the area damaged in the majority of animals. 1, Butter (1969); 2, Izquierdo et al. (2004); 3, Butter (1969); 4, Kazama and Bachevalier (2009); 5, Depicts region that was lesioned in the majority of animals, Ferry et al., (2000); 6, Depicts largest lesion, Chudasama and Robbins (2003); 7, Depicts representative lesion, Schoenbaum et al., (2003); 8, Depicts smallest and largest lesion, McAlonan and Brown (2003).

(Fuchs et al., 2004). In addition, of particular relevance to the present discussion, the early studies of Butter and colleagues described different effects on reversal learning and extinction following lesions of lateral (area 12), anteromedial (areas 10 and 11), and posteromedial (areas 13/insula) orbitofrontal regions (Butter, 1969). Thus, while it is tempting to search for a single, unifying function of the OFC that may explain the entire repertoire of behavioral deficits associated with OFC damage, it is more likely that they are due to a number of related, but distinct processes, dependent upon specific regions of the OFC.

Indeed, evidence for differentiable functions within the OFC, while limited, raises the possibility that impaired reversal learning may itself be the product of multiple deficits. Thus, the most profound reversal learning impairments in rhesus monkeys occur following global ablations of the entire OFC (including areas 10,11,13,14, 47/12 and parts of area 45; Jones and Mishkin, 1972). In contrast, more selective deficits occur following ablations of 11/13/14 versus area 47/12 (Fig. 10.1a), which differ with respect to whether the deficits are relatively short-lasting, i.e., occur over the first one or two reversals only, and perseverative (persistent responding to the previously rewarded stimulus), or longer lasting i.e., present over seven or more reversals, and primarily non-perseverative in nature (Butter, 1969; Iversen and Mishkin, 1970; Izquierdo et al., 2004). This particular difference is quite striking and suggests that distinct processing within the lateral, versus more medial, regions of OFC are contributing differentially to reversal learning performance. However, area 47/12 not only encompasses cortex on the orbital surface but extends up into the inferior prefrontal convexity. Consequently it is unknown whether the reversal deficit in the Iversen and Mishkin study is indeed due to damage to the orbital part of area 47/12. This has not been resolved by functional neuroimaging studies of reversal learning as activations, specifically related to shifting responding from one stimulus to another following reversal of the contingencies, have been reported in both lateral OFC (O'Doherty et al., 2003; Hampshire and Owen, 2006), and more dorsally in the inferior prefrontal convexity (Cools et al., 2002; Budhani et al., 2007). Moreover, given the recent finding that a lesion of area 11/13 does not disrupt reversal learning (Kazama and Bachevalier, 2009), the deficit associated with damage to areas 11/13 and 14 combined (Iversen and Mishkin, 1970; Izquierdo et al., 2004), requires further investigation. Whilst the reversal deficit may be due to damage specifically to area 14, the region not included in the lesion of Kazama and Bachevalier (2009), an alternative explanation is that the deficit is only apparent following damage to all three regions. The latter would be consistent with the hypothesis that there are a number of different psychological processes that can contribute to reversal learning, including: (1) outcome prediction— both the incentive value of the outcome *and* the precise contingent relationship between the stimulus and the outcome (Ostlund and Balleine, 2007); (2) aspects of contextual integration that enable an animal to maintain multiple representations of a stimulus that has more than one meaning, as is the case for stimuli within a visual discrimination reversal task (Rescorla, 2001; Bouton, 2004); (3) the tracking and evaluation of outcomes associated with different stimuli across multiple trials, presumably dependent upon working memory processes (Walton et al., this volume); as well as (4) sensitivity to negative feedback, including non-reward. Reversal learning may only be impaired following OFC damage if a critical number of these processes are compromised.

Another relevant issue to this debate is the type of errors made on reversal learning tasks following OFC lesions, and whether they provide insight into the nature of the underlying impairment. As described above, Iversen and Mishkin (1970) were the first to demonstrate that a distinctive pattern of reversal deficits was associated with lesions of two neighboring regions on the orbitofrontal surface, including the inferior prefrontal convexity. We would suggest that such differences between error types are most informative for identifying the underlying mechanism of a reversal deficit, when comparing neural manipulations within (Iversen and Mishkin, 1970), or between, studies (Clarke et al., 2004, 2007, 2008) in which all other behavioral/task parameters, including the method of error analysis, are kept constant. Since the study by Iversen and Mishkin, there have been numerous studies reporting either perseverative or non-perseverative impairments in reversal learning following permanent damage to various sectors of the OFC in humans (Rolls et al., 1994; Fellows and Farah, 2003; Hornak et al., 2004), rhesus monkeys (Meunier et al., 1997; Izquierdo et al., 2004), marmosets (Dias et al., 1996; Clarke et al., 2008), and rats (Ferry et al., 2000; Chudasama and Robbins, 2003; McAlonan and Brown, 2003; Kim and Ragozzino, 2005; Boulougouris et al., 2007). However, in many cases, comparison has been difficult due to differences in (1) sensory modality (e.g. object/pattern, odor, spatial location), (2) task parameters (e.g. reversal within or between sessions; reversal embedded within an attentional set-shifting task or not), (3) overall task difficulty (e.g. errors made to learn the original discrimination can vary an order of magnitude between studies; compare Chudasama and Robbins, 2003; with McAlonan and Brown, 2003) and (4) classification of error types (ranging from statistical to non-statistical-based, e.g., compare Clarke et al. (2008) and Chudasama and Robbins (2003) with Boulougouris et al. (2007), Kim and Ragozzino (2005) and Ghods-Sharifi et al. (2008); it should be noted that where overall errors to criterion are quite low, then statistical methods cannot easily be used). The fact that reversal impairments are seen following OFC lesions in studies using different species, different sensory modalities, different tasks, and often differences in the overall location of the lesion within the OFC (see Fig. 10.1b for variation of OFC lesions in rats), highlights the overall robustness of the impairment, but it also adds further support to the hypothesis that reversal impairments may be the product of multiple deficits. However, the differences in the underlying pattern of errors between studies cannot easily be explained solely in terms of variations in lesion location, although the latter may well act as a contributory factor. An additional factor may be that of context. Thus, a loss of OFC function(s) can result in the emergence of perseverative responses that are inappropriate to the current situation and may well occur as a consequence of the loss of top-down regulation of subcortical response systems. The precise nature of the perseverative responses that emerge may depend upon which responses are the strongest in the context of a particular study and so, whilst they may be responses to the previously rewarded stimulus (Chudasama and Robbins, 2003; Boulougouris et al., 2007), they may instead be perseverative responses to a particular location (spatial response bias) or to a previously rewarded cue from an alternative perceptual dimension (Ghods-Sharifi et al., 2008). In addition, when perseverative responding to the previously rewarded stimulus is present on a two-stimulus discrimination reversal task, it may be due either to failure to inhibit responding to the previously rewarded stimulus, or alternatively, to marked avoidance of the previously unrewarded, but currently rewarded, stimulus, i.e., learned avoidance or learned non-reward (Clarke et al., 2007; Tait and Brown, 2007). The latter, however, may also be seen as "perseverative behavior" but in this case, perseveration of a previously learned avoidance response. Whether such perseverative responses are seen at all may also depend upon whether other regions of the prefrontal cortex, involved in behavioral regulation and top-down control, govern behavioral output in the absence of the OFC.

In summary, OFC lesion-induced reversal learning impairments may be the product of deficits in multiple psychological processes, including: (1) prediction of outcome value; (2) prediction of stimulus-outcome contingencies; (3) contextual processes supporting multiple stimulus representations; (4) working memory processes to track reinforcement across trials; and (5) sensitivity to negative feedback. There is limited evidence that loss of distinct functions within the OFC may cause distinct patterns of errors but this needs further investigation by direct comparison of selective lesions within OFC on the same reversal task. Where differences in error types are reported across different reversal tasks, difficulties in interpretation may be due, in part, to overall differences in task designs affecting which inappropriate responses emerge following a loss of top-down control. However, it is argued that, where differences in error type between two neural manipulations are seen in the same task and study, then this will provide insight into the differential contribution of those two neural manipulations. When stimulus bound, perseverative-like responding is seen, it will not only provide insight into the neural mechanisms underlying the top-down regulatory control of behavior, but also into the etiology and treatment of disease states in which perseverative responding is a symptom. It is the context in which perseverative responding is seen following OFC lesions that we turn to next.

10.3 Perseverative responding following OFC lesions in marmosets

Excitotoxic lesions of the OFC in marmosets do produce a reversal impairment that is primarily perseverative in nature (Dias et al., 1996; Clarke et al., 2008). Quinolinic acid lesions that targeted area 11 and anterior regions of area 13, as defined by Burman and Rosa (2009), impaired the ability of marmosets to learn a compound visual discrimination following reversal of the reward contingencies (Dias et al., 1996, 1997). The two discriminanda in these studies were each composed of two perceptual dimensions, blue shapes and white lines, but only exemplars from one of the dimensions was relevant to the task. For example, a response to one of the lines resulted in reward and a response to the other did not, whilst the shape exemplars were irrelevant. Whilst lesions of the OFC did not disrupt the ability of marmosets to perform an attentional shift, i.e., learn a new discrimination in which the previously relevant dimension became irrelevant, e.g., lines, and the previously irrelevant dimension became relevant, e.g., shapes, they did disrupt the ability to reverse responding between two exemplars from within a dimension (Dias et al., 1996, 1997). This reversal learning deficit was seen regardless of whether the reversal occurred before or after the animals had performed an attentional shift (Dias et al., 1997), was perseverative in nature, and was only seen when performing a reversal for the first time. Subsequent reversals, involving new stimuli, were not impaired. More recently, the effects of the same lesions have been investigated on a series of reversals of a pattern discrimination presented on a touch-sensitive computer screen. Here, signal detection theory (Macmillan and Creelman, 1991) was used to establish subjects' ability to discriminate correct from incorrect stimuli. The discrimination measure d' was calculated and the normal cumulative distribution function (CDF) compared with the criterion values of a two-tailed Z test (each tail $P = 0.05$) to determine the classification of each session (or part of a session) as perseveration, chance, or learning. Sessions in which CDF(d') ≤ 0.05 were classified as perseverative; sessions in which CDF(d') ≥ 0.95 were classified as learning, and sessions in which $0.05 \geq$ CDF(d') ≤ 0.95 were classified as chance (Clarke et al., 2004). This approach confirmed that overall, OFC-lesioned marmosets made significantly more perseverative, but not non-perseverative (chance or learning), errors to the previously-rewarded stimulus, compared to controls across all four reversals; although the deficit did appear to decline by the fourth reversal (Fig. 10.2a; Clarke et al., 2008).

In addition to discrimination reversal learning, the subsequent use of more naturalistic object-retrieval tasks, in which the animal has to modify the tendency to reach directly for a reward, have extended the view that the OFC causes a loss of stimulus-driven flexibility (Dias et al., 1996, 1997; Roberts and Wallis, 2000). Two types of such tasks have been investigated in the marmoset: the detour reaching and incongruent discrimination tasks. Unlike reversal learning, the detour-reaching task does not involve an alteration in the contingent relationship between the conditioned object/stimulus and reward. Instead the monkey is presented with a clear Perspex box containing a visible marshmallow reward. Access to the reward is at the side of the box and the monkey, therefore, has to learn this

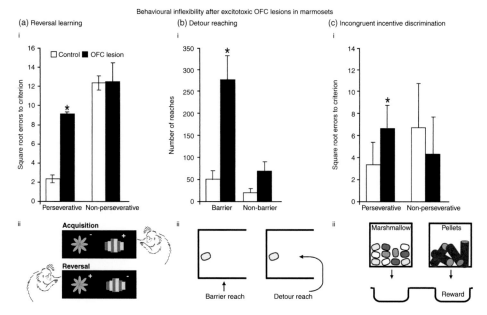

Behavioural inflexibility after excitotoxic OFC lesions in marmosets

(a) Reversal learning

(b) Detour reaching

(c) Incongruent incentive discrimination

Fig. 10.2 (a) Reversal learning. (a.i) Depicts the mean number of perseverative and non-perseverative errors (± SEM) made by monkeys with OFC lesions ($n = 3$) and control monkeys ($n = 4$) across a series of four serial reversals. In this task (a.ii), monkeys were required to respond to two abstract colored stimuli on a touch-sensitive computer screen. Through trial and error they learnt that a response to one stimulus ("+") earned reward, while a response to the other ("−") earned nothing. Once criterion was attained, the reward contingency was reversed and in order to continue gaining reward, marmosets were required to switch responding to the previously-incorrect stimulus and to cease responding to the previously-correct stimulus. They received four such reversals. Marmosets with OFC lesions persisted in responding to the previously-correct stimulus for much longer than controls, despite gaining no reward (*$P<0.05$), but did not differ in the number of non-perseverative errors. Adapted from figure 6, Clarke et al. (2008). (b) Detour reaching. (b.i) Depicts the mean number of "barrier" and "non-barrier" reaches (± SEM) made by monkeys with OFC lesions ($n = 6$) and control monkeys ($n = 6$) before they made two consecutive correct responses (detour reaches). In this task (b.ii), monkeys were required to inhibit the prepotent response to reach directly towards food reward in a transparent box (barrier reach), and instead to make a detour reach around the open side of the box in order to retrieve the food. A reach around the "closed" side of the box was a non-barrier reach. The OFC-lesioned group made significantly more barrier reaches (*$P<0.05$) but not more non-barrier reaches than controls. Reprinted by permission from John Wiley and Sons: European *Journal of Neuroscience*, 1797–1808, Wallis J.D., Dias, R., Robbins T.W., et al. Dissociable contributions of the orbitofrontal and lateral prefrontal cortex of the marmoset to performance on a detour reaching task copyright 2001. (c) Incongruent discrimination task. (c.i) Depicts the mean number of perseverative and non-perseverative errors (± SEM) made by OFC-lesioned ($n = 3$) and control monkeys ($n = 4$) prior to reaching criterion on the discrimination. In this task (c. ii), marmosets must learn to overcome a prepotent response tendency to reach for a Perspex box containing high-incentive marshmallows, and instead choose a box containing low-incentive lab chow in order to gain an alternative, high incentive reward. Excitotoxic OFC-lesioned monkeys made many more perseverative responses to the high-incentive food choice (marshmallow) than controls (*$P<0.01$). R. Cools, et al., The Role of the Orbitofrontal Cortex and Medial Striatum in the Regulation of Preotent Responses to Food Rewards, *Cerebral Cortex*, 2009 19(4) by permission of Oxford University Press.

Perseverative and non-perseverative errors were defined using the same method of classification as that used for the reversal learning task (see text for details).

detour reach and to inhibit making a direct reach along its line of sight. The sight and smell of the food itself acts as the conditioned stimulus in this task and animals have to overcome a prepotent response tendency to reach directly for the food, and instead learn an alternative response to obtain the food. In the incongruent discrimination task, marmosets must learn to inhibit responding to a Perspex box containing high-incentive marshmallows, and instead choose a box containing low-incentive lab chow in order to gain an alternative high-incentive reward, syrup bread. Here, the sight of high-incentive food is the conditioned stimulus, and the marmosets have to overcome a prepotent response tendency to reach for their favored food (marshmallow) and select an intrinsically lower value alternative (lab chow) in order to gain reward. Consistent with the reversal learning task, excitotoxic OFC lesions impaired performance in both tasks, resulting in an increased number of line-of-sight reaches on the detour-reaching task (Fig. 10.2b; Wallis et al., 2001) and high-incentive food choices on the incongruent discrimination task (Fig. 10.2c; Wallis et al., 2001; Man et al., 2009). Thus, in both cases, OFC lesions disrupted performance when animals were required to learn a new response, guided by the specific relationship between external cues and reward, but in the presence of an inappropriate, prepotent response alternative. In the same way that OFC lesions do not affect acquisition of a novel, two-pattern/object visual discrimination, OFC lesions did not affect the ability to learn to make a detour reach around a barrier in order to gain access to food reward, if the food reward was within an opaque Perspex box and thus was hidden from view (Wallis et al., 2001).

10.4 Role of the OFC in adapting the emotional response

In the majority of examples discussed so far, the contribution of the OFC has been investigated in the context of adaptation of an instrumental response. However, although the instrumental response is one easily quantifiable result of the overall adaptation that is occurring as a consequence of such environmental changes, this particular behavioral output is only one component of a multifaceted adaptive response that also includes emotional and motivational changes in autonomic and endocrine output. Indeed, the continuum of emotional responses stretches from unlearnt reflexes and fixed action patterns, through Pavlovian learning in which novel stimuli come to elicit conditioned responses, to instrumental behavior whereby the organism takes active control of the environment to satisfy motivational and emotional requirements. Thus, stimuli in the environment, by virtue of their association with a rewarding or punishing outcome, elicit conditioned behavioral, autonomic, and endocrine responses, that together provide an integrated conditioned output in anticipation of an outcome, which can then be used to guide instrumental actions. In the case of a rewarding outcome, Pavlov showed that dogs learned to salivate to a bell signaling the arrival of food, and ceased to salivate when the bell no longer signaled food (Pavlov, 1927). Presumably, if Pavlov had measured the behavioral response he would have shown that behavior during the bell waxed and waned too, according to whether food was anticipated or not. Anatomical evidence shows that the OFC has the relevant connections with structures at the level of the amygdala, hypothalamus, and brainstem involved in controlling the endocrine and autonomic systems (Barbas, 2007; Ghashghaei et al., 2007). But, despite the OFC's importance in behavioral adaptation of motivated responding, few studies have investigated the contribution of the OFC to the adaptation of the other aspects of the motivated/emotional response. Consequently, Roberts and colleagues developed a novel paradigm in the marmoset to investigate the autonomic and behavioral correlates of the anticipation and consumption of high-incentive foods during Pavlovian conditioning, and its subsequent reversal.

Marmosets are implanted with a small telemetric probe into the descending aorta that allows the measure of heart rate and blood pressure while the animal is freely moving in the test chamber. Initial findings have shown a rise in blood pressure (systolic and diastolic) and heart rate to the sight of high, but not low, incentive food, in anticipation of getting access to the food a short time afterwards (Braesicke et al., 2005; Roberts et al., 2007a). In addition, marmosets show a greater amount of conditioned approach behavior to the sight of preferred vs non-preferred food that is consistent with the arousing properties of the preferred food. This approach behavior, whilst correlated with the rise in blood pressure, is not causal, since post-training lesions of the amygdala, including central and basolateral nuclei, disrupt the conditioned autonomic activity, but leave the conditioned behavior intact (Braesicke et al., 2005). More recently, arbitrary auditory stimuli have been used to predict access to either high-incentive foods or an empty food box, and similar increases in cardiovascular activity and associated conditioned orienting responses have been reported during the presentation of the stimulus (CS^+) associated with the high-incentive food. Whilst the expression of the conditioned autonomic, but not behavioral, responses are dependent upon an intact amygdala (Braesicke et al., 2005), neither are affected by post-training lesions of the OFC (targeting area 11 and anterior 13), indicating that once learned, the OFC is not required for the expression of such CRs (Reekie et al., 2008).

The OFC does, however, contribute to the adaptation of these CRs. Thus, upon reversal of the reward contingencies, OFC-lesioned monkeys took many more trials than controls to re-direct their conditioned increases in blood pressure to the newly-rewarded, but previously-unrewarded CS^+, thereby demonstrating that the OFC contributes to the adaptation of autonomic, as well as behavioral, processes (Fig. 10.3a, b). Moreover, while the reversal of the conditioned blood pressure response in control animals was accompanied by a reversal of the conditioned orienting behaviors, no such behavioral reversal accompanied the autonomic reversal of OFC-lesioned monkeys (inset to Fig. 10.3b). Indeed, in some cases a monkey with an OFC lesion was exhibiting conditioned autonomic responses to the currently rewarded stimulus, whilst displaying behavioral orienting towards the previously-rewarded, but currently unrewarded stimulus (see open and filled arrowheads in Fig. 10.3a and b). Consistent with this finding, the strong coupling between conditioned blood pressure and orienting behaviors apparent in controls during reversal learning (Fig. 10.3c) was absent in OFC-lesioned monkeys (Fig. 10.3d), suggesting that the OFC is important in integrating the conditioned autonomic and somatic (behavioral) elements of the peripheral response. Whether the OFC acts to co-ordinate

Fractionation of the emotional response by lesions of the OFC during reversal learning

a. Conditioned systolic BP during pavlovian reversal.

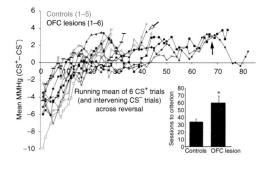

b. Conditioned behaviour during pavlovian revesal.

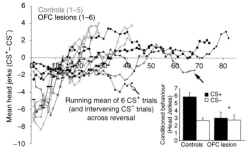

c. Coupling of conditioned BP and behavior in controls.

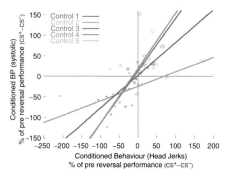

d. Uncoupling of conditioned BP and behavior in OFC lesions.

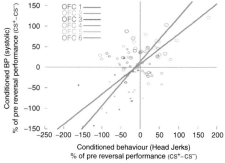

Fig. 10.3 Difference between (a) the conditioned systolic blood pressure (BP) response and (b) conditioned CS-directed behavior (i.e., head jerks) to the new CS$^+$ and CS$^-$ over the entire reversal phase for individual animals. The difference score was calculated as a running mean of six consecutive CS$^+$ trials and intervening CS$^-$ trials (6–14), i.e., means were calculated for CS$^+$ trials 1–6, 2–7, 3–8, etc. Animals were considered to have reversed successfully (reversal criterion) when their mean systolic BP response across 6 consecutive CS$^+$ trials was significantly greater than that for the intervening CS$^-$ trials at $P<0.02$. At the beginning of reversal learning, responses to the new CS$^+$ were initially low, i.e., below baseline, as their responses were still high to the previous CS$^+$. Compared to controls, OFC-lesioned monkeys took more trials to reverse their conditioned rise in systolic BP (inset in "a") and one OFC-lesioned monkey still hadn't reversed after 90 trials. In addition, while the CS-directed behavior of all control monkeys was significantly greater to the new CS$^+$ than the new CS$^-$ at this BP reversal criterion, this was not the case for the OFC-lesioned animals (inset "b"). Indeed, two OFC-lesioned monkeys (open and closed arrows) were still showing CS-directed responding towards the previously rewarded CS$^+$ (current CS-; b) while their conditioned rise in systolic BP was to the current CS$^+$ (a). Numbers on the x-axis represent the first session of the group of sessions that together contain the 6 CS$^+$ trials and intervening CS$^-$ trials that make up each data point. Graphs depicting the correlations between the CS-directed behavior (head jerks) and conditioned systolic BP for (c) control and (d) OFC-lesioned monkeys, across the reversal. The data points are difference measures between CS$^+$ and CS$^-$ responses during the reversal, calculated as a percentage of pre reversal performance. Each circle reflects the mean of approximately five sessions with small and large circles reflecting performance earlier and later in reversal, respectively. Points in the lower-left quadrant indicate that both the conditioned behavioral and BP responses reflect the pre-reversal contingencies, and points in the upper-right quadrant indicate successful reversal of both conditioned responses. Control monkeys show points largely restricted to these two quadrants, which indicates strong coupling between the two response outputs during reversal. Lines represent significant correlations between behavior and BP in individual animals. In contrast, OFC-lesioned monkeys show points scattered across all four quadrants, which indicates uncoupling of the two response outputs during reversal.

Reprinted by permission from National Academy of Sciences, *Proc Nat Acad Sci*, Reekie YL, Braesicke K, Man MS, Roberts AC, Uncoupling of behavioural and automatic responses after lesions of the primate orbitofrontal cortex, Copyright (2008), National Academy of Sciences, USA.

the different response outputs directly or, alternatively, co-ordination is an emergent property of emotional circuits regulated by the OFC, remains to be determined. Regardless of the precise mechanism, such uncoupling could lead to ambiguous peripheral signals that may affect overall emotionality. Thus, interoceptive feedback from the somatic and autonomic systems is a core feature of many theories of emotion, linked primarily to subjective emotional experience of "feelings" (Craig, 2002; Damasio, 2003). Consistent with such theories, recent evidence implicates peripheral feedback in emotional processing (Critchley et al., 2004; Nicotra et al., 2006), although the extent to which it is implicated may depend on a subject's overall interoceptive awareness (Critchley et al., 2007). Ambiguous peripheral signaling may, therefore, contribute to the emotional and behavioral biases seen in a variety of psychiatric disorders, including OCD, schizophrenia, depression, autism, and anxiety (Pantelis et al., 1999; Saxena and Rauch, 2000; Bachevalier and Loveland, 2006; Paulus and Stein, 2006; Drevets, 2007; Chamberlain et al., 2008). Consistent with this hypothesis, an uncoupling of autonomic responses and activations in emotion-specific brain regions, following the presentation of a variety of negatively valenced facial expressions, has been reported in schizophrenic patients (Williams et al., 2007) and has been suggested to contribute to their paranoid symptoms. In addition, the hyper- or hypo-responsive autonomic system apparent in autistic children may lead to the development of certain stereotyped behaviors (Hirstein et al., 2001). Exaggerated differences between the observed and expected body state in individuals prone to anxiety has also been proposed to trigger an increase in anxious affect (Paulus and Stein, 2006). Since disrupted processing within the OFC is associated with schizophrenia (Baare et al., 1999), autism (Bachevalier and Loveland, 2006), and anxiety disorders (Milad and Rauch, 2007), the present results identify OFC dysfunction as a contributory cause of emotional uncoupling in these disorders.

10.5 Monoamines and adaptive responding in the OFC

In many of the above-mentioned neuropsychiatric disorders involving compromised OFC function and impaired adaptive responding, the ascending monoaminergic systems have been implicated. Thus, successful treatment with selective serotonin reuptake inhibitors (SSRIs) normalizes both symptoms and OFC/medial PFC dysfunction in depression and OCD (Brody et al., 1999; Saxena and Rauch, 2000; Drevets, 2001; Mayberg, 2003). In contrast, the primary target of the antipsychotic drug treatment of schizophrenia is dopamine, although the enhanced efficacy of the newer "atypical" antipsychotics is increasingly being allied to their greater serotonergic activity (Ichikawa and Meltzer, 1999; Ichikawa et al., 2001). Alterations in 5-HT and dopamine have also been reported in drug addiction. 5-HT metabolites (5-hydroxyindoleacetic acid; 5-HIAA) are reduced in the OFC of methamphetamine abusers postmortem (Wilson et al., 1996), while cocaine addicts show alterations in striatal dopamine-receptor binding that correlates with OFC hypoactivity (Volkow and Fowler, 2000). Moreover, cocaine addicts (Ersche et al., 2008) and schizophrenics (Elliott et al., 1995; Pantelis et al., 1999; Waltz and Gold, 2007; McKirdy et al., 2008; Murray et al., 2008) are impaired on the discrimination reversal-task, and

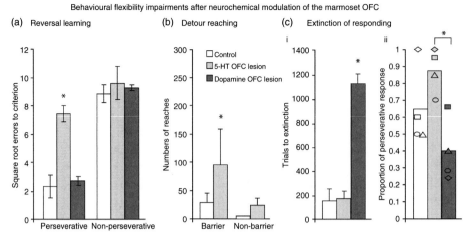

Fig. 10.4 (a) Reversal learning depicts the mean number of perseverative and non-perseverative errors (± SEM) made by monkeys with selective 5-HT OFC depletions (*n* = 4), selective dopamine OFC depletions (*n* = 4), and control monkeys (*n* = 4) across a series of four reversals (see Fig. 10.2a for task description). In contrast to both control and dopamine-lesioned monkeys, monkeys with 5-HT OFC depletions made many more perseverative responses to the previously-correct stimulus after a reversal (*P<0.001), but did not differ in the number of non-perseverative errors. Adapted from figure 3, Clarke et al. (2007). (b) Detour reaching depicts the mean number of barrier and non-barrier reaches (± SEM) made by monkeys with 5-HT OFC lesions (*n* = 4) and controls (*n* = 4) before they made two consecutive correct responses (detour reaches). 5-HT OFC-lesioned monkeys made many more barrier reaches than control monkeys but did not differ in the number of non-barrier reaches. (*P<0.01) (see Fig. 10.2b for task description). Adapted from figure 1, Walker et al. (2006). (c) Extinction of responding. As in the reversal learning task, monkeys on the extinction task were initially required to learn a discrimination between two abstract, colored stimuli on a touch-sensitive computer screen, where a response to one stimulus earned reward and a response to the other earned nothing. However, unlike reversal learning, when criterion was attained, both stimuli became unrewarded and the monkeys were allowed to respond freely for 40 trials every session until responding was considered extinguished, i.e., less than 10 responses/session for two consecutive sessions. (c.i) Depicts the mean trials to extinction (± SEM) for monkeys with selective 5-HT OFC depletions (*n* = 4), selective dopamine OFC depletions (*n* = 4), and controls (*n* = 4). Dopamine-lesioned monkeys took significantly more trials to extinguish responding than control or 5-HT-lesioned monkeys (*P<0.01). (c.ii) Depicts the proportion of extinction responses that were classified as perseverative (individual data represented by filled shapes). 5-HT depleted monkeys made a significantly higher proportion of perseverative responses to the previously-correct stimulus than dopamine-lesioned monkeys (*P<0.01), and showed a trend towards significance compared to controls. Adapted from figure 4, Walker et al. (2008).

OFC hypoactivity is associated with impaired reversal learning performance in OCD patients and their first-degree relatives (Remijnse et al., 2006; Chamberlain et al., 2008; Valerius et al., 2008; Remijnse et al., 2009). Thus, an understanding of how dopamine and serotonin contribute to the functions of the OFC is long overdue.

Clarke et al. (2004) used the selective serotonergic neurotoxin 5, 7-dihydroxytryp-tamine (5,7-DHT) combined with dopamine and noradrenaline protectors to induce a selective loss of 5-HT throughout marmoset prefrontal cortex (PFC). The specificity of the neurochemical lesion was confirmed with both in vivo microdialysis and postmortem tissue measurements using high-pressure liquid chromatography. Compared to controls, monkeys with depletions of prefrontal 5-HT were profoundly impaired at serial reversals, displaying repetitive, perseverative responding to the previously-correct stimulus (Fig. 10.4a)—comparable to that seen after excitotoxic lesions of the marmoset OFC. A similar perseverative deficit in reversal learning, and an increased number of line-of-sight reaches on the detour reaching task (Fig. 10.4b) were associated with serotonergic depletions of just the ventral PFC, including orbitofrontal and lateral prefrontal cortices (Clarke et al., 2005; Walker et al., 2006). Since, the perseveration could be due to (1) continued responding to the previously-rewarded stimulus due to stimulus-bound behavior or, (2) avoidance of the previously-unrewarded stimulus (termed "learned avoidance") that would also result in continuing responding to the other, previously-correct stimulus, a new task was designed to fractionate these options. Upon reversal of the reward contingencies, the previously rewarded or unrewarded stimulus was replaced by a novel stimulus. If presented with the previously-correct stimulus and a novel stimulus, any perseveration to the previously-correct stimulus would not be due to "learned avoidance." Conversely, if presented with the previously-incorrect stimulus and a novel stimulus there is no opportunity for stimulus-bound behavior and learned avoidance would manifest itself as a bias of responding away from the previously-incorrect stimulus. Comparison of these two conditions revealed that 5-HT depletions within the ventral PFC only disrupted reversal learning when the previously-rewarded stimulus was still present and perseverative responding to the previously rewarded stimulus was still possible (Clarke et al., 2007).[1]

In contrast to discrimination reversal learning, the ability to switch attentional sets or rules, which is dependent upon the lateral PFC, and not the OFC (Dias et al., 1996), was unaffected by PFC 5-HT depletions, highlighting the functional selectivity of the actions of 5-HT (Clarke et al., 2005). Perhaps more surprisingly, 5-HT depletion within the ventral PFC also failed to affect the overall rate of response extinction. As in reversal learning, successful extinction performance in the face of no reward relies on the ability to learn that a previously-rewarded stimulus is no longer rewarded, and is impaired by lesions of the OFC (Izquierdo and Murray, 2005). However, whereas reversal learning requires a redirection of responding to the newly-correct stimulus, extinction involves the cessation of responding, altogether. In the majority of studies, extinction is investigated in the context of an animal learning that one particular rewarded stimulus and/or one rewarded response is no longer rewarded (Butter, 1969; Izquierdo and Murray, 2005). In contrast,

---

[1] It should be noted that a bias towards the previously-rewarded stimulus, but not away from the previously-unrewarded stimulus, may be a consequence of the rewarded stimulus driving learning in this task. If responding to the unrewarded stimulus received an explicit punishment, then the punished stimulus may drive learning via an avoidance response and a different result may have been obtained.

we investigated it in the context of a two-choice visual discrimination task, comparable to that of reversal learning, except that, instead of the contingency reversing once the visual discrimination was learned, both stimuli became unrewarded. Marmosets with 5-HT reductions within the ventral PFC, including the OFC, extinguished their responding as rapidly as controls, demonstrating that the perseverative impairment on the serial reversal task does not reflect a deficit in response extinction per se. However, these same animals did show a far greater choice of the previously-rewarded stimulus than controls (Walker et al., 2008). Thus, whilst the preference for the previously-rewarded stimulus soon disappeared in the control group, and responding between the two stimuli became random, the 5-HT depleted animals did not lose their preference for the previously-rewarded stimulus, before their responding extinguished (Fig. 10.4b; Walker et al., 2008). Moreover, they also showed stimulus-bound responding in a task that required animals to discriminate between two visual stimuli, based on their association with a conditioned reinforcer. Here, there were no competing stimulus–reward associations but, initially, the responding of all subjects was determined by a perceptual bias towards, what appeared to be, the more visually salient of the two stimuli. However, whereas control animals were able to overcome this bias and use new learning about the association between visual stimuli and a conditioned reinforcer to guide responding, 5-HT depleted monkeys were not. This perseveration could not be explained solely in terms of a deficit in using the conditioned reinforcer to guide responding, because monkeys with OFC dopamine depletion were impaired at using the conditioned reinforcer to guide responding but, unlike 5-HT depleted animals, they overcame their perceptual bias, equivalently to controls.

Taken together, these findings highlight the importance of 5-HT within OFC in overcoming competing response biases to sensory stimuli, whether driven by past associations with reward (as in reversal learning and extinction) or by the intrinsic perceptual properties of stimuli, and thus, either directly, or indirectly, in promoting exploratory behavior. They also identify serotonin dysfunction within the OFC as a likely contributor to some of the deficits in flexibility associated with disorders such as schizophrenia, drug addiction, and OCD. More recently, OFC serotonin dysfunction has been implicated in certain forms of stress-induced flexibility. Chronic, intermittent cold stress in rats reduces extracellular levels of serotonin in the OFC and impairs discrimination reversal learning; an impairment that is ameliorated by an acute treatment with the SSRI citalopram (Lapiz-Bluhm et al., 2008). Since stress is a major risk factor in many neuropsychiatric disorders, these results illustrate the close interaction between stress, serotonin, and OFC that may lead to behavioral inflexibility in these disorders.

Such attentional processing biases following 5-HT depletion may be akin to those reported in depressed patients performing an emotional go/no-go task (Murphy et al., 1999), that are associated with an increased BOLD response in the OFC (Elliott et al., 2002). Of more direct relevance to 5-HT are the findings of Hitsman et al. (2007) showing that acute tryptophan depletion increases the attentional salience of smoking-related cue words in smokers, independent of any change in mood. It remains to be determined whether these effects are best explained by the hypothesized role of serotonin in processing negative information (Daw et al., 2002) or in modulating the drive to withdraw from environmental stimulation (Tops et al., 2009).

In contrast to 5-HT's actions within the OFC, selective depletions of OFC dopamine do not disrupt discrimination reversal performance (Fig. 10.4a; Clarke et al., 2007), despite peripheral manipulations of dopaminergic activity having been shown to modulate reversal learning. Administration of the dopaminergic precursor L-dopa to Parkinson's disease patients is found to impair probabilistic reversal learning (Swainson et al., 2000; Cools et al., 2001), while Mehta et al. (2001) found that a similar, non-perseverative deficit was induced in normal people by low doses of the D2 dopamine-receptor agonist, bromocriptine. Such effects may be due to the actions of dopamine at the level of the striatum, rather than the OFC. Although DA depletions in the striatum have proved inconclusive with respect to reversal learning (marmoset caudate nucleus,: Crofts et al., 2001; rat dorsomedial striatum: O'Neill and Brown, 2007), both systemic and intra-accumbens manipulation of D2 receptors have been shown to impair reversal learning (Lee et al., 2007; Haluk and Floresco, 2009), suggesting the involvement of striatal dopamine. At the level of the OFC, dopamine has been implicated in specific aspects of reward processing, including incentive motivation in rats, as measured by responding on a progressive ratio schedule of reinforcement (Schultz, 2002; Cetin et al., 2004; Kheramin et al., 2004). Similarly, in marmosets, OFC dopamine has been implicated in the mechanisms by which the conditioned reinforcing properties of visual stimuli can guide responding (Walker et al., 2008). Based upon these findings we have proposed that, in much the same way as dopamine has been hypothesized to stabilize the internal representations of task-relevant sensory stimuli in dorsolateral PFC (Goldman-Rakic, 1987; Durstewitz et al., 2000), dopamine in the OFC may act to stabilize the internal representation of the CS–outcome relationship (Robbins and Roberts, 2007). In addition, and of particular relevance to the present discussion, is the prolonged instrumental responding, displayed by marmosets with OFC dopamine depletions, in the absence of reward.

Unlike OFC 5-HT depletions, OFC DA depletions markedly prolonged responding during extinction, with three out of four monkeys failing to extinguish their responding after 40 daily sessions of 40 trials (Fig. 10.4c). Such prolonged responding in the presence of non-reward could be due solely to a weakening of expected reward representations within the OFC. However, an up-regulation of dopamine function in the striatum may also be contributing. Depletion of dopamine in the PFC in both rats and marmosets increases striatal dopamine function (Mitchell and Gratton, 1992; Roberts et al., 1994; King et al., 1997), although the specific effects of orbitofrontal dopamine loss on striatal dopamine are as yet unknown. This up-regulation is hypothesized to be due to removal of the inhibitory influence of PFC dopamine on the glutamate containing projection neurons of the PFC. The resulting excitatory glutamatergic effect on the striatum is thought to lead to tonic dopamine release (Pycock et al., 1980). In addition, activation of D2 receptors by tonic increases in dopamine has been shown to attenuate prefrontal inputs (Goto and Grace, 2005) and peripheral administration of the D2 receptor agonist, quinpirole, increases responding in extinction (Kurylo and Tanguay, 2003). Thus, a loss of OFC dopamine may not only disrupt OFC functioning directly, but may also cause a loss of prefrontal control at the level of the striatum, as a result of increased tonic dopamine stimulation of D2 receptors, one consequence of which may be a potentiation of habitual responding. The transition from goal-directed to habitual responding has been proposed to reflect a transfer of the control of behavior between distinct prefronto-striatal loops (Everitt and Robbins, 2005), and lesions of the dorsolateral striatum disrupt habit formation (Yin et al., 2004), as do lesions of the nigrostriatal pathway (Faure et al., 2005). Thus, disruption of OFC may expedite the transition from goal-directed to habitual behavior, specifically modulated by DA, accounting for the over-responding of OFC dopamine-depleted monkeys following extinction of a visual discrimination.

Such effects downstream in the striatum may not only contribute to the loss of behavioral regulation seen following DA depletions within the OFC, but may also contribute to the effects of 5-HT dysfunction in the OFC. Whilst there is, as yet, no direct evidence for such effects, indirect evidence includes the finding that excitotoxic lesions of the OFC result in an increase in the density of the striatal serotonin transporter (Joel et al., 2005). Moreover, the inverse correlation between 5-HT_{2A} receptor density in medial PFC and emotion-related amygdala reactivity (Fisher et al., 2009) suggests interactions between prefrontal 5-HT and the amygdala. These findings highlight the dynamic interaction between the OFC and downstream structures, such as the striatum and amygdala, and it is to these downstream structures that we now turn our attention.

10.6 The role of the striatum and amygdala in reversal learning

Only recently has the role of the striatum and amygdala in discrimination reversal learning begun to be elucidated. Although both electrolytic lesions of the macaque caudate nucleus and human imaging have implicated the ventral caudate nucleus in visual discrimination reversal learning (Divac et al., 1967; Rogers et al., 2000), the majority of studies utilizing excitotoxic lesions have proved inconclusive, due to differences in lesion location, e.g., nucleus accumbens (Schoenbaum and Setlow, 2003) versus ventral or medial striatum (Ferry et al., 2000) and behavioral paradigm, e.g., discrimination go/no-go (Ferry et al., 2000) or rule switching (Reading and Dunnett, 1991; Block et al., 2007). Consequently, the effects of excitotoxic lesions of the marmoset striatum on reversal learning have been compared directly to the effects of excitotoxic lesions of both the OFC and amygdala. Striatal lesions were confined to the medial caudate and nucleus accumbens—those regions known to receive inputs from the OFC in marmosets (Roberts et al., 2007b). In contrast to both control and amygdala-lesioned monkeys, both OFC- and striatally-lesioned monkeys were impaired at reversal learning (Fig. 10.5a) and both groups displayed perseverative responding towards the previously-correct stimulus (Clarke et al., 2008). Although it is not clear whether the deficit following striatal damage is due primarily to the caudate nucleus or accumbens, the former is most likely, as lesions restricted to the nucleus accumbens in rats do not selectively disrupt discrimination reversal (Annett et al., 1989; Schoenbaum and Setlow, 2003). A similar pattern of impairment following medial striatal lesions in marmosets has also been seen in the incongruent

Behavioural flexibility after excitotoxic lesions of the medial striatum and amygdala

(a) Reversal Learning: overall performance (b) Incongruent incentive discrimination

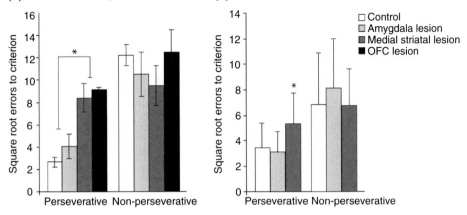

(c) Reversal learning: response to feedback

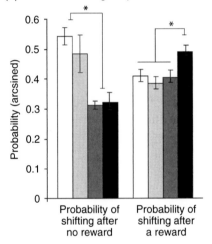

Fig. 10.5 (a) Reversal learning depicts the mean number of perseverative and non-perseverative errors (± SEM) made by monkeys with selective excitotoxic lesions of the amygdala ($n = 3$), medial striatum ($n = 3$), or control monkeys ($n = 4$) across a series of four reversals. The OFC-lesion data are the same as depicted in Fig. 10.2a.i (see Fig. 10.2a.ii for task description). Monkeys with both OFC and medial striatal lesions made significantly more perseverative errors than either controls or amygdala-lesioned monkeys (*$P<0.05$). Non-perseverative errors were not affected. Adapted from figure 6, Clarke et al. (2008). (b) Incongruent discrimination depicts the mean number of perseverative and non-perseverative errors (± SEM) made by amygdala-lesioned ($n = 3$), medial striatal-lesioned ($n = 3$), and control monkeys ($n = 4$) prior to reaching criterion on the discrimination. See Fig. 10.2c.ii for task description. Excitotoxic medial striatal-lesioned monkeys made more perseverative responses to the high-incentive food choice (marshmallow) than controls or amygdala-lesioned monkeys (*$P<0.01$). Adapted from figure 3, Man et al. (2009). (c) Reversal learning depicts the mean probabilities (± SEM) of the monkeys shifting their responding to the other stimulus after a positive (rewarded) or negative

Fig. 10.5 (*Contd*). (non-rewarded) outcome on the previous trial. Both OFC- and medial striatally-lesioned monkeys were less likely to shift responding after an incorrect choice than controls or amygdala-lesioned monkeys, indicating insensitivity to negative feedback. In contrast, only OFC-lesioned monkeys showed an increased likelihood of shifting after a correct response, indicative of insensitivity to positive feedback (*$P<0.05$). Adapted from figure 7, Clarke et al. (2008).

discrimination task, whereby both OFC- and striatally-lesioned, but not amygdala-lesioned, monkeys showed impairments at the acquisition (Fig. 10.5b) and reversal of the incongruent discrimination (Man et al., 2009). Whilst the effects on detour reaching in marmosets have not been investigated, perseverative impairments in detour reaching have been seen in baboons with selective degeneration of the caudate and putamen (Palfi et al., 1996). Together, these findings highlight the similarity of the effects of damage to both the OFC and medial striatum on response flexibility. However, differences between OFC- and striatally-lesioned monkeys have been revealed on the discrimination reversal task when taking into account their likelihood of repeating or changing their response on the next trial, following negative or positive feedback. Both were less likely than controls to alter their subsequent response following negative feedback, but only the OFC-lesioned monkeys were also less likely to repeat their response on the subsequent trial following positive feedback (Clarke et al., 2008). The latter is consistent with the finding that the OFC represents both positive and negative outcome expectancies (Schoenbaum et al., 1998; O'Doherty et al., 2001), while the relatively selective effect of striatal lesions on sensitivity to negative feedback (i.e., loss of expected reward) may relate to its involvement in reward prediction error signaling (Pagnoni et al., 2002; Seymour et al., 2007).

In contrast to the OFC and striatum, lesions of the amygdala had no effect on reversal learning (Fig. 10.5a) or the incongruent incentive discrimination task (Fig. 10.5b). This lack of involvement of the amygdala is consistent with other studies in which excitotoxic amygdala lesions have been shown not to impair reversal learning paradigms (Izquierdo and Murray, 2007) (but see Schoenbaum et al., 2003). However, a recent study by Stalnaker et al. (2007), showing that combined excitotoxic lesions of the OFC and the amygdala abolish the reversal deficits seen after OFC lesions alone, suggests that the amygdala does contribute to the OFC-induced reversal deficits. This result has a number of implications for our understanding of the neural circuitry underlying reversal learning. It clearly shows that, under certain circumstances, other regions of the forebrain can implement reversal learning, without orbitofronto-basolateral amygdala circuitry. As discussed by ourselves (Roberts, 2006), and others (Izquierdo et al., 2004), associations between the stimulus and the sensory, non-affective properties of the food, rather than its incentive value, can guide behavior in many versions of the discrimination reversal task. Thus, it may be that brain regions involved in these other forms of associative learning may also guide behavior, one example being the rhinal cortex, lesions of which also disrupt reversal learning (Murray et al., 1998). In all cases, however, the final common pathway for rapid reversal learning may be the striatum. We suggest that the orbitofronto-basolateral amygdala circuitry may only be both necessary and sufficient for rapid reversal learning when only incentive value guides the response.

Altogether, these findings emphasize the importance of looking at the processes of behavioral adaptation as the manifestation of circuit-based processing. Clearly, reversal learning performance is the product of a neural interaction that includes the OFC, striatum, and amygdala and imbalances within this circuit will disrupt performance. As mentioned above, one cause of that imbalance may be a disturbance in its monoaminergic innervation that may increase or decrease the relative influence that the OFC has over striatal and amygdala output. Whilst relatively little is known about the relationship between the OFC and striatal or amygdala activity, interactions between other PFC areas and these downstream structures have been described. Thus, the extent of amygdala-medial prefrontal coupling, as indicated by correlated activity derived from BOLD fMRI data, has been shown to vary with serotonin transporter genetic variation (Heinz et al., 2005). In addition, of special relevance to the current discussion, rhesus monkey carriers of the short allele of this polymorphism show impaired serial discrimination reversal performance (Izquierdo et al., 2007), suggesting that the OFC, along with the medial PFC and the amygdala, is also compromised, either in addition to, or as a consequence of such circuit-level uncoupling (Hariri et al., 2002). Similarly, dopamine can affect the relative impact of medial prefrontal inputs on both ventral striatal (Goto and Grace, 2005) and amygdala (Rosenkranz and Grace, 2001) activity. Thus both DA and 5-HT may be in a position to determine the extent to which perceptual, cognitive, affective, and contextual information streams impact upon current behavioral flexibility processes (Goto and Grace, 2005; Goto et al., 2007). Consequently, in addition to determining the effects of neurochemical manipulation on a given structure, future research must also investigate the implications that such manipulations have for the rest of the circuit.

10.7 Conclusions

The integrity of the OFC is fundamental to successful reversal learning. However, differences between studies in the discrimination task used, the lesion location and the method of error analysis has meant that uncertainty still remains as to whether the OFC provides a single or multiple contribution to reversal learning. What is clear is that the OFC is part of a more widespread circuit that includes not only the striatum and amygdala, but also other regions involved in the processing of emotional and peripheral information that together contribute to such flexible responding. Indeed, the importance of the OFC for emotional regulation may be highly relevant to our understanding of disorders in which emotional uncoupling and the proposed resulting anxiety could lead to symptomatic behavioral inflexibility.

Although the monoamines are implicated in the integration of emotional and peripheral information into the decision-making process, their precise contribution remains to be determined. Nevertheless, progress is being made in elucidating the contributions of serotonin and dopamine to OFC-dependent behavior. OFC serotonin appears to modulate attentional focus, with reductions in serotonin narrowing that focus and reducing environmental interactions, leading to perseverative responding. In contrast, OFC dopamine appears to mediate specific aspects of reward processing, and we have suggested that it may act to stabilize internal representations of stimulus–outcome relationships. An understanding of these monoamines, however, cannot be complete without considering their overall modulation of OFC-striatal and OFC-amygdala circuitry. Their ability to alter the balance of information flow through the striatum and amygdala, and, in particular, their influence on prefrontal regulation of striatal and amygdala activity, is key. Future studies investigating the behavioral consequences of these interactions will be important in determining how healthy, flexible behavior is mediated, and will hopefully shed light on the causes of behavioral inflexibility.

Acknowledgments

This work was supported by a Wellcome Trust program Grant 076274/z/04/z awarded to T.W. Robbins, B.J. Everitt, A.C. Roberts, and B.J. Sahakian, and a Medical Research Council (MRC) Programme Grant awarded to A.C. Roberts. It was conducted within the University of Cambridge Behavioural and Clinical Neuroscience Institute, supported by a joint award from the MRC and the Wellcome Trust. HFC was further supported by a Wellcome Trust Prize Studentship, the Newton Trust, Cambridge, a Network Grant from the McDonnell Foundation and a Junior Research Fellowship from Newnham College, Cambridge.

References

Annett, L.E., McGregor, A., Robbins, T.W. (1989). The effects of ibotenic acid lesions of the nucleus accumbens on spatial learning and extinction in the rat. *Behav Brain Res*, **31**: 231–42.

Azmitia, EC., Whitaker-Azmitia, P.M. (1995). Anatomy, cell biology and maturation of the serotonergic system: neurotrophic implications for the actions of psychotropic drugs. In: *Psychopharmacology, fourth generation of progress* (Bloom FE, Kupfer DJ, eds). New York: Raven Press. Accessed July 2009 from http:\\www.acnp.org/publications/psycho4generation.aspx.

Baare, WF., Hulshoff Pol, H.E., Hijman, R., Mali, W.P., Viergever, M.A., Kahn, R.S. (1999). Volumetric analysis of frontal lobe regions in schizophrenia: relation to cognitive function and symptomatology. *Biol Psychiatry*, **45**: 1597–605.

Bachevalier, J., Loveland, K.A. (2006). The orbitofrontal-amygdala circuit and self-regulation of social-emotional behavior in autism. *Neurosci Biobehav Rev*, **30**: 97–117.

Barbas, H. (2007). Flow of information for emotions through temporal and orbitofrontal pathways. *J Anat*, **211**: 237–49.

Blair, R.J., Colledge, E., Mitchell, D.G. (2001). Somatic markers and response reversal: is there orbitofrontal cortex dysfunction in boys with psychopathic tendencies? *J Abnorm Child Psychol*, **29**: 499–511.

Block, AE., Dhanji, H., Thompson-Tardif, S.F., Floresco, S.B. (2007). Thalamic-prefrontal cortical-ventral striatal circuitry mediates dissociable components of strategy set shifting. *Cereb Cortex*, **17**: 1625–36.

Boulougouris, V., Dalley, J.W., Robbins, T.W. (2007). Effects of orbitofrontal, infralimbic and prelimbic cortical lesions on serial spatial reversal learning in the rat. *Behav Brain Res*, **179**: 219–28.

Bouton, M.E. (2004). Context and behavioral processes in extinction. *Learn Mem*, **11**: 485–94.

Braesicke, K., Parkinson, J.A., Reekie, Y., Man, M.S., Hopewell, L., Pears, A. et al. (2005). Autonomic arousal in an appetitive context in primates: a behavioral and neural analysis. *Eur J Neurosci*, **21**: 1733–40.

Brody, A,L., Saxena, S., Silverman, D.H.S., Alborzian, S., Fairbanks, L.A., Phelps, M.E. et al. (1999). Brain metabolic changes in major depressive disorder from pre- to post-treatment with paroxetine. *Psychiatry Research-Neuroimaging*, **91**: 127–39.

Budhani, S., Blair, R.J. (2005). Response reversal and children with psychopathic tendencies: success is a function of salience of contingency change. *J Child Psychol Psychiatry*, **46**: 972–81.

Budhani, S., Marsh, A.A., Pine, D.S., Blair, R.J. (2007). Neural correlates of response reversal: considering acquisition. *Neuroimage*, **34**: 1754–65.

Burman, K.J., Rosa, M.G. (2009). Architectural subdivisions of medial and orbital frontal cortices in the marmoset monkey (*Callithrix jacchus*). *J Comp Neurol*, **514**: 11–29.

Butter, C.M. (1969). Perseveration in extinction and in discrimination reversal tasks following selective frontal ablations in *Macaca mulatta*. *Physiology and Behavior*, **4**: 163–71.

Carmichael, S.T., Price, J.L. (1994). Architectonic subdivision of the orbital and medial prefrontal cortex in the macaque monkey. *Journal of Comparative Neurology*, **346**: 366–402.

Celada, P., Puig, M.V., Casanovas, J.M., Guillazo, G., Artigas, F. (2001). Control of dorsal raphe serotonergic neurons by the medial prefrontal cortex: Involvement of serotonin-1A, GABA(A), and glutamate receptors. *J Neurosci*, **21**: 9917–29.

Cetin, T., Freudenberg, F., Fuchtemeier, M., Koch, M. (2004). Dopamine in the orbitofrontal cortex regulates operant responding under a progressive ratio of reinforcement in rats. *Neurosci Lett*, **370**: 114–7.

Chamberlain, S.R., Menzies, L., Hampshire, A., Suckling, J., Fineberg, N.A., del Campo, N. et al. (2008). Orbitofrontal dysfunction in patients with obsessive-compulsive disorder and their unaffected relatives. *Science*, **321**: 421–2.

Chudasama, Y., Robbins, T.W. (2003). Dissociable contributions of the orbitofrontal and infralimbic cortex to pavlovian autoshaping and discrimination reversal-learning: further evidence for the functional heterogeneity of the rodent frontal cortex. *J Neurosci*, **23**: 8771–80.

Clarke, H.F., Dalley, J.W., Crofts, H.S., Robbins, T.W., Roberts, A.C. (2004). Cognitive inflexibility after prefrontal serotonin depletion. *Science*, **304**: 878–80.

Clarke, H.F., Walker, S.C., Crofts, H.S., Dalley, J.W., Robbins, T.W., Roberts, A.C. (2005). Prefrontal serotonin depletion affects reversal learning but not attentional set shifting. *J Neurosci*, **25**: 532–38.

Clarke, H.F., Walker, S.C., Dalley, J.W., Robbins, T.W., Roberts, A.C. (2007). Cognitive inflexibility after prefrontal serotonin depletion is behaviorally and neurochemically specific. *Cereb Cortex*, **17**: 18–27.

Clarke, H.F., Robbins, T.W., Roberts, A.C. (2008). Lesions of the medial striatum in monkeys produce perseverative impairments during reversal learning similar to those produced by lesions of the orbitofrontal cortex. *J Neurosci*, **28**: 10972–82.

Cools, R., Barker, R.A., Sahakian, B.J., Robbins, T.W. (2001). Enhanced or impaired cognitive function in Parkinson's disease as a function of dopaminergic medication and task demands. *Cereb Cortex*, **11**: 1136–43.

Cools, R., Clark, L., Owen, A.M., Robbins, T.W. (2002). Defining the neural mechanisms of probabilistic reversal learning using event-related functional magnetic resonance imaging. *J Neurosci*, **22**: 4563–67.

Cowen, P.J. (2008). Serotonin and depression: pathophysiological mechanism or marketing myth? *Trends Pharmacol Sci*, **29**: 433–36.

Craig, A.D. (2002). How do you feel? Interoception: the sense of the physiological condition of the body. *Nat Rev Neurosci*, **3**: 655–66.

Critchley, H.D., Wiens, S., Rotshtein, P., Ohman, A., Dolan, R.J. (2004). Neural systems supporting interoceptive awareness. *Nat Neurosci*, **7**: 189–95.

Critchley, H.D., Lewis, P.A., Orth, M., Josephs, O., Deichmann, R., Trimble, M.R., Dolan, R.J. (2007). Vagus nerve stimulation for treatment-resistant depression: behavioral and neural effects on encoding negative material. *Psychosom Med,* **69**: 17–22.

Crofts, H.S., Dalley, J.W., Collins, P., Van Denderen, J.C., Everitt, B.J., Robbins, T.W., Roberts, A.C. (2001). Differential effects of 6-OHDA lesions of the frontal cortex and caudate nucleus on the ability to acquire an attentional set. *Cereb Cortex,* **11**: 1015–26.

Damasio, A. (2003). Feelings of emotion and the self. *Ann NY Acad Sci* **1001**: 253–61.

Daw, N.D., Kakade, S., Dayan, P. (2002). Opponent interactions between serotonin and dopamine. *Neural Netw,* **15**: 603–16.

Dias, R., Robbins, T.W., Roberts, A.C. (1996). Dissociation in prefrontal cortex of affective and attentional shifts. *Nature,* **380**: 69–72.

Dias, R., Robbins, T.W., Roberts, A.C. (1997). Dissociable forms of inhibitory control within prefrontal cortex with an analog of the Wisconsin Card Sort Test: restriction to novel situations and independence from "on-line" processing. *Journal of Neuroscience,* **17**: 9285–97.

Divac. I., Rosvold, H.E., Szwarcbart, M.K. (1967). Behavioral effects of selective ablation of the caudate nucleus. *J Comp Physiol Psychol,* **63**: 184–90.

Drevets, W.C. (2001). Neuroimaging and neuropathological studies of depression: implications for the cognitive-emotional features of mood disorders. *Curr Opin Neurobiol,* **11**: 240–49.

Drevets, W.C. (2007). Orbitofrontal cortex function and structure in depression. *Ann NY Acad Sci,* **1121**: 499–527.

Durstewitz, D., Seamans, J.K., Sejnowski, T.J. (2000). Dopamine-mediated stabilization of delay-period activity in a network model of prefrontal cortex. *J Neurophysiol,* **83**: 1733–50.

Elliott, R., McKenna, P.J., Robbins, T.W., Sahakian, B.J. (1995). Neuropsychological evidence for frontostriatal dysfunction in schizophrenia. *Psychol Med,* **25**: 619–30.

Elliott, R., Rubinsztein, J.S., Sahakian, B.J., Dolan, R.J. (2002). The neural basis of mood-congruent processing biases in depression. *Arch Gen Psychiatry,* **59**: 597–604.

Ersche, K.D., Roiser, J.P., Robbins, T.W., Sahakian, B.J. (2008). Chronic cocaine but not chronic amphetamine use is associated with perseverative responding in humans. *Psychopharmacology (Berl),* **197**: 421–31.

Everitt, B.J., Robbins, T.W. (2005). Neural systems of reinforcement for drug addiction: from actions to habits to compulsion. *Nat Neurosci,* **8**: 1481–89.

Faure, A., Haberland, U., Conde, F., El Massioui, N. (2005). Lesion to the nigrostriatal dopamine system disrupts stimulus-response habit formation. *J Neurosci,* **25**: 2771–80.

Fellows, L.K., Farah, M.J. (2003). Ventromedial frontal cortex mediates affective shifting in humans: evidence from a reversal learning paradigm. *Brain,* **126**: 1830–37.

Ferry, A.T., Lu, X.C., Price, J.L. (2000). Effects of excitotoxic lesions in the ventral striatopallidal—thalamocortical pathway on odor reversal learning: inability to extinguish an incorrect response. *Exp Brain Res,* **131**: 320–35.

Fisher, P.M., Meltzer, C.C., Price, J.C., Coleman, R.L., Ziolko, S.K., Becker, C. et al. (2009). Medial prefrontal cortex 5-HT2A density is correlated with amygdala reactivity, response habituation, and functional coupling. *Cereb Cortex,* **19**(11) 2499–507.

Floresco, S.B., Zhang, Y., Enomoto, T. (2008). Neural circuits subserving behavioral flexibility and their relevance to schizophrenia. *Behav Brain Res,* **204**(2) 396–409.

Fuchs, R.A., Evans, K.A., Parker, M.P., See, R.E. (2004). Differential involvement of orbitofrontal cortex subregions in conditioned cue-induced and cocaine-primed reinstatement of cocaine seeking in rats. *J Neurosci,* **24**: 6600–10.

Gallagher, M., McMahan, R.W., Schoenbaum, G. (1999). Orbitofrontal cortex and representation of incentive value in associative learning. *J Neurosci,* **19**: 6610–14.

Gaykema, R.P., van Weeghel, R., Hersh, L.B., Luiten, P.G. (1991). Prefrontal cortical projections to the cholinergic neurons in the basal forebrain. *J Comp Neurol*, **303**: 563–83.

Ghashghaei, H.T., Hilgetag, C.C., Barbas, H. (2007). Sequence of information processing for emotions based on the anatomic dialogue between prefrontal cortex and amygdala. *Neuroimage*, **34**: 905–23.

Ghods-Sharifi, S., Haluk, D.M., Floresco, S.B. (2008). Differential effects of inactivation of the orbitofrontal cortex on strategy set-shifting and reversal learning. *Neurobiol Learn Mem*, **89**: 567–73.

Goldman-Rakic, P. (1987). Circuitry of primate prefrontal cortex and regulation of behavior by representational memory. In: *Handbook of physiology: the nervous system* (Mountcastle V, Plum F, Geiger S, eds) pp. 373–417. Bethesda, MD: American Physiological Society.

Goto, Y., Grace, A.A. (2005). Dopaminergic modulation of limbic and cortical drive of nucleus accumbens in goal-directed behavior. *Nat Neurosci*, **8**: 805–12.

Goto, Y., Otani, S., Grace, A.A. (2007). The Yin and Yang of dopamine release: a new perspective. *Neuropharmacology*, **53**: 583–87.

Haluk, D.M., Floresco, S.B. (2009). Ventral striatal dopamine modulation of different forms of behavioral flexibility. *Neuropsychopharmacology*, **34**: 2041–52.

Hampshire, A., Owen, A.M. (2006). Fractionating attentional control using event-related fMRI. *Cereb Cortex*, **16**: 1679–89.

Hariri, A.R., Mattay, V.S., Tessitore, A., Kolachana, B., Fera, F., Goldman, D. et al. (2002). Serotonin transporter genetic variation and the response of the human amygdala. *Science*, **297**: 400–3.

Heinz, A., Braus, D.F., Smolka, M.N., Wrase, J., Puls, I., Hermann, D. et al. (2005). Amygdala-prefrontal coupling depends on a genetic variation of the serotonin transporter. *Nat Neurosci*, **8**: 20–1.

Hirstein, W., Iversen, P., Ramachandran, V.S. (2001). Autonomic responses of autistic children to people and objects. *Proc Biol Sci* **268**: 1883–8.

Hitsman, B., Spring, B., Pingitore, R., Munafo, M., Hedeker, D. (2007). Effect of tryptophan depletion on the attentional salience of smoking cues. *Psychopharmacology (Berl)*, **192**: 317–24.

Holets, V.R. (1990). The anatomy and function of noradrenaline in the mammalian brain. In: *The pharmacology of noradrenaline in the central nervous system* (Heal DJ, Marsden CA, eds), pp 1–40. Oxford: Oxford University Press.

Hornak, J., O'Doherty, J., Bramham, J., Rolls, E.T., Morris, R.G., Bullock, P.R., Polkey, C.E. (2004). Reward-related reversal learning after surgical excisions in orbito-frontal or dorsolateral prefrontal cortex in humans. *J Cogn Neurosci*, **16**: 463–78.

Ichikawa, J., Meltzer, H.Y. (1999). Relationship between dopaminergic and serotonergic neuronal activity in the frontal cortex and the action of typical and atypical antipsychotic drugs. *Eur Arch Psychiatry Clin Neurosci*, **249** Suppl 4: 90–8.

Ichikawa, J., Ishii, H., Bonaccorso, S., Fowler, W.L., O'Laughlin, I.A., Meltzer, H.Y. (2001). 5-HT(2A) and D(2) receptor blockade increases cortical DA release via 5-HT(1A) receptor activation: a possible mechanism of atypical antipsychotic-induced cortical dopamine release. *J Neurochem*, **76**: 1521–31.

Iversen, S.D., Mishkin, M. (1970). Perseverative interference in monkeys following selective lesions of the inferior prefrontal convexity. *Experimental Brain Research*, **11**: 376–86.

Izquierdo, A., Murray, E.A. (2005). Opposing effects of amygdala and orbital prefrontal cortex lesions on the extinction of instrumental responding in macaque monkeys. *Eur J Neurosci*, **22**: 2341–46.

Izquierdo, A., Murray, E.A. (2007). Selective bilateral amygdala lesions in rhesus monkeys fail to disrupt object reversal learning. *J Neurosci*, **27**: 1054–62.

Izquierdo, A., Suda, R.K., Murray, E.A. (2003). Effects of selective amygdala and orbital prefrontal cortex lesions on object reversal learning in monkeys. *Society for Neuroscience Abstracts*, **90**.2.

Izquierdo, A., Suda, R.K., Murray, E.A. (2004). Bilateral orbital prefrontal cortex lesions in rhesus monkeys disrupt choices guided by both reward value and reward contingency. *J Neurosci*, **24**: 7540–48.

Izquierdo, A., Newman, T.K., Higley, J.D., Murray, E.A. (2007). Genetic modulation of cognitive flexibility and socioemotional behavior in rhesus monkeys. *Proc Natl Acad Sci USA,* **104**: 14128–33.

Jodo, E., Chiang, C., Aston-Jones, G., (1998). Potent excitatory influence of prefrontal cortex activity on noradrenergic locus coeruleus neurons. *Neuroscience,* **83**: 63–79.

Joel, D., Doljansky, J., Roz, N., Rehavi, M. (2005). Role of the orbital cortex and of the serotonergic system in a rat model of obsessive compulsive disorder. *Neuroscience,* **130**: 25–36.

Jones, B., Mishkin, M. (1972). Limbic lesions and the problem of stimulus—reinforcement associations. *Exp Neurol,* **36**: 362–77.

Kazama, A., Bachevalier, J. (2009). Selective aspiration or neurotoxic lesions of orbital frontal areas 11 and 13 spared monkeys' performance on the object discrimination reversal task. *J Neurosci,* **29**: 2794–804.

Kheramin, S., Body, S., Ho, M.Y., Velazquez-Martinez, D.N., Bradshaw, C.M., Szabadi, E. et al. (2004). Effects of orbital prefrontal cortex dopamine depletion on inter-temporal choice: a quantitative analysis. *Psychopharmacology* (Berl), **175**: 206–14.

Kim, J., Ragozzino, M.E. (2005). The involvement of the orbitofrontal cortex in learning under changing task contingencies. *Neurobiol Learn Mem,* **83**: 125–33.

King, D., Zigmond, M.J., Finlay, J.M. (1997). Effects of dopamine depletion in the medial prefrontal cortex on the stress-induced increase in extracellular dopamine in the nucleus accumbens core and shell. *Neuroscience,* **77**: 141–53.

Kurylo, D.D., Tanguay, S. (2003). Effects of quinpirole on behavioral extinction. *Physiol Behav,* **80**: 1–7.

Lapiz-Bluhm, M.D., Soto-Piña, A.E., Hensler, J.G., Morilak, D.A. (2009). Chronic intermittent cold stress and serotonin depletion induce deficits of reversal learning in an attentional set-shifting test in rats. *Psychopharmacology,* **202**: 329–41.

Lee, B., Groman, S., London, E.D., Jentsch, J.D. (2007). Dopamine D2/D3 receptors play a specific role in the reversal of a learned visual discrimination in monkeys. *Neuropsychopharmacology,* **32**: 2125–34.

Macmillan, N.A., Creelman, C.D. (1991). *Detection theory: a user's guide.* Cambridge University Press.

Man, MS., Clarke, HF., Roberts, A.C. (2009). The role of the orbitofrontal cortex and medial striatum in the regulation of prepotent responses to food rewards. *Cereb Cortex,* **19**: 899–906.

Mayberg, H.S. (2003). Modulating dysfunctional limbic-cortical circuits in depression: towards development of brain-based algorithms for diagnosis and optimised treatment. *Br Med Bull,* **65**: 193–207.

McAlonan, K., Brown, V.J. (2003). Orbital prefrontal cortex mediates reversal learning and not attentional set shifting in the rat. *Behav Brain Res,* **146**: 97–103.

McKirdy, J., Sussmann, J.E., Hall, J., Lawrie, S.M., Johnstone, E.C., McIntosh, A.M. (2008). Set shifting and reversal learning in patients with bipolar disorder or schizophrenia. *Psychol Med,*: 1–5.

Mehta, M.A., Swainson, R., Ogilvie, A.D., Sahakian, J., Robbins, T.W. (2001). Improved short-term spatial memory but impaired reversal learning following the dopamine D(2) agonist bromocriptine in human volunteers. *Psychopharmacology (Berl),* **159**: 10–20.

Meltzer, H.Y., Li, Z., Kaneda, Y., Ichikawa, J. (2003). Serotonin receptors: their key role in drugs to treat schizophrenia. *Prog Neuropsychopharmacol Biol Psychiatry,* **27**: 1159–72.

Menzies, L., Achard, S., Chamberlain, S.R., Fineberg, N., Chen, C.H., del Campo, N. et al. (2007) Neurocognitive endophenotypes of obsessive-compulsive disorder. *Brain,* **130**: 3223–36.

Mesulam, M.M., Geula, C. (1992). Overlap between acetylcholinesterase-rich and choline acetyltransferase-positive (cholinergic) axons in human cerebral cortex. *Brain Res,* **577**: 112–20.

Meunier, M., Bachevalier, J., Mishkin, M. (1997). Effects of orbital frontal and anterior cingulate lesions on object and spatial memory in rhesus monkeys. *Neuropsychologia,* **35**: 999–1015.

Milad, M.R., Rauch, S.L. (2007). The role of the orbitofrontal cortex in anxiety disorders. *Ann NY Acad Sci,* **1121**: 546–61.

Mitchell, J.B., Gratton, A. (1992). Partial dopamine depletion of the prefrontal cortex leads to enhanced mesolimbic dopamine release elicited by repeated exposure to naturally reinforcing stimuli. *J Neurosci,* **12**: 3609–3618.

Murphy, F.C., Sahakian, B.J, Rubinsztein, J.S, Michael, A., Rogers, R.D, Robbins, T.W, Paykel, E.S. (1999). Emotional bias and inhibitory control processes in mania and depression. *Psychol Med,* **29**: 1307–21.

Murray, E.A., Baxter, M.G., Gaffan, D. (1998). Monkeys with rhinal cortex damage or neurotoxic hippocampal lesions are impaired on spatial scene learning and object reversals. *Behav Neurosci,.* **112**: 1291–303.

Murray, G.K., Cheng, F., Clark, L., Barnett, J.H., Blackwell, A.D., Fletcher, P.C. et al. (2008). Reinforcement and reversal learning in first-episode psychosis. *Schizophr Bull,* **34**: 848–55.

Nicotra, A., Critchley, H.D., Mathias, C.J., Dolan, R.J. (2006). Emotional and autonomic consequences of spinal cord injury explored using functional brain imaging. *Brain,* **129**: 718–28.

O'Doherty, J., Kringelbach, M.L., Rolls, E.T., Hornak, J., Andrews, C. (2001). Abstract reward and punishment representations in the human orbitofrontal cortex. *Nat Neurosci,* **4**: 95–102.

O'Doherty, J., Critchley, H., Deichmann, R., Dolan, R.J. (2003). Dissociating valence of outcome from behavioral control in human orbital and ventral prefrontal cortices. *J Neurosci,* **23**: 7931–39.

O'Neill, M., Brown, V.J. (2007). The effect of striatal dopamine depletion and the adenosine A2A antagonist KW-6002 on reversal learning in rats. *Neurobiol Learn Mem,* **88**: 75–81.

Ongur, D., Price, J.L. (2000). The organization of networks within the orbital and medial prefrontal cortex of rats, monkeys and humans. *Cerebral Cortex,* **10**: 206–19.

Ostlund, S.B., Balleine, B.W. (2007). Orbitofrontal cortex mediates outcome encoding in Pavlovian but not instrumental conditioning. *J Neurosci,* **27**: 4819–25.

Pagnoni, G., Zink, C.F., Montague, P.R., Berns, G.S. (2002). Activity in human ventral striatum locked to errors of reward prediction. *Nat Neurosci,* **5**: 97–8.

Palfi, S., Ferrante, R.J., Brouillet, E., Beal, M.F., Dolan, R., Guyot, M.C. et al. (1996). Chronic 3-nitro-propionic acid treatment in baboons replicates the cognitive and motor deficits of Huntington's disease. *J Neurosci,* **16**: 3019–25.

Pantelis, C., Barber, F.Z., Barnes, T.R., Nelson, H.E., Owen, A.M., Robbins, T.W. (1999). Comparison of set-shifting ability in patients with chronic schizophrenia and frontal lobe damage. *Schizophr Res,* **37**: 251–70.

Paulus, M.P., Stein, M.B. (2006). An insular view of anxiety. *Biol Psychiatry,* **60**: 383–7.

Pavlov, I.P., (1927). *Conditioned reflexes.* Oxford: Oxford University Press.

Paxinos, G., Watson, C.. (1997). *The rat brain in stereotaxic coordinates,* 2nd edn. Sydney: Academic.

Petrides, M., Pandya, D.N. (1994). Comparative architectonic analysis of the human and the macaque frontal cortex. In: *Handbook of nuropsychology* (Boller F, Grafman J, eds), pp 17–58. Amsterdam: Elsevier Science BV.

Pickens, C.L., Saddoris, M.P., Setlow, B., Gallagher, M., Holland, P.C., Schoenbaum, G. (2003). Different roles for orbitofrontal cortex and basolateral amygdala in a reinforcer devaluation task. *J Neurosci,* **23**: 11078–84.

Pickens, C.L., Saddoris, M.P., Gallagher, M., Holland, P.C. (2005). Orbitofrontal lesions impair use of cue-outcome associations in a devaluation task. *Behav Neurosci,* **119**: 317–22.

Porrino, L.J., Goldman-Rakic, P.S. (1982). Brainstem innervation of prefrontal and anterior cingulate cortex in the rhesus monkey revealed by retrograde transport of HRP. *J Comp Neurol,* **205**: 63–76.

Preuss, T.M., (1995). Do rats have prefrontal cortex? The Rose-Woolsey-Akert programme reconsidered. *J Cog Neurosci,* **7**: 1–24.

Pycock, C.J., Kerwin, R.W., Carter, C.J., (1980). Effect of lesion of cortical dopamine terminals on subcortical dopamine receptors in rats. *Nature,* **286**: 74–76.

Reading, P.J., Dunnett, S.B. (1991). The effects of excitotoxic lesions of the nucleus accumbens on a matching to position task. *Behav Brain Research,* **46**: 17–29.

Reekie, Y.L., Braesicke, K., Man, M.S., Roberts, A.C. (2008). Uncoupling of behavioral and autonomic responses after lesions of the primate orbitofrontal cortex. *Proc Natl Acad Sci USA,* **105**: 9787–92.

Remijnse, P.L., Nielen, M.M., van Balkom, A.J., Cath, D.C., van Oppen, P., Uylings, H.B., Veltman, D.J. (2006). Reduced orbitofrontal-striatal activity on a reversal-learning task in obsessive-compulsive disorder. *Arch Gen Psychiatry,* **63**: 1225–36.

Remijnse, P.L., Nielen, M.M., van Balkom, A.J., Hendriks, G.J., Hoogendijk, W.J., Uylings, H.B., Veltman, D.J. (2009). Differential frontal-striatal and paralimbic activity during reversal learning in major depressive disorder and obsessive-compulsive disorder. *Psychol Med,* **39**: 1503–18.

Rescorla, R.A. (2001). Experimental extinction. In: *Handbook of contemporary learning theories* (Mowrer RR, Klein SB, eds), pp 119–54. Mahwah: Lawrence Erlbaum Associates.

Robbins, T.W., Roberts, A.C. (2007). Differential regulation of fronto-executive function by the monoamines and acetylcholine. *Cereb Cortex,* **17** Suppl1:i151–60.

Roberts, A.C. (2006). Primate orbitofrontal cortex and adaptive behavior. *TICS,* **10**: 83–90.

Roberts, A.C., Wallis, J.D. (2000). Inhibitory control and affective processing in the prefrontal cortex: neuropsychological studies in the common marmoset. *Cereb Cortex,* **10**: 252–62.

Roberts, A.C., De Salvia, M.A., Wilkinson, L.S., Collins, P., Muir, J.L., Everitt, B.J., Robbins, T.W. (1994). 6-Hydroxydopamine lesions of the prefrontal cortex in monkeys enhance performance on an analog of the Wisconsin Card Sort Test: possible interactions with subcortical dopamine. *J Neurosci,* **14**: 2531–44.

Roberts, A.C., Reekie, Y., Braesicke, K. (2007a). Synergistic and regulatory effects of orbitofrontal cortex on amygdala-dependent appetitive behavior. *Ann NY Acad Sci,* **1121**: 297–319.

Roberts, A.C., Tomic DL, Parkinson, C.H., Roeling, T.A., Cutter, D.J., Robbins, T.W., Everitt, B.J. (2007b). Forebrain connectivity of the prefrontal cortex in the marmoset monkey (*Callithrix jacchus*): an anterograde and retrograde tract-tracing study. *J Comp Neurol,* **502**: 86–112.

Rogers, R.D., Andrews, T.C., Grasby, P.M., Brooks, D.J., Robbins, T.W. (2000). Contrasting cortical and subcortical activations produced by attentional-set shifting and reversal learning in humans. *J Cogn Neurosci,* **12**: 142–62.

Rolls, E.T., Hornak, J., Wade, D., McGrath, J. (1994). Emotion-related learning in patients with social and emotional changes associated with frontal lobe damage. *J Neurol Neurosurg Psychiatry,* **57**: 1518–24.

Rosenkranz, J.A., Grace, A.A. (2001). Dopamine attenuates prefrontal cortical suppression of sensory inputs to the basolateral amygdala of rats. *J Neurosci,* **21**: 4090–103.

Saxena, S., Rauch, S.L. (2000). Functional neuroimaging and the neuroanatomy of obsessive-compulsive disorder. *Psychiatr Clin North Am,* **23**: 563–86.

Saxena, S., Brody, A.L., Maidment, K.M., Dunkin, J.J., Colgan, M., Alborzian, S., et al. (1999). Localized orbitofrontal and subcortical metabolic changes and predictors of response to paroxetine treatment in obsessive-compulsive disorder. *Neuropsychopharm,* **21**: 683–93.

Schoenbaum, G., Setlow, B. (2003). Lesions of nucleus accumbens disrupt learning about aversive outcomes. *J Neurosci,* **23**: 9833–41.

Schoenbaum, G., Chiba, A.A., Gallagher, M. (1998). Orbitofrontal cortex and basolateral amygdala encode expected outcomes during learning. *Nat Neurosci,* **1**: 155–9.

Schoenbaum, G., Nugent, S.L., Saddoris, M.P., Setlow, B. (2002). Orbitofrontal lesions in rats impair reversal but not acquisition of go, no-go odor discriminations. *Neurorep,* **13**: 885–90.

Schoenbaum, G., Setlow, B., Nugent, S.L., Saddoris, M.P., Gallagher, M. (2003). Lesions of orbitofrontal cortex and basolateral amygdala complex disrupt acquisition of odor-guided discriminations and reversals. *Learn Mem,* **10**: 129–40.

Schoenbaum, G., Saddoris, M.P., Stalnaker, T.A. (2007). Reconciling the roles of orbitofrontal cortex in reversal learning and the encoding of outcome expectancies. *Ann NY Acad Sci,* **1121**: 320–35.

Schultz, W. (2002). Getting formal with dopamine and reward. *Neuron,* **36**: 241–63.

Sesack, S.R., Deutch, A.Y., Roth, R.H., Bunney, B.S. (1989). Topographical organization of the efferent projections of the medial prefrontal cortex in the rat: an anterograde tract-tracing study with Phaseolus vulgaris leucoagglutinin. *J Comp Neurol,* **290**: 213–42.

Seymour, B., Daw, N., Dayan, P., Singer, T., Dolan, R. (2007). Differential encoding of losses and gains in the human striatum. *J Neurosci,* **27**: 4826–31.

Stalnaker, T.A., Franz, T.M., Singh, T., Schoenbaum, G. (2007). Basolateral amygdala lesions abolish orbitofrontal-dependent reversal impairments. *Neuron,* **54**: 51–58.

Swainson, R., Rogers, R.D., Sahakian, B.J., Summers, B.A., Polkey, C.E., Robbins, T.W. (2000). Probabilistic learning and reversal deficits in patients with Parkinson's disease or frontal or temporal lobe lesions: possible adverse effects of dopaminergic medication. *Neuropsychologia,* **38**: 596–612.

Tait, D.S., Brown, V.J. (2007). Difficulty overcoming learned non-reward during reversal learning in rats with ibotenic acid lesions of orbital prefrontal cortex. *Ann NY Acad Sci,* **1121**: 407–20.

Thorpe, S.J., Rolls, E.T., Maddison, S. (1983). The orbitofrontal cortex: neuronal activity in the behaving monkey. *Exp Brain Res,* **49**: 93–115.

Tops, M., Russo, S., Boksem, M.A., Tucker, D.M. (2009). Serotonin: Modulator of a drive to withdraw. *Brain Cogn,* **71**(3): 427–36.

Tremblay, L., Schultz, W. (2000). Reward-related neuronal activity during go-nogo task performance in primate orbitofrontal cortex. *J Neurophysiol,* **83**: 1864–76.

Uylings, H.B.M., Groenewegen, H.J., Kolb, B. (2003). Do rats have a prefrontal cortex? *Behav Brain Res,* **146**: 3–17.

Valerius, G., Lumpp, A., Kuelz, A.K., Freyer, T., Voderholzer, U. (2008). Reversal learning as a neuropsychological indicator for the neuropathology of obsessive compulsive disorder? A behavioral study. *J Neuropsychiatry Clin Neurosci,* **20**: 210–8.

Volkow, N.D., Fowler, J.S. (2000). Addiction, a disease of compulsion and drive: involvement of the orbitofrontal cortex. *Cereb Cortex,* **10**: 318–25.

Walker, S.C., Robbins, T.W., Roberts, A.C. (2009). Differential contributions of dopamine and serotonin to orbitofrontal cortex function in the marmoset. *Cereb Cortex,* **19**: 889–98.

Walker, S.C., Mikheenko, Y.P., Argyle, L.D., Robbins, T.W., Roberts, A.C. (2006). Selective prefrontal serotonin depletion impairs acquisition of a detour-reaching task. *Eur J Neurosci,* **23**: 3119–23.

Wallis, J.D., Dias, R., Robbins, T.W., Roberts, A.C. (2001). Dissociable contributions of the orbitofrontal and lateral prefrontal cortex of the marmoset to performance on a detour reaching task. *Eur J Neurosci,* **13**: 1797–808.

Waltz, J.A., Gold, J.M. (2007). Probabilistic reversal learning impairments in schizophrenia: further evidence of orbitofrontal dysfunction. *Schizophr Res,* **93**: 296–303.

Williams, L.M., Das, P., Liddell, B.J., Olivieri, G., Peduto, A.S., David, A.S., Gordon, E., Harris, A.W. (2007). Fronto-limbic and autonomic disjunctions to negative emotion distinguish schizophrenia subtypes. *Psychiatry Res,* **155**: 29–44.

Wilson, J.M., Kalasinsky, K.S., Levey, A.I., Bergeron, C., Reiber, G., Anthony, R.M., Schmunk, G.A., Shannak, K., Haycock, J.W., Kish, S.J. (1996). Striatal dopamine nerve terminal markers in human, chronic methamphetamine users. *Nat Med,* **2**: 699–703.

Yin, H.H., Knowlton, B.J., Balleine, B.W. (2004). Lesions of dorsolateral striatum preserve outcome expectancy but disrupt habit formation in instrumental learning. *Eur J Neurosci,* **19**: 181–9.

Zaborszky, L., Gaykema, R.P., Swanson, D.J., Cullinan, W.E. (1997). Cortical input to the basal forebrain. *Neurosci,* **79**: 1051–78.

Chapter 11

Cingulate and orbitofrontal contributions to valuing knowns and unknowns in a changeable world

Mark E. Walton, Peter H. Rudebeck,
Timothy E. J. Behrens, and
Matthew F. S. Rushworth

Abstract

The world that we and other animals inhabit is frequently stochastic, uncertain, and changeable and it is imperative that our brains are able to evaluate and keep track of varying contingencies. While behavioral ecologists have long researched how animals operate in such natural environments, investigations into aspects of higher cognition in the psychology laboratory have tended to focus on controlled, static situations in which the experimenter determines that some responses are clearly more correct than others. Over the last few years, there has been increasing interest in the roles of two parts of the frontal lobe—the sulcal region of the dorsal anterior cingulate cortex (ACCs) and orbitofrontal cortex (OFC)—when outcome information indicates a need for a change in behavior. Here we review some recent lesion and functional imaging studies that have compared the contributions of these regions in guiding beneficial choice behavior in uncertain, changeable situations. In particular, we demonstrate that in such task environments, both regions are not simply important for detecting mistakes and updating behavior, but instead play dissociable roles in the continuous assessment of outcome value in terms of its relationship with predictors in the world, with different courses of action, and the usefulness of information to guide subsequent decision making.

11.1 Introduction

In the stable, predictable world of many laboratory experiments, learning what responses are best to make can seem a relatively straightforward process. This is not to suggest that the tasks themselves are not taxing. There can be difficulties imposed by memory or attentional demands or by the insertion of distracting information, any of which may prompt an erroneous response. Moreover, there may be complex conditional response rules, which require that actions selected are based on the overall context of a situation and not merely on simple learned stimulus-response mappings. Nonetheless, from an objective standpoint, on each trial there is a "correct" response among the set available, one option that will clearly result in the best outcome, and such an optimal response can be rapidly uncovered by the subject undertaking the task, often within a single trial if the number of possible of options is constrained, and can be repeated on subsequent trials with equal success.

The demands of operating in an uncertain, stochastic world are, however, somewhat different. In particular, the outcome of any one particular choice may not be a particularly good guide as to what the best response to make is as even low probability events can occur on some occasions and, conversely, likely events do not always have to happen. Therefore, it is imperative to integrate across several choices and outcomes both to build up an accurate representation of the underlying likelihood, and hence the risk, of a particular outcome and to minimise the uncertainty in this estimate (Platt and Huettel, 2008; Rushworth and Behrens, 2008). So long as this task environment is stable, meaning that the choice–outcome associations remain unchanged during a session, and, particularly, if the outcome of one option is informative about the outcome that would have been available for taking an alternative (for instance, if it is known that only one option will be rewarded in any one instance), it will still be possible to discover which is the best available option, even if this will require an increased sampling of choices and outcomes that in a deterministic situation.

However, the environment that we and all animals are required to navigate through on a daily basis is not only stochastic but also changeable and uncertain. This leads to two particular difficulties. First, whichever course of action may appear the best available at one point in time may not remain so in the future. This means there is a constant requirement to monitor fluctuations in outcomes to work out what response to make, rather than always relying on a straightforward and cognitively undemanding strategy of choosing what was previously the best option. Such fluctuations will not only inform estimates of the expected value of an outcome (either in terms of likelihood of occurrence, quantity, quality, or any combination of these), but also confidence in these estimates as a function of the variability in the outcomes and how often they have been sampled. Second, the outcome gained for the chosen response may not necessarily be a good predictor of what might have happened if an alternative decision had been taken. On some occasions, the value of these alternative possibilities is available to the decision maker and several lines of evidence show that these can strongly modulate people's choices, both by allowing updating of value estimates of all other options and, at least in humans, by causing regret (or even the anticipation of future regret) (Camille et al., 2004; Mellers, 2000; Montague et al., 2006). More commonly, the consequences of taking alternative courses of action remain ambiguous or there are too many possible options to make such a strategy feasible, meaning that alternative courses of action need actively to be explored and outcomes experienced. Overall, the value of gaining information has constantly to be weighed against what is known about the expected reward values of the options (Aston-Jones and Cohen, 2005; Daw et al., 2006; Gittins, 1979; Krebs et al., 1978).

Many of the psychological processes important for performing well in more complex deterministic situations described in the opening paragraph—selective attention, working memory, strategy selection—have been associated with frontal lobe function, particularly the regions on the lateral surface (Bunge, 2004; Desimone and Duncan, 1995; Miller and Cohen, 2001). However, while similar functions have, on occasion, also been linked with medial and orbital parts of the frontal lobe (Bush et al., 2000; Mesulam, 1999; Petit et al., 1998), evidence from interference-based studies frequently shows that these regions are not directly necessary in order to select between appropriate strategies or hold information over delays so long as the correct stimulus–response–outcome mappings are static (Baxter et al., 2007; Fellows and Farah, 2005; Mishkin, 1957; Murray et al., 1989; Pribram and Fulton, 1954; Rushworth et al., 2003). Instead, numerous studies have implicated both orbitofrontal (OFC) and anterior cingulate cortex (ACC) as critical for guiding behavior, only when the environment affords uncertainty about outcomes, particularly in situations when the most appropriate response changes during a testing session (Murray et al., 2007; Roberts, 2006; Rushworth et al., 2007; Walton et al., 2007). Both the ACC and OFC share reciprocal projections, as well as having connections with other frontal lobe regions, and both have access to a variety of outcome information through connections with limbic areas such as the amygdala and ventral striatum, and by being recipients of dense innervation from midbrain monoaminergic cells (Amaral and Price, 1984; Carmichael and Price, 1996; Gaspar et al., 1989; Williams and Goldman-Rakic, 1998). Both also project to evolutionarily old subcortical structures involved with control of basic motivational states and responses such as the hypothalamus and periacqueductal gray (An et al., 1998; Ongur et al., 1998). They, therefore, both have access to the type of information that would be critical to allow animals to keep track of their history of choices and outcomes plus also, importantly, to be able to assess the value of that outcome in terms of the animal's present state.

Although the OFC and ACC have been implicated in guiding, evaluating, and altering choices on the basis of outcome information, their precise contribution to performance-monitoring and decision making in uncertain, changeable environments remains contentious. Many neuroimaging studies of reward-guided choice behavior and outcome evaluation find activations in both regions (e.g., Coricelli et al., 2005; Elliott et al., 2000a; O'Doherty et al., 2003a; Rolls et al., 2008). By contrast, the majority of animal studies, using either electrophysiological and lesion methodologies, have either focused on one of the regions alone or have compared either ACC or OFC function against another region, such as the amygdala or striatum, making it difficult to determine precisely how the functions of the OFC and ACC might differ (Clarke et al., 2008; e.g., Izquierdo et al., 2004; Kennerley et al., 2006; Kepecs et al., 2008; Quilodran et al., 2008; Roesch et al., 2007). Moreover, few studies have investigated choice behavior using tasks that closely mimic the challenges faced in the natural environment, namely selecting a response when outcomes are uncertain, probabilistic, and changeable.

The purpose of the present chapter is twofold. First, we will review recent studies from our laboratory and from others, which have explicitly investigated the functions of the OFC and ACC in primates using analogous reward-guided decision-making situations, with particular emphasis on determining how these regions participate when animals or humans have to track outcome value in a changeable situation. This will attempt to demonstrate that, while both of these regions play vital roles in allowing animals to alter their behavior in this type of environment, one of their specific *functions* is likely not to be in actually implementing the change or inhibiting previously rewarded actions, but may instead be related to more fundamental learning processes that enable animals to ascribe the appropriate value to options. Moreover, there appears a fundamental dissociation between the types of information-processing that these regions are preferentially engaged in, with OFC being particularly important for monitoring outcomes of externally-guided, stimulus-based choices and ACCs with outcomes connected with internally-guided actions. Second, we will discuss the factors that animals might use to assess the value of an outcome and to decide when to acquire new information about available alternatives, and how these might be implemented in these frontal regions. Here again there appears a subtle but important dissociation between the roles of these two regions, with ACCs being involved with evaluating the significance of an outcome for guiding learning and future choices, whereas OFC is more important for determining aspects of specific stimulus–outcome association in environments where there are multiple stimuli. While both OFC and ACC have been shown to play a role, both in choosing responses and monitoring their consequences, we will concentrate largely on the latter process while acknowledging that any separation of outcome evaluation and learning from consequent decision making may be somewhat artificial in practice.

To aid cross-species comparison, our focus here will be on studies comparing OFC with dorsal, supracallosal ACC, which will be referred to throughout as ACCs, denoting the tissue in the cingulate sulcus in macaque monkeys and what is believed to be the homologous part in the human brain, a perigenual region of ACC lying anterior to the AC–PC line (a theoretical line perpendicular to one traversing the anterior and posterior commissures) (Picard and Strick, 1996; Ridderinkhof et al., 2004; Zilles et al., 1996), as few investigations in monkeys have extended outside of this ACC region (Fig. 11.1A). Anatomical studies have demonstrated that this part of the ACC has direct connections with the motor system, as well as access to outcome information (Beckmann et al., 2009; He et al., 1995; Morecraft and Van Hoesen, 1998; Wang et al., 2001). While the OFC is a large and anatomically heterogeneous region, with lateral OFC regions having somewhat different anatomical connectivity than medial parts and more anterior regions having different cytoarchitecture from posterior ones (Croxson et al., 2005; Ongur and Price, 2000), and possibly separable functions (e.g., Elliott et al., 2000b), for the sake of simplicity we have here chosen to treat the structure as a whole, though restricted to the dysgranular and homotypical portions of areas 11, 13, and 14 (Murray and Izquierdo, 2007) (Fig. 11.1A).

11.2 Stimulus- or action-guided reversal learning

In order to be able to survive in a changeable world, animals need to be able to keep track of whether or not expected outcomes were received and, if not, to decide whether to persist with the current response or adjust their behavior accordingly. The simplest model of such an environment in the laboratory utilizes task-switching or reversal-learning paradigms. In these types of tasks, several response options are typically presented, one of which is rewarded at a much higher probability than the others on any given trial (the best option is often rewarded deterministically, always giving reward, while the alternatives never do). However, at certain points during a session the outcome contingencies completely reverse, so that the previously highly rewarding option now has a low likelihood of giving reward and one of the other alternatives now has a high probability of resulting in reward. Such changes in contingency can be explicitly signaled by an external, contextual or conditional cue, which indicates that the outcome associations have changed prior to any decision being made. There is little direct evidence of a role for the OFC in this type of explicit rule- or cue-guided switching behavior (Aron et al., 2004; though see Shallice et al., 2007), and while neuroimaging studies of this type of explicit task-switching frequently have shown activations in dorsomedial parts of the frontal lobe, including in the ACCs (Crone et al., 2006; Liston et al., 2006; Rushworth et al., 2002), lesions or inactivations of this region do not cause an impairment directly related to the cued changing of behavior when the rules have been taught prior to the interference (Rushworth et al., 2003; Shima and Tanji, 1998).

Instead, what links together the long literature of studies in several species implicating both the ACCs and OFC in this type of flexible behavior is a dependence on the alterations in contingency being evident only once the outcome of a choice has been revealed (Butter, 1969; Dias et al., 1996; Fellows and Farah, 2003; Iversen and Mishkin, 1970; Izquierdo et al., 2004; Kennerley et al., 2006; O'Doherty et al., 2001; Schoenbaum et al., 2003; Shima and Tanji, 1998). For instance, in a two-choice deterministic reinforcement-guided reversal task using objects as stimuli, where only one of the stimuli was ever associated with reward at any one time and a reversal was signaled by the sudden absence of reward for the previously reinforced stimulus, monkeys with selective OFC lesions (including areas 11 and 13 on the orbital surface, though sparing more lateral area 12) were significantly less likely than controls to update their behavior and choose the correct response following a reversal, even though their initial learning of which stimulus to choose was intact (Fig. 11.1B) (Izquierdo et al., 2004). These animals had particular deficits not at switching away from the previously reinforced object, but at consolidating their learning of the new association, making significantly more errors in the stage when performing around chance levels. Post-operatively, monkeys with ACCs lesions were also impaired following a reversal (as well as prior to it—see below for details) on a two-choice deterministic reinforcement-guided reversal task using a joystick response, where again correct behavior was guided solely by the presence or absence of reward (Kennerley et al., 2006) (Fig. 11.1C). However, when the same ACCs-lesioned animals were tested on a similar task to that given to the OFC-lesioned animals in the study by Izquierdo and colleagues, where the animals chose between visual stimuli on a touchscreen, rather than joystick movements, intriguingly these animals now showed no clear deficit in performance (Rudebeck et al., 2006a) (Fig. 11.1E).

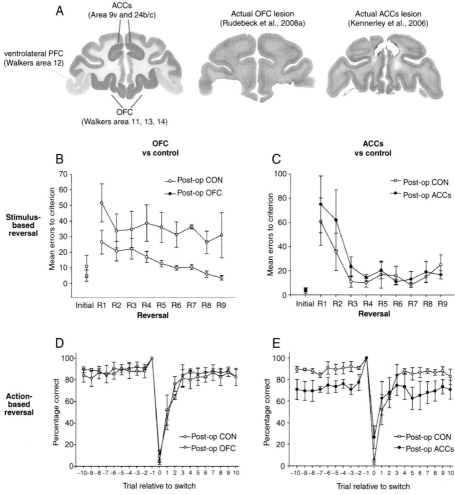

Fig. 11.1 Location of OFC and ACCs, and performance of OFC- and ACCs-lesioned monkeys on stimulus- or action-based reversal tasks. (A) Coronal schematic of macaque OFC (green) and ACCs (red) discussed in the current article, along with individual examples of OFC (centre panel) and ACCs lesions (right panel). The OFC region targeted centered on Walker's areas 11 and 13, but largely spared more lateral parts of Walker's area 12. From *Science*, P.H. Rudebeck, M.J. Buckley, M.E. Walton, and M.F.S. Rushworth, A Role for the Macaque Anterior Cingulate Gyrus in Social Valuation, Copyright 2006. Reprinted with permission from AAAS. (B) OFC lesions cause significant reversal impairments on a stimulus-based reversal task, while the animals are unimpaired at learning the novel associations (C) ACCs lesions do not result significant reversal impairments on a stimulus-based reversal task (D) OFC lesions do not impair reversal learning on a action-based joystick reversal task (E) ACCs lesions, however, are significantly impaired on the action-based joystick reversal task (Kennerley et al., 2006). (B–E) Reprinted from *Journal of Neuroscience*, 17; 28(51), 13775–85 Rudebeck PH; Behrens TE, Kennerley SW, Baxter MG, Buckley MJ, Walton ME, Rushworth MF, Frontal cortex subregions play distinct roles in choices between actions and stimuli, Copyright 2008. Reprinted with permission from the Society of Neuroscience.

This highlights an important facet of decision making, namely that there are likely several distinct valuation signals that influence the selection of an action (Rangel et al., 2008a). The evidence from the aforementioned studies hints that the OFC and ACCs may be involved in guiding and altering choices based on the expected value associated, respectively, with an external stimulus or with an internally-generated action in the absence of any guiding cues (Rushworth et al., 2007). To test this directly, Rudebeck and colleagues (2008) recently studied the effects of OFC lesions in monkeys carrying out the joystick-based two-choice reinforcement-guided reversal task learned prior to surgery, which animals with ACCs lesions had been impaired at performing (Kennerley et al., 2006). Post-operatively, OFC-lesioned animals exhibited none of the deficits observed in the ACCs-lesioned group and were just as able as unoperated control animals, in this action-based task, to update their responses when signaled by a change in reinforcement (Fig. 11.1D). Such a distinction between using stimulus- compared to action-reinforcement associations to update behavior is bolstered by an important anatomical difference between the OFC and ACCs, with the former receiving much more prominent afferents from sensory association areas on the temporal lobes, whereas only the latter is able directly to elicit movements through projections to primary motor cortex and the spinal cord (Beckmann et al., 2009; Carmichael and Price, 1996; Croxson et al., 2005; He et al., 1995; Wang et al., 2001).

11.3 Changing choices or learning the value of actions?

Reversal tasks have been important tools for allowing investigation of flexible behavior in a changeable environment and how different brain circuits may be involved in updating choice–outcome associations. However, they also represent a somewhat extreme, and ecologically unlikely, circumstance whereby a previously rewarded option suddenly no longer yields any positive outcome from which an inference needs to be made that the poorly rewarded alternative will now always deliver reward. It has been pointed out that humans, at least, can perform even slightly more demanding probabilistic reinforcement-based reversal tasks by inferring the higher order structure, rather than solely using reinforcement learning to guide choices (Hampton et al., 2006). Therefore, an important question arises as to whether the reason that ACCs and OFC frequently show activity around the time of a reversal, and lesions to these regions selectively impair different types of deterministic reinforcement-guided reversal tasks, reflects their importance in allowing animals to change behavior, in interpreting the task structure or instead other processes involved in assigning the appropriate value according to the choices made. Even though OFC lesions in humans, monkeys, or rats do not affect choice behavior when initially learning novel associations in deterministic reversal tasks (Fellows and Farah, 2003; Izquierdo et al., 2004; Schoenbaum et al., 2003), cells in OFC consistently have been shown to adjust their firing rates when animals learn the expected reinforcement associated with a stimulus (Hosokawa et al., 2005; Tremblay and Schultz, 2000; Wallis and Miller, 2003). Moreover, lesions to this region in rats selectively impair stimulus–outcome encoding without affecting the expression of action–outcome associations (Ostlund and

Balleine, 2007). Similarly, it has been shown that there are increases in cell firing and BOLD signal activity in ACCs when subjects are learning novel action–outcome associations, as well as when they are updating them, and that this occurs both when presented with positive, as well as with negative feedback (Matsumoto et al., 2007; Quilodran et al., 2008; Walton et al., 2004).

Moreover, while, as mentioned above, ACCs lesions do impair overall performance on the joystick-based reversal task, inspection of Fig. 11.1E shows that the monkeys' choices are equally poor on the trials running up to a reversal, as on those just subsequent to it, suggesting no cardinal deficit at the time of the response reversal. Indeed, further analyses demonstrated that the lesioned animals were just as good as controls at updating performance immediately after making an erroneous response and, instead, seemed unable to integrate across a history of outcomes to gain evidence to persist with the correct response (Kennerley et al., 2006) (Fig. 11.1D). A similar pattern has recently been shown in OFC-lesioned animals performing the object-guided reversal learning task (Izquierdo et al., 2004), with these animals having a particular inability to use reward information to guide and persist with subsequent choices (Rudebeck and Murray, 2008) (Fig. 11.2A). A comparable difference between control and OFC groups was not observed for responses after extended runs of unrewarded responses, demonstrating that the effect of OFC lesions seemed specific to integrating positive evidence to guide choices. Indeed, although the ACCs-lesioned monkeys were just as able to update their choices as controls in the stimulus-based reversal task, even here the ACCs group did exhibit a subtle initial deficit at using reward information following an error to persist with the correct response (this impairment was, however, significantly less marked than that observed on the action-based reversal task) (Fig. 11.2B). Although these deterministic reversal tasks had clear correct and incorrect responses that can be evaluated and updated in a single trial, intriguingly, all animals performed as if weighing evidence for choosing one option or the other, having approximately only a 50% likelihood of updating their behavior when receiving no reward and then being increasingly likely to select the correct response as positive reinforcement for that option accumulated (Kennerley et al., 2006; Rudebeck and Murray, 2008) (Fig. 11.2A–D).

In order to investigate response selection in a task environment that *required* animals to integrate across outcomes by making the reward associations probabilistic, monkeys with lesions of either OFC or ACCs were tested on two different two-choice discrete trial dynamic matching tasks. These tasks differ from the reversal tasks in two important ways. First, the likelihood of obtaining a reward associated with each option was chosen prior to the start of testing and remained fixed throughout the session. This meant that there were no explicit points in testing when the values of the options reversed. Second, rewards were assigned on each trial to both options *independently*, according to the imposed probabilities, and any reward assigned for an option that was not selected on the current trial remains available for collection as soon as this alternative is chosen on some subsequent trial. Take the example if the two options, A and B, were set to be associated with giving reward at probabilities of 0.75 and 0.25 and on trial N a reward was allocated for

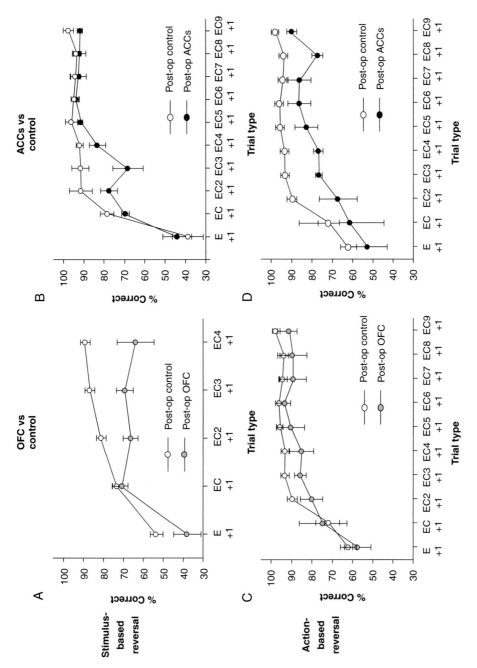

Fig. 11.2 Use of reward information as evidence for selecting the correct response. E+1 = performance on a trial after an error; EC+1 = performance on a trial following a single correct response after an error; EC(N)+1 = performance on a trial following N correct responses after an error. Data are included for each trial type for which every animal had at least 10 instances (which is why there are fewer trial types in the analysis of the stimulus-based reversal task in Rudebeck and Murray, 2008, panel C). (A) Effect of OFC lesions on using reinforcement

Fig. 11.2 (*Contd*). information in the stimulus-based reversal task. Reprinted from *Journal of Neuroscience*, 13, 28(33), 8338–43 Rudebeck, PH and Murry, EA, Amygdala and Orbitofrontal cortex lesions differentially influence choices during object reversal leaning, Copyright 2008. Reprinted with permission from the Society of Neuroscience. (B) Effect of ACCs lesions on using reinforcement information in the stimulus-based reversal task (unpublished data). There was a significant group × trial type interaction ($F_{9,45} = 2.45$, $P = 0.028$, Huynh-Feldt corrected), caused by the ACCs group being less likely to persist with the correct response following reinforcement in the trials following an error. However, this effect was significantly less prominent than in the action-based joystick reversal task (panel D) (controls vs ACCs: group × task interaction: $F_{1,5} = 15.47$, $P = 0.011$; ACCs: main effect of task: $F_{1,2} = 17.85$, $P = 0.05$; controls: no main effect of task: $P>0.1$). (C) Effect of OFC lesions on using reinforcement information in the action-based joystick reversal task. (D) Effect of ACCs lesions on using reinforcement information in the action-based joystick reversal task (Kennerley et al., 2006). (C and D) Reprinted from *Journal of Neuroscience*, 13; 28(51), 13775–85 Rudebeck, PH Behrers, TE, Kennerley, SW, Baxter, MG, Buckley, MJ, Walton, ME, Frontal cortex subregions play distinct notes in choices between actions and stimuli, Copyright 2008. Reprinted by permission from the Society of Neuroscience.

both responses. If the monkey chooses option A, it will receive the reward but the reward on the option B remains unharvested (there is no counterfactual evidence available to the animal, such as the visual presence or absence of reward, to show what would have been received for the alternative response). On the immediately subsequent trial N+1, therefore, the likelihoods of gaining reward for A and B are now 0.75 and 1.0, as the previously allocated reward remains available for capture on B. Once B is chosen and the reward is gained, however, its likelihood of giving reward then returns on subsequent trials to 0.25. Therefore, to perform the task optimally and gain the most rewards possible, it is necessary, on occasion, to sample the option with a lower allocated probability as the carryover of unobtained rewards will make this option have a higher expected value than the high probability alternative after several trials on which it is not selected (Herrnstein et al., 1997; Staddon et al., 1981; Sugrue et al., 2004). Moreover, this means that the animals should monitor both their history of outcomes and their history of choices to perform optimally, as the structure of the environment means that the expected value of each option will depend partly on their recent choice history (Lau and Glimcher, 2005).

In keeping with the reversal study, monkeys with either ACCs or OFC lesions were tested on two versions of the dynamic matching task, one where the choices were between two visual stimuli presented on a touchscreen, the location of which changed from trial to trial (meaning that stimulus value was not associated with any one particular response: stimulus-matching task), the other where choices were made between two joystick movements (action-matching task). The probability of gaining reward for the two options in two conditions of both matching tasks was also analogous—high probability to low probability ratios of 0.75:0.25 or 0.5:0.2 (in the action matching, 0.5:0.18 in the stimulus matching) (the action-matching task also had two extra conditions with 1.0:0.0 and 0.4:0.1 reward ratios).

Mirroring the previous findings in the reversal tasks, there was a striking double-dissociation in the abilities of the lesioned animals to reach optimal performance in the two tasks (defined as the proportion of responses that would yield at least 97% of the maximum rate of reward). In the stimulus-matching task, the OFC group was significantly slower to reach this optimal ratio of choices in the stimulus-matching task than control animals, while the ACCs group showed no comparable impairment (Fig. 23A and C). In the action-matching task, by contrast, it was the ACCs group who took significantly more trials to reach optimal performance in the conditions with probabilistic outcomes, whereas the OFC-lesioned animals learned at a similar rate to the controls (Kennerley et al., 2006; Rudebeck et al., 2008a) (Fig. 11.3B and D). All three groups performed comparably in the action-matching task when the options were rewarded deterministically (1.0:0.0), even though the best option was always the reverse of the previous session.

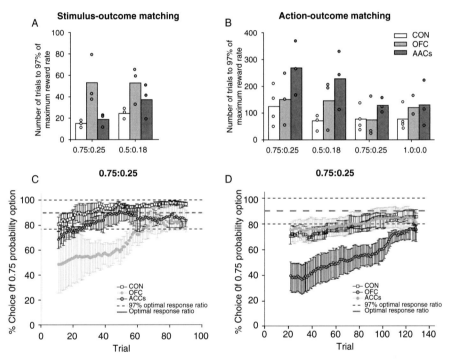

Fig. 11.3 Performance on OFC- and ACCs-lesioned monkeys on stimulus- or action-based dynamic matching tasks. (A) OFC but not ACCs lesions cause animals to be significantly slower to attain a near-optimal level of performance on the stimulus-based matching task. (B) ACCs but not OFC lesions cause animals to be significantly slower on all probabilistic schedules to attain a near-optimal level of performance on the action-based joystick matching task. There was no difference on the deterministic (1.0:0.0) schedule. (C) High-value stimulus choices of OFC, ACCs, and control animals post-operatively, averaged over two sessions, across the 0.75:0.25 session in the stimulus-based matching task. (D) High-value action choices of OFC, ACCs, and control groups post-operatively, averaged over two sessions, across the 0.75:0.25 session in the action-based matching task. Reprinted from *Journal of Neuroscience*, 25; Izquiedo A, Suda RK, and Murray RA, Bilateral orbital prefrontal cortex lesions in rhesus monkeys disrupt choices guided by both reward value and reward contingency, Copyright 2004. Reprinted with permission from the Society of Neuroscience.

While matching tasks do not contain an explicit requirement to change responses as found in response reversal tasks, owing to the aforementioned carrying over of allocated rewards on the unchosen option, it is sometimes necessary to switch to the low-probability option to perform optimally. However, this did not seem to be the primary cause of the impairment as both the OFC-lesioned animals in the stimulus-matching and the ACCs-lesioned animals in the action-matching task were just as likely, overall, to switch between the two options, regardless of the outcome of the trial.

In contrast to the reversal tasks, the availability of allocated but unchosen rewards on subsequent trials means that immediate outcome information on its own is not an adequate guide as to when to change or when to persist with a response (for instance, using a "win-stay, lose-shift strategy," a simple but efficient heuristic often adopted by primates, which may be used for learning associations or even when playing certain economic games (Genovesio et al., 2005; Nowak and Sigmund, 1993; Seo and Lee, 2008). Take the example of a monkey optimally performing the 0.5:0.2 condition. This hypothetical animal will only sample the low-probability option sparsely, on ~20% of trials, and if these choices are well-spaced apart, then they are likely often to result in reward being delivered. However, to gather the maximum number of rewards, it is important to interpret this positive outcome information in the context of the task, meaning that animals should be less likely to choose the same option again after gaining a reward for selecting the low- compared to the high-probability option. Equally, the monkeys should be more likely to persist with a response option after not receiving a reward for selecting the high- rather than the low-probability option. This is exactly the pattern of reinforcement-guided choices displayed by the control animals, suggesting that they may, at least partly, be able to interpret the value of the outcome information in the context of the task. However, such a pattern of performance was significantly less evident in the OFC-lesioned animals during the stimulus-matching task and, conversely, in the ACC-lesioned animals compared to controls in the action-matching task. Taken together, this demonstrates again that the OFC and ACCs are critical for making beneficial decisions when directed by reward associations with either stimuli or actions, respectively, and that their roles in directing flexible reinforcement-guided decisions are not limited to occasions when animals make errors and receive no reward, requiring new courses of action to be adopted.

11.4 What influences how valuable outcome information is?

One consistent finding from all of the above studies is that animals performing tasks in which outcomes are uncertain or the reinforcement structure changes, in the latter case even sometimes when outcomes are deterministic, categorize receipt or omission of reward as a piece of evidence to help guide behavior, rather than a categorical cue as to what to choose. Moreover, the value of this reward will depend highly on the context in which it is received. From an ecological point of view, this may seem entirely unsurprising. To a foraging animal, a piece of food found when resources are sparse and it is hungry has a great deal more value than the same food discovered in a state of satiation or when there is bountiful choice as to what to eat. However, it is not simply how overall metabolically or homeostatically useful an option is that can give it value for a foraging animal (see Stephens and Krebs, 1986). In dynamic, changeable environments, it is important to continuously monitor the likelihoods of outcomes occurring and be able to evaluate the usefulness of each new piece of information in the context of the structure of the environment to guide future decisions. As mentioned, in the matching tasks, there is a predictable increase in the likelihood of an option yielding a positive outcome when it has not recently been chosen and the overall value function is a product of both reward and choice history. Similarly, in the deterministic reversal tasks, the frequent and partially predictable switches of the consequences associated with each alternative means that recent experience will be a better guide to future response selection than outcomes that were attained far in the past.

One powerful tool that has been used to model the process of step-by-step learning about the value of options based on experience has been reinforcement learning (Sutton and Barto, 1998). In its simplest form, each option is associated with a value function representing the estimated upcoming reward for selecting that option in a given state. These functions are updated by reward prediction errors, the discrepancy between the current estimate and the received reward, which is scaled by the learning rate representing the expected usefulness of this current information to accurately modify this estimate (Dayan et al., 2000; Sutton and Barto, 1998). Although signaling of such prediction errors and their effect on learning has been particularly connected with the dopamine system (Schultz et al., 1997; Waelti et al., 2001), such quantitative prediction error-like signals have also been observed in several other regions, including striatum, OFC, and ACCs (Amiez et al., 2005; Hare et al., 2008; Matsumoto et al., 2007; O'Doherty et al., 2003b; Tobler et al., 2006).

While such simple reinforcement learning provides stable, prudent, experience-based assessments of the likely value of available options, it has often been pointed out that such trial-and-error learning without modification may be less efficient at guiding beneficial behavior when the likelihood of reward is liable to change radically and/or predictably, such as in reversal learning or dynamic matching situations (Daw et al., 2005; Hampton et al., 2006; Sutton and Barto, 1998). Moreover, most reinforcement learning as applied to neuroscientific data has focused on how responses are chosen on the basis of each option's expected values and how these values are updated, and much less on how reliable these estimates are in the first place. For instance, if a monkey decides to forage in a particular nearby patch on two occasions, once which resulted in some reward and once not, it might be possible to say that the expected value of that option was 0.5 (reward × probability) and then use that value to compare against other available alternatives. However, after only two samples, the animal's uncertainty in its estimate should also be extremely high, as the actual underlying probability of reward can only be deduced to be anywhere greater than 0 and less than 1. In such situations, or in circumstances where uncertainty is brought about by being in a rapidly changeable, volatile environment, outcomes, whether positive or negative, have important value for minimizing uncertainty (Daw et al., 2006; Yu and Dayan, 2005). In particular, such uncertainty should affect the learning rate, meaning that recently acquired information will have a greater impact on the estimated value of an option and, therefore, on subsequent behavior (Behrens et al., 2007; Dayan and Niv, 2008).

One example of this is in the behavior of the monkeys in the joystick reversal task where contingencies reversed relatively frequently (every time the animal had harvested 25 rewards). Following a reversal, these animals showed an increasing tendency to continue with the correct response with increasing numbers of reward and analysis of this effect showed that their current decisions were influenced in a graded manner by the previous four outcomes (with the most recent outcome having most influence, the fourth the least). Such reward history effects have also been calculated in other similar two-choice studies in macaques in which the likelihood of reward on each option, while probabilistic, changes less often (every 100–200 trials) and, interestingly, in these more stable environments, outcomes from further in the past (between 7 to as far as 30 trials back) had influence on current behavior (Bayer and Glimcher, 2005; Corrado et al., 2005; Lau and Glimcher, 2005).

While the above evidence is suggestive of a link between the structure of the reward environment and the way in which past outcomes influence current behavior, it is difficult to reach firm conclusions on the basis of comparisons made across different studies. Therefore, to investigate in the same task whether human subjects are sensitive to the structure of the reward environment and to use this to work out the value of each outcome in determining future behavior, Behrens and colleagues (2007) tested subjects on a two-choice probabilistic task, where in one part of the task (120 trials), the identity of the most likely option was stable, its likelihood fixed at 0.75 at yielding reward, and in the other part (170 trials), the identity of the most likely option was volatile and reversed on five occasions (every 30–40 trials) (Fig. 11.4A). The magnitude of the reward available for either option differed from trial to trial, meaning that the highest value option (as defined by expected reward × estimated probability) was sometimes the less likely one. As predicted, subjects had significantly higher learning rates and, therefore, were more responsive to outcome information during the latter part of the volatile phase, after they had experienced at least two reversals in probability, than during the comparable part of the stable phase. This demonstrates that individual subjects, within the same task situation and the space of 100 trials, can dynamically adjust their learning rates according to the structure of their reinforcement history. Moreover, behavior matched closely that produced by an optimal Bayesian learner, which uses only the statistics of the outcome information to guide future responses and, unlike most reinforcement learning models, contains no free parameters that need to be tuned and fitted (Fig. 11.4B). These data show that not only are humans able to accumulate evidence about what responses to make, but also they can use information about the structure of the environment to determine optimally how informative each outcome is, given their state of uncertainty about the likelihood of future outcomes.

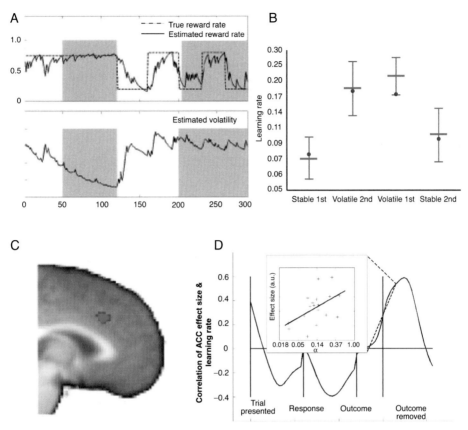

Fig. 11.4 Effect of the volatility of the reward environment on behavior and the BOLD signal. (A) Reward schedule during the task along with the estimated reward rate for an optimal Bayesian learner (upper panel) along with the optimal estimates of the volatility during the task (lower panel). Gray blocks are the periods analyzed for the effects of the reward environment on subjects' learning rates and, subsequently, BOLD signal. The reward rate was stable for the first 120 trials and volatile during the latter 180 trials for half the subjects (depicted here) and the opposite for the other half. (B) Learning rates during the periods when the reward rate was stable or volatile in the behavioral experiment when either the stable period came first (two left-hand sets of data) or second in the task (two right-hand sets of data). Red and black bars depict the mean (and SEM) learning rates for the human subjects, blue dots show the optimal learning rates derived from the behavior of the optimal Bayesian learner. (C) Activity in ACCs when the outcome is revealed is modulated by subjects' estimates of volatility. (D) Effect size in this ACCs region is significantly correlated with subjects' learning rate, demonstrating that the size of the ACCs signal is related to how useful each piece of information is for updating estimates of the likelihood of reward. Reprinted by permission from Macmillan Publishers Ltd: *Nature Neuroscience*, 10(9), 1214–21, Behrens TE, Woolrich MW, Walton ME, Rushworth MF, Learning the value of information in an uncertain world, Copyright 2007.

11.5 **Different components of outcome value in OFC and ACCs**

Several lines of evidence have shown that the significance of an outcome, in terms of its informative value for guiding future choices rather than its calorific worth, may be an important determinant of activity particularly in the ACCs. Following lesions, ACC animals performing the joystick reversal task only seemed significantly influenced by the immediately preceding outcome alone, rather than the four previous outcomes that the normal animals took into consideration, suggesting that this region may play a role in using information about the task environment to guide how to learn from outcomes (Kennerley et al., 2006). Both human fMRI and monkey electrophysiological studies have demonstrated that signals in the ACCs are correlated both with generating responses to discover what the most appropriate available course of action is and with how useful outcome information is to guide future decisions, particularly when the outcome of a choice resolves uncertainty about which upcoming responses should be selected (Matsumoto et al., 2007; Quilodran et al., 2008; Walton et al., 2004; Yoshida and Ishii, 2006). Conversely, inactivation of ACCs in both monkeys and rats can make animals insensitive to the value of an outcome in the context of a task, causing them to return to previously rewarded responses, even if other options would subsequently result in greater benefits (Amiez et al., 2006; Seamans et al., 1995).

To test the degree to which ACCs activation is modulated by how useful outcome information is for guiding future choices, Behrens and colleagues examined fMRI responses while subjects performed the stable/volatile task described above, adapted for the scanning environment (Behrens et al., 2007). When subjects were observing the outcome of their choice, regardless of its valence or the phase of the task, there was activity in a large part of rostral ACCs, as well as in several other temporal lobe and subcortical structures. Importantly, however, one part of this ACCs region, but no other brain structures at the corrected significance level used, showed a significant interaction between outcome monitoring and subjects' estimates of the volatility of the environment (Fig. 11.4C). Moreover, this ACCs signal in turn significantly predicted subjects' learning rates, showing that there was a strong link between the size of the ACCs signal during the outcome phase and the amount to which this recent outcome information would be used to modify ongoing value estimates (Fig. 11.4D). This activation was separate to the magnitude of the outcome, the prediction error on each trial at the time of the outcome, whether subjects were exploring the alternative option on the present trial, and also the likelihood that reward would be received.

In spite of using scanning parameters that minimized signal dropout in the OFC, no part of this structure was modulated by the usefulness of the outcome, or even by the outcome, irrespective of the point during the task. This may seem unexpected given that, as discussed in this chapter, there is a wealth of evidence implicating the OFC in outcome monitoring and certain types of value processing assessed by tasks such as stimulus reversal learning, as well as by others not discussed here such as reinforcer devaluation (Izquierdo et al., 2004). However, unlike the ACCs region, OFC cells do not always simply respond to the informative nature of the outcome but also to reinforcement, even when a task is well learned (Tremblay and Schultz, 2000), an effect in humans that may be particularly prominent in medial OFC regions (Kim et al., 2006). Nonetheless, it is important to remember that "significance" is only one facet that makes up the overall value of an outcome and several aspects of reported affective value coding appear more prominently in the OFC than in ACCs. First, there is converging evidence that OFC is strongly involved in processing taste and flavor and, more generally, the affective value of nutritious items. Neurons in OFC have been shown to respond to different food groups and to different sensory properties of food and liquid (Rolls et al., 1989; Verhagen et al., 2003). Moreover, while there is debate over whether it is represented in absolute or relative terms, OFC seems to code for the subjective value of received rewards, as well as specific sensory properties of these items (Padoa-Schioppa and Assad, 2008; Tremblay and Schultz, 1999). Functional imaging studies in humans have also shown changes in activation in the OFC associated with alterations in satiety or overfeeding on a pleasant substance to aversion correlating with subjective preference measures (although there are also some reports of activation in parts of the ACC including ACCs) (Hinton et al., 2004; Kringelbach et al., 2003; Small et al., 2001). Both OFC and ACCs have anatomical connections with several nuclei in the hypothalamus (Floyd et al., 2001; Ongur et al., 1998) and both have been implicated in processing aspects of the internal energy content of food (De Araujo and Rolls, 2004; Teves et al., 2004).

Similarly, the value of an item will depend not only on the eventual payoff, but also on how costly, in terms of an animal's limited metabolic resources, an option is. Again, both the OFC and ACCs have been shown to play important, dissociable roles in rats, monkeys, and humans in allowing animals to evaluate different costs, with the former being particularly important when there is a requirement to generate and maintain a reward expectation across a delay and the latter critical for processing effort costs and allowing an animal to overcome effort-related constraints conditional on the response (Croxson et al., 2009; Kennerley et al., 2008; Kheramin et al., 2002; Roesch et al., 2006; Rudebeck et al., 2006b; Winstanley et al., 2004). Interestingly, some cells in rat OFC explicitly appear to code for delay costs independently of reward magnitude (and therefore also behavior) (Roesch et al., 2006) and a region of posterior OFC in humans, which may be a homologous region in primates to rodent OFC (Wise, 2008), has also recently been shown to code for expected reward independent of effort costs (Croxson et al., 2009).

While these are factors that will play an important role at the decision stage, this does not necessarily speak to how outcomes are valued in these regions. However, there is recent evidence that not only do cells in ACCs track progress through a schedule of responses towards reward (Amiez et al., 2005; Shidara and Richmond, 2002), but also many more cells in this region than the OFC explicitly encode outcomes, not only as a function of reward magnitude and likelihood, but also of the response costs entailed to gain the outcome (Kennerley and Wallis, 2009). When they do show outcome-specific activity, OFC cells, by contrast, tend to be more concerned simply with the size or likelihood of the outcome.

Taken together, this demonstrates that the value of an outcome consists of more than merely whether or not it occurs or its absolute size. Instead, both intrinsic and extrinsic variables can influence how rewards are assessed, in terms of its immediate and long-term homeostatic benefit to the animal and the usefulness of the information in minimizing uncertainty about the likely upshot of embarking on a particular course of action. For this latter function, ACCs appears to be in a prime position to monitor ongoing behavior and to assess each new piece of information not simply in terms of its absolute deviance from expectation, but instead in the context of the variability of outcomes over a longer time period, allowing it to help guide how to interpret the influence of the current information on future decisions.

11.6 Learning what to do in a complex changeable environment

While there might not be good evidence that the OFC plays an important role in simple discrimination learning or interpreting the value of outcome information for determining future behavior, this is not to imply that the OFC has no role in guiding reinforcement learning and subsequent choices. There is evidence that OFC and adjacent regions may play an important role in reporting the confirmation of specific perceptual expectations (Summerfield and Koechlin, 2008), again linking the OFC to processing the likely outcome based on associations with stimuli rather than according to the statistics of the reward environment or the means to achieve a particular outcome. In their analysis of the visual reversal task, Rudebeck and Murray (2008) showed that the OFC-lesioned animals had an inability to persist with the correct response following a series of positive reinforcements. Similarly, as observed in the stimulus-based dynamic matching task, OFC deficits were not simply caused by an inability to change responses, as has been observed in reversal learning tasks in rats and marmosets with OFC lesions or in macaques where the lesion extends to include parts of the inferior convexity ventral to the principal sulcus (Chudasama and Robbins, 2003; Clarke et al., 2008; Iversen and Mishkin, 1970; Jones and Mishkin, 1972), but instead to a difficulty using the outcome information to learn which stimulus had the highest likelihood of giving reward (Rudebeck et al., 2008a).

One difficulty with interpreting the role of the OFC in using outcome information to guide learning and decision making has been that most studies in animals and humans to date have used paradigms that have constrained the number of available options to two, making it often difficult to determine why one option has been chosen over the other. Moreover, in these tasks, the best option has usually been clearly evident owing to a wide disparity in the expected values of the alternatives and the fact that any changes are usually categorical reversals in value. Therefore, while there have been several studies reporting no affects on choice behavior of OFC lesions in simple discrimination-learning paradigms, this may have been that these tasks did not require subjects ever to integrate outcome information and there was little doubt about how the stimuli and outcomes should be associated together.

To investigate this question, Rudebeck and colleagues (2008a) tested monkeys both before and after OFC lesions on a three-stimulus probabilistic learning task. The likelihood that selection of an option would result in reward was calculated independently for each one according to a predetermined schedule (though there was no carryover of unharvested rewards as happened in the matching tasks) (Fig. 11.5A). This schedule was interleaved with another comparable three-option probabilistic schedule (not reported here) and animals were presented with entirely novel stimuli at the start of each testing session, meaning they could only determine which option was best by sampling the three alternatives and learning their values based on the received outcomes, rather than using prior information about task structure or stimulus values to guide choice behavior. Moreover, as the values of all the options drifted throughout the 300-trial session, and the option most likely to lead to reward changed approximately every 100 trials, the animals had constantly to keep track of values to gain the most benefit.

Given that the monkeys have constantly to weigh up exploiting what they know about the values of the options against exploring what may have changed since they last sampled the alternatives, there is no clear optimal solution as to how to perform this task. Nonetheless, both in terms of what is objectively the best option (as defined by highest probability option across the task schedule) or in terms of the subjective best value to the monkey (the highest probability based on the outcome information the animal has received for the choices it made), the animals prior to surgery were able to perform this complex task well, learning to find the option with the highest probability of reward within the first 100 trials and, on average, switching to find the highest value option when the identity of the best option changed in the second and third 100 trials. Across the whole schedule, the animals chose the option with both the objective and subjective highest probability of reward significantly more often than chance, demonstrating that they

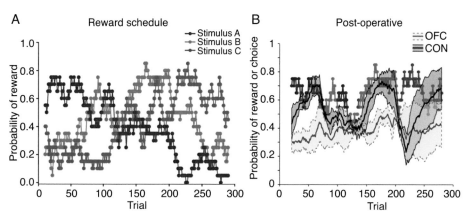

Fig. 11.5 Performance of OFC-lesioned monkeys on a 3 choice probabilistic learning task. (A) The reward schedule showing the likelihood that choosing each of the three options would result in reward across the 300-trial session. (B) Post-operative choice performance following OFC-lesions showing animals were significantly impaired at learning and tracking the values of the options in order to be able to choose the stimulus with the highest probability of giving reward.

could learn and track outcome likelihoods and use this information to guide beneficial decision making.

Following OFC lesions, however, the animals became notably worse at learning and tracking the best option, choosing this stimulus on significantly fewer trials, whether defined objectively or subjectively (Fig. 11.5B). Once again, while there was both an explicit requirement to alter choices as the identity of the stimulus with the highest probability changed across the schedule, as well as an implicit one based on the need for exploration, a switching deficit did not appear to be the sole determinant of the lesion effect, as the OFC group were also impaired at discovering the best stimulus at the start of the session when the identity of the best option remained unchanged. Moreover, throughout the task, the lesion group was just as likely to alter their behavior as controls, showing that their impairment was not caused by simple perseveration or a failure to explore the available options. Importantly also, it did not appear as if the OFC-lesioned animals were responding randomly, as they showed a comparable pattern of alternative choices when not selecting the subjectively highest value option as controls.

This finding demonstrates that the OFC does play a vital role in aspects of stimulus–outcome learning, which is particularly evident in uncertain, probabilistic environments that require outcome information to be integrated and tracked across time to build up an accurate estimate of the reward likelihoods associated with several stimuli. While the fact that the task involved associating values to stimuli would suggest that the ACCs would not be required to perform normally in this task, it remains to be tested whether this region would play some role in this more complex environment requiring constant evaluation of the probabilities and uncertainty in these estimates in order to decide whether to persist with the current option or explore the alternatives. As observed in the deterministic stimulus-based reversal task, even though the ability to update choice behavior was intact, the ACCs-lesioned animals nonetheless appeared not to evaluate the positive reinforcement following an error, indicating a need to persist with the current response, in the same manner as controls.

11.7 **Conclusions**

Throughout this chapter, we have presented evidence that illustrates how novel insights into frontal function can be gained by employing tasks which, in their requirement for animals to deal with multiple options, probabilities, uncertainty, and changes in value, replicate some of the issues faced by animals in their natural physical environment. In particular, we have hoped to demonstrate that animals frequently do not interpret outcomes as either categorically correct or incorrect, clearly determining what subsequent behavior should be, but instead as pieces of evidence that needed to be weighed up before they can guide one course of action or another. While many psychologists and economists assume there must eventually be some common scale on which we compare all values, it is becoming increasingly clear that there are also numerous aspects of outcome processing that occur, at least partially independently, at the neural level, including that associated with stimuli and actions, and in terms of subjective preference and the information gained about the world, as well as aspects not touched on here, such as social value (Rangel et al., 2008; Rudebeck et al., 2008b; Rushworth et al., 2007; Watson and Platt, 2008).

Rather than having a specific function involved with detecting when contingencies alter or incorrect responses are made, the roles of OFC and ACCs in performance monitoring can be better understood by considering how these regions use outcome information to learn and update the values of the available options when the consequences of taking one course of action or another is uncertain and changeable. Both OFC and ACCs are involved in constantly tracking and evaluating outcomes, the former particularly involved when considering the predicted value of external stimuli and the latter for the value associated with internally-generated actions, which can then be used to guide subsequent response selection. More explicitly, OFC appears to play a crucial role in linking the specific reinforcement associated with a particular stimulus, whereas the ACCs appears crucial for calculating the net worth of an outcome in terms of how valuable it was in the context of the overall task. These are properties that will be particularly relevant for performance in complex environments, where there are multiple options without fixed outcome associations. However, they are also likely to play a role in several other simpler environments that require choices to be guided by outcome associations, rather than by specific, pre-learned rules or explicit cues. While the information processing in these regions is at least partially dissociable, based on whether stimulus- or action-based associations have guided a choice, it is likely that both OFC and ACCs contribute to help guide beneficial decision making in most complex naturalistic settings. Moreover, these regions undoubtedly interact with several interconnected structures, such as the amygdala, parts of the striatum, and other frontal and temporal cortical areas, in order to guide learning and choice behavior. Whether and when such contributions are cooperative or competitive, and how their processing affects the coding in other interconnected regions remain open questions for future research.

Acknowledgments

This work was supported by the Medical Research Council (TEJB, PHR, MFSR) and the Wellcome Trust (MEW). We would like to thank Dr. Betsy Murray for providing the data from Izquierdo et al. (2004) and for helpful comments about our interpretation of these results.

References

Amaral, D.G. and Price, J.L. (1984). Amygdalo-cortical projections in the monkey (Macaca fascicularis). *J Comp Neurol*, **230**(4), 465–96.

Amiez, C., Joseph, J.P., and Procyk, E. (2005). Anterior cingulate error-related activity is modulated by predicted reward. *Eur J Neurosci*, **21**(12), 3447–52.

Amiez, C., Joseph, J.P., and Procyk, E. (2006). Reward encoding in the monkey anterior cingulate cortex. *Cereb Cortex*, **16**(7), 1040–55.

An, X., Bandler, R., Ongur, D., and Price, J.L. (1998). Prefrontal cortical projections to longitudinal columns in the midbrain periaqueductal gray in macaque monkeys. *J Comp Neurol*, **401**(4), 455–79.

Aron, A.R., Monsell, S., Sahakian, B.J., and Robbins, T.W. (2004). A componential analysis of task-switching deficits associated with lesions of left and right frontal cortex. *Brain,* 127(Pt 7), 1561–73.

Aston-Jones, G. and Cohen, J.D. (2005). An integrative theory of locus coeruleus-norepinephrine function: adaptive gain and optimal performance. *Annu Rev Neurosci,* 28, 403–50.

Baxter, M.G., Gaffan, D., Kyriazis, D.A., and Mitchell, A.S. (2007). Orbital prefrontal cortex is required for object-in-place scene memory but not performance of a strategy implementation task. *J Neurosci,* 27(42), 11327–33.

Bayer, H.M. and Glimcher, P.W. (2005). Midbrain dopamine neurons encode a quantitative reward prediction error signal. *Neuron,* 47(1), 129–41.

Beckmann, M., Johansen-Berg, H., and Rushworth, M.F. (2009). Connectivity-based parcellation of human cingulate cortex and its relation to functional specialization. *J Neurosci,* 29(4), 1175–90.

Behrens, T.E., Woolrich, M.W., Walton, M.E., and Rushworth, M.F. (2007). Learning the value of information in an uncertain world. *Nat Neurosci,* 10(9), 1214–21.

Bunge, S.A. (2004). How we use rules to select actions: a review of evidence from cognitive neuroscience. *Cogn Affect Behav Neurosci,* 4(4), 564–79.

Bush, G., Luu, P., and Posner, M.I. (2000). Cognitive and emotional influences in anterior cingulate cortex. *Trends Cogn Sci,* 4(6), 215–22.

Butter, C.M. (1969). Perseveration in extinction and in discrimination reversal tasks following selective prefrontal ablations in Macaca mulatta. *Physiol Behav,* 4, 163–71.

Camille, N., Coricelli, G., Sallet, J., Pradat-Diehl, P., Duhamel, J.R., and Sirigu, A. (2004). The involvement of the orbitofrontal cortex in the experience of regret. *Science,* 304(5674), 1167–70.

Carmichael, S.T. and Price, J.L. (1996). Connectional networks within the orbital and medial prefrontal cortex of macaque monkeys. *J Comp Neurol,* 371(2), 179–207.

Chudasama, Y. and Robbins, T.W. (2003). Dissociable contributions of the orbitofrontal and infralimbic cortex to pavlovian autoshaping and discrimination reversal learning: further evidence for the functional heterogeneity of the rodent frontal cortex. *J Neurosci,* 23(25), 8771–80.

Clarke, H.F., Robbins, T.W., and Roberts, A.C. (2008). Lesions of the medial striatum in monkeys produce perseverative impairments during reversal learning similar to those produced by lesions of the orbitofrontal cortex. *J Neurosci,* 28(43), 10972–82.

Coricelli, G., Critchley, H.D., Joffily, M., O'Doherty, J.P., Sirigu, A., and Dolan, R.J. (2005). Regret and its avoidance: a neuroimaging study of choice behavior. *Nat Neurosci,* 8(9), 1255–62.

Corrado, G.S., Sugrue, L.P., Seung, H.S., and Newsome, W.T. (2005). Linear-Nonlinear-Poisson models of primate choice dynamics. *J Exp Anal Behav,* 84(3), 581–617.

Crone, E.A., Wendelken, C., Donohue, S.E., and Bunge, S.A. (2006). Neural evidence for dissociable components of task-switching. *Cereb Cortex,* 16(4), 475–86.

Croxson, P.L., Johansen-Berg, H., Behrens, T.E., Robson, M.D., Pinsk, M.A., Gross, C.G., et al. (2005). Quantitative investigation of connections of the prefrontal cortex in the human and macaque using probabilistic diffusion tractography. *J Neurosci,* 25(39), 8854–66.

Croxson, P.L., Walton, M.E., O'Reilly, J.X., Behrens, T.E., and Rushworth, M.F. (2009). Effort-based cost-benefit valuation and the human brain. *J Neurosci,* 29(14), 4531–41.

Daw, N.D., Niv, Y., and Dayan, P. (2005). Uncertainty-based competition between prefrontal and dorsolateral striatal systems for behavioral control. *Nat Neurosci,* 8(12), 1704–11.

Daw, N.D., O'Doherty, J.P., Dayan, P., Seymour, B., and Dolan, R.J. (2006). Cortical substrates for exploratory decisions in humans. *Nature,* 441(7095), 876–79.

Dayan, P. and Niv, Y. (2008). Reinforcement learning: the good, the bad and the ugly. *Curr Opin Neurobiol,* 18(2), 185–96.

Dayan, P., Kakade, S., and Montague, P.R. (2000). Learning and selective attention. *Nat Neurosci*, **3** Suppl, 1218–23.

De Araujo, I.E. and Rolls, E.T. (2004). Representation in the human brain of food texture and oral fat. *J Neurosci*, **24**(12), 3086–93.

Desimone, R. and Duncan, J. (1995). Neural mechanisms of selective visual attention. *Annu Rev Neurosci*, **18**, 193–222.

Dias, R., Robbins, T.W., and Roberts, A.C. (1996). Dissociation in prefrontal cortex of affective and attentional shifts. *Nature*, **380**(6569), 69–72.

Elliott, R., Friston, K.J., and Dolan, R.J. (2000a). Dissociable neural responses in human reward systems. *J Neurosci*, **20**(16), 6159–65.

Elliott, R., Dolan, R.J., and Frith, C.D. (2000b). Dissociable functions in the medial and lateral orbitofrontal cortex: evidence from human neuroimaging studies. *Cereb Cortex*, **10**(3), 308–17.

Fellows, L.K. and Farah, M.J. (2003). Ventromedial frontal cortex mediates affective shifting in humans: evidence from a reversal learning paradigm. *Brain*, **126**(Pt 8), 1830–37.

Fellows, L.K. and Farah, M.J. (2005). Is anterior cingulate cortex necessary for cognitive control? *Brain*, **128**(Pt 4), 788–96.

Floyd, N.S., Price, J.L., Ferry, A.T., Keay, K.A., and Bandler, R. (2001). Orbitomedial prefrontal cortical projections to hypothalamus in the rat. *J Comp Neurol*, **432**(3), 307–28.

Gaspar, P., Berger, B., Febvret, A., Vigny, A., and Henry, J.P. (1989). Catecholamine innervation of the human cerebral cortex as revealed by comparative immunohistochemistry of tyrosine hydroxylase and dopamine-beta-hydroxylase. *J Comp Neurol*, **279**(2), 249–71.

Genovesio, A., Brasted, P.J., Mitz, A.R., and Wise, S.P. (2005). Prefrontal cortex activity related to abstract response strategies. *Neuron*, **47**(2), 307–20.

Gittins, J.C. (1979). Bandit processes and dynamic allocation indices. *J. R. Stat. Soc. B.*, **41**, 148–77.

Hampton, A.N., Bossaerts, P., and O'Doherty, J.P. (2006). The role of the ventromedial prefrontal cortex in abstract state-based inference during decision making in humans. *J Neurosci*, **26**(32), 8360–67.

Hare, T.A., O'Doherty, J., Camerer, C.F., Schultz, W., and Rangel, A. (2008). Dissociating the role of the orbitofrontal cortex and the striatum in the computation of goal values and prediction errors. *J Neurosci*, **28**(22), 5623–30.

He, S.Q., Dum, R.P., and Strick, P.L. (1995). Topographic organization of corticospinal projections from the frontal lobe: motor areas on the medial surface of the hemisphere. *J Neurosci*, **15**(5 Pt 1), 3284–3306.

Herrnstein, R.-J. (1997). In: Rachlin, H. and Laibson, D.I. (eds.) *The matching law: papers in psychology and economics*. Cambridge, MA: Harvard University Press.

Hinton, E.C., Parkinson, J.A., Holland, A.J., Arana, F.S., Roberts, A.C., and Owen, A.M. (2004). Neural contributions to the motivational control of appetite in humans. *Eur J Neurosci*, **20**(5), 1411–8.

Hosokawa, T., Kato, K., Inoue, M., and Mikami, A. (2005). Correspondence of cue activity to reward activity in the macaque orbitofrontal cortex. *Neurosci Lett*, **389**(3), 146–51.

Iversen, S.D. and Mishkin, M. (1970). Perseverative interference in monkeys following selective lesions of the inferior prefrontal convexity. *Exp Brain Res*, **11**(4), 376–86.

Izquierdo, A., Suda, R.K., and Murray, E.A. (2004). Bilateral orbital prefrontal cortex lesions in rhesus monkeys disrupt choices guided by both reward value and reward contingency. *J Neurosci*, **24**(34), 7540–8.

Jones, B. and Mishkin, M. (1972). Limbic lesions and the problem of stimulus—reinforcement associations. *Exp Neurol*, **36**(2), 362–77.

Kennerley, S.W. and Wallis, J.D. (2009). Evaluating choices by single neurons in the frontal lobe: outcome value encoded across multiple decision variables. *Eur J Neurosci*, **29**(10), 2061–73.

Kennerley, S.W., Walton, M.E., Behrens, T.E., Buckley, M.J., and Rushworth, M.F. (2006). Optimal decision making and the anterior cingulate cortex. *Nat Neurosci*, **9**(7), 940–47.

Kennerley, S.W., Dahmubed, A.F., Lara, A.H., and Wallis, J.D. (2009). Neurons in the frontal lobe encode the value of multiple decision variables. *J Cogn Neurosci*, **21**(6), 1162–78.

Kepecs, A., Uchida, N., Zariwala, H.A., and Mainen, Z.F. (2008). Neural correlates, computation and behavioral impact of decision confidence. *Nature*, **455**(7210), 227–31.

Kheramin, S., Body, S., Mobini, S., Ho, M.Y., Velazquez-Martinez, D.N., Bradshaw, C.M., et al. (2002). Effects of quinolinic acid-induced lesions of the orbital prefrontal cortex on inter-temporal choice: a quantitative analysis. *Psychopharmacology (Berl)*, **165**(1), 9–17.

Kim, H., Shimojo, S., and O'Doherty, J.P. (2006). Is avoiding an aversive outcome rewarding? Neural substrates of avoidance learning in the human brain. *PLoS Biol*, **4**(8), e233.

Krebs, J.R., Kacelnik, A., and Taylor, A. (1978). Tests of optimal sampling by foraging great tits. *Nature*, **275**, 27–31.

Kringelbach, M.L., O'Doherty, J., Rolls, E.T., and Andrews, C. (2003). Activation of the human orbitofrontal cortex to a liquid food stimulus is correlated with its subjective pleasantness. *Cereb Cortex*, **13**(10), 1064–71.

Lau, B. and Glimcher, P.W. (2005). Dynamic response-by-response models of matching behavior in rhesus monkeys. *J Exp Anal Behav*, **84**(3), 555–79.

Liston, C., Matalon, S., Hare, T.A., Davidson, M.C., and Casey, B.J. (2006). Anterior cingulate and posterior parietal cortices are sensitive to dissociable forms of conflict in a task-switching paradigm. *Neuron*, **50**(4), 643–53.

Matsumoto, M., Matsumoto, K., Abe, H., and Tanaka, K. (2007). Medial prefrontal cell activity signaling prediction errors of action values. *Nat Neurosci*, **10**(5), 647–56.

Mellers, B.A. (2000). Choice and the relative pleasure of consequences. *Psychol Bull*, **126**(6), 910–24.

Mesulam, M.M. (1999). Spatial attention and neglect: parietal, frontal and cingulate contributions to the mental representation and attentional targeting of salient extrapersonal events. *Philos Trans R Soc Lond B Biol Sci*, **354**(1387), 1325–46.

Miller, E.K. and Cohen, J.D. (2001). An integrative theory of prefrontal cortex function. *Annu Rev Neurosci*, **24**, 167–202.

Mishkin, M. (1957). Effects of small frontal lesions on delayed alternation in monkeys. *J Neurophysiol*, **20**(6), 615–22.

Montague, P.R., King-Casas, B., and Cohen, J.D. (2006). Imaging valuation models in human choice. *Annu Rev Neurosci*, **29**, 417–48.

Morecraft, R.J. and Van Hoesen, G.W. (1998). Convergence of limbic input to the cingulate motor cortex in the rhesus monkey. *Brain Res Bull*, **45**(2), 209–32.

Murray, E.A. and Izquierdo, A. (2007). Orbitofrontal cortex and amygdala contributions to affect and action in primates. *Ann N Y Acad Sci*, **1121**, 273–96.

Murray, E.A., Davidson, M., Gaffan, D., Olton, D.S., and Suomi, S. (1989). Effects of fornix transection and cingulate cortical ablation on spatial memory in rhesus monkeys. *Exp Brain Res*, **74**(1), 173–86.

Murray, E.A., O'Doherty, J.P., and Schoenbaum, G. (2007). What we know and do not know about the functions of the orbitofrontal cortex after 20 years of cross-species studies. *J Neurosci*, **27**(31), 8166–69.

Nowak, M. and Sigmund, K. (1993). A strategy of win-stay, lose-shift that outperforms tit-for-tat in the Prisoner's Dilemma game. *Nature*, **364**(6432), 56–8.

O'Doherty, J., Kringelbach, M.L., Rolls, E.T., Hornak, J., and Andrews, C. (2001). Abstract reward and punishment representations in the human orbitofrontal cortex. *Nat Neurosci*, **4**(1), 95–102.

O'Doherty, J.P., Critchley, H., Deichmann, R., and Dolan, R.J. (2003a). Dissociating valence of outcome from behavioral control in human orbital and ventral prefrontal cortices. *J Neurosci*, **23**(21), 7931–39.

O'Doherty, J.P., Dayan, P., Friston, K., Critchley, H., and Dolan, R.J. (2003b). Temporal difference models and reward-related learning in the human brain. *Neuron*, **38**(2), 329–37.

Ongur, D. and Price, J.L. (2000). The organization of networks within the orbital and medial prefrontal cortex of rats, monkeys and humans. *Cereb Cortex*, **10**(3), 206–19.

Ongur, D., An, X., and Price, J.L. (1998). Prefrontal cortical projections to the hypothalamus in macaque monkeys. *J Comp Neurol*, **401**(4), 480–505.

Ostlund, S.B., and Balleine, B.W. (2007). Orbitofrontal cortex mediates outcome encoding in Pavlovian but not instrumental conditioning. *J Neurosci*, **27**(18), 4819–25.

Padoa-Schioppa, C. and Assad, J.A. (2008). The representation of economic value in the orbitofrontal cortex is invariant for changes of menu. *Nat Neurosci*, **11**(1), 95–102.

Petit, L., Courtney, S.M., Ungerleider, L.G., and Haxby, J.V. (1998). Sustained activity in the medial wall during working memory delays. *J Neurosci*, **18**(22), 9429–37.

Picard, N. and Strick, P.L. (1996). Motor areas of the medial wall: a review of their location and functional activation. *Cereb Cortex*, **6**(3), 342–53.

Platt, M.L. and Huettel, S.A. (2008). Risky business: the neuroeconomics of decision making under uncertainty. *Nat Neurosci*, **11**(4), 398–403.

Pribram, K.H. and Fulton, J.F. (1954). An experimental critique of the effects of anterior cingulate ablations in monkey. *Brain*, **77**, 34–44.

Quilodran, R., Rothe, M., and Procyk, E. (2008). Behavioral shifts and action valuation in the anterior cingulate cortex. *Neuron*, **57**(2), 314–25.

Rangel, A., Camerer, C., and Montague, P.R. (2008). A framework for studying the neurobiology of value-based decision making. *Nat Rev Neurosci*, **9**(7), 545–56.

Ridderinkhof, K.R., Ullsperger, M., Crone, E.A., and Nieuwenhuis, S. (2004). The role of the medial frontal cortex in cognitive control. *Science*, **306**(5695), 443–7.

Roberts, A.C. (2006). Primate orbitofrontal cortex and adaptive behavior. *Trends Cogn Sci*, **10**(2), 83–90.

Roesch, M.R., Taylor, A.R., and Schoenbaum, G. (2006). Encoding of time-discounted rewards in orbitofrontal cortex is independent of value representation. *Neuron*, **51**(4), 509–20.

Roesch, M.R., Stalnaker, T.A., and Schoenbaum, G. (2007). Associative encoding in anterior piriform cortex versus orbitofrontal cortex during odor discrimination and reversal learning. *Cereb Cortex*, **17**(3), 643–52.

Rolls, E.T., Sienkiewicz, Z.J., and Yaxley, S. (1989). Hunger modulates the responses to gustatory stimuli of single neurons in the caudolateral orbitofrontal cortex of the macaque monkey. *Eur J Neurosci*, **1**(1), 53–60.

Rolls, E.T., McCabe, C., and Redoute, J. (2008). Expected value, reward outcome, and temporal difference error representations in a probabilistic decision task. *Cereb Cortex*, **18**(3), 652–63.

Rudebeck, P.H., and Murray, E.A. (2008). Amygdala and orbitofrontal cortex lesions differentially influence choices during object reversal learning. *J Neurosci*, **28**(33), 8338–43.

Rudebeck, P.H., Buckley, M.J., Walton, M.E., and Rushworth, M.F. (2006a). A role for the macaque anterior cingulate gyrus in social valuation. *Science*, **313**(5791), 1310–2.

Rudebeck, P.H., Walton, M.E., Smyth, A.N., Bannerman, D.M., and Rushworth, M.F. (2006b). Separate neural pathways process different decision costs. *Nat Neurosci*, **9**(9), 1161–8.

Rudebeck, P.H., Behrens, T.E., Kennerley, S.W., Baxter, M.G., Buckley, M.J., Walton, M.E., et al. (2008a). Frontal cortex subregions play distinct roles in choices between actions and stimuli. *J Neurosci*, **28**(51), 13775–85.

Rudebeck, P.H., Bannerman, D.M., and Rushworth, M.F. (2008b). The contribution of distinct subregions of the ventromedial frontal cortex to emotion, social behavior, and decision making. *Cogn Affect Behav Neurosci*, 8(4), 485–97.

Rushworth, M.F. and Behrens, T.E. (2008). Choice, uncertainty and value in prefrontal and cingulate cortex. *Nat Neurosci*, 11(4), 389–97.

Rushworth, M.F., Hadland, K.A., Paus, T., and Sipila, P.K. (2002). Role of the human medial frontal cortex in task switching: a combined fMRI and TMS study. *J Neurophysiol*, 87(5), 2577–92.

Rushworth, M.F., Hadland, K.A., Gaffan, D., and Passingham, R.E. (2003). The effect of cingulate cortex lesions on task switching and working memory. *J Cogn Neurosci*, 15(3), 338–53.

Rushworth, M.F., Behrens, T.E., Rudebeck, P.H., and Walton, M.E. (2007). Contrasting roles for cingulate and orbitofrontal cortex in decisions and social behavior. *Trends Cogn Sci*, 11(4), 168–76.

Schoenbaum, G., Setlow, B., Nugent, S.L., Saddoris, M.P., and Gallagher, M. (2003). Lesions of orbitofrontal cortex and basolateral amygdala complex disrupt acquisition of odor-guided discriminations and reversals. *Learn Mem*, 10(2), 129–40.

Schultz, W., Dayan, P., and Montague, P.R. (1997). A neural substrate of prediction and reward. *Science*, 275(5306), 1593–99.

Seamans, J.K., Floresco, S.B., and Phillips, A.G. (1995). Functional differences between the prelimbic and anterior cingulate regions of the rat prefrontal cortex. *Behav Neurosci*, 109(6), 1063–73.

Seo, H. and Lee, D. (2008). Cortical mechanisms for reinforcement learning in competitive games. *Philos Trans R Soc Lond B Biol Sci,* 363(1511), 3845–57.

Shallice, T., Stuss, D.T., Picton, T.W., Alexander, M.P., and Gillingham, S. (2007). Multiple effects of prefrontal lesions on task-switching. *Front Hum Neurosci*, 1, 2.

Shidara, M. and Richmond, B.J. (2002). Anterior cingulate: single neuronal signals related to degree of reward expectancy. *Science*, 296(5573), 1709–1711.

Shima, K. and Tanji, J. (1998). Role for cingulate motor area cells in voluntary movement selection based on reward. *Science*, 282(5392), 1335–8.

Small, D.M., Zatorre, R.J., Dagher, A., Evans, A.C., and Jones-Gotman, M. (2001). Changes in brain activity related to eating chocolate: from pleasure to aversion. *Brain*, 124(Pt 9), 1720–33.

Staddon, J.E., Hinson, J.M., and Kram, R. (1981). Optimal choice. *J Exp Anal Behav*, 35(3), 397–412.

Stephens, D. W. and Krebs, J. R. (1986). *Foraging theory*. Princeton: Princeton University Press.

Sugrue, L.P., Corrado, G.S., and Newsome, W.T. (2004). Matching behavior and the representation of value in the parietal cortex. *Science,* 304(5678), 1782–87.

Summerfield, C. and Koechlin, E. (2008). A neural representation of prior information during perceptual inference. *Neuron*, 59(2), 336–47.

Sutton, R. S. and Barto, A. G. (1998). *Reinforcement learning: an introduction*. London: MIT Press.

Teves, D., Videen, T.O., Cryer, P.E., and Powers, W.J. (2004). Activation of human medial prefrontal cortex during autonomic responses to hypoglycemia. *Proc Natl Acad Sci USA*, 101(16), 6217–21.

Tobler, P.N., O'Doherty J, P., Dolan, R.J., and Schultz, W. (2006). Human neural learning depends on reward prediction errors in the blocking paradigm. *J Neurophysiol*, 95(1), 301–10.

Tremblay, L. and Schultz, W. (1999). Relative reward preference in primate orbitofrontal cortex. *Nature*, 398(6729), 704–8.

Tremblay, L. and Schultz, W. (2000). Modifications of reward expectation-related neuronal activity during learning in primate orbitofrontal cortex. *J Neurophysiol*, 83(4), 1877–85.

Verhagen, J.V., Rolls, E.T., and Kadohisa, M. (2003). Neurons in the primate orbitofrontal cortex respond to fat texture independently of viscosity. *J Neurophysiol*, 90(3), 1514–25.

Waelti, P., Dickinson, A., and Schultz, W. (2001). Dopamine responses comply with basic assumptions of formal learning theory. *Nature*, 412(6842), 43–48.

Wallis, J.D. and Miller, E.K. (2003). Neuronal activity in primate dorsolateral and orbital prefrontal cortex during performance of a reward preference task. *Eur J Neurosci,* **18**(7), 2069–81.

Walton, M.E., Devlin, J.T., and Rushworth, M.F. (2004). Interactions between decision making and performance monitoring within prefrontal cortex. *Nat Neurosci,* **7**(11), 1259–65.

Walton, M.E., Croxson, P.L., Behrens, T.E., Kennerley, S.W., and Rushworth, M.F. (2007). Adaptive decision making and value in the anterior cingulate cortex. *Neuroimage,* **36 Suppl 2**, T142–154.

Wang, Y., Shima, K., Sawamura, H., and Tanji, J. (2001). Spatial distribution of cingulate cells projecting to the primary, supplementary, and pre-supplementary motor areas: a retrograde multiple labeling study in the macaque monkey. *Neurosci Res,* **39**(1), 39–49.

Watson, K.K. and Platt, M.L. (2008). Neuroethology of reward and decision making. *Philos Trans R Soc Lond B Biol Sci,* **363**(1511), 3825–35.

Williams, S.M. and Goldman-Rakic, P.S. (1998). Widespread origin of the primate mesofrontal dopamine system. *Cereb Cortex,* **8**(4), 321–45.

Winstanley, C.A., Theobald, D.E., Cardinal, R.N., and Robbins, T.W. (2004). Contrasting roles of basolateral amygdala and orbitofrontal cortex in impulsive choice. *J Neurosci,* **24**(20), 4718–22.

Wise, S.P. (2008). Forward frontal fields: phylogeny and fundamental function. *Trends Neurosci.*

Yoshida, W. and Ishii, S. (2006). Resolution of uncertainty in prefrontal cortex. *Neuron,* **50**(5), 781–89.

Yu, A.J. and Dayan, P. (2005). Uncertainty, neuromodulation, and attention. *Neuron,* **46**(4), 681–92.

Zilles, K., Schlaug, G., Geyer, S., Luppino, G., Matelli, M., Qu, M., et al. (1996). Anatomy and transmitter receptors of the supplementary motor areas in the human and nonhuman primate brain. In: H. O. Luders (ed.), *Supplementary sensorimotor area* (pp. 29–43). Philadelphia: Lippincott-Raven.

Neural systems of emotion, reward, and learning

Chapter 12

Dissociating encoding of attention, errors, and value in outcome-related neural activity

(Tutorial Review)

Matthew R. Roesch and Geoffrey Schoenbaum

Abstract

In numerous brain areas, neuronal activity varies according to reward predictability. In many of these areas this activity is thought to represent errors in reward prediction, as has been described for dopamine neurons; however, it might alternatively be related to the animal's enhanced behavioral state, which may include surprise or changes in arousal or attention. Unfortunately, few studies have examined firing in these areas in the context of the same behavioral task, making it difficult to dissociate different types of encoding. Here we compare neural correlates in these areas to that of dopamine neurons in the same behavioral task. We show that while activity in dopamine neurons appears to signal prediction errors, similar activity in orbitofrontal cortex, basolateral amygdala, and ventral striatum does not. Instead, increased firing in basolateral amygdala to unexpected outcomes likely reflects attention, whereas activity in orbitofrontal cortex and ventral striatum is unaffected by prior expectations and may provide information on outcome expectancy. These results have important implications for how these areas interact to facilitate learning and guide behavior.

12.1 Introduction

Outcome-related neural activity in a large and growing number of brain areas has been shown to signal unexpected outcomes. Initially reported in midbrain dopamine neurons, such neural correlates have now been reported, using either brain imaging or single-unit recording, in a variety of areas, including prefrontal cortex, orbitofrontal cortex, ventral striatum, amygdala, habenula, and putamen (Nobre et al., 1999; Schultz and Dickinson 2000; Knutson et al., 2003; McClure et al., 2003; Satoh et al., 2003; Nakahara et al., 2004; Ramnani et al., 2004; Bayer and Glimcher 2005; Tobler et al., 2005; Tobler et al., 2006; Yacubian et al., 2006; Belova et al., 2007; Knutson and Wimmer 2007; Matsumoto and

Hikosaka 2007; Roesch et al., 2007a; D'Ardenne et al., 2008). These correlates are typically cited as evidence that these regions "encode" or signal reward prediction errors—or the difference between expected and actual outcomes.

Yet BOLD signal and single-unit activity have very different origins, and often evidence from the two modalities differs dramatically. Moreover, there are a number of other interpretations for changes (increases or decreases) in neural activity to an unexpected outcome, including most prominently surprise or changes in attention or motivation. Both prediction errors and these other factors, which we will refer to as attentional factors for short, are thought to play a critical role in learning (Holland and Gallagher 1993a, b; Gallagher and Holland 1994; Gallagher and Schoenbaum 1999).

Although most associative learning models agree that attention to a cue is necessary for learning, simple prediction error models, such as those suggested by Rescorla and Wagner (1972) or proponents of temporal-difference reinforcement learning (Sutton and Barto 1998) treat it as a static or fixed quantity. By contrast, other models, including that proposed by Pearce and Hall (1980; Hall and Pearce 1982; Pearce et al., 1982) have treated attention to the cue as a variable quantity that varies with experience. Attention increases when the cue does a poor job predicting a reward and decreases when the cue does a good job predicting reward. The better the cue predicts reward, the less attention the animal pays to it, and the less learning is possible. Following this basic rule, Pearce and Hall proposed that attention on the current trial would reflect attention on the prior trial plus the absolute value of the summed error in reward prediction—the surprise—on the preceding trial.

Theoretically signaling of attentional factors and prediction errors should be dissociable. Specifically, error signaling should differ when outcomes are better versus worse than expected. This is evident in reports on the phasic firing of midbrain dopamine neurons, which are generally acknowledged to signal reward-prediction errors. These neurons increase firing when a reward is delivered unexpectedly, an outcome that is better than expected, and suppress firing when an expected reward is omitted, an outcome that is worse than expected. By contrast, neural activity correlated with changes in factors affecting attention should change similarly in these two circumstances, at least initially, because both would be expected to increase attention and associability. And, of course, areas signaling the value of the outcome should not differ.

Here we will look for this dissociation of error and attentional signaling and value in single-unit data from a number of areas mentioned above: ventral tegmental area, orbitofrontal cortex, ventral striatum, and basolateral amygdala (Roesch et al., 2007a). By analyzing changes in firing in response to unexpected reward and reward omission we will argue that activity in response to unexpected outcomes in VTA and ABL reflects encoding of prediction errors and attention, respectively. Moreover, we will also demonstrate that similar firing single-unit activity in OFC and VS, two areas prominently cited as signaling prediction errors by fMRI studies, does not correlate with either prediction errors or attentional factors (McClure et al., 2003; Ramnani et al., 2004; Tobler et al., 2006; D'Ardenne et al., 2008). Instead, we will suggest that error-related activity reported in these regions likely reflects inputs from these other structures (VTA and ABL) and that output from these areas—evident in single-units—actually provides information bearing on the state value.

12.2 **Dopamine neurons encode prediction errors**

Dopamine neurons in midbrain have been widely reported to signal reward-prediction errors (Mirenowicz and Schultz 1994; Montague et al., 1996, Hollerman and Schultz 1998; Waelti et al., 2001; Fiorillo et al., 2003; Tobler et al., 2003; Nakahara et al., 2004; Bayer and Glimcher 2005; Pan et al., 2005; Morris et al., 2006; D'Ardenne et al., 2008). The evidence supporting this is clear and comes from multiple labs, species, and tasks. Most importantly, these studies show clearly that a large proportion of the dopamine neurons exhibit bidirectional changes in activity in response to rewards that are better or worse than expected. As we have noted, this is a cardinal feature that should distinguish error signaling from signaling of attentional factors.

Thus, our first goal was to demonstrate that we could replicate these basic findings in rats. We recorded from single neurons in VTA, while rats performed a task in which we unexpectedly delivered or omitted reward by altering the timing or number of rewards delivered (task details in Fig. 12.1).

As expected, we found that most DA neurons reported errors in reward prediction. This is illustrated by the single-cell example in Fig. 12.2. Note activity is high or low, depending on whether reward was unexpectedly delivered (positive prediction error) or omitted (negative prediction error), respectively. These effects were significant across the population and in counts of single neurons (Fig. 12.3).

Consistent with the notion that activity in midbrain DA neurons signal prediction errors, we found that activity was also high for delayed reward (Fig. 12.4). In our task, delayed reward was unpredictable, as indicated by the rats' inability to precisely time their licking prior to delivery of delayed reward. The fact that DA neurons fire to unexpected reward in this circumstance further suggests that DA neurons are truly reporting errors in reward prediction (Roesch et al., 2007a; Fiorillo et al., 2008; Kobayashi and Schultz 2008; Takahashi et al., 2009).

Of course, prediction error encoding is not limited to reward delivery; unpredicted cues should also elicit prediction errors. Accordingly, the same dopamine neurons that fired to unpredictable reward also fired to the odor cues in our task, and this activity was higher when the odor cues predicted the more valuable reward (Fig. 12.5; immediate >delayed, big>small). Thus, several features of DA firing are entirely consistent with prediction error encoding (Roesch et al., 2007a).

12.3 **Neural activity in basolateral amygdala signals shifts in attention**

Recently we have recorded from ABL in the same task described above (Roesch et al., 2010). As in VTA, activity of many single neurons increased firing when unexpected reward was delivered (Fig. 12.6). Although these results in ABL are entirely consistent with prediction error signaling (as described above for DA), other aspects of firing in ABL

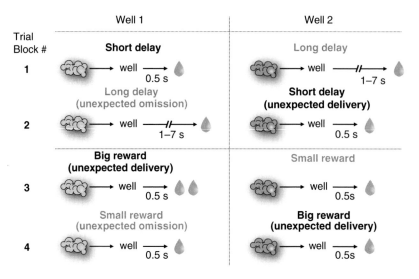

Fig. 12.1 Behavioral task. Figure shows sequence of events in each trial in four blocks in which we manipulated the time to reward or the size of reward. Trials were signaled by illumination of the panel lights inside the box. When these lights were on, nosepoke into the odor port resulted in delivery of the odor cue to a small hemicylinder located behind this opening. One of three different odors was delivered to the port on each trial, in a pseudorandom order. At odor offset, the rat had 3 s to make a response at one of the two fluid wells located below the port. One odor instructed the rat to go to the left to get a reward, a second odor instructed the rat to go to the right to get a reward, and a third odor indicated that the rat could obtain a reward at either well. At the start of each recording session one well was randomly designated as short (a 0.5-s delay before reward) and the other long (a 1–7-s delay before reward) (block 1). In the second block of trials these contingencies were switched (block 2). In blocks 3–4, we held the delay constant, while manipulating the number of the rewards delivered. Expected rewards were thus omitted on long-delay trials at the start of block 2 and small reward conditions at the start of blocks 3 and 4, and rewards were delivered unexpectedly on short-delay trials and big-reward trials at the start of blocks 2 and block 3–4, respectively (Roesch et al., 2006; Roesch et al., 2007a,b).

clearly do not support this claim. First and foremost, activity in ABL was not significantly inhibited by omission of an expected reward (Figs. 12.6 and 12.7). Instead, activity was actually slightly stronger during reward omission. In fact, those neurons that tended to fire more strongly for unexpected reward delivery also tended to fire more strongly under unexpected reward omission, which is inconsistent with bidirectional encoding of prediction errors. This impression was confirmed by analysis of the individual neurons across a population of outcome-selective ABL neurons, which fired more strongly at the start than at the end of these. Second, even though activity in ABL resembled a putative positive prediction error signal, it failed to represent prediction errors in other circumstances. For example, not a single ABL neuron whose activity was higher for unexpected reward also fired significantly more strongly during the delivery of the delayed (unpredictable) reward (Fig. 12.8), nor did any of these neurons transfer firing to stimuli predicting the more valued outcome. Together these observations suggest that activity during

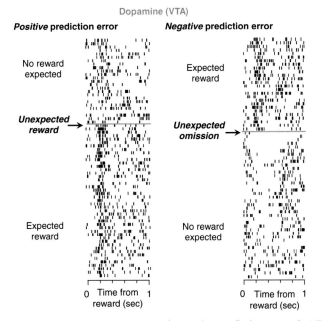

Fig. 12.2 Single cell example showing positive and negative prediction errors in VTA. *Left panel:* Example of error signaling (positive prediction error) when reward was unexpectedly instituted during the transition from a "small" to "big" block (*black arrow*). *Right panel:* Example of error signaling (negative prediction error) in the same cell shown to the left when an expected reward was unexpectedly omitted during the transition between a "big" to "small" block (*black arrow*). Activity is aligned to the onset of reward. Consistent with encoding of errors, activity changes were transient, diminishing as the rats learned to expect the new reward contingencies (Roesch et al., 2007a; Takahashi et al., 2009).

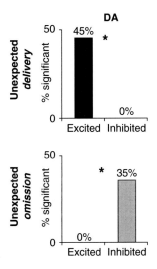

Fig. 12.3 Percent cells significantly modulated by unexpected reward delivery and omission in VTA (DA). Effects illustrated in Fig. 12.2 are quantified during reward delivery (top panel) and reward omission (bottom panel) for reward-responsive punitive dopamine neurons ($n = 20$) in VTA by comparing the average firing rate of each neuron early (unexpected reward) versus late (expected reward) in trials blocks (t-test; $P < 0.05$). This analysis includes both size and delay blocks (Fig. 12.1). Asterisks indicate results of chi-square tests comparing number of neurons increasing or decreasing firing during the trial block after delivery and omission (Roesch et al., 2007a; Takahashi et al., 2009).

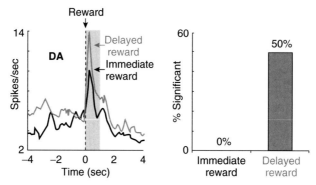

Fig. 12.4 Cells in VTA fired more for delayed unpredictable reward. Average firing rate for all reward-responsive neurons in VTA (DA) on the last 10 trials during immediate (light gray) and delayed (dark gray) reward after learning. Height of bars indicate the percent of cells in VTA (DA) that fired significantly more (dark gray) or less (light gray) strongly (t-test; $P<0.05$) for delayed reward (Roesch et al., 2007a; Takahashi et al., 2009).

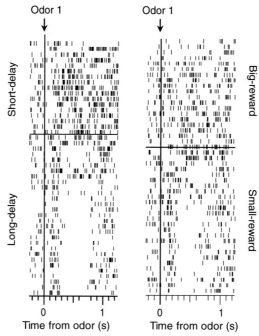

Fig. 12.5 Cue-evoked activity in reward-responsive dopamine neurons reflects prediction errors. Single-unit example of cue-evoked activity in dopamine neurons on forced-choice trials. Initially, the odor predicted that the reward would be delivered immediately ("short"). Subsequently, the same odor predicted a delayed reward ("long"), an immediate but large reward ("big"), and, finally, an immediate but small reward ("small"). Note, "short" and "small" conditions were identical (1 bolus of reward after 500 ms) but differed in their relative value because "short" was paired against "long" in the opposite well, whereas "small" was paired against "big" (Roesch et al., 2007a).

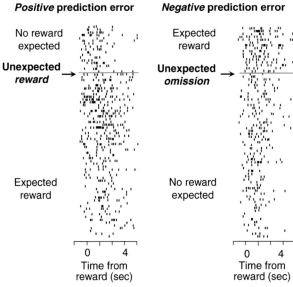

Basolateral amygdala

Positive prediction error   *Negative* prediction error

No reward expected

Expected reward

Unexpected reward →

Unexpected omission →

Expected reward

No reward expected

0   4
Time from reward (sec)

0   4
Time from reward (sec)

Fig. 12.6 Single cell example showing increased activity during unexpected reward delivery in ABL. Conventions the same as in Fig. 12.2 (Roesch et al., 2010).

unexpected reward delivery, though remarkably similar to activity in midbrain DA neurons, is not encoding positive errors in reward prediction.

So what are these ABL neurons signaling? We would suggest the changes in activity in these neurons are more closely related to the animal's enhanced behavioral state, reflecting changes in attention. Like errors, such changes are also thought to affect associative learning; however, unlike errors, activity related to attention should not be inhibited by unexpected decrements in reward.

Allocation of attention should also be temporally dissociable from simple prediction errors. In other words, attentional changes might not necessarily be strongest when reward is most unexpected, as should be the case for prediction errors. This dissociation seems to be evident in a comparison of activity in dopamine versus ABL neurons. Firing in dopamine neurons is strongest on the first encounter with an unexpected reward and then declines (Fig. 12.9; diamonds), paralleling changes in choice performance (Fig. 12.9; triangles). Activity in the ABL neurons does not follow this pattern, instead it increases more slowly, over several trials on which expectancies are violated (Fig. 12.9; squares). This change does not correlate with changes in choice performance and instead parallels changes in the rats' latency to initiate trials (Fig. 12.9; circles). Latency to initiate trials cannot reflect upcoming reward, since the rats don't know what odor is coming, and might therefore be a measure of general attention to the task. Rather, changes in odor-port approach latency might reflect variations in the strength of conditioned orienting behavior directed at the odors. Similar orienting responses have been shown to follow the predictions by the Pearce–Hall model for attentional changes in various learning settings (Kaye and Pearce 1984; Pearce et al., 1988; Swan and Pearce 1988), and have come to be accepted as a behavioral index for attention in associative learning.

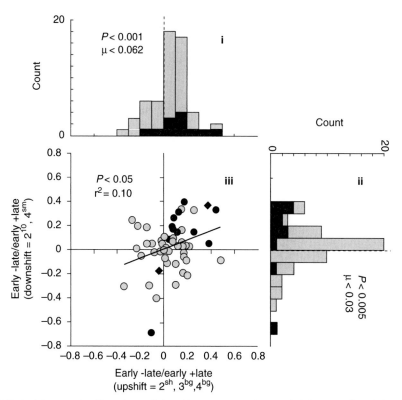

Fig. 12.7 Activity was significantly modulated by unexpected reward delivery and omission in ABL. Distribution of indices (early-late/early+late) representing the difference in firing to reward delivery and omission during the last 10 trials (late) after (i) up-shifts (2^{sh}, 3^{bg} and 4^{bg}) and (ii) down-shifts (2^{lo} and 4^{sm}). Filled bars in distribution plots (i, ii) indicate the number of cells that showed a main effect ($P<0.05$) of learning (early vs late). (iii) Correlation between contrast indices shown in (i) and (ii). Filled points in scatter plot (iii) indicate the number of cells that showed a main effect ($P<0.05$) of learning (early vs late). Black diamonds indicate those neurons that also showed an interaction with shift-type (up vs. down-shift). Analysis and figures shown here include both free- and forced-choice trials. P values for distributions are derived from Wilcoxon test (Roesch et al., 2010).

Interestingly, this slow change suggests that attention—and effects on learning rate—need not be locked to the size of the prediction error. Indeed, the putative attentional measure was unrelated to the reward-related firing of the dopamine neurons (Fig. 12.9 and 12.10). This decoupling would allow ABL to influence learning based in part on the reliability of new circumstances or contingencies. In other words, ABL would provide the adaptive ability to continue to increase learning, even as the size of the prediction error declines, as occurs when the change is highly reliable (as in our task). Alternatively, it would also serve to modulate or slow learning in the face of large errors in reward prediction, when those changes were highly unreliable.

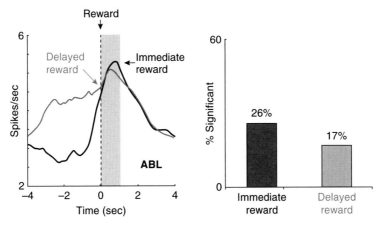

Fig. 12.8 Cells in ABL fired less for delayed unpredictable reward. Conventions the same as in Fig. 12.4, but for all outcome-selective ABL neurons (Roesch et al., 2010).

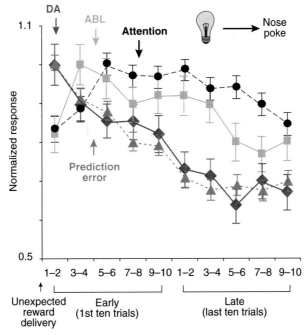

Fig. 12.9 Comparison of activity in ABL and DA to behavioral measures of prediction errors and attention. *Light gray triangles:* The probability of choosing of the low-value reward during the first and last 10 trials in blocks 2–4 normalized to the maximum. *Dark gray circles:* Attention as measured by increase in speed at which rats initiated trials after house light illumination during the first and last 10 trials in blocks 2–4 normalized to the maximum. Thus, the higher the value on the y-axis, the faster the latency to respond. Average firing rate (500 ms after reward delivery) in DA (*diamonds*) and ABL (*squares*) during the first and last 10 trials in blocks 2–4 normalized to the maximum (Roesch et al., 2010).

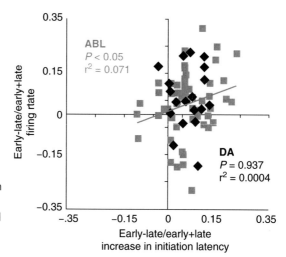

Fig. 12.10 Correlation between firing rate and behavioral measure of attention described in Fig. 12.9 (Roesch et al., 2010).

Of course activity in VTA signaling prediction errors and in ABL signaling attentional factors would presumably interact at some level. Thus any decoupling would not be complete. For example, error signaling by the DA system may initiate changes in activity related to attentional factors in ABL, enhancing representations of outcomes to maximize learning when they are unexpected. This is supported by the finding that activity related to unexpected reward in VTA preceded changes in reward-related activity in ABL by several trials (Fig. 12.9). It would also be intuitively consistent, given that recognition of an error or discrepancy between expected and actual outcomes presumably must precede changes in attention. It is also possible that activity in ABL may feedback directly on to midbrain areas to regulate prediction error signaling. This counter-intuitive possibility would also explain the observation that attention and ABL firing increased as prediction errors and DA firing decreased. Perhaps, once attention is being paid to unexpected rewards, prediction error signals are less necessary.

Another possibility is that ABL and VTA do not influence each other directly, but rather interact via independent influences on downstream areas that encode representations of value critical in optimizing long-term behavior. Support for this hypothesis comes from lesion/inactivation studies that have shown that elimination of these signals impacts encoding of associative information in downstream areas, such as OFC and VS (Schoenbaum et al., 2003; Ambroggi et al., 2008). If single-unit activity in ABL encodes such a potent learning signal, then the role of the ABL in a variety of learning processes may need to be reconceptualized, or at least modified to include attention. For example, ABL appears to be critical for encoding associative information in other areas. This can be interpreted as reflecting an initial role in acquiring the simple associative representations (Pickens et al., 2003). However an alternative account—not mutually exclusive—is that ABL may also augment the allocation of attentional resources to directly drive acquisition of the same associative information in other areas. In other words, the signal in ABL, identified here, may serve to augment or amplify the associability of cue-representations in downstream regions, so that these cues are more "associable" or "salient" on subsequent trials.

12.4 Orbitofrontal cortex and ventral striatum do not signal prediction errors

Speculation that attentional and error related signals from VTA and ABL may influence signaling in OFC and VS is intriguing because both of these areas are strongly implicated in encoding of reward-prediction errors (McClure et al., 2003; Ramnani et al., 2004; Tobler et al., 2006; D'Ardenne et al., 2008). Numerous human brain-imaging studies have shown that BOLD signal in VS and OFC is elevated in response to unexpected rewards, and a fairly large number have reported that BOLD in various subregions within these areas is directly correlated with regressors based on positive and negative reward-prediction errors. This is equivalent to showing, in single-unit data, that activity increases when outcomes are better than expected and is suppressed when outcomes are worse than expected, and thus provides strong evidence that signals that impact metabolic activity in these areas reflect this information.

However single-unit studies in these areas rarely look for neural correlates of reward-prediction errors. As a result, it is unclear whether spiking activity in OFC and VS, which represents potential output of these areas, signals prediction errors, or whether the BOLD correlates might instead reflect inputs to these regions (and not functional output). To address this issue we performed the identical analysis described above on single-unit activity in OFC and VS recorded in the same task. In contrast to the evidence from BOLD signal, we found that counts of neurons in OFC and VS showing a significant increase in activity during delivery of unexpected reward was no more than chance (Fig. 12.11; chi-square; $P > 0.05$) (Takahashi et al., 2009). Furthermore roughly equal numbers of neurons in VS and OFC showed the opposite effect, firing less during unexpected than expected reward delivery (Fig. 12.11; chi-square; $P > 0.2$). These data show that spiking activity in VS and OFC reflects neither attention nor reward-prediction errors. Thus the BOLD signal observed in other studies is highly unlikely to reflect output from these regions to other areas and almost surely reflects inputs. Notably, both the midbrain dopamine system and amygdala project strongly to both VS and OFC, thus there is a ready source to explain these input signals (Groenewegen et al., 1987; Groenewegen et al., 1990; Berger et al., 1991; McDonald 1991a; McDonald 1991b; Johnson et al., 1994; Haber et al., 1995; Wright et al., 1996; Schultz 2002; Schoenbaum and Roesch 2005; Schoenbaum et al., 2006). Such inputs might facilitate the function of these areas (see below) but they cannot logically be that function, if they are not represented in spiking activity.

12.5 Orbitofrontal cortex and ventral striatum signal state values

So what is the function of these areas in the context of learning? One possibility is that VS and OFC signal information regarding the value of the current state. This has been

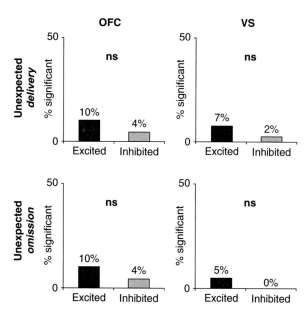

Fig. 12.11 Percent cells significantly modulated by unexpected reward delivery and omission in OFC and VS. Effects illustrated in Fig. 12.2 are quantified during reward delivery (top panels) and reward omission (bottom panels) for reward-responsive neurons in OFC (left panels; $n = 69$) and VS (right panels; $n = 41$) by comparing the average firing rate of each neuron early (unexpected reward) versus late (expected reward) in trials blocks. Analysis is the same as in Roesch et al. (2007). Asterisks indicate results of chi-square tests comparing number of neurons increasing or decreasing firing during the trial block after delivery and omission (Roesch et al., 2006; Takahashi et al., 2009).

proposed previously for ventral striatum in the so-called actor–critic models (Joel et al., 2002; Takahashi et al., 2008). According to this hypothesis, VS is proposed to act as the critic, signaling the expected value of the current state, which can then be used by areas like VTA to generate error signals. We would propose that OFC serves a similar role. Consistent with this, activity in both regions fires in anticipation of expected rewards. Moreover we have shown recently that OFC plays a critical role in learning driven by reward-prediction errors (Takahashi et al., 2009). Specifically, OFC must be online when errors are generated in order for changes in behavior to be observed later. This role appears to depend on connections with VTA. These data are consistent with the proposal that OFC is providing information regarding state value.

We would speculate that OFC and VS may signal state values based on different types of information. OFC is most strongly implicated in signaling information about predicted outcomes—their specific features and value—whereas VS is more clearly implicated in signaling information about the general affect or emotion that a particular outcome shares with other outcomes. According to this hypothesis, OFC would serve as an outcome-specific critic, whereas VS would serve as a general-affect critic. These roles should be dissociable using manipulations that independently manipulate the value and identity of expected rewards. Indeed, we have already shown that learning in a setting in which only outcome identity changes is critically dependent on OFC (Takahashi et al., 2009).

12.6 **Conclusions**

We conclude that delivery of unexpected reward sets in motions two distinct processes. One, manifest in the activity of midbrain dopamine neurons, involves signaling of prediction errors. The other, manifest in the activity of ABL neurons, involves modulation of attention during learning when reward unexpectedly changes. It is unclear how these two neural signals interact to drive learning in downstream areas or if other brain areas serve similar functions; however, careful consideration should be taken to dissociate signals related to prediction errors and those related to behavioral state changes, such as attention. These results also suggest that we must re-examine the role of ABL in attention, a function that is typically ascribed to CN.

Additionally we would suggest that special attention needs to be paid to the concordance, or lack thereof, between single-unit and brain-imaging studies. Discrepant findings should be particularly revealing about the relationship between inputs and outputs in a particular region. This is certainly the case for OFC and VS, where a comparison of data from the two approaches suggests a model in which inputs from VTA and ABL influence encoding of state values, which OFC and VS then broadcast to other regions to influence behavior and subsequent learning.

References

Ambroggi, F., Ishikawa, A., Fields, H.L., and Nicola, S.M. Basolateral amygdala neurons facilitate reward-seeking behavior by exciting nucleus accumbens neurons. *Neuron,* **59,** 648–61 (2008).

Bayer, H.M. and Glimcher, P.W. Midbrain dopamine neurons encode a quantitative reward prediction errorreward-prediction error signal. *Neuron,* **47,** 129–41 (2005).

Belova, M.A., Paton, J.J., Morrison, S.E., and Salzman, C.D. Expectation modulates neural responses to pleasant and aversive stimuli in primate amygdala. *Neuron,* **55,** 970–84 (2007).

Berger, B., Gaspar, P., and Verney, C. Dopaminergic innervation of the cerebral cortex: unexpected differences between rodents and primates. *Trends Neurosci,* **14,** 21–7 (1991).

D'Ardenne, K., McClure, S.M., Nystrom, L.E., and Cohen, J.D. BOLD responses reflecting dopaminergic signals in the human ventral tegmental area. *Science,* **319,** 1264–7 (2008).

Fiorillo, C.D., Tobler, P.N. and Schultz, W. Discrete coding of reward probability and uncertainty by dopamine neurons. *Science,* **299,** 1856–902 (2003).

Fiorillo, C.D., Newsome, W.T., and Schultz, W. The temporal precision of reward prediction in dopamine neurons. *Nat Neurosci,* **11,** 966–73 (2008).

Gallagher, M. and Holland, P.C. The amygdala complex: multiple roles in associative learning and attention. *Proc Natl Acad Sci USA* **91,** 11771–6 (1994).

Gallagher, M. and Schoenbaum, G. Functions of the amygdala and related forebrain areas in attention and cognition. *Ann N Y Acad Sci,* **877,** 397–411 (1999).

Groenewegen, H.J., Vermeulen-Van der Zee, E., te Kortschot, A., and Witter, M.P. Organization of the projections from the subiculum to the ventral striatum in the rat. A study using anterograde transport of Phaseolus vulgaris leucoagglutinin. *Neuroscience,* **23,** 103–20 (1987).

Groenewegen, H.J., Berendse, H.W., Wolters, J.G., and Lohman, A.H. The anatomical relationship of the prefrontal cortex with the striatopallidal system, the thalamus and the amygdala: evidence for a parallel organization. *Prog Brain Res, 85*, 95–116 discussion 116–8 (1990).

Haber, S.N., Kunishio, K., Mizobuchi, M., and Lynd-Balta, E. The orbital and medial prefrontal circuit through the primate basal ganglia. *J Neurosci, 15*, 4851–67 (1995).

Hall, G. and Pearce, J. M. in *Quantitative Analyses of Behavior* (eds, Commons, M. L., Herrnstein, R. J., and Wagner, A. R.), pp. 221–39. Ballinger, Cambridge, MA (1982).

Holland, P.C. and Gallagher, M. Amygdala central nucleus lesions disrupt increments, but not decrements, in conditioned stimulus processing. *Behav Neurosci, 107*, 246–53 (1993a).

Holland, P.C. and Gallagher, M. Effects of amygdala central nucleus lesions on blocking and unblocking. *Behav Neurosci, 107*, 235–45 (1993b).

Hollerman, J.R. and Schultz, W. Dopamine neurons report an error in the temporal prediction of reward during learning. *Nature Neuroscience, 1*, 304–9 (1998).

Joel, D., Niv, Y., and Ruppin, E. Actor-critic models of the basal ganglia: new anatomical and computational perspectives. *Neural Netw, 15*, 535–47 (2002).

Johnson, L.R., Aylward, R.L., Hussain, Z., and Totterdell, S. Input from the amygdala to the rat nucleus accumbens: its relationship with tyrosine hydroxylase immunoreactivity and identified neurons. *Neuroscience, 61*, 851–65 (1994).

Kaye, H. and Pearce, J.M. The strength of the orienting response during Pavlovian conditioning. *Journal of Experimental Psychology: Animal Behavior Processes, 10*, 90–109 (1984).

Knutson, B. and Wimmer, G. E. Splitting the difference: how does the brain code reward episodes? *Ann N Y Acad Sci, 1104*, 54–69 (2007).

Knutson, B., Fong, G.W., Bennett, S.M., Adams, C.M., and Hommer, D. A region of mesial prefrontal cortex tracks monetarily rewarding outcomes: characterization with rapid event-related fMRI. *Neuroimage, 18*, 263–72 (2003).

Kobayashi, S. and Schultz, W. Influence of reward delays on responses of dopamine neurons. *J Neurosci, 28*, 7837–46 (2008).

Matsumoto, M. and Hikosaka, O. Lateral habenula as a source of negative reward signals in dopamine neurons. *Nature, 447*, 1111–5 (2007).

McClure, S.M., Berns, G.S., and Montague, P.R. Temporal prediction errors in a passive learning task activate human striatum. *Neuron, 38*, 339–46 (2003).

McDonald, A.J. Organization of amygdaloid projections to the prefrontal cortex and associated striatum in the rat. *Neuroscience, 44*, 1–14 (1991a).

McDonald, A.J. Topographical organization of amygdaloid projections to the caudatoputamen, nucleus accumbens, and related striatal-like areas of the rat brain. *Neuroscience, 44*, 15–33 (1991b).

Mirenowicz, J. and Schultz, W. Importance of unpredictability for reward responses in primate dopamine neurons. *Journal of Neurophysiology, 72*, 1024–27 (1994).

Montague, P.R., Dayan, P., and Sejnowski, T.J. A framework for mesencephalic dopamine systems based on predictive hebbian learning. *Journal of Neuroscience, 16*, 1936–47 (1996).

Morris, G., Nevet, A., Arkadir, D., Vaadia, E., and Bergman, H. Midbrain dopamine neurons encode decisions for future action. *Nat Neurosci, 9*, 1057–63 (2006).

Nakahara, H., Itoh, H., Kawagoe, R., Takikawa, Y., and Hikosaka, O. Dopamine neurons can represent context-dependent prediction error. *Neuron, 41*, 269–80 (2004).

Nobre, A.C., Coull, J.T., Frith, C.D., and Mesulam, M.M. Orbitofrontal cortex is activated during breaches of expectation in tasks of visual attention. *Nat Neurosci, 2*, 11–2 (1999).

Pan, W.X., Schmidt, R., Wickens, J.R., and Hyland, B.I. Dopamine cells respond to predicted events during classical conditioning: evidence for eligibility traces in the reward-learning network. *J Neurosci, 25*, 6235–42 (2005).

Pearce, J.M. and Hall, G. A model for Pavlovian learning: variations in the effectiveness of conditioned but not of unconditioned stimuli. **87**, 532–52 (1980).

Pearce, J. M., Kaye, H., and Hall, G. in *Quantitative analyses of behavior* (eds, **Commons, M. L.**, **Herrnstein, R. J.**, and **Wagner, A. R.**), pp. 241–55. Ballinger, Cambridge, MA (1982).

Pearce, J.M., Wilson, P., and Kaye, H. The influence of predictive accuracy on serial conditioning in the rat. *Quarterly Journal of Experimental Psychology*, **40B**, 181–98 (1988).

Pickens, C.L. , Saddoris, M.P., Setlow, B., Gallagher, M., Holland, P.C., and Schoenbaum, G. Different roles for orbitofrontal cortex and basolateral amygdala in a reinforcer devaluation task. *Journal of Neuroscience*, **23**, 11078–84 (2003).

Ramnani, N., Elliott, R., Athwal, B.S. and Passingham, R.E.; Prediction error for free monetary reward in the human prefrontal cortex. *Neuroimage*, **23**, 777–86 (2004).

Rescorla, R. A. and Wagner, A. R. in *Classical conditioning II: current research and theory* (eds, **Black, A. H.** and **Prokasy, W. F.**), pp. 64–99. Appleton-Century-Crofts, New York (1972).

Roesch, M.R., Taylor, A.R., and Schoenbaum, G. Encoding of time-discounted rewards in orbitofrontal cortex is independent of value representation. *Neuron*, **51**, 509–20 (2006).

Roesch, M.R., Calu, D.J., and Schoenbaum, G. Dopamine neurons encode the better option in rats deciding between differently delayed or sized rewards. *Nat Neurosci*, **10**, 1615–24 (2007a).

Roesch, M.R., Calu, D.J., Burke, K.A., and Schoenbaum, G. Should I stay or should I go? Transformation of time-discounted rewards in orbitofrontal cortex and associated brain circuits. *Ann NY Acad Sci*, **1104**, 21–34 (2007b).

Roesch, M.R., Calu, D.J., Esber, G.R., and Schoenbaum, G. Neural correlates of variations in event processing during learning in basolateral amygdala. *J Neurosci*, **30**, 2464–71(2010).

Satoh, T., Nakai, S., Sato, T., and Kimura, M. Correlated coding of motivation and outcome of decision by dopamine neurons. *J Neurosci*, **23**, 9913–23 (2003).

Schoenbaum, G. and Roesch, M. Orbitofrontal cortex, associative learning, and expectancies. *Neuron*, **47**, 633–6 (2005).

Schoenbaum, G., Setlow, B., Saddoris, M.P., and Gallagher, M. Encoding predicted outcome and acquired value in orbitofrontal cortex during cue sampling depends upon input from basolateral amygdala. *Neuron*, **39**, 855–67 (2003).

Schoenbaum, G., Roesch, M.R., and Stalnaker, T.A. Orbitofrontal cortex, decision-making and drug addiction. *Trends Neurosci*, **29**, 116–24 (2006).

Schultz, W. and Dickinson, A. Neuronal coding of prediction errors. *Annu Rev Neurosci*, **23**, 473–500 (2000).

Schultz, W. Getting formal with dopamine and reward. *Neuron*, **36**, 241–63 (2002).

Sutton, R. S. and Barto, A. G. *Reinforcement learning: an introduction.* MIT Press, Cambridge MA (1998).

Swan, J.A. and Pearce, J.M. The orienting response as an index of stimulus associability in rats. *Journal of Experimental Psychology: Animal Behavior Processes*, **14**, 292–301 (1988).

Takahashi, Y., Schoenbaum, G., and Niv, Y. Silencing the critics: understanding the effects of cocaine sensitization on dorsolateral and ventral striatum in the context of an actor/critic model. *Front Neurosci*, **2**, 86–99 (2008).

Takahashi, Y.K., Roesch, M.R., Stalnaker, T.A., Harey, R.Z., Calu, D.J., Taylor, A.R., et al. The orbitofrontal cortex and ventral tegmental area are necessary for learning from unexpected outcomes. *Neuron*, **62**, 269–80 (2009).

Tobler, P.N., Dickinson, A., and Schultz, W. Coding of predicted reward omission by dopamine neurons in a conditioned inhibition paradigm. *Journal of Neuroscience*, **23**, 10402–10 (2003).

Tobler, P.N., Fiorillo, C.D., and Schultz, W. Adaptive coding of reward value by dopamine neurons. *Science*, **307**, 1642–5 (2005).

Tobler, P.N., O'Doherty J, P., Dolan, R.J., and Schultz, W. Human neural learning depends on reward prediction errorreward-prediction errors in the blocking paradigm. *J Neurophysiol*, **95**, 301–10 (2006).

Waelti, P., Dickinson, A., and Schultz, W. Dopamine responses comply with basic assumptions of formal learning theory. *Nature*, **412**, 43–48 (2001).

Wright, C.I., Beijer, A.V., and Groenewegen, H.J. Basal amygdaloid complex afferents to the rat nucleus accumbens are compartmentally organized. *J Neurosci*, **16**, 1877–93 (1996).

Yacubian, J., Gläscher, J., Schnoeder, K., Sommer, T., Braus, D.F., and Büchel, C. Dissociable systems for gain- and loss-related value predictions and errors of prediction in the human brain. *J Neurosci* **26**, 9530–7 (2006).

Chapter 13

The striatum and beyond: contributions of the hippocampus to decision making

G. Elliott Wimmer and Daphna Shohamy

Abstract

Recent research on the neural bases of decision making has focused on the role of the striatum and dopamine in learning to predict and obtain rewards. These studies have illuminated the processes by which repeated experiences of choice and reward feedback lead to the updating of value representations, allowing an organism to use past experience to improve choices when encountering the same situation. However, in a constantly changing environment, choices may not repeat themselves. Instead, decisions often involve novel contexts and options, requiring flexible generalization of past experience to novel choices. Extensive evidence from studies of the neural bases of learning and memory suggests that flexible use of learned knowledge depends on a "declarative" memory system in the hippocampus. Investigations of the neural bases of decision making and of memory systems have developed largely independently of each other. However, there are a number of important links between them, at both the brain and behavioral levels. Here, we briefly review these two literatures and propose a critical role for the hippocampus in decision making when past experience must be flexibly generalized to new situations. Further, we suggest that dopamine modulates learning in both the striatum and the hippocampus, with these two systems working together to adaptively guide choices. Finally, we present behavioral evidence from a novel paradigm designed to probe the role of hippocampal-dependent memory in decision making. The findings demonstrate that past experience can flexibly guide decision making in novel contexts, indicating a possible cooperation between reinforcement history and declarative memories in guiding decision making.

13.1 Introduction

There has been a recent surge of interest in the brain mechanisms underlying decision making. This has been motivated primarily by significant advances in understanding the neurophysiological, neurochemical, and neurocomputational properties of dopamine-containing midbrain neurons and their striatal targets (e.g., Bayer and Glimcher, 2005; Beiser and Houk, 1998; Daw and Doya, 2006; Daw et al., 2005; Schultz et al., 1997). Collectively, these studies suggest that *midbrain dopamine neurons are critical for learning to predict reward*. Together with numerous studies suggesting an important role for the striatum and dopamine in reinforcement-based learning in humans (e.g. Aron et al., 2004; Delgado et al., 2000; Frank et al., 2004; Hare et al., 2008; Kirsch et al., 2003; Knutson et al., 2001; McClure et al., 2004; O'Doherty, 2004; Pessiglione et al., 2006; Shohamy et al., 2004a), this literature emphasizes that decision making and learning are highly interconnected—that dopamine modulation of the striatum allows past experiences to drive future choices.

Importantly, midbrain dopamine neurons also project to other brain systems that are important for learning, such as the hippocampus and surrounding medial temporal lobe (MTL) cortices (Gasbarri et al., 1994)—regions known to play a key role in long-term memory (Cohen and Eichenbaum, 1993; Eichenbaum and Cohen, 2001; Eichenbaum et al., 2007; Gabrieli, 1998; Paller and Wagner, 2002; Squire, 1987, 1992; Wagner et al., 1998). Traditionally, the hippocampus and the striatum were thought to play distinct and independent roles in learning, supporting two independent "memory systems" (Eichenbaum and Cohen, 2001; Gabrieli, 1998; Schacter, 1990; Schacter and Graf, 1986). However, the common input from midbrain dopamine neurons poses a challenge to this view, and suggests that both regions may contribute to learning-based decision making. Thus, a critical question is whether memory processes subserved by the hippocampus also contribute to decision making, and if so, what is the unique contribution of each system?

Here we review existing data regarding the role of the hippocampus and the striatum in learning, and their modulation by dopamine, in order to provide a broader understanding of how learning guides decision making. In particular, we suggest that, while the striatum supports decisions based on gradual stimulus–response learning, the hippocampus supports decisions that depend upon episodic, contextual information and mnemonic flexibility. Finally, we describe an experiment with a novel paradigm that investigates the role of hippocampal-dependent memory processes in decision making, and demonstrate that representational processes characteristic of episodic memory emerge in the context of a reward-based decision-making task.

13.2 Multiple mechanisms for memory-guided choice

Choices are often thought to be driven by value. For example, deciding between eating at a restaurant that serves sushi or one that serves tapas may involve accessing associated values, comparing the values, and selecting the option with the highest value (Rangel et al., 2008). A central question is how values are impacted by past experience.

One way in which past experience may modulate value associations is simply by the history of outcomes associated with a particular event. If a given restaurant has usually provided a rewarding experience, we are likely to choose it again. Recent studies of the neural bases of decision making have focused on this type of learning, exploring how past repeated encounters with a stimulus influence its neural and cognitive representations and the likelihood of choosing the stimulus again (Montague et al., 2006; Rangel et al., 2008). These studies have shown that midbrain dopamine and its modulation of the striatum play a critical role in driving both learning and choice. In particular, converging evidence from animals and humans suggests that midbrain dopamine neurons code for a *prediction error*—the extent to which a received reward deviates from what would be expected, given past experience (Schultz et al., 1997). Computationally, this type of learning is well described by temporal difference (TD) reinforcement learning models, a class of models that employ reward prediction error signals to make predictions about the value of stimuli (Dayan and Abbott, 2001; Sutton and Barto, 1998).

However, past experience may impact choices, even when considering options that have never been directly experienced. For example, decisions in novel settings are often driven by *generalizing* from the past—by applying past knowledge towards future novel situations (Cohen and Eichenbaum, 1993; Eichenbaum, 2000; Shohamy and Wagner, 2008). In such cases, decisions may be guided by the context, by the relationship between novel choices and past ones, or by an abstract ability to imagine each choice and its likely outcome (Gilbert and Wilson, 2007). In all of these situations, decisions are driven *not* by the value associated with a single, previously encountered stimulus, but by structured representation of the relations between multiple stimuli and the context in which they were experienced.

As reviewed below, there is ample evidence to suggest that that such memory-guided choice is dependent on representational processes in the hippocampus. To understand how this view emerges from existing literature, we first review evidence regarding the distinct contribution of the striatum and the hippocampus to different forms of learning and memory, with a focus on bridging between mnemonic and decision-making processes. We then turn more specifically to a discussion of dopamine modulation of the hippocampus and the possible role of episodic memory processes in decision making.

13.3 Multiple memory systems in the brain

Decades of research into the neural bases of learning and memory suggest that these different forms of memory-guided choice depend on representations formed by distinct cognitive and neural systems. Extensive evidence indicates that the MTL (particularly the hippocampus and surrounding cortices) supports the rapid acquisition of long-term, explicit memories for events or episodes—often described as "declarative" memory (Cohen and Eichenbaum, 1993; Eichenbaum and Cohen, 2001; Schacter and Wagner, 1999; Squire, 1987, 1992). The striatum, by contrast, is thought to support an independent and dissociable system for gradual learning of stimulus–response associations over many trials—a form of non-declarative memory often referred to as "procedural" or "habit" learning (Gabrieli, 1998; Knowlton et al., 1996; Robbins, 1996; White, 1997).

The idea that there are different forms of memory that are subserved by different systems has been prominent in the cognitive and neural sciences for decades (Eichenbaum and Cohen, 2001; Gabrieli, 1998; Schacter, 1990; Schacter and Graf, 1986). Much of the evidence in favor of this view comes from the demonstration of a dissociation in the pattern of memory impairments following damage to the MTL and damage to the striatum, in both humans and animals. In humans, striatal disruption (such as occurs in Parkinson's disease) impairs performance on a variety of incremental, stimulus–response learning tasks (Downes et al., 1989; Knowlton et al., 1996; Owen et al., 1993; Saint-Cyr et al., 1988; Shohamy et al., 2004a, 2004b, 2005, 2006; Swainson et al., 2000), but spares performance on tasks that involve declarative memory (Knowlton et al., 1996). The opposite pattern is observed following damage to the MTL: striking declarative memory deficits, but spared incremental learning of stimulus–response associations (Gabrieli, 1998; Knowlton et al., 1996).

Animal lesion studies provide further support for the multiple memory systems framework. Combining lesions of either the MTL or the striatum with behavioral tasks that probe either spatial-relational learning or habit learning, these studies have shown that an intact MTL is essential for the former, while the striatum (specifically, the caudate) is essential for the latter (Kesner et al., 1993; McDonald and White, 1993; Packard, 1999; Packard et al., 1989; Packard and McGaugh, 1996); see Poldrack and Packard, 2003 for review). These animal studies have additionally shown that inactivating one system, in some cases, improves the performance of the type of memory supported by the other system (Lee et al., 2008; Poldrack and Packard, 2003), suggesting that these two systems not only support different kinds of learning, but also that in some situations the learning processes supported by the striatum and MTL competitively interact.

13.3.1 The striatum and feedback-based, incremental learning

Recent studies have sought to provide a more direct link between the role of the striatum in stimulus–response learning and the evidence that dopamine neurons encode a reward prediction error (Montague et al., 1996; Schultz et al., 1997), an essential learning signal used to update estimates of value. Building on this theoretical and electrophysiological research, studies have indicated that the striatum may be particularly important for learning that involves repeated reward feedback (including feedback that may rapidly shift, as in reversal) (Aron et al., 2004; Cools et al., 2002; Poldrack et al., 2001; Schonberg et al.; Shohamy et al., 2004a, 2005) or learning the correct sequences of choices that lead to reward (Nagy et al., 2007; Schendan et al., 2003; Shohamy et al., 2005; Suri and Schultz, 1998).

More specific insight into the role of dopamine in learning comes from studies examining the effect of dopaminergic medication on learning in Parkinson's patients. In such studies, patients are tested on the same learning task either "on" or "off" dopamine-replacement therapy. Consistent with computational models of dopamine and the striatum, these studies reveal that dopamine may have differential effects on learning, depending on whether or not learning depends heavily on response-contingent feedback (Shohamy et al., 2004a, 2006), and more specifically, depending on whether learning is driven by reward vs. punishment (Cools et al., 2006; Frank et al., 2004; Moustafa et al.,

2008; Palminteri et al., 2009). These studies suggest that patients tested "off" medication showed improvements in learning from punishment, but impairment in learning from reward, relative to controls, while patients "on" medication exhibit the opposite pattern (Frank et al., 2004).

Functional imaging (fMRI) studies in humans similarly suggest that the fMRI BOLD signal (henceforth, "activation") in the ventral striatum reflects the magnitude of anticipated reward (Delgado et al., 2000; Knutson et al., 2001) and deviations from expected reward outcomes, i.e. a reward prediction error signal (Delgado et al., 2005b; McClure et al., 2003; O'Doherty et al., 2003; Pessiglione et al., 2006) that is thought to originate in the phasic firing of striatum-projecting midbrain dopamine neurons (D'Ardenne et al., 2008; Knutson and Gibbs, 2007; Zaghloul et al., 2009). The dopaminergic prediction error signal then updates values associated with stimuli, these representations may reside in the ventral or orbital prefrontal cortex or in the striatum itself (Hare et al., 2008; Padoa-Schioppa and Assad, 2006; Samejima et al., 2005). Subsequent decisions, informed by recent reward experience (e.g., reversal learning) or by pre-existing value associations (e.g., purchasing products) have been shown to be predicted from BOLD activity in the ventral striatum, anterior cingulate, and ventromedial prefrontal cortex—regions hypothesized to represent value (Hampton and O'Doherty J, 2007; Knutson et al., 2007; Plassmann et al., 2007).

13.3.2 The hippocampus and episodic, relational learning

Extensive, converging evidence indicates that the hippocampus and surrounding medial temporal cortices subserve the rapid formation of memories for single episodes (Cohen and Eichenbaum, 1993; Eichenbaum and Cohen, 2001; Eichenbaum et al., 2007; Gabrieli, 1998; Paller and Wagner, 2002; Squire, 1987, 1992; Wagner et al., 1998). In humans, damage to the MTL results in a highly specific memory deficit that renders new episodic learning impaired while sparing other learning processes (Cohen and Squire, 1980, 1981; Eichenbaum and Cohen, 2001; Gabrieli, 1998; Squire, 1992). Similarly, in animals, damage to the MTL leads to specific impairments in rapid learning of arbitrary associations between co-occurring stimuli, while gradual learning of stimulus–response associations remains intact (e.g., (Eichenbaum et al., 1990; Squire, 1987, 1992). Functional imaging studies in healthy individuals further indicate a tight link between MTL activation and the formation of episodic memories. For example, fMRI studies have demonstrated that memory for single-trial events relates to neural activity occurring during encoding of those events (Brewer et al., 1998; Kirchhoff et al., 2000; Otten et al., 2001; Schacter and Wagner, 1999; Wagner et al., 1998).

Extensive evidence from humans and animals suggests that MTL-based episodic memories have two key characteristics. First, the memory representations are *relational*, in that they contain information about spatial, temporal, or associative relations between multiple stimuli (Eichenbaum and Cohen, 2001; Eichenbaum et al., 2007; Staresina and Davachi, 2009). A second key feature of MTL-based memory is *representational flexibility*— MTL-based memories can be accessed, transferred, and used in novel contexts (Cohen, 1984; Cohen and Eichenbaum, 1993; Eichenbaum, 2000). For example, animals and humans are able to learn associations with overlapping features (e.g., A→B and B→C), and can subsequently transfer this knowledge when tested on a novel pairing (A→C). Importantly, MTL damage specifically impairs the ability to perform such transfer, without significantly impacting the ability to learn the individual associations (Buckmaster et al., 2004; Bunsey and Eichenbaum, 1996; Dusek and Eichenbaum, 1997; Eichenbaum and Cohen, 2001). Damage to the striatum results in the opposite pattern—impaired feedback-based learning of the individual associations, but spared transfer (Myers et al., 2003; Shohamy et al., 2006).

Complementing these lesion data, a recent brain-imaging study in humans further suggests a specific role for the hippocampus in such transfer, and highlights a possible mechanism by which such transfer takes place. In this study, participants learned a series of associations using trial and error. Each of the associations in the series was learned individually; however, the associations sometimes overlapped between stimuli. For example, participants learned that A→X, B→X, and A→Y. Participants were tested on transfer of this knowledge to a novel association (B→Y). The results indicated that, during the learning phase, when individual associations were being experienced, the hippocampus was engaged and predictive of subsequent transfer (Shohamy and Wagner, 2008). Thus, consistent with prior reports, these results support a role for the hippocampus in flexible transfer (Heckers et al., 2004; Preston et al., 2004).

These findings also provide insight into a possible mechanism by which transfer takes place. By demonstrating that hippocampal activity during the learning itself predicts subsequent transfer, the findings raise the possibility that associative mechanisms in the hippocampus continuously integrate episodes as they are being experienced. This suggests that hippocampal-dependent transfer is essentially a form of generalization, emerging from mnemonic links between learned representations driven by the overlap between them.

The role of the hippocampus in supporting flexible transfer of knowledge provides important insight into one putative mechanism by which the hippocampus contributes to decision making. In particular, beyond the obvious role of explicit memories in modulating value and choice, these data indicate that *for long-term memories to adaptively guide future actions and decisions, they must provide a flexible and generalizable representation of the environment.*

Interestingly, in the fMRI study described above, successful generalization was also correlated with activation in a midbrain region consistent with the ventral tegmental area (VTA), a region rich in dopamine-containing neurons known to play a role in reward prediction. Further, during learning, activation in the VTA and the hippocampus was highly correlated, suggesting a cooperative interaction between them. Thus, it is possible that dopamine may modulate learning and decision making in situations requiring flexibility and where reward predictions may play only a small role. This highlights a second putative mechanism by which the hippocampus may contribute to decision making: by directly interacting with midbrain dopamine regions to both enhance and to modulate mnemonic representations of value.

13.4 **Dopamine and the hippocampus**

The novel demonstration of a functional interaction of the dopaminergic midbrain and the hippocampus in successful generalization is not a surprise. In fact, there are several reasons to consider the involvement of the hippocampus in reward-related learning and decision making. Although most research on dopamine in learning has focused on striatal targets, midbrain dopamine neurons also project to the hippocampus (Fuxe, 1965; Gasbarri et al., 1994; Lindvall and Bjorklund, 1974; Swanson, 1982). Dopamine has been shown to modulate cellular learning. For example, dopamine agonists promote long-term plasticity in the hippocampus (Huang and Kandel, 1995; Otmakhova and Lisman, 1996), while dopamine antagonists prevent it (Frey et al., 1990). Indicating the behavioral importance of hippocampal dopamine in learning, lesions to the mesolimbic tract have been shown to impair spatial memory (Gasbarri et al., 1996), and dopamine in the hippocampus has been shown to be necessary for long-lasting maintenance of fear memories (Rossato et al., 2009).

13.4.1 **Novelty, reward, and memory**

Dopamine may play a central role in modulating hippocampal-dependent memory for novel episodes. A recent theory suggests that the hippocampus may encode novel events, in part by activating this dopamine response to novelty (Lisman and Grace, 2005), which is consistent with findings that the hippocampus responds to novel stimuli, as do midbrain dopamine neurons (Fyhn et al., 2002; Ljungberg et al., 1992). The model builds on the idea that the hippocampus detects novelty by comparing incoming sensory information with existing stored memory representations. Then, when novel information is detected, the hippocampus sends a signal to dopamine neurons in the VTA (relayed through intermediate ventral striatal circuitry). By way of projections from the dopamine neurons back to the hippocampus, the novelty-driven activation of VTA dopamine neurons increases dopamine levels in the hippocampus, facilitating the encoding of the novel information (Huang and Kandel, 1995). In support of this idea, studies demonstrate that increased hippocampal plasticity in response to a novel environment depends on the activation of dopamine receptors (Granado et al., 2008; Lemon and Manahan-Vaughan, 2006; Li et al., 2003). Dopamine D1-type receptor knockout also alters the ability of hippocampal place cells to adapt coding to a new environment (Tran et al., 2008).

In contrast to the notion that the hippocampus and the striatum serve as independent systems, the hippocampus has been shown to exert some control over the striatal dopamine and striatal activity. For example, stimulation of the ventral hippocampus has been shown to enhance the number of spontaneously activated dopamine neurons in the VTA, resulting in significantly greater dopamine release in the ventral striatum (Legault and Wise, 1999; Lodge and Grace, 2006, 2008). Neuroanatomical studies have shown that the hippocampus projects directly to the ventral striatum, forming a component of the "reward-related" ventral corticostriatal loop (Cohen et al., 2009; Haber et al., 2006; Haber and Knutson, 2010). Neurophysiological studies suggest that this connection underlies functional interactions between these two regions (Lansink et al., 2009; van der Meer and

Redish, 2009). Recent human fMRI research provides further evidence for a functional interaction between the hippocampus and midbrain dopamine system. Intriguingly, several studies have shown that both the MTL and midbrain dopamine regions respond to various forms of novelty (Bunzeck and Duzel, 2006; Krebs et al., 2009; Wittmann et al., 2007), consistent with the theoretical model of hippocampal-dopamine interactions in detecting and encoding novel stimuli (Lisman and Grace, 2005).

Other data indicate that interactions between the hippocampus and the midbrain may be essential for successful memory formation. A functional coupling between the MTL and midbrain dopamine regions has been shown to support successful reward-motivated memory formation in humans (Adcock et al., 2006). Furthermore, enhanced midbrain BOLD activity is related to better long-term memory for novel stimuli, for associations between stimuli, and for reward-related stimuli (Schott et al., 2006; Schott et al., 2004; Wittmann et al., 2005).

13.4.2 "Episodic" prediction errors in the hippocampus

The studies reviewed above suggest that midbrain dopamine neurons and the hippocampus respond to novelty, and that a functional interaction between these systems may promote memory, particularly when there is reward-induced motivation to do so (Lisman and Grace, 2005). The responses to novelty in both the hippocampus and in midbrain dopamine neurons, share characteristics with dopamine neuronal responses to reward. As discussed, evidence points to a role for dopamine neurons in coding deviations from reward expectations—the occurrence of an unexpected reward, or differences between an expected reward and the received reward (Schultz et al., 1997). Similarly, studies in animals and brain-imaging studies in humans suggest that the hippocampus and midbrain dopamine neurons also respond to deviations in the *content* of an experience, outside of reward, such as signaling the occurrence of a novel and unexpected event, or the non-occurrence of an expected one (Lisman and Grace, 2005; Wittmann et al., 2007).

This raises the intriguing hypothesis that dopamine may code for an "episodic" prediction error. Consistent with this notion, human functional imaging studies demonstrate greater responses in the hippocampus to novel arrangements of stimuli and also to violations of expected sequences of events (Kumaran and Maguire, 2006, 2007). These results suggest that the hippocampus may have a special role in recognizing and encoding novel information (Kumaran and Maguire, 2009). Emerging data suggest that the novelty response is not only broadly reminiscent of the reward prediction error signal in midbrain dopamine neurons, but that it may be anatomically and physiologically intertwined with it.

Collectively, these studies support a tight linkage between the midbrain dopamine system and the hippocampus in episodic memory formation. Thus, dopamine, which has been primarily associated with stimulus–response learning and value-based decision making, may play an essential role in hippocampal dependent episodic memory.

13.5 Episodic representations and transfer of value

How does episodic memory interact with learned value associations to guide decisions? The hippocampus is thought to be particularly important for rapid, relational encoding of single events and episodes, and in the deployment of this information in making flexible decisions. Neurophysiological and functional imaging data suggest that reward-related signals in midbrain dopamine neurons modulate hippocampal function, with important implications for episodic memory and for generalization of learned knowledge towards decisions in novel contexts. If there is indeed a cooperative interaction between learned value and relational knowledge, one prediction is that value may come to be associated not only with stimuli that are directly predictive of reward, but may also flexibly transfer or generalize to *related* stimuli.

The generalization of information to novel contexts has been demonstrated in several recent experiments. In one example, generalization across stimuli was observed to guide decisions based on the similarity of reward history between stimuli (Daw and Shohamy, 2008), much as has been reported for generalization based on associative links (Shohamy and Wagner, 2008). This study adapted a typical monetary decision-making task (e.g., Daw et al., 2006) to include yoked reinforcement histories between stimuli and found that participants indeed use reward information associated with one stimulus to inform choices about another (related) stimulus (Daw and Shohamy, 2008). This suggests that the human brain has the capability to generalize reward information across stimuli that are similar in terms of their recent reward history, an effect not predicted by simple reinforcement learning models that take into account only the reward history of each stimulus independently.

Decisions may also be more broadly influenced by relations among stimuli established *prior* to learning. For example, Walther (2002) investigated the transfer of associations through social relations, using a learning paradigm that probes the generalization of attractiveness. In the study, after rating the attractiveness of a set of face pictures, participants were asked to observe a series of faces. Unbeknownst to the participants, the series included sequential pairs of neutrally rated faces. Participants were then presented with another series of faces, but this time, previously seen neutral faces predicted the appearance of either attractive or unattractive faces. Similar to Pavlovian conditioning, this manipulation was expected to alter attractiveness ratings of the predictive face. Post-experiment liking ratings for the predictive faces indeed shifted in the direction of their associated face. More importantly, they found that this change of value also spread to the paired neutral faces from the first series that had only been seen in a neutral context (Walther, 2002).

13.6 Brain mechanisms of preference via value transfer

Relational representations can serve as the basis for flexible generalization of value associations that are learned later, as shown in the above study. This transfer of newly learned value to stimuli that have a pre-established relational representation has been called sensory preconditioning (Brogden, 1939). A value transfer paradigm involves three phases: (1) pairing of stimuli, (2) conditioning of one member of the pair, and (3) testing the response to both the conditioned stimulus and the stimulus related to it via pairing.

In the original animal sensory preconditioning experiments, relations between two stimuli are established by the simultaneous presentation of stimuli, such as a light and a tone.

Subsequently, one member of the pair, such as the tone, is associated with a valued event, such as a foot shock. After conditioning, the animal shows an aversion to the tone. Critically, the animal displays the same aversion to the light. Thus, the value of the conditioned stimulus, learned via repeated stimulus–reward associations, has been transferred to the neutral, paired stimulus. This endows the paired stimulus with the ability to elicit a similar response as the conditioned stimulus, even though it has never been associated with a valued event. After early research by Brogden and Prodkopaev in dogs (Brogden, 1939; Kimmel, 1977), successful demonstrations of value transfer using this paradigm have been shown in multiple other species, including humans (Barr et al., 2003; Brogden, 1947; Hall and Suboski, 1995; Karn, 1947; Kojima et al., 1998; Muller et al., 2000).[1]

What memory systems are involved in value transfer, and how can these systems bias decision making? Value transfer offers an opportunity to study the function and interaction of memory systems, as it involves both relational and stimulus–reward learning processes. The prominent role of relational pairing in the first phase would suggest the involvement of the MTL, given the importance of the MTL in encoding relational information. In the second phase, the repetition of stimulus–reward associations may be expected to engage the striatum and the midbrain dopamine system. Finally, the value acquired via the striatal system must impact the representation of the paired stimulus in some way, shifting its value toward that of the conditioned stimulus, which hints at a functional interaction between these two memory systems.

In support of the idea that the MTL is an essential brain area for successful value transfer, studies have shown that impacting the function of the MTL impairs sensory preconditioning. Animal-lesion studies have demonstrated that lesions to the entire MTL, the perirhinal cortex, or the fimbria, an essential output pathway of the hippocampus, all abolish value transfer in sensory preconditioning, while primary conditioning is left intact (Nicholson and Freeman, 2000; Port et al., 1987; Port and Patterson, 1984; Talk et al., 2002; Ward-Robinson et al., 2001; but see Ward-Robinson et al., 2001). Thus, without a functioning MTL, the ability to form the relational representation between the two initially neutral stimuli is impaired, eliminating the capacity for subsequent value transfer. Computational models of memory systems further support a role of the MTL in sensory preconditioning (Gluck and Myers, 1993).

The striatum, by contrast, is important for learning value association in sensory preconditioning. As reviewed above, the striatum and its dopaminergic afferents play an important role in reward learning. Animals with impaired striatal functioning cannot learn simple instrumental or Pavlovian reward associations, while it has been shown that phasic dopamine signaling in the striatum is sufficient for conditioning (Robinson et al., 2007; Smith-Roe and Kelley, 2000; Tsai et al., 2009).

---

[1] "Value transfer" is used here as a concise description of the long-established findings from sensory preconditioning paradigms. This usage is similar in spirit, but distinct from, the "value transfer theory" of von Fersen (1991), which was suggested as an alternative account of transitive inference performance in pigeons (von Fersen, 1991; Wynne, 1992).

A conditioning paradigm similar to value transfer suggests that the sequence of the experimental phases in learning paradigms is also important in determining what memory systems are engaged. Second-order conditioning depends on a pairing phase to transfer value from one stimulus to another, as does sensory preconditioning. Critically, in second-order conditioning, the pairing phase occurs after value learning, when a neutral stimulus is paired with a conditioned stimulus (Gewirtz and Davis, 2000), thus transferring value to the neutral stimulus. In second-order conditioning, the transfer of positive or negative value to a neutral stimulus paired with a conditioned stimulus relies on the basolateral amygdala (Gewirtz and Davis, 1997; Hatfield et al., 1996; Setlow et al., 2002a) and connections between the amygdala and the ventral striatum (Setlow et al., 2002b), but not the MTL. In sensory preconditioning, however, relations involve neutral stimuli and are formed prior to conditioning, and amygdala lesions have no impact on learning or transfer (Dwyer and Killcross, 2006). In addition to demonstrating the role of the MTL in choice, the dependence of value transfer on an intact MTL and striatum suggests that coordination between these memory systems may be necessary for successful value transfer.

13.6.1 Value transfer in sensory preconditioning

We developed a novel experimental paradigm to test the influence of value transfer on economic decision making in humans. Our aim in this experiment was to address the fundamental question of whether value can transfer and then influence decision making for items that themselves have no reward history. Based on the findings on sensory preconditioning reviewed above, we predicted that paired presentation of stimuli would establish relations between them. During subsequent conditioning, where one member of the pair became a predictor of monetary reward, the pair relation could then support the transfer of value from the conditioned stimulus to the other member of the pair. At test, gamble choices involving the conditioned stimuli would be predicted by their value associations during conditioning. Critically, choices involving the incidentally paired stimuli should be biased in the direction predicted by the newly acquired value of their associated conditioned stimulus, even though these paired stimuli themselves had no experienced association with value.

13.6.1.1 Participants

Data are reported from 22 healthy adults (13 females; ages 18–32 years); all were native English speakers. Participants received $12/h plus experimental winnings for participation, with the experiment lasting approximately 1h. Informed written consent was obtained from all participants in accordance with procedures approved by the institutional review board at Columbia University.

13.6.1.2 Procedure

The experiment consisted of three phases (Fig. 13.1a–c):

(1) *Incidental pairing phase*, during which subjects were exposed to stimulus pairs composed of sequentially presented scene and fractal images;

(2) *Conditioning phase*, during which the fractal stimuli predicted monetary outcome (gain money, lose money, or neither); and

(3) *Test phase*, in which participants were asked to place a gamble on one of two presented stimuli, which were novel combinations of fractals or scenes.

As an additional test measure, stimulus liking ratings were also collected before and after the experiment.

13.6.1.3 Incidental pairing phase

In the incidental pairing phase, subjects were exposed to five pairs of sequentially presented scene-fractal stimuli (Fig. 13.1a). On each trial, a scene stimulus was presented centrally for 2 s, followed by a 2 s fixation, a 2 s fractal stimulus, and finally a 4 s intertrial fixation. Subjects were not instructed about the pairing relation but were exposed to the pairs while performing a separate task, detecting a "target" yellow scene (the target was followed by a unique fractal not subsequently used). The scene-fractal pairs and the target pair each appeared 10 times in a pseudo-random order.

13.6.1.4 Conditioning phase

To establish value associations with one member of the incidentally paired stimuli, we employed a classical conditioning procedure (Fig. 13.1b; following O'Doherty,

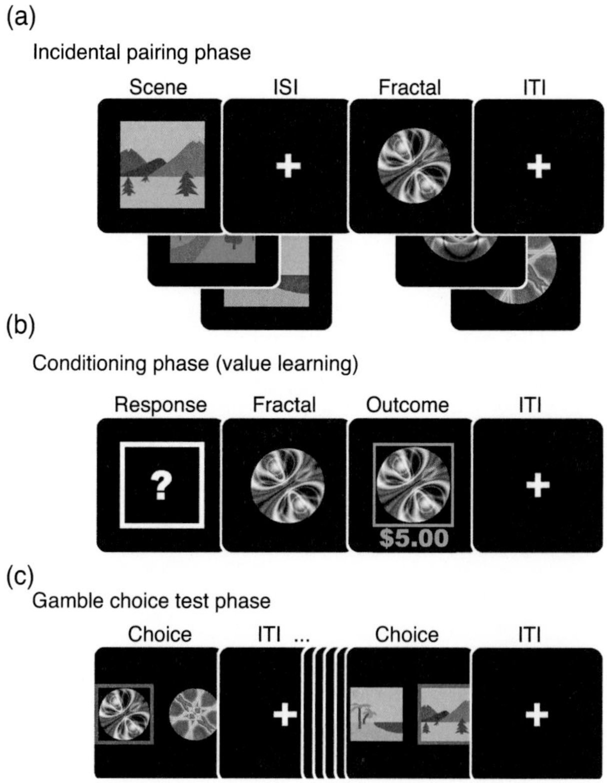

Fig. 13.1 Experimental paradigm. (a) Incidental pairing phase: mere exposure to stimulus pairings establish associations between the scene and fractal images. (b) Conditioning phase: fractals reliably predict monetary gain, loss, or neutral outcome ($5.00, –$4.00, and $0.00, respectively). (c) Test phase: scene–scene and fractal–fractal combinations are presented on gamble trials where participants choose the stimulus on which they prefer to place a $1 gamble.

Dayan et al. 2003). Fractal stimuli were used as predictors of monetary reinforcement: a reward-predicting fractal was followed by a gain of $5.00 on 79% of trials (11/14), a punishment-predicting fractal was followed by a loss of $4.00 on 75% of trials (12/16; losses were presented 12 times to reach average total winnings of $7), and two neutral fractal stimuli were always followed by a neutral $0.00 outcome. On each trial, a question mark was displayed during a 2 s response period. Subjects were instructed to respond to the question mark with a button press. After the response, one of the four fractal stimuli was presented for 2 s, after which the amount of monetary outcome of that trial appeared below the fractal for 2 s (Fig. 13.1b). If the subject did not initiate the trial during the 2 s response period (mean 2.3±3.4 trials per subject), the screen displayed "TOO LATE! –$0.10" and the next trial would begin. Subjects were instructed that all outcomes in the conditioning phase, including those in a brief practice block, would be paid in full at the end of the experiment.

13.6.1.5 Test phase

After the incidental pairing and conditioning phases, we assessed subjects' learned and transferred preferences using a two-alternative gamble choice test phase. Fractal–fractal or scene–scene stimulus combinations were presented (Fig. 13.1c), and subjects were instructed to choose the stimulus on which they would prefer to place a gamble for a chance of winning $1.00 if making the correct choice. Subjects were instructed that one stimulus in each combination was more "lucky" and more likely to win, and that the goal was to pick the stimulus they thought was luckier and that they liked more. On each trial, the choice stimulus combination was presented on the screen for 3 s, during which the subject indicated her preferred stimulus (left–right stimulus screen position was randomized). The chosen image was then framed for 2 s, followed by a 3 s inter-trial fixation. If no response was made during the response period, both stimuli disappeared and were replaced by the text "TOO LATE! –$0.10." To avoid new learning of stimulus–reward associations, gamble outcomes were not presented during the test phase. However, subjects were instructed that five gamble choices would be randomly selected at the end of the experiment to be played for real. All pairings within each stimulus class, including those with the "non-conditioned" fractal and its paired scene, were presented for 2–5 repetitions in a pseudo-random order, yielding 56 gamble test trials.

Finally, as an additional test of learning and transfer, we examined the change in fractal and scene liking ratings over the course of the experiment. We collected liking ratings for all the stimuli at the beginning of the experiment and again after the gamble choice test phase. On each rating trial, a stimulus was individually presented above an unmarked line labeled with "Strong Dislike" on the left and "Strong Like" on the right. Subjects used a computer mouse to indicate their degree of liking for a stimulus. Liking ratings, in arbitrary pixel units, were converted to percent of maximum liking for display. Finally, subjects completed a post-task questionnaire that assessed explicit knowledge of the experimental hypotheses, awareness of the stimulus-pairing contingencies, choice strategy in the gamble test phase, and memory for the scene-fractal pairs from the incidental pairing phase (here, subjects were instructed to match the scene and fractal stimuli that "seem to go together").

13.6.1.6 Results

Gamble choices

The value-transfer paradigm included two test measures to examine the effect of value learning and possible value transfer to the paired scene stimuli. First, participants made gambling decisions where they chose to place a gamble on one of two presented fractal stimuli or one of two presented scene stimuli. The percentage of choices to gamble on a stimulus was interpreted as a reflection of the learned preference for that stimulus. For both the fractal and scene stimuli, we performed planned t-tests comparing choice preference for the reward-predicting (or "reward-associated" for the scene stimulus) vs. neutral stimuli to choice preference for the punishment-predicting (-associated) vs. neutral stimuli. We also compared general preference for the reward-predicting (-associated) stimulus vs. all other stimuli to chance (50%), and similarly for the punishment-predicting (-associated) stimulus (see Fig. 13.2). Gamble choices involving the fractals exhibited a robust effect of conditioning. Preferences for the reward-predicting vs. neutral fractals compared to punishment-predicting vs. neutral fractals were significantly different $(t(21) = 4.26, P<0.001)$, and similar results were found when comparing vs. the non-conditioned stimulus instead of the neutral stimulus. Participants showed a general preference for the reward-predicting fractal, making significantly more gamble choices on it than would be predicted by chance $(t(21) = 8.84, P<0.001;$ Fig. 13.2). Participants also avoided the punishment-predicting fractal, making significantly fewer gamble choices on it than predicted by chance $(t(21) = -3.16, P<0.01;$ the preference for the reward-predicting fractal was significantly greater than the preference to avoid the punishment-predicting fractal, $t(21) = 2.56, P<0.05)$.

Next, we tested the transfer of value to the scene stimuli that were incidentally paired with the fractal stimuli prior to conditioning. Overall, preference for the scene stimuli paralleled the preferences shown for the fractal stimuli, with gamble choices biased toward the direction predicted by the respective related fractal stimulus. Gamble choices for the scene associated with the reward-predicting fractal in the pairing phase vs. the neutral scene, compared to choices for the punishment-related scene vs. the neutral scene, were significantly different $(t(21) = 2.85, P<0.01)$, and similar results were obtained when comparing choices of the reward-related and punishment-related scenes vs. the scene paired with the non-conditioned fractal. Participants also generally gambled significantly more than chance on the scene associated with the reward-predicting fractal vs. all other stimuli $(t(21) = 5.11, P<0.001;$ Fig. 13.2), and, conversely, participants gambled significantly less on the punishment-related scene $(t(21) = -1.76, P<0.05$ one-tailed; Fig. 13.2; gamble preferences showed a trend toward being greater for the reward-associated scene $t(21) = 1.92, P<0.10)$.

Liking ratings

Liking ratings, the second measure of value learning and transfer, also exhibited significant shifts in fractal and scene values. Liking ratings were analyzed in a valenceXtimeXstimulus type ANOVA and two separate valenceXtime ANOVAs for the

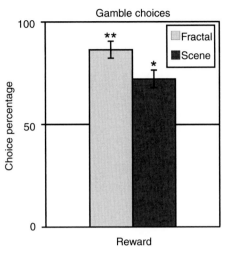

Fig. 13.2 Value transfer test phase gamble choices. Fractal stimuli were directly associated with monetary outcomes, while scene stimuli were only incidentally paired with the fractal stimuli prior to conditioning mean of choices for the reward-associated versus all other stimuli; *P<.01; **P<.001.

scene and fractal stimuli. We found a predicted interaction of valence and time (F = 15.56, P<0.001), reflecting successful increases and decreases in liking due to value learning and transfer of value (Fig. 13.3), as well as a full interaction (F = 11.34, P<0.01), likely driven by the expectedly weaker change in liking for the scene stimuli (but we found no main effect of stimulus type, P>0.1). Within fractal stimuli, a separate valenceXtime ANOVA revealed a significant interaction(F = 7.54, P<0.05; Fig. 13.3a). Planned t-tests revealed that the change in liking ratings from pre- to post-conditioning for both the reward-predicting and the punishment-predicting stimulus were significant (t(21) = 3.73, P<0.001, t(21) = −3.73, P<0.001, respectively).

Supporting the value transfer that was found in the gamble test phase, liking ratings for scene stimuli revealed a trend toward the predicted interaction (F = 3.16, P<0.09; Fig. 13.3b). Planned t-tests showed a significant increase in liking ratings for the reward-related scene stimulus (t(21) = 2.00, P<0.05, 1-tailed). The change in liking ratings for the punishment-related stimulus was in the predicted direction but did not reach significance.

Finally, we examined whether participants acquired explicit knowledge of the pair relationships in the incidental pairing phase and any other knowledge of the task relationships. Participants did not recall the scene-fractal pairings from the first phase, as post-task scene-fractal matching performance was at chance (mean 19.0%±19.9). Further, responses to various multiple-choice and free-response questions indicated no awareness of the pairing manipulation or experimental hypothesis. While we found no evidence of pairing knowledge, if participants did utilize some memory of the pairs to strategically guide test-phase choices, reaction times for scene-gamble choices would be expected to be longer than reaction times for fractal-gamble choices. However, reaction times for scene-gamble choices and fractal-gamble choices differed by less than 80ms (1,250 ms versus 1,327 ms, P<0.05), and while significant, this difference allows little additional time for strategic reasoning. These results collectively suggest that value transfer may not be the result of a

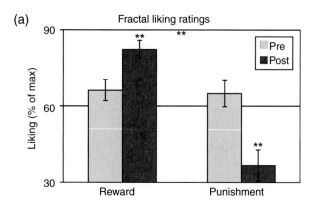

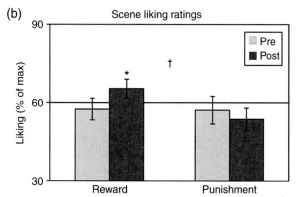

Fig. 13.3 Pre- and post-conditioning liking ratings for the scene stimuli, which were incidentally paired with fractals during the first phase of the experiment (a), and the fractal stimuli, which were subject to conditioning (b) ($P<0.10^{\dagger}$, $P<0.01^{*}$, $P<0.001^{**}$).

test-phase mechanism but may instead be the result of learning processes operating during the pairing and conditioning phases of the experiment.

13.6.1.7 Discussion

This experiment demonstrates that relational learning can impact subsequent value-based decision making. Neutral stimuli were incidentally paired during a relational learning phase, and subsequently, one member of the pair was associated with a monetary value (gain or loss). In a test phase gamble choice task, participants preferred the stimulus that predicted winning money over the stimulus that predicted losing money. Critically, this preference transferred to the neutral stimuli that were only incidentally paired with these predictive stimuli in the first phase, demonstrating a transfer, or generalization, of value. Value transfer was found across two separate measures—gambling choices and changes in stimulus liking—and was found for gain and loss associations.

The present results provide an initial demonstration of the use of relational representations in value-based decision making. Future studies will be necessary to explore the boundary conditions of the effect. While value transfer is robust during the time period of the experiment, it is an open question how long this effect can significantly influence behavior. Also, it is not known how many related representations can be updated via value transfer—does value spread only to a few strong relations, or to many incidentally experienced relations? Finally, the current value-transfer paradigm formed relations between stimuli through sequential presentation, but other relational connections, such as spatial associations (e.g., items within a room or a maze), might be predicted to show similar transfer effects, as suggested by past research on temporal and spatial relational encoding in the MTL (Davachi, 2006; Kumaran and Maguire, 2009).

13.6.1.8 Models of how the hippocampus may contribute to value transfer

What is the mechanism underlying value transfer in sensory preconditioning? Transfer could be driven by several distinct mechanisms operating in different phases of the experimental paradigm. First, value transfer could arise purely in the test phase during the presentation of the neutral stimuli, where transfer could be strategic or mediated via flexible associative recollection. While the existence of value transfer in a wide range of animals suggests that a complicated inferential mechanism does not underlie transfer (in these species, at least), the alternative test-phase associative process could be a more broadly applicable mechanism, biasing preference by activating a representation of the reward-associated stimulus and thus the reward. Indeed, a similar mechanism operating in the MTL at test is believed to underlie some types of information generalization in humans (Preston et al., 2004). However, experimental evidence on value transfer in animals, as well as data from the present experiment, argues against such a mechanism in this case. Ward-Robinson and Hall (1996) utilized a "backwards" sensory preconditioning paradigm, where the first of the incidentally paired stimuli serves as the reward-predicting stimulus, instead of the second. In this manipulation, because of the reversed temporal ordering of the reward associated and neutral pair members, a test-phase transfer mechanism linking the paired stimulus to the reward would require an unlikely series of backwards and forwards associations (Hall, 1996; Ward-Robinson and Hall, 1996). Further, in the present experiment, a test-phase mechanism is not supported by the minimal reaction time difference between test-phase fractal choices and scene choices. Also, after the completion of the experiment, participants exhibited a complete lack of knowledge of the pairing relationships. Thus, while definitive experimental data in humans or animals are not yet available, existing data suggest that value transfer is not likely to occur during the test phase.

Value transfer may instead rely on a learning mechanism operating during the earlier incidental pairing or value-learning phases. In one such mechanism, value transfer relies primarily on learning that occurs during the pairing phase. The pairing phase establishes a representation of the neutral stimulus–stimulus pair as a unitary item (Gluck and Myers, 1993; Rescorla, 1980). Then, during the conditioning phase, reward presentation would simultaneously affect both members of the unitary pair representation. If so, successful transfer would be predicted by the degree of stimulus–stimulus binding and associated hippocampal activity during the pairing phase.

Alternatively, value transfer in sensory preconditioning could rely on learning during the conditioning phase. After pair representations are established in the incidental pairing phase, presentation of one stimulus would be able to associatively reactivate a representation of the other member of the pair. Thus, during the subsequent conditioning phase, the lone presentation of one stimulus would reactivate the representation of its pair at the same time that reward feedback is being received. A re-encoding process would then be able to associate the reward value with both of the active stimulus representations (Hall, 1996). At the same time, this re-learning process may be aided by the known activation of the hippocampus by unexpected events (Kumaran and Maguire, 2006)—the surprising lone presentations of the reward associated stimulus. The hippocampal response to this unexpected and novel event, resembling a kind of prediction error, may be part of a circuit that facilitates re-encoding (Lisman and Grace, 2005). This conditioning-phase reactivation and re-encoding mechanism is similar to the "integrative encoding" mechanism that was proposed to account for a strong correlation between associative generalization and learning phase activation in the hippocampus and VTA (Shohamy and Wagner, 2008). Similarly, in sensory preconditioning, successful transfer may be predicted by hippocampal activation during the conditioning phase.

Studies in animals have offered conflicting results on the learning mechanisms guiding transfer across a variety of paradigms. In experimental and theoretical work, transfer has been argued to be driven by reinforcement learning alone (Couvillon and Bitterman, 1992), reinforcement learning augmented with model-based components (Frank et al., 2003; von Fersen et al., 1991), or primarily relational learning (Dusek and Eichenbaum, 1997). In the past, these mechanisms were tested in paradigms where putative reinforcement and relational learning processes could happen at the same time, i.e., feedback-based learning of overlapping associations was itself the basis for building any relations across associations. By contrast, the sensory preconditioning paradigm is unique in that learning of stimulus–stimulus relations takes place first (with no reinforcement), followed by a phase of learning stimulus–outcome associations (with no relational overlap between the stimuli). Thus, this paradigm provides a unique opportunity to tease out reinforcement and relational learning processes and to probe their interaction. In particular, by recording activation across the whole brain in the different phases of sensory preconditioning, functional imaging studies in humans may be uniquely positioned to address some of these controversial questions that have emerged from animal studies.

13.7 General discussion

13.7.1 The MTL and decision making

Research in the cognitive neuroscience of decision making has been focused in large part on how people learn value associations from rewards and punishments, and then use this information to inform future choices (Rangel et al., 2008). In particular, as reviewed here, extraordinary advances have been made in understanding the role of the striatum and midbrain dopamine neurons in feedback-driven learning (Schultz, 2006). A separate area of research has focused on how the hippocampus encodes a different type of information, building flexible memories of specific episodes. Emerging findings suggest that both of these learning systems may jointly guide adaptive future behavior: learning values from reinforcement and learning relations from experience are in this sense both "memory in service of the future."

Here, we sought to emphasize emerging data indicating that the hippocampus may also contribute to decision making, in two ways. First, given its role in relational, episodic encoding, the hippocampus may be critical for guiding decisions in situations requiring flexible relational representations to make decisions in novel contexts (Myers et al., 2003; Shohamy and Wagner, 2008). Second, the hippocampus, like the striatum, is modulated by dopamine neuron projections from the midbrain. Thus, the hippocampus is well positioned to build adaptive memory representations that are modulated by reward and motivation. The hippocampus also projects back to the midbrain, suggesting that episodic memories for the past may help modulate reward related activity in midbrain neurons (Lisman and Grace, 2005). Consistent with this idea, both reward and novelty increase activity in both the hippocampus and midbrain dopamine regions, facilitating subsequent episodic memory (Adcock et al., 2006; Wittmann et al., 2007).

Recent research has begun to show how relational representations can be used to adaptively guide decisions. In everyday life, an organism encounters countless "episodes" consisting of associative relations within and between episodes and of associations with value. The research on value transfer in sensory preconditioning suggests that relational learning can form the basis for the transfer of value to related stimuli that are not present at the time of value learning: "[t]he experience of two contiguous sensory stimuli completely divorced from any phasic activity is frequent to any organism. If one of these stimuli becomes the signal for the response of a given reaction-pattern, the other will then elicit a similar response." (Brogden, 1939). Thus, factors in addition to simple reinforcement learning can strongly modulate value associations and guide economic decisions, effects that likely rely on cooperation between the striatum and the hippocampus (Port et al., 1987).

13.7.2 Future explorations of the MTL in generalization

The demonstration, in numerous studies, reviewed above, that relational learning processes can bias behavior suggest numerous future questions. Further exploration of the role of the MTL in decision making can further our understanding of the nature and dynamics of the relations established and the neural systems that underlie these effects. For instance, how persistent is generalization? Can extinction diminish the value of paired stimuli, similar to conditioned stimuli?

Although value learning and decision making is the primary focus of this review, it may also be of interest to explore whether the transfer via relational encoding extends to decisions beyond those guided by value. For example, if the incidental pairing were followed instead by categorization learning (e.g., person 1 is paired with person 2; person 1 prefers chocolate ice cream; what about person 2?), it might be expected that these associations will also generalize (Shohamy and Wagner, 2008). Interestingly, in support of the flexibility of the transfer effect shown here, the original report of sensory preconditioning in humans used button responses, not value, as the dependent variable (Brogden, 1947).

Can the extent of relational learning modulate value transfer? While research suggests that the hippocampus is responsible for encoding relations between stimuli, after extensive training this response could become more "habitual" and more dependent on the dorsal striatum. Repetitions during the pairing phase could eventually impair the relational flexibility underlying transfer, which would diminish the sensory preconditioning effect. Intriguingly, prior research suggests that the amount of relational learning eventually decreases value transfer in animals (Hoffeld et al., 1960), and increased repetition of relational pairs may also decrease the generalization of overlapping associations in humans (Clement et al., 2008).

Social decisions and evaluations may also be influenced by generalization mechanisms. Recent experiments set in social exchange contexts have explored the development of trust, as well as the influence of reputation information, on behavior and brain activation in the striatum (Delgado et al., 2005a; King-Casas et al., 2005). However, it is possible that social decisions are also influenced by the flexible associations characteristic of the MTL. Most recently, Walther (2002) demonstrated the transfer of liking in a series of elegant behavioral experiments. Attractiveness spread from an inherently valenced face to a neutral face directly associated with it, and critically, attractiveness also spread to a face only incidentally related to the conditioned face earlier in the experiment (Walther, 2002). It is an interesting question whether generalization can occur for associations that carry value in interpersonal relations, such as good or bad reputations. For example, after the incidental-pairing phase, positive and negative social attributions for particular people could be introduced (e.g., Delgado et al., 2005a); these reputations might be expected to spread by mere association to the paired person.

13.7.3 Other roles for the MTL in decision making

We have emphasized the importance of the hippocampus in decisions that depend on mnemonic flexibility and generalization, but a growing number of studies are exploring other complementary ways that the hippocampus may contribute to decision making. Explicit memory representations may bias economic choices. For example, in an experiment where participants decide between a sooner reward or a later, larger reward, the order and content of accessed memory representations (e.g. "What could you do with the money later?") can eliminate discounting of future rewards (Weber et al., 2007). Another important body of research is exploring how the flexibility of hippocampal representations can support thinking about novel future situations. Patients with damage to the hippocampus are impaired at imaging detailed future scenarios (Hassabis et al., 2007; Tulving et al., 1988), and human brain-imaging studies have consistently shown that the hippocampus is activated when participants imagine future scenarios (Addis et al., 2007; Botzung et al., 2008; Buckner et al., 2008; Szpunar et al., 2007). This ability to plan and make decisions about the future has been captured by computational models. Recent proposals suggest that the hippocampus may work in concert with a planning-oriented system in the prefrontal cortex or even as its own decision system (Daw et al., 2005; Lengyel and

Dayan, 2005; Zilli and Hasselmo, 2008). A major challenge for future research is to provide a unified account of how the hippocampus supports decisions in all of these situations.

The current review emphasizes the importance of different memory systems in decision making. In particular, we focused on how a relational memory system based in the hippocampus and surrounding medial temporal cortices may be essential for flexibly deploying knowledge in future decisions. Experimental results from our value-transfer paradigm suggest that relational learning can also influence economic decisions, such as gambling. Although many different types of information can be used to guide novel decisions, this generalization mechanism may be an important influence. Experience often involves learning new relations or recognizing old relational associations, while rewarding events may be fewer and farther in between. By learning relational representations that can serve as a basis for generalizing related value experiences, the brain may be able to take advantage of relational learning to flexibly apply knowledge in novel decisions.

In conclusion, studies of reward learning and decision making have shed light on the important role of the striatum and dopamine in these processes, but many open questions and unexplored areas remain. In everyday experience, we often flexibly use episodic experience to guide our decisions, especially in novel situations, which suggests a prominent role for the hippocampus in decision making. Intriguingly, the hippocampus interacts strongly with the dopamine system to facilitate encoding novel and reward-related stimuli. In some decision situations, this interaction may underlie successful generalization of learning to novel situations. However, the role of a relational hippocampus-based memory system in decision making has so far received little attention. A full understanding of how the brain learns from experience and makes future decisions is a pressing issue in psychology and neuroscience, as understanding these capacities can help us understand everyday actions, and, most importantly, make progress in treating dysfunctions of behavior caused by addiction, disease, and psychiatric disorders. Here, we hope to illuminate one direction for expanding our understanding of flexible decision making, by exploring how learning and memory systems beyond the striatum, such as the hippocampus, can guide our choices.

Acknowledgments

We would like to thank Nathan Clement, Nathaniel Daw, and Karin Foerde for helpful comments on the manuscript and Michael Frank for helpful discussion of the ideas presented here.

References

Adcock, R.A., Thangavel, A., Whitfield-Gabrieli, S., Knutson, B., Gabrieli, J.D. (2006). Reward-motivated learning: mesolimbic activation precedes memory formation. *Neuron*, 50, 507–17.

Addis, D.R., Wong, A.T., and Schacter, D.L. (2007). Remembering the past and imagining the future: Common and distinct neural substrates during event construction and elaboration. *Neuropsychologia*, 45, 1363–77.

Aron, A.R., Shohamy, D., Clark, J., Myers, C., Gluck, M.A., and Poldrack, R.A. (2004). Human midbrain sensitivity to cognitive feedback and uncertainty during classification learning. *J Neurophysiol*, 92, 1144–52.

Barr, R., Marrott, H., and Rovee-Collier, C. (2003). The role of sensory preconditioning in memory retrieval by preverbal infants. *Learn Behav*, **31**, 111–23.

Bayer, H.M. and Glimcher, P.W. (2005). Midbrain dopamine neurons encode a quantitative reward prediction error signal. *Neuron*, **47**, 129–41.

Beiser, D.G. and Houk, J.C. (1998). Model of cortical-basal ganglionic processing: encoding the serial order of sensory events. *J Neurophysiol*, **79**, 3168–88.

Botzung, A. Denkova, E., and Manning, L. (2008). Experiencing past and future personal events: functional neuroimaging evidence on the neural bases of mental time travel. *Brain Cogn*, **66**, 202–12.

Brewer, J.B., Zhao, Z., Desmond, J.E., Glover, G.H., and Gabrieli, J.D. (1998). Making memories: brain activity that predicts how well visual experience will be remembered. *Science*, **281**, 1185–87.

Brogden, W.J. (1939). Sensory pre-conditioning. *J Exp Psychol*, **25**, 323–32.

Brogden, W.J. (1947). Sensory pre-conditioning of human subjects. *J Exp Psychol*, **37**, 527–39.

Buckmaster, C.A., Eichenbaum, H., Amaral, D.G., Suzuki, W.A., and Rapp, P.R. (2004). Entorhinal cortex lesions disrupt the relational organization of memory in monkeys. *J Neurosci*, **24**, 9811–25.

Buckner, R.L., Andrews-Hanna, J.R., and Schacter, D.L. (2008). The brain's default network: anatomy, function, and relevance to disease. *Ann NY Acad Sci*, **1124**, 1–38.

Bunsey, M. and Eichenbaum, H. (1996). Conservation of hippocampal memory function in rats and humans. *Nature*, **379**, 255–57.

Bunzeck, N. and Duzel, E. (2006). Absolute coding of stimulus novelty in the human substantia nigra/VTA. *Neuron* **51**, 369–79.

Clement, N., Foerde, K., and Shohamy, D. (2008). Quantity vs. Quality: Practice affects medial temporal lobe and basal ganglia contributions to learning and generalization In Society for Neuroscience (Washington, DC).

Cohen, N.J. (1984). *Preserved learning capacity in amnesia: evidence for multiple memory systems.* (New York: Guilford).

Cohen, N.J. and Eichenbaum, H. (1993). *Memory, amnesia, and the hippocampal system.* (Cambridge, MA: MIT Press).

Cohen, N.J. and Squire, L.R. (1980). Preserved learning and retention of pattern-analyzing skill in amnesia: dissociation of knowing how and knowing that. *Science* **210**, 207–10.

Cohen, N.J. and Squire, L.R. (1981). Retrograde amnesia and remote memory impairment. *Neuropsychologia*, **19**, 337–56.

Cohen, M.X., Schoene-Bake, J.C., Elger, C.E., and Weber, B. (2009). Connectivity-based segregation of the human striatum predicts personality characteristics. *Nat Neurosci*,**12**, 32–4.

Cools, R., Clark, L., Owen, A.M., and Robbins, T.W. (2002). Defining the neural mechanisms of probabilistic reversal learning using event-related functional magnetic resonance imaging. *J Neurosci*, **22**, 4563–67.

Cools, R., Altamirano, L., and D'Esposito, M. (2006). Reversal learning in Parkinson's disease depends on medication status and outcome valence. *Neuropsychologia*, **44**, 1663–73.

Couvillon, P.A. and Bitterman, M.E. (1992). A conventional conditioning analysis of "transitive inference" in pigeons. *J Exp Psychol Anim Behav Process*, **18**, 308–310.

D'Ardenne, K., McClure, S.M., Nystrom, L.E., and Cohen, J.D. (2008). BOLD responses reflecting dopaminergic signals in the human ventral tegmental area. *Science*, **319**, 1264–67.

Davachi, L. (2006). Item, context and relational episodic encoding in humans. *Curr Opin Neurobiol*, **16**, 693–700.

Daw, N.D. and Doya, K. (2006). The computational neurobiology of learning and reward. *Curr Opin Neurobiol*, **16**, 199–204.

Daw, N.D., Niv, Y., and Dayan, P. (2005). Uncertainty-based competition between prefrontal and dorsolateral striatal systems for behavioral control. *Nat Neurosci*, **8**, 1704–1711.

Daw, N.D. and Shohamy, D. (2008). The cognitive neuroscience of motivation and learning. *Soc Cogn,* **26,** 593–620.

Dayan, P. and Abbott, L.F. (2001). *Theoretical neuroscience* (Cambridge, MA: MIT Press).

Delgado, M.R., Nystrom, L.E., Fissell, C., Noll, D.C., and Fiez, J.A. (2000). Tracking the hemodynamic responses to reward and punishment in the striatum. *J Neurophysiol,* **84,** 3072–77.

Delgado, M.R., Frank, R.H., and Phelps, E.A. (2005a). Perceptions of moral character modulate the neural systems of reward during the trust game. *Nat Neurosci,* **8,** 1611–18.

Delgado, M.R., Miller, M.M., Inati, S., and Phelps, E.A. (2005b). An fMRI study of reward-related probability learning. *Neuroimage,* **24,** 862–73.

Downes, J.J., Roberts, A.C., Sahakian, B.J., Evenden, J.L., Morris, R.G., and Robbins, T.W. (1989). Impaired extra-dimensional shift performance in medicated and unmedicated Parkinson's disease: evidence for a specific attentional dysfunction. *Neuropsychologia,* **27,** 1329–43.

Dusek, J.A. and Eichenbaum, H. (1997). The hippocampus and memory for orderly stimulus relations. *Proc Natl Acad Sci USA,* **94,** 7109–14.

Dwyer, D.M. and Killcross, S. (2006). Lesions of the basolateral amygdala disrupt conditioning based on the retrieved representations of motivationally significant events. *J Neurosci,* **26,** 8305–309.

Eichenbaum, H. (2000). A cortical-hippocampal system for declarative memory. *Nat Rev Neurosci,* **1,** 41–50.

Eichenbaum, H. and Cohen, N.J. (2001). *From conditioning to conscious recollection: memory systems of the brain* (New York: Oxford University Press).

Eichenbaum, H., Stewart, C., and Morris, R.G. (1990). Hippocampal representation in place learning. *J Neurosci,* **10,** 3531–42.

Eichenbaum, H., Yonelinas, A.P., and Ranganath, C. (2007). The medial temporal lobe and recognition memory. *Annu Rev Neurosci,* **30,** 123–52.

Frank, M.J., Rudy, J.W., and O'Reilly, R.C. (2003). Transitivity, flexibility, conjunctive representations, and the hippocampus. II. A computational analysis. *Hippocampus,* **13,** 341–54.

Frank, M.J., Seeberger, L.C., and O'Reilly R, C. (2004). By carrot or by stick: cognitive reinforcement learning in parkinsonism. *Science,* **306,** 1940–43.

Frey, U., Schroeder, H., and Matthies, H. (1990). Dopaminergic antagonists prevent long-term maintenance of posttetanic LTP in the CA1 region of rat hippocampal slices. *Brain Res,* **522,** 69–75.

Fuxe, K. (1965). Evidence for the existence of monoamine neurons in the central nervous System. Iv. Distribution of monoamine nerve terminals in the central nervous system. *Acta Physiol Scand Suppl,* SUPPL 247:37+.

Fyhn, M., Molden, S., Hollup, S., Moser, M.B., and Moser, E. (2002). Hippocampal neurons responding to first-time dislocation of a target object. *Neuron,* **35,** 555–66.

Gabrieli, J.D. (1998). Cognitive neuroscience of human memory. *Annu Rev Psychol,* **49,** 87–115.

Gasbarri, A., Packard, M.G., Campana, E., and Pacitti, C. (1994). Anterograde and retrograde tracing of projections from the ventral tegmental area to the hippocampal formation in the rat. *Brain Res Bull,* **33,** 445–52.

Gasbarri, A., Sulli, A., Innocenzi, R., Pacitti, C., and Brioni, J.D. (1996). Spatial memory impairment induced by lesion of the mesohippocampal dopaminergic system in the rat. *Neuroscience,* **74,** 1037–44.

Gewirtz, J.C. and Davis, M. (1997). Second-order fear conditioning prevented by blocking NMDA receptors in amygdala. *Nature,* **388,** 471–74.

Gewirtz, J.C. and Davis, M. (2000). Using pavlovian higher-order conditioning paradigms to investigate the neural substrates of emotional learning and memory. *Learn Mem,* **7,** 257–66.

Gilbert, D.T. and Wilson, T.D. (2007). Prospection: experiencing the future. *Science,* **317,** 1351–54.

Gluck, M.A. and Myers, C.E. (1993). Hippocampal mediation of stimulus representation: a computational theory. *Hippocampus,* **3,** 491–516.

Granado, N., Ortiz, O., Suarez, L.M., Martin, E.D., Cena, V., Solis, J.M., and Moratalla, R. (2008). D1 but not D5 dopamine receptors are critical for LTP, spatial learning, and LTP-Induced arc and zif268 expression in the hippocampus. *Cereb Cortex*, 18, 1–12.

Haber, S.N. and Knutson, B. (2010). The reward circuit: linking primate anatomy and human imaging. *Neuropsychopharmacology* 35, 4–26.

Haber, S.N., Kim, K.S., Mailly, P., and Calzavara, R. (2006). Reward-related cortical inputs define a large striatal region in primates that interface with associative cortical connections, providing a substrate for incentive-based learning. *J Neurosci*, 26, 8368–76.

Hall, D. and Suboski, M.D. (1995). Sensory preconditioning and secord-order conditioning of alarm reactions in zebra danio fish *(Brachydanio rerio)*. *J Comp Psych*, 109, 76–84.

Hall, G. (1996). Learning about associatively activated stimulus representations: Implications for acquired equivalence and perceptual learning. *Anim Learn Beh*, 24, 233–55.

Hampton, A.N. and O'Doherty J, P. (2007). Decoding the neural substrates of reward-related decision making with functional MRI. *Proc Natl Acad Sci USA*, 104, 1377–82.

Hare, T.A., O'Doherty, J., Camerer, C.F., Schultz, W., and Rangel, A. (2008). Dissociating the role of the orbitofrontal cortex and the striatum in the computation of goal values and prediction errors. *J Neurosci*, 28, 5623–30.

Hassabis, D., Kumaran, D., Vann, S.D., and Maguire, E.A. (2007). Patients with hippocampal amnesia cannot imagine new experiences. *Proc Natl Acad Sci USA*, 104, 1726–31.

Hatfield, T., Han, J.S., Conley, M., Gallagher, M., and Holland, P. (1996). Neurotoxic lesions of basolateral, but not central, amygdala interfere with Pavlovian second-order conditioning and reinforcer devaluation effects. *J Neurosci*, 16, 5256–65.

Heckers, S., Zalesak, M., Weiss, A.P., Ditman, T., and Titone, D. (2004). Hippocampal activation during transitive inference in humans. *Hippocampus*, 14, 153–62.

Hoffeld, D.R., Kendall, S.B., Thompson, R.F., and Brogden, W.J. (1960). Effect of amount of preconditioning training upon the magnitude of sensory preconditioning. *J Exp Psychol*, 59, 198–204.

Huang, Y.Y. and Kandel, E.R. (1995). D1/D5 receptor agonists induce a protein synthesis-dependent late potentiation in the CA1 region of the hippocampus. *Proc Natl Acad Sci USA*, 92, 2446–50.

Karn, H.W. (1947). Sensory pre-conditioning and incidental learning in human subjects. *J Exp Psychol*, 37, 540–44.

Kesner, R.P., Bolland, B.L., and Dakis, M. (1993). Memory for spatial locations, motor responses, and objects: triple dissociation among the hippocampus, caudate nucleus, and extrastriate visual cortex. *Exp Brain Res*, 93, 462–70.

Kimmel, H.D. (1977). Notes from "Pavlov's Wednesdays": sensory preconditioning. *Am J Psychol*, 90, 319–21.

King-Casas, B., Tomlin, D., Anen, C., Camerer, C.F., Quartz, S.R., and Montague, P.R. (2005). Getting to know you: reputation and trust in a two-person economic exchange. *Science*, 308, 78–83.

Kirchhoff, B.A., Wagner, A.D., Maril, A., and Stern, C.E. (2000). Prefrontal-temporal circuitry for episodic encoding and subsequent memory. *J Neurosci*, 20, 6173–80.

Kirsch, P., Schienle, A., Stark, R., Sammer, G., Blecker, C., Walter, B., Ott, U., Burkart, J., and Vaitl, D. (2003). Anticipation of reward in a nonaversive differential conditioning paradigm and the brain reward system: an event-related fMRI study. *Neuroimage*, 20, 1086–95.

Knowlton, B.J., Mangels, J.A., and Squire, L.R. (1996). A neostriatal habit learning system in humans. *Science*, 273, 1399–1402.

Knutson, B. and Gibbs, S.E. (2007). Linking nucleus accumbens dopamine and blood oxygenation. *Psychopharmacology (Berl)*, 191, 813–22.

Knutson, B., Adams, C.M., Fong, G.W., and Hommer, D. (2001). Anticipation of increasing monetary reward selectively recruits nucleus accumbens. *J Neurosci*, 21, RC159.

Knutson, B., Rick, S., Wimmer, G.E., Prelec, D., and Loewenstein, G. (2007). Neural predictors of purchases. *Neuron,* 53, 147–56.

Kojima, S., Kobayashi, S., Yamanaka, M., Sadamoto, H., Nakamura, H., Fujito, Y., Kawai, R., Sakakibara, M., and Ito, E. (1998). Sensory preconditioning for feeding response in the pond snail, Lymnaea stagnalis. *Brain Res,* 808, 113–115.

Krebs, R.M., Schott, B.H., and Duzel, E. (2009). Personality traits are differentially associated with patterns of reward and novelty processing in the human substantia nigra/ventral tegmental area. *Biol Psychiatry,* 65, 103–110.

Kumaran, D. and Maguire, E.A. (2006). An unexpected sequence of events: mismatch detection in the human hippocampus. *PLoS Biol,* 4, e424.

Kumaran, D. and Maguire, E.A. (2007). Match mismatch processes underlie human hippocampal responses to associative novelty. *J Neurosci,* 27, 8517–24.

Kumaran, D. and Maguire, E.A. (2009). Novelty signals: a window into hippocampal information processing. *Trends Cogn Sci,* 13, 47–54.

Lansink, C.S., Goltstein, P.M., Lankelma, J.V., McNaughton, B.L., and Pennartz, C.M. (2009). Hippocampus leads ventral striatum in replay of place-reward information. *PLoS Biol,* 7, e1000173.

Lee, A.S., Duman, R.S., and Pittenger, C. (2008). A double dissociation revealing bidirectional competition between striatum and hippocampus during learning. *Proc Natl Acad Sci USA,* 105, 17163–68.

Legault, M. and Wise, R.A. (1999). Injections of N-methyl-D-aspartate into the ventral hippocampus increase extracellular dopamine in the ventral tegmental area and nucleus accumbens. *Synapse,* 31, 241–49.

Lemon, N., and Manahan-Vaughan, D. (2006). Dopamine D1/D5 receptors gate the acquisition of novel information through hippocampal long-term potentiation and long-term depression. *J Neurosci,* 26, 7723–29.

Lengyel, M. and Dayan, P. (2005). Hippocampal contributions to control: the third way. In *Advances in neural information processing systems 20,* J. Platt, D. Koller, Y. Singer, and S. Roweis, eds. (Cambridge, MA: MIT Press).

Li, S., Cullen, W.K., Anwyl, R., and Rowan, M.J. (2003). Dopamine-dependent facilitation of LTP induction in hippocampal CA1 by exposure to spatial novelty. *Nat Neurosci,* 6, 526–31.

Lindvall, O. and Bjorklund, A. (1974). The organization of the ascending catecholamine neuron systems in the rat brain as revealed by the glyoxylic acid fluorescence method. *Acta Physiol Scand Suppl,* 412, 1–48.

Lisman, J.E. and Grace, A.A. (2005). The hippocampal-VTA loop: controlling the entry of information into long-term memory. *Neuron,* 46, 703–13.

Ljungberg, T., Apicella, P., and Schultz, W. (1992). Responses of monkey dopamine neurons during learning of behavioral reactions. *J Neurophysiol,* 67, 145–63.

Lodge, D.J. and Grace, A.A. (2006). The hippocampus modulates dopamine neuron responsivity by regulating the intensity of phasic neuron activation. *Neuropsychopharmacology,* 31, 1356–61.

Lodge, D.J. and Grace, A.A. (2008). Amphetamine activation of hippocampal drive of mesolimbic dopamine neurons: a mechanism of behavioral sensitization. *J Neurosci,* 28, 7876–82.

McClure, S.M., Berns, G.S., and Montague, P.R. (2003). Temporal prediction errors in a passive learning task activate human striatum. *Neuron,* 38, 339–46.

McClure, S.M., Li, J., Tomlin, D., Cypert, K.S., Montague, L.M., and Montague, P.R. (2004). Neural correlates of behavioral preference for culturally familiar drinks. *Neuron,* 44, 379–87.

McDonald, R.J. and White, N.M. (1993). A triple dissociation of memory systems: hippocampus, amygdala, and dorsal striatum. *Behav Neurosci,* 107, 3–22.

Montague, P.R., Dayan, P., and Sejnowski, T.J. (1996). A framework for mesencephalic dopamine systems based on predictive Hebbian learning. *J Neurosci,* 16, 1936–47.

Montague, P.R., King-Casas, B., and Cohen, J.D. (2006). Imaging valuation models in human choice. *Annu Rev Neurosci*, **29**, 417–48.

Moustafa, A.A., Cohen, M.X., Sherman, S.J., and Frank, M.J. (2008). A role for dopamine in temporal decision making and reward maximization in Parkinsonism. *J Neurosci*, **28**, 12294–304.

Muller, D., Gerber, B., Hellstern, F., Hammer, M., and Menzel, R. (2000). Sensory preconditioning in honeybees. *J Exp Biol*, **203**, 1351–64.

Myers, C.E., Shohamy, D., Gluck, M.A., Grossman, S., Kluger, A., Ferris, S., Golomb, J., Schnirman, G., and Schwartz, R. (2003). Dissociating hippocampal versus basal ganglia contributions to learning and transfer. *J Cogn Neurosci*, **15**, 185–93.

Nagy, H., Keri, S., Myers, C.E., Benedek, G., Shohamy, D., and Gluck, M.A. (2007). Cognitive sequence learning in Parkinson's disease and amnestic mild cognitive impairment: dissociation between sequential and non-sequential learning of associations. *Neuropsychologia*, **45**, 1386–92.

Nicholson, D.A. and Freeman, J.H., Jr (2000). Lesions of the perirhinal cortex impair sensory preconditioning in rats. *Behav Brain Res*, **112**, 69–75.

O'Doherty, J.P. (2004). Reward representations and reward-related learning in the human brain: insights from neuroimaging. *Curr Opin Neurobiol*, **14**, 769–76.

O'Doherty, J.P., Dayan, P., Friston, K., Critchley, H., and Dolan, R.J. (2003). Temporal difference models and reward-related learning in the human brain. *Neuron*, **38**, 329–37.

Otmakhova, N.A., and Lisman, J.E. (1996). D1/D5 dopamine receptor activation increases the magnitude of early long-term potentiation at CA1 hippocampal synapses. *J Neurosci*, **16**, 7478–86.

Otten, L.J., Henson, R.N., and Rugg, M.D. (2001). Depth of processing effects on neural correlates of memory encoding: relationship between findings from across- and within-task comparisons. *Brain*, **124**, 399–412.

Owen, A.M., Beksinska, M., James, M., Leigh, P.N., Summers, B.A., Marsden, C.D., Quinn, N.P., Sahakian, B.J., and Robbins, T.W. (1993). Visuospatial memory deficits at different stages of Parkinson's disease. *Neuropsychologia*, **31**, 627–44.

Packard, M.G. (1999). Glutamate infused posttraining into the hippocampus or caudate-putamen differentially strengthens place and response learning. *Proc Natl Acad Sci USA*, **96**, 12881–86.

Packard, M.G. and McGaugh, J.L. (1996). Inactivation of hippocampus or caudate nucleus with lidocaine differentially affects expression of place and response learning. *Neurobiol Learn Mem*, **65**, 65–72.

Packard, M.G., Hirsh, R., and White, N.M. (1989). Differential effects of fornix and caudate nucleus lesions on two radial maze tasks: evidence for multiple memory systems. *J Neurosci*, **9**, 1465–72.

Padoa-Schioppa, C. and Assad, J.A. (2006). Neurons in the orbitofrontal cortex encode economic value. *Nature*, **441**, 223–26.

Paller, K.A. and Wagner, A.D. (2002). Observing the transformation of experience into memory. *Trends Cogn Sci*, **6**, 93–102.

Palminteri, S., Lebreton, M., Worbe, Y., Grabli, D., Hartmann, A., and Pessiglione, M. (2009). Pharmacological modulation of subliminal learning in Parkinson's and Tourette's syndromes. *Proc Natl Acad Sci USA*.

Pessiglione, M., Seymour, B., Flandin, G., Dolan, R.J., and Frith, C.D. (2006). Dopamine-dependent prediction errors underpin reward-seeking behaviour in humans. *Nature*, **442**, 1042–45.

Plassmann, H., O'Doherty, J., and Rangel, A. (2007). Orbitofrontal cortex encodes willingness to pay in everyday economic transactions. *J Neurosci*, **27**, 9984–88.

Poldrack, R.A., Clark, J., Pare-Blagoev, E.J., Shohamy, D., Creso Moyano, J., Myers, C., and Gluck, M. (2001). Interactive memory systems in the human brain. *Nature*, **414**, 546–50.

Poldrack, R.A. and Packard, M.G. (2003). Competition among multiple memory systems: converging evidence from animal and human brain studies. *Neuropsychologia*, **41**, 245–51.

Port, R.L. and Patterson, M.M. (1984). Fimbrial lesions and sensory preconditioning. *Behav Neurosci,* **98**, 584–89.

Port, R.L., Beggs, A.L., and Patterson, M.M. (1987). Hippocampal substrate of sensory associations. *Physiol Behav,* **39**, 643–47.

Preston, A.R., Shrager, Y., Dudukovic, N.M., and Gabrieli, J.D. (2004). Hippocampal contribution to the novel use of relational information in declarative memory. *Hippocampus,* **14**, 148–52.

Rangel, A., Camerer, C., and Montague, P.R. (2008). A framework for studying the neurobiology of value-based decision making. *Nat Rev Neurosci* **9**, 545–56.

Rescorla, R.A. (1980). Simultaneous and successive associations in sensory preconditioning. *J Exp Psychol Anim Behav Process,* **6**, 207–16.

Robbins, T.W. (1996). Refining the taxonomy of memory. *Science,* **273**, 1353–54.

Robinson, S., Rainwater, A.J., Hnasko, T.S., and Palmiter, R.D. (2007). Viral restoration of dopamine signaling to the dorsal striatum restores instrumental conditioning to dopamine-deficient mice. *Psychopharmacology (Berl),* **191**, 567–78.

Rossato, J.I., Bevilaqua, L.R., Izquierdo, I., Medina, J.H., and Cammarota, M. (2009). Dopamine controls persistence of long-term memory storage. *Science,* **325**, 1017–20.

Saint-Cyr, J.A., Taylor, A.E., and Lang, A.E. (1988). Procedural learning and neostriatal dysfunction in man. *Brain,* 111 (Pt 4), 941–59.

Samejima, K., Ueda, Y., Doya, K., and Kimura, M. (2005). Representation of action-specific reward values in the striatum. *Science,* **310**, 1337–40.

Schacter, D.L. (1990). Perceptual representation systems and implicit memory. Toward a resolution of the multiple memory systems debate. *Ann NY Acad Sci,* **608**, 543–67; discussion 567-571.

Schacter, D.L. and Graf, P. (1986). Preserved learning in amnesic patients: perspectives from research on direct priming. *J Clin Exp Neuropsychol* **8**, 727–43.

Schacter, D.L. and Wagner, A.D. (1999). Medial temporal lobe activations in fMRI and PET studies of episodic encoding and retrieval. *Hippocampus* **9**, 7–24.

Schendan, H.E., Searl, M.M., Melrose, R.J., and Stern, C.E. (2003). An FMRI study of the role of the medial temporal lobe in implicit and explicit sequence learning. *Neuron,* **37**, 1013–25.

Schonberg, T., O'Doherty, J.P., Joel, D., Inzelberg, R., Segev, Y., and Daw, N.D. Selective impairment of prediction error signaling in human dorsolateral but not ventral striatum in Parkinson's disease patients: evidence from a model-based fMRI study. *Neuroimage,* **49**, 772–81.

Schott, B.H., Sellner, D.B., Lauer, C.J., Habib, R., Frey, J.U., Guderian, S., Heinze, H.J., and Duzel, E. (2004). Activation of midbrain structures by associative novelty and the formation of explicit memory in humans. *Learn Mem,* **11**, 383–87.

Schott, B.H., Seidenbecher, C.I., Fenker, D.B., Lauer, C.J., Bunzeck, N., Bernstein, H.G., Tischmeyer, W., Gundelfinger, E.D., Heinze, H.J., and Duzel, E. (2006). The dopaminergic midbrain participates in human episodic memory formation: evidence from genetic imaging. *J Neurosci,* **26**, 1407–1417.

Schultz, W. (2006). Behavioral theories and the neurophysiology of reward. *Annu Rev Psychol,* **57**, 87–115.

Schultz, W., Dayan, P., and Montague, P.R. (1997). A neural substrate of prediction and reward. *Science,* **275**, 1593–99.

Setlow, B., Gallagher, M., and Holland, P.C. (2002a). The basolateral complex of the amygdala is necessary for acquisition but not expression of CS motivational value in appetitive Pavlovian second-order conditioning. *Eur J Neurosci,* **15**, 1841–53.

Setlow, B., Holland, P.C., and Gallagher, M. (2002b). Disconnection of the basolateral amygdala complex and nucleus accumbens impairs appetitive pavlovian second-order conditioned responses. *Behav Neurosci,* **116**, 267–75.

Shohamy, D. and Wagner, A.D. (2008). Integrating memories in the human brain: hippocampal-midbrain encoding of overlapping events. *Neuron, 60*, 378–89.

Shohamy, D., Myers, C.E., Grossman, S., Sage, J., Gluck, M.A., and Poldrack, R.A. (2004a). Corticostriatal contributions to feedback-based learning: converging data from neuroimaging and neuropsychology. *Brain, 127*, 851–59.

Shohamy, D., Myers, C.E., Onlaor, S., and Gluck, M.A. (2004b). Role of the basal ganglia in category learning: how do patients with Parkinson's disease learn? *Behav Neurosci, 118*, 676–86.

Shohamy, D., Myers, C.E., Grossman, S., Sage, J., and Gluck, M.A. (2005). The role of dopamine in cognitive sequence learning: evidence from Parkinson's disease. *Behav Brain Res, 156*, 191–99.

Shohamy, D., Myers, C.E., Geghman, K.D., Sage, J., and Gluck, M.A. (2006). L-dopa impairs learning, but spares generalization, in Parkinson's disease. *Neuropsychologia, 44*, 774–84.

Smith-Roe, S.L. and Kelley, A.E. (2000). Coincident activation of NMDA and dopamine D1 receptors within the nucleus accumbens core is required for appetitive instrumental learning. *J Neurosci, 20*, 7737–42.

Squire, L.R. (1987). The organization and neural substrates of human memory. *Int J Neurol, 21-22*, 218–22.

Squire, L.R. (1992). Memory and the hippocampus: a synthesis from findings with rats, monkeys, and humans. *Psychol Rev, 99*, 195–231.

Staresina, B.P. and Davachi, L. (2009). Mind the gap: binding experiences across space and time in the human hippocampus. *Neuron, 63*, 267–76.

Suri, R.E. and Schultz, W. (1998). Learning of sequential movements by neural network model with dopamine-like reinforcement signal. *Exp Brain Res, 121*, 350–54.

Sutton, R.S. and Barto, A.G. (1998). *Reinforcement learning: an introduction* (Cambridge, MA: MIT Press).

Swainson, R., Rogers, R.D., Sahakian, B.J., Summers, B.A., Polkey, C.E., and Robbins, T.W. (2000). Probabilistic learning and reversal deficits in patients with Parkinson's disease or frontal or temporal lobe lesions: possible adverse effects of dopaminergic medication. *Neuropsychologia, 38*, 596–612.

Swanson, L.W. (1982). The projections of the ventral tegmental area and adjacent regions: a combined fluorescent retrograde tracer and immunofluorescence study in the rat. *Brain Res Bull, 9*, 321–53.

Szpunar, K.K., Watson, J.M., and McDermott, K.B. (2007). Neural substrates of envisioning the future. *Proc Natl Acad Sci USA, 104*, 642–47.

Talk, A.C., Gandhi, C.C., and Matzel, L.D. (2002). Hippocampal function during behaviorally silent associative learning: dissociation of memory storage and expression. *Hippocampus, 12*, 648–56.

Tran, A.H., Uwano, T., Kimura, T., Hori, E., Katsuki, M., Nishijo, H., and Ono, T. (2008). Dopamine D1 receptor modulates hippocampal representation plasticity to spatial novelty. *J Neurosci, 28*, 13390–400.

Tsai, H.C., Zhang, F., Adamantidis, A., Stuber, G.D., Bonci, A., de Lecea, L., and Deisseroth, K. (2009). Phasic firing in dopaminergic neurons is sufficient for behavioral conditioning. *Science, 324*, 1080–84.

Tulving, E., Schacter, D.L., McLachlan, D.R., and Moscovitch, M. (1988). Priming of semantic autobiographical knowledge: a case study of retrograde amnesia. *Brain Cogn, 8*, 3–20.

van der Meer, M.A. and Redish, A.D. (2009). Covert Expectation-of-Reward in Rat Ventral Striatum at Decision Points. *Front Integr Neurosci, 3*, 1.

von Fersen, L., Wynne, C.D.L., Delius, J.D., and Staddon, J.E.R. (1991). Transitive inference in pigeons. *J Exp Psychol Anim Behav Process, 17*, 334–41.

Wagner, A.D., Schacter, D.L., Rotte, M., Koutstaal, W., Maril, A., Dale, A.M., Rosen, B.R., and Buckner, R.L. (1998). Building memories: remembering and forgetting of verbal experiences as predicted by brain activity. *Science, 281*, 1188–91.

Walther, E. (2002). Guilty by mere association: evaluative conditioning and the spreading attitude effect. *J Pers Soc Psychol*, **82**, 919–34.

Ward-Robinson, J., Coutureau, E., Good, M., Honey, R.C., Killcross, A.S., and Oswald, C.J. (2001). Excitotoxic lesions of the hippocampus leave sensory preconditioning intact: implications for models of hippocampal function. *Behav Neurosci*, **115**, 1357–62.

Ward-Robinson, J. and Hall, G. (1996). Backward sensory preconditioning. *J Exp Psychol Anim Behav Processes*, **22**, 395–404.

Weber, E.U., Johnson, E.J., Milch, K.F., Chang, H., Brodscholl, J.C., and Goldstein, D.G. (2007). Asymmetric discounting in intertemporal choice: a query-theory account. *Psych Science*, **18**, 516–23.

White, N.M. (1997). Mnemonic functions of the basal ganglia. *Curr Opin Neurobiol*, **7**, 164–69.

Wittmann, B.C., Bunzeck, N., Dolan, R.J., and Duzel, E. (2007). Anticipation of novelty recruits reward system and hippocampus while promoting recollection. *Neuroimage*, **38**, 194–202.

Wittmann, B.C., Schott, B.H., Guderian, S., Frey, J.U., Heinze, H.J., and Duzel, E. (2005). Reward-related FMRI activation of dopaminergic midbrain is associated with enhanced hippocampus-dependent long-term memory formation. *Neuron*, **45**, 459–67.

Wynne, C.D.L., Ferser, L., and Von Staddon, J.E.R. (1992). Pigeons' inferences are transitive and the outcome of elementary conditioning principles: a response. *J Exp Psychol Anim Behav Proc*, **18**, 313–15.

Zaghloul, K.A., Blanco, J.A., Weidemann, C.T., McGill, K., Jaggi, J.L., Baltuch, G.H., and Kahana, M.J. (2009). Human substantia nigra neurons encode unexpected financial rewards. *Science*, **323**, 1496–99.

Zilli, E.A., and Hasselmo, M.E. (2008). Modeling the role of working memory and episodic memory in behavioral tasks. *Hippocampus*, **18**, 193–209.

Chapter 14

The neural basis of positive and negative emotion regulation: implications for decision making

Laura N. Martin and Mauricio R. Delgado

Abstract

Emotions can influence our behaviors in many beneficial ways important for human survival. At times, however, emotions can also promote maladaptive responses, such as drug-seeking behaviors, carried out after intense feelings of cravings. One way to cope with irregularities in emotional responding is the use of cognitive strategies that attempt to modulate emotions that are anticipated or experienced. Research has demonstrated that the successful application of cognitive emotion regulation strategies can effectively enhance and attenuate emotion, irrespective of its valence (i.e., negative or positive). Such cognitive regulation techniques are thought to be dependent on cortical modulation of subcortical regions typically linked with affective learning and emotional-related responses, such as the amygdala and the striatum. In this chapter, we review recent advances in neuroimaging research, probing the efficacious application of emotion regulation strategies on both negative and positive emotions. Further, we consider potential extensions of this research that focus on the influence of emotion regulation on decision making, probing a mechanism for changing maladaptive behaviors.

14.1 Introduction

Emotions color and enrich our lives, signal when something is important, enhance memory, and prime us to engage in approach or avoidance behaviors (Panksepp, 1998). From an evolutionary perspective, emotions are defined as adaptive behavioral and physiological response tendencies initiated by salient situations or stimuli (James, 1894). Negative emotions, such as fear and anxiety, can be important indicators of the need for attention and vigilance. For example, imagine driving at high speeds on an unfamiliar highway when sudden feelings of anxiety, accompanied by autonomic changes, are experienced. This emotion is deemed protective, signaling potential caution in behavior. Yet, emotions can also influence decision making in maladaptive ways. A surge of anxious symptoms while driving, for instance, could lead to an overwhelming stressful response with dangerous consequences on the road. Thus, at times, the need to exert cognitive control over our emotions is necessary to facilitate goal-directed behavior.

Humans are afforded the unique ability to try to cognitively control the way they feel via methods commonly known as emotion regulation strategies. Effective use of regulation strategies allows individuals to alter the emotions they experience and express (Gross, 1998b). In addition to these short-term effects of emotion regulation, habitual use of regulation affects personal well-being and interpersonal relationships (Gross and John, 2003). Finally, dysfunctional emotion regulation capability is a hallmark of psychiatric disorders, such as panic disorder and depression (Johnstone et al., 2007).

Given their prominence and potential clinical significance, negative emotions have historically been the target of emotion regulation research. The goal of this research has been to understand the behavioral and neural mechanisms through which cognitive strategies effectively decrease the intensity of anticipated or experienced negative affect. In contrast, less research exists focusing on the neural structures responsible for efficient control of more positive emotions, such as desires, cravings, and excitement, which can influence decision making in maladaptive ways (e.g., drug-seeking behavior due to intense cravings). In this chapter, we consider the growing body of research aimed at investigating the cognitive neuroscience of emotion regulation, while emphasizing recent findings pertaining to the regulation of positive emotions and its association to decision making.

14.2 Working definitions of emotion and emotion regulation

This chapter adopts James' view of emotions as adaptive response tendencies (1894). Conceptualizing emotions as malleable tendencies is the foundation of theories of emotion regulation; if emotions were not susceptible to change, strategies for regulation of emotion could not exist. The whole course of emotion generation can be described with a process model (Gross, 1998a). In this model emotion consists of three major components: emotional cues, emotional response tendencies, and emotional responses. Even more specifically, the model can be divided into four time points: situations, aspects, meanings, and responses (Gross, 2002). Emotion regulation strategies can be engaged at five different points in this model, beginning just before the first time point in the model. Strategies initiated at different times have goals and methods that vary appropriately with the stage of the emotion-generation process.

Based on the time course of emotion, two major types of cognitive regulation have been postulated: antecedent- and response-focused strategies (Gross, 2002; see Fig. 14.1). Antecedent-focused strategies act early in the emotion-generation process to change the nature of the experienced and expressed emotion (Gross, 2002). Alternatively, response-focused strategies take effect after onset of emotion and aim to alter only the expression of emotion (Gross, 2002). The main response-focused technique is suppression, in which individuals inhibit the outward expression of emotion (e.g., facial expressions) in response to a situation or stimulus. The use of suppression techniques, however, have been reported to negatively affect cognitive performance (e.g., memory accuracy;

Richards and Gross, 2000) while increasing autonomic responses (Gross, 1998a). Moreover, habitual use of suppression has been associated with adverse effects on well-being (increased negative emotion and decreased positive emotion experienced) and interpersonal relationships (Gross and John, 2003) bringing this technique to question as an effective long-term mechanism of control.

Antecedent-focused techniques are typically more efficient and flexible than response-focused techniques. The most dynamic antecedent-focused strategies are cognitive change techniques, which involve directing and monitoring conscious thoughts in order to alter emotional experiences (Gross, 1998a). One type of cognitive change strategy is reappraisal, in which individuals reevaluate the meaning of a situation or stimulus, thereby altering their emotional response. For example, if the affective stimulus is a photograph of a man who appears bruised and injured, one could reduce the negative emotions elicited by the image by thinking that the man is an actor in makeup and that he is not really hurt at all. This example describes a situation-focused reappraisal method; to decrease emotion in a situation-focused way, the initial evaluation of the stimulus must be altered such that it can be perceived as not as bad as it seemed at first (Ochsner et al., 2004). Reappraisal can also be achieved through more self-focused cognitions, for instance distancing oneself from the stimulus by taking the perspective of a detached observer (Ochsner et al., 2004). Perhaps because of the thoughtful, cognitive nature of reappraisal it is particularly effective with complex emotional stimuli, such as films (see Gross, 1998b for a review). The efficacy of reappraisal in altering emotion experience and expression, without the cognitive impairments associated with suppression, has generated much interest, making reappraisal and other antecedent cognitive strategies the focus of many recent neuroimaging studies of emotion regulation. For these reasons, this chapter will primarily focus on antecedent cognitive regulation strategies, such as reappraisal.

Roughly 10 years ago, emotion regulation was described as an "emerging field" encompassing methods of anxiety regulation in psychoanalysis and insights from the stress and coping literature (Gross, 1998b). Initial efforts to understand how to control our emotions focused on negative affective experiences and modern emotion regulation techniques have been heavily influenced by this work, as well as a myriad of sub-disciplines of psychology (for an historical review of emotion regulation, see Gross, 1998b). As this topic of study continues to develop, new strategies, techniques, and

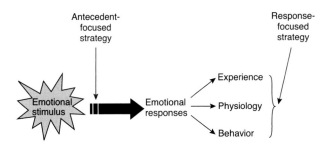

Fig. 14.1 Schematic of the time course of the emotion-generation process indicating the onsets of the two major types of emotion regulation strategies: antecedent-focused and response-focused strategies.

methodologies have surfaced, allowing for further explorations of the efficacy of emotion regulation.

14.3 Methodological considerations

Emotion regulation studies utilize various methodologies and an assortment of stimuli, which reliably evoke emotional responses. The type of emotion studied varies from the very specific, basic emotions identified by Ekman (happiness, sadness, surprise, anger, disgust, and fear; Ekman and Friesen, 1971) to more complex types of emotion (e.g., anxious feelings, desires). Many investigations have bypassed discrete emotion distinctions and instead employed more general labels, such as negative and positive (e.g., Kim and Hamann, 2007; Ochsner et al., 2002; Phan et al., 2005; Schaefer et al., 2002; Urry et al., 2006). Despite variability in the type of emotion studied, research using cognitive regulatory strategies has primarily focused on negative emotions, typically evoked by visual stimuli.

The most common stimuli used in emotion regulation studies are pictures, particularly the validated set presented by the International Affective Picture System (IAPS; Lang et al., 1993). Affective pictures are practical stimuli for use in studies of regulation through reappraisal, because they reliably evoke emotional responses and automatically prompt the viewer to generate a descriptive narrative, which can be altered with reappraisal. While pictures are easy to employ in emotion regulation studies, they do not have as much ecological validity as other types of stimuli, such as movie clips (e.g. Beauregard et al., 2001). Recently, researchers have expanded the range of affective stimuli used in regulation studies by employing conditioning procedures to attach value to previously neutral stimuli and testing the efficacy of emotion regulation at altering emotional response to these conditioned cues (Delgado et al., 2008a, 2008b). Regardless of the type of affective stimulus used, researchers have demonstrated that using emotion regulation techniques results in modulation of emotional responses, suggesting that successful regulation is not specific to one type of stimulus.

The efficacy of cognitive regulation techniques is typically characterized by the observed changes in emotional experience and responses. Most studies of emotion regulation rely on self-report ratings of emotion (i.e., emotion intensity) to detect changes in experienced emotion. Self-report is an important tool for understanding an individual's emotional response, as emotional content is inherently subjective (Barrett et al., 2007). However, social desirability may affect self-report data by leading responses to conform to the expected results, making self-reports potentially unreliable (Crowne and Marlowe, 1960). The time of self-report administration may also affect its validity, as research has shown that current emotions are perceived as more intense than previous emotions (Van Boven et al., 2009).

Other measures of affective responses have been used to supplement self-reports. For instance, expressive behavior captured by video-taping participants during the experiment and then coding their facial behavior has been used to assess fluctuations in emotion (Giuliani et al., 2008; Goldin et al., 2008). Further, autonomic measures, such as skin conductance responses (SCRs), can assess arousal levels and provide a measure of one component of the emotional response. Such measures depend on sympathetic nervous system activity increases in response to motivationally significant stimuli (e.g., affective stimuli), which, in the case of SCRs, results in greater levels of sweat excretion and increased conductivity of the skin (Critchley, 2002). However, interpretation of SCRs are limited by the observation that sympathetic arousal can be caused by not just emotional changes, but also fluctuations in cognition or attention (Critchley, 2002). Other physiological measures, such as heart rate (e.g., Kalisch et al., 2005), blood pressure (e.g., Giuliani et al., 2008), finger temperature (e.g., Giuliani et al., 2008), and startle response (e.g., Dillon and LaBar, 2005) have also been used as indexes of emotional changes. These physiological measures typically affirm self-reports of emotional shifts with regulation.

Brain-imaging techniques are a useful counterpart to the physiological and behavioral assessments described above, as neuroimaging can highlight the potential neural circuitry involved in emotion perception, experience, expression, and regulation. Functional magnetic resonance imaging (fMRI), for example, can be used to detect and contrast brain activity during the natural experience of emotion (for a review see Kober et al., 2008) and during the experience of emotion under regulation (for a review see Ochsner and Gross, 2008). The efficacy of emotion regulation techniques can be inferred from shifts in activity with regulation, although inferences must be made with caution, as the level of brain activity is not a direct index of the intensity of experienced emotion. The goal of neuroimaging studies of emotion regulation is to complement and extend behavioral and physiological measures of emotion to probe the underlying neural circuits that mediate how cognitive control processes exert their influence on emotional responses. Given the strengths and limitations of all of these possible techniques for measuring emotion, the convergence of multiple assessments provides an ideal experimental situation that allows for the examination of individual differences in emotional responses.

14.4 General neural processes underlying emotion regulation

How do emotion regulation processes manifest changes in the neural circuitry involved in emotion? The consensus in the literature on emotion regulation, specifically anteced-ent-focused strategies, is that prefrontal regions involved in cognitive control influence processing in emotion-related brain regions such as the amygdala (for reviews see Green and Malhi, 2006; Ochsner and Gross, 2008). Manipulating and reevaluating situations and stimuli involve prefrontal brain regions important in cognitive control, response selection, working memory, and keeping task demands online (Miller and Cohen, 2001). More specifically, cognitive reappraisal is thought to involve working memory and selective attention mediated by the dorsal prefrontal cortex (PFC), inhibition initiated by the ventral PFC (including ventral lateral PFC, vlPFC; Lieberman et al., 2007), regulation of control processes by the dorsal anterior cingulate cortex (ACC), and consideration of the emotional states of oneself or another mediated by the medial PFC (Ochsner and Gross, 2008). The dorsolateral region of PFC (dlPFC) is believed to play an important, but somewhat indirect, role in emotion regulation due to the fact that it does not have direct connections to brain regions such as the amygdala (Delgado et al., 2008b; Ochsner and Gross, 2008; Quirk and Beer, 2006). Indeed, the dlPFC has been shown to be involved in a broad spectrum of cognitive tasks (Miller and Cohen, 2001), supporting the notion of its role as a domain-general system. The function of the dlPFC during emotion regulation is likely to keep regulation goals online and maintain an active representation of task demands.

Successful emotion regulation does not result solely from recruitment of prefrontal regions; modulation of activity in regions involved in emotional learning, such as the amygdala, striatum, and insula, has been linked to regulation success (Ochsner and Gross, 2008). These regions have direct and indirect anatomical connections to various prefrontal sites and have been previously implicated in affective processing and motivation, with both negative and positive stimuli (Amaral and Price, 1984; Cardinal et al., 2002). Additionally, a recent functional connectivity analysis determined that prefrontal cortex activity during emotion regulation, covaried with amygdala activity, and reductions in negative emotion varied with the strength of functional connectivity between prefrontal regions (orbitofrontal cortex and dorsal medial PFC) and the amygdala (Banks et al., 2007). In a related study, a formal mediation analysis revealed that vlPFC disrupted or partially inhibited activity in the amygdala via the medial PFC (Lieberman et al., 2007), which is anatomically connected to both the vlPFC and amygdala (Ghashghaei and Barbas, 2002). These cortical–subcortical relationships will be described further in the following sections, in which we will discuss how neuroimaging studies have advanced our knowledge of the neural basis of emotion regulation by examining how cognitive strategies can attenuate or enhance emotional responses.

14.5 **Regulation of negative emotions**

One of the first investigations into the neural underpinnings of emotion regulation relied on the antecedent-focused strategy of reappraisal, where a negative stimulus that elicits an emotional response is reinterpreted in a less negative or more neutral context (Ochsner et al., 2002). In this experiment, participants were presented with negative emotional pictures and cued to either respond naturally or to actively engage in reappraisal to decrease the intensity of negative emotion they experienced. As assessed by online self-reports, subjective ratings of negative affect were decreased when regulation strategies were used. Further, reappraisal techniques, compared to a natural response condition, led to increased responses in cortical regions such as the dorsal and ventral lateral PFC and medial PFC, and decreased activity in the amygdala and medial orbitofrontal cortex (OFC). Although other studies at this time were reporting modulation of amygdala and prefrontal cortex by conscious cognitive effort (Schaefer et al., 2002), this was one of the first reports demonstrating that the explicit use of an emotion regulation strategy attenuates negative emotion and modulates activity in cortical and amygdala regions. Numerous studies investigating the neural correlates underlying successful reappraisal of negative emotions evoked by pictures followed. Across research reports, the common theme has been that successful application of emotion regulation strategies leads to increased activity in the PFC and decreased activity in regions mediating an emotional response, such as the amygdala (e.g., Harenski and Hamann, 2006; Kim and Hamann, 2007; Ochsner and Gross, 2008; Ochsner et al., 2004; Phan et al., 2005; Urry et al., 2006).

Antecedent regulation of negative emotions can also be achieved with strategies other than reappraisal (e.g., detaching oneself from the emotional context) and stimuli other than pictures (e.g., movies). For example, while viewing sad film clips, participants who successfully distanced themselves from the film decreased their self-reported subjective feelings of sadness (Levesque et al., 2003). Sadness ratings during blocks of active emotion detachment correlated with increases in BOLD signals in the right OFC and dlPFC. While there are discrepancies in the loci within the prefrontal cortex identified across these and other emotion regulation studies, these differences are likely due to variations in the type of emotion elicited (e.g., disgust), affective stimuli used (e.g., photos, films), or the type of regulation strategy employed (Ochsner and Gross, 2008).

Regulation techniques can also be applied with negative emotional responses, such as pain and fear, potentially providing a translational window to the treatment of anxiety disorders. Detachment strategies have been shown to successfully decrease physiological arousal (e.g., SCRs) elicited by the anticipation of pain (electric pulses), while engaging anterolateral PFC (Kalisch et al., 2005). Interestingly, attempts to distract oneself during the anticipation of pain did not successfully reduce subjective feelings of anxiety (Kalisch et al., 2006), suggesting some types of emotional responses may require specific regulation strategies to achieve reductions in emotion intensity.

Imagery-focused techniques have been used to regulate physiological and neural responses to conditioned fear (Delgado et al., 2008b). In traditional fear-conditioning studies, a previously neutral stimulus (e.g., a blue square) elicits a conditioned response (e.g., increased arousal as indexed by SCRs) due to repeated associations with an aversive outcome (e.g., an electric shock, the unconditioned stimulus). Across species, variations of this paradigm consistently anoint the amygdala as a key structure in the acquisition and expression of fears (for review see Delgado et al., 2006; Phelps and LeDoux, 2005). The use of imagery techniques that promote detachment (e.g., "think of something blue in nature that calms you down") decreased conditioned responses (SCRs) to a conditioned stimulus (CS, the blue square), when compared to a control condition where participants reacted naturally upon presentation of the CS (Delgado et al., 2008b). Successful emotion regulation led to increases in the BOLD response in the left dlPFC, while attenuation of the amygdala response to the presentation of the CS was observed. Notably, a connectivity analysis suggested that the influence of dlPFC on the amygdala response could be indirectly mediated by the ventromedial prefrontal cortex (vmPFC, Fig. 14.2), a region previously linked with the extinction of fears in both rodents (Milad and Quirk, 2002) and humans (Phelps et al., 2004; Fig. 14.2). Together, these findings, and those of Kalisch and colleagues, suggest that emotion regulation strategies may be useful in controlling one's response to painful stimuli or fear, perhaps by co-opting pre-existing mechanisms of fear extinction.

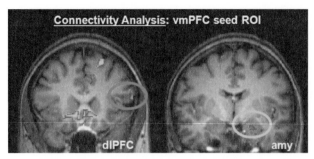

Fig. 14.2 Emotion regulation of conditioned fear. An area in the vmPFC identified during emotion regulation trials was used as the seed region for a connectivity analysis. The time course of activity in vmPFC throughout the entire experiment correlated with the time course in dlPFC (green circle) and amygdala (yellow circle) suggesting a potential circuitry through which conditioned fear can be diminished with cognitive strategies.
Reprinted from *Neuron*, 59(5), 829–38, M. R. Delgado, K. I. Nearing, J. E. LeDoux, and E. A. Phelps (2008) Neural circuitry underlying the regulation of conditioned fear and its relation to extinction. Copyright (2008) with permission from Elsevier.

Amidst the variety of stimuli and strategies, research in emotion regulation has started to focus on the time course in which these strategies can be effective and the neural networks that potentially mediate their success. A recent study investigated the time course of neural activity associated with the use of reappraisal during exposure to 15 s disgust film clips (Goldin et al., 2008). As participants began using reappraisal during early time periods (0–4.5 s), increases in PFC activity were observed (specifically, the medial, dorsolateral, ventrolateral and lateral OFC regions). At later time periods (10.5–15 s), BOLD responses in the amygdala and left insula were decreased, suggested by the authors to be a function of the earlier increase in PFC activity. Interestingly, the use of a response-focused strategy, suppression, led to increases in PFC only during later time periods and no corresponding decreases in amygdala and insula. This study and others serve as further support for the emotion regulation model proposed earlier, in which strategy use recruits PFC regions, which then modulates subcortical regions involved in affective processing. A recent test of this mediation hypothesis suggests that the relationship between PFC activity (i.e., right vlPFC) during reappraisal and reported decreases in emotion is mediated by activity in subcortical regions (Wager et al., 2008). Specifically, increased activity in the nucleus accumbens is associated with greater decreases in negative emotion, while increased activity in the amygdala is associated with increases in negative emotion.

To summarize this review of neuroimaging studies of the regulation of negative emotions it is informative to consider several studies that do not involve emotion regulation per se, but that provide information about how regulatory processes may be working. The basis of emotion regulation may be in the labels, words, or imagery one generates. A recent study examined the effect of supplying subjects with negative or neutral verbal descriptions prior to the presentation of negative pictures (Foti and Hajcak, 2008). After receiving neutral descriptions, participants showed decreased neural electrophysiological responses and lower ratings of unpleasantness and arousal, as compared to images preceded by negative descriptions. Another interpretation is that the negative descriptions increased neural responding and arousal; however, a similar study also suggested that the verbal processes of interpretation and labeling underlie changes in emotional responding (Hariri et al., 2000). When subjects matched pictures of angry or fearful faces the authors observed increased activity in the amygdala bilaterally. In contrast, when subjects assigned written labels to these emotional faces the authors found decreased activity in the amygdala, which correlated with increased activity in the right PFC. This finding was replicated and extended to suggest PFC-amygdala associations during labeling to be mediated by a region of medial PFC (Lieberman et al., 2007). Thus, the simple cognitive process of verbally labeling emotional stimuli can lead to reductions in the involvement of brain areas involved in emotion, coupled with recruitment of prefrontal regions. While these studies do not involve a specific regulation strategy, they demonstrate at a more basic level what may be the functional underpinnings of the successful regulation of negative emotion.

14.6 Regulation of positive emotions

Research over the last few years has successfully highlighted the potential neural correlates underlying successful regulation of negative emotions but only more recently have investigations begun to probe if similar strategies (e.g., reappraisal, Giuliani et al., 2008) and neural underpinnings also mediate the control of positive emotions. The arousing feelings associated with craving and excitement are some examples of positive emotions that can trigger approach behaviors that become detrimental to well-being if not controlled (e.g., higher than normal consumption of appetitive stimuli like food or drugs). Thus, an understanding of the neural and behavioral processes underlying successful emotion regulation of positive emotions not only bolsters our understanding of general cognitive control processes, it also has beneficial implications.

There is evidence suggesting overlap in the cortical loci implicated in the successful regulation of positive and negative emotions. Similar to previous studies of negative emotions (e.g., Levesque et al., 2003), increases in BOLD responses in PFC regions, such as dlPFC and ACC, have been reported to be associated with diminished feelings of positive arousal (elicited by films) when using regulation strategies (Beauregard et al., 2001). Additionally, a direct within-subjects comparison of use of reappraisal with positive and negative affective pictures revealed that both positive and negative regulation involve cortical regions, such as the right lateral PFC, dorsomedial PFC, medial PFC, and bilateral lateral OFC (Kim and Hamann, 2007). Notably, greater activation in PFC regions was observed when participants attempted to regulate negative emotions, suggesting that while regulation of positive and negative emotions may recruit similar cortical structures, the extent and level of cortical activity may differ between the emotion types, as will the specific subcortical targets of regulation.

The expectation of a potential reward can bring about positive emotions and promote approach behaviors, with the caveat that such behaviors can be risky and detrimental to one's well-being (Potenza and Winters, 2003). The striatum, a subcortical region involved

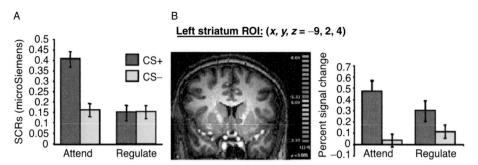

Fig. 14.3 Physiological and neural changes associated with emotion regulation of reward expectation. (A) SCRs from 15 participants shows an interaction between type of conditioned stimulus (CS+, CS–) and type of instruction cue (Attend, Regulate; ± SEM). (B) Activation of the striatum identified by the contrast of attend CS+ and CS– trials (reward expectation). Mean beta weights from both striatum ROIs (left striatum ROI graph depicted) showed an interaction between type of conditioned stimulus (CS+, CS–) and instruction (attend, regulate; ± SEM). Reprinted from *Neuron*, 59(5), 829–838, M.R. Delgado, K.I. Nearing, J.E. LeDoux, E.A. Phelps, Neural circuitry underlying the regulation of conditioned fear and its relation to extinction, Copyright (2008) with permission from Elsevier.

in reward-related processing and affective learning, is a potential target for cortical modulation via cognitive strategies, given its key role in reward prediction and expectations elicited by conditioned reinforcers (for review see Delgado, 2007; Knutson and Cooper, 2005; O'Doherty, 2004) and correlations with drug-specific cravings (Breiter et al., 1997; Sinha et al., 2005). Regulation of positive emotion associated with the expectation of reward has been recently investigated using a conditioning design that varied the type of conditioned stimulus (paired with a monetary reinforcer, CS+, or paired with no reinforcer, CS–) and type of instruction (attend to natural emotions or regulate via imagery techniques; Delgado et al., 2008a). Physiological responses, measured by SCRs, demonstrated the effectiveness of the regulation strategy as the heightened response to the CS+ observed during natural responding was diminished during regulation (Fig. 14.3A). A similar decrease was observed in BOLD signals in the striatum; that is, striatum signals were reduced when a regulation strategy was used with a stimulus that predicted a potential reward (Fig. 14.3B). In contrast, increases during emotion regulation trials were observed in dlPFC as participants used the imagery technique. The combination of increased prefrontal and decreased striatum activity may be the positive analog of increased PFC and decreased amygdala activity systematically observed in studies of negative regulation. As understanding the regulation of conditioned fear has important implications for anxiety disorders, understanding the regulation of conditioned reward may inform research on addiction.

14.7 **Emotion regulation and decision making**

While historically, research in psychology may have segregated emotion and cognition, it is now accepted that these domains largely overlap (e.g., Blair et al., 2007; Gray, 2004), and the emotions we experience can have considerable influence on our decisions (Bechara et al., 2000). Emotions induced via subliminal methods have been shown to influence valuation and decision making; for example, thirsty participants were willing to pay greater amounts, and wanted, poured, and drank more of a sugary beverage, after being unconsciously exposed to happy faces (Winkielman et al., 2005). The opposite pattern occurred after unconscious exposure to angry faces, demonstrating differential effects of positive and negative emotions. Of course, explicit emotions can also affect decision making, as evidenced by emotion inductions via video clips disrupting typically observed economic decision-making patterns, such as the endowment effect, where sellers assign higher prices to owned items (Lerner et al., 2004). Specifically, disgust inductions were associated with an absence of the endowment effect and sadness inductions with a reversal of it. Beyond emotion inductions, the existence of a negative emotional state, e.g., acute stress, can influence cognition at both the behavioral (e.g., Patil et al., 1995) and neural levels (e.g., Arnsten and Goldman-Rakic, 1998). Further, acute stress modulates financial decision making (Porcelli and Delgado, 2009) and may put those who cannot cope with stress at risk of poor decision making, as illustrated by addiction relapse (Sinha, 2007). It is plausible that employing cognitive emotion regulation strategies to control these emotions may foster better, more goal-directed decision making. Thus, the role of emotion regulation in decision-making contexts is likely to be among the most important topics in future emotion regulation research.

Some studies on self-control help provide insight into the potential mechanisms involved in cognitive control of decision making. Having depleted self-regulatory resources, for example, has been shown to lead to greater impulse buying behaviors (Vohs and Faber, 2007), suggesting that self-control mechanisms are important for making advantageous decisions. Moreover, the successful use of self-control by dieters when making choices about food consumption recruits cortical mechanisms (Hare et al., 2009). Activity in the vmPFC in this population reflected both taste and health information of displayed food items, while activity in this region in non-self-controllers reflected only taste information, suggesting different appraisal mechanisms for food items in self-controllers compared to non-self-controllers. Taken together, these studies provide evidence that greater self-control promotes decision making in line with long-term goals (e.g., saving money, weight loss).

A recent study directly tested the effect of emotion regulation on monetary decision making in which participants were faced with choices between a gamble and a guaranteed amount (Sokol-Hessner et al., 2009). For the emotion regulation strategy, participants were instructed to think about each decision as if they were a trader assembling a portfolio, thus diminishing the importance of each individual decision. As a control condition, participants thought of each decision in isolation. On average, the emotion regulation strategy significantly reduced a behavioral measure of loss aversion and the physiological response to losses as compared to gains (as assessed by SCRs). Further, the authors identified individual differences, such that only half of the 30 subjects showed significantly reduced loss aversion. These 15 "regulators" showed reduced skin conductance responses during regulation trials compared to control trials, while the "non-regulators" did not differ in their skin conductance responses across regulation and control trials.

Neuroimaging investigations of emotion regulation and decision making are in their infancy. One investigation asked participants to imagine a relaxing scene when faced with a stimulus that predicted a monetary decision between a risky (50% chance of $20) and a safe (100% chance of $5) option (Martin et al., 2007; Fig. 14.4A), extending previous use of this imagery regulation technique from conditioned stimuli to decision making (Delgado et al., 2008a). Using regulation decreased risky decision making (i.e., participants picked the safe option more often during regulation trials; Fig. 14.4B). While the results demonstrate a potential role for emotion regulation in altering decision making, the financial decision options were simple, repetitive, and not equated in terms of value, and this study did not probe shifts in neural activity during the time of decision. Given that prior studies of positive emotion regulation with the same imagery regulation strategy (Delgado et al., 2008a) and with a detachment-focused strategy (Staudinger et al., 2009) found that regulation decreased striatum activity during reward-processing, future work may focus on modulation of neural responses in the striatum during decision making and its impact on shifting behavior.

A more recent study examined regulation of craving in cigarette smokers (Kober et al., 2010). Smokers were presented with cigarette-related images and were cued either to regulate their feelings of craving by focusing on the long-term consequences of smoking or to focus on the immediate sensory experience of smoking (no regulation). Regulation was

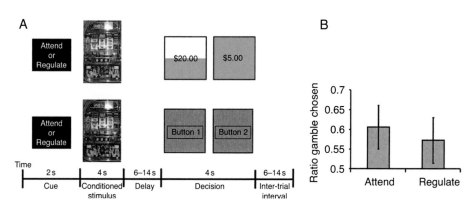

Fig. 14.4 Paradigm and behavioral results of potential influence of emotion regulation strategies on decision making. (A) Participants were presented with two conditioned stimuli: (CS), colorful slot-machine (top image, CS+); and grayscale slot-machine (bottom image, CS–), that represented an upcoming monetary reward opportunity and no reward, respectively. Prior to presentation of the CS, the cues "Attend" and "Regulate" instructed participants to respond naturally ("Attend") or use emotion regulation ("Regulate"). After the CS+ presentation, participants were faced with a financial decision between a risky option (gamble, 50% chance of winning $20) and a safe option (100% chance of winning $5). After the CS– presentation, participants made a choice between two different buttons of no monetary value. (B) Behavioral results from 17 participants showed a decrease in gambling behavior (i.e., picking the risky option) with emotion regulation (± SEM).

associated with increased activity in prefrontal regions and decreased activity in craving-related brain regions, such as ventral striatum and ACC (Kober et al., 2009). While early work with emotion regulation targeted negative emotions, these two studies are indicative of a shift in the focus of research on emotion regulation towards the regulation of positive emotions in the context of decision making, driven in large part due to their crucial role in the maladaptive approach behavior exhibited in addiction.

14.8 Future directions in emotion regulation research

The last decade of research on emotion regulation has characterized the efficacy of cognitive regulation strategies at changing emotion experience and the neural basis of these processes. The next step is to understand the full extent of the benefits of regulation, that is, how does regulation enable more beneficial behavior, and what brain systems support these changes? As discussed in the previous section, a potential merit of emotion regulation use is that it can promote shifts in decision making. However, emotional responses typically serve as important tools to guide behavior (Bechara and Damasio, 2005), thus it is essential that future emotion regulation research identify the contexts in which emotion regulation will be necessary and advantageous, and those in which it will do more harm than good. Very few neuroimaging studies of emotion regulation and decision making have been conducted thus far, highlighting the need for additional studies that test the effect of both positive (e.g., craving) and negative (e.g., anxious feelings) emotion regulation on behavior (e.g., making choices about food consumption). Additionally, future studies of emotion regulation and decision making may target more complex decisions, such as those involving inter-temporal choices, when one must choose between an immediate smaller reward and a delayed larger reward, which can be linked to impulsive behaviors (e.g., making food choices without regard for long term health) and addiction.

Another topic of substantial interest in the emotion regulation literature is the issue of individual differences. The experience of emotion is different from person to person; therefore, the efficacy of emotion regulation strategies will also differ across individuals. One important category for differences may be gender, as men and women differ in the experience and expression of emotion (Kring and Gordon, 1998). Many studies of emotion regulation have sidestepped the gender issue by including participants of one gender (usually women). A recent investigation of gender differences in the cognitive reappraisal of negative images did not observe any behavioral differences between men and women (ratings of emotional intensity), although neural differences were apparent (McRae et al., 2008). During reappraisal, men showed less PFC activity than women, but greater decreases in amygdala activity, while women showed greater ventral striatum activity than men; the authors suggested that these results may indicate that men are more efficient regulators or that women may generate positive emotion during reappraisal of negative emotion.

Categories other than gender are also useful for identifying differences. Neural differences in emotion processing have been identified and linked to personality traits, genotypes, and dispositional affect (Hamann and Canli, 2004). Research has begun specifically targeting individual differences in habitual use of two main regulation strategies, reappraisal and suppression (Gross and John, 2003). Frequent use of reappraisal leads to more positive and less negative emotional experiences compared to individuals who typically use suppression. Differences in regulation-related neural activity may be better understood by considering certain traits, for instance a tendency to focus on negative aspects of oneself (Ray et al., 2005). To date, a few studies have begun to tackle the issue of individual differences in emotion regulation, but consideration and characterization of these factors are an important aim of future research on emotion regulation as unpacking these differences may reveal a clearer picture of the effects of regulation and its potential clinical applications (e.g., using regulation strategies to increase chronically reduced dlPFC activity observed in unipolar depression; Siegle et al., 2007).

Acknowledgments

This work was supported by a National Institute on Drug Abuse grant (DA027764-01) to M.R.D. and a predoctoral fellowship (DA025426–01) to L.N.M. The authors would like to acknowledge Peter Sokol-Hessner for constructive feedback and Mike Niznikiewicz for assistance with figures.

References

Amaral, D. G., and Price, J. L. (1984). Amygdalo-cortical projections in the monkey (Macaca fascicularis). *Journal of Comparative Neurology, 230*(4), 465–96.

Arnsten, A. F. and Goldman-Rakic, P. S. (1998). Noise stress impairs prefrontal cortical cognitive function in monkeys: evidence for a hyperdopaminergic mechanism. *Archives of General Psychiatry, 55*(4), 362–68.

Banks, S. J., Eddy, K. T., Angstadt, M., Nathan, P. J., and Phan, K. L. (2007). Amygdala-frontal connectivity during emotion regulation. *Social Cognitive and Affective Neuroscience, 2*(4), 303–312.

Barrett, L. F., Mesquita, B., Ochsner, K. N., and Gross, J. J. (2007). The experience of emotion. *Annual Review of Psychology, 58*, 373–403.

Beauregard, M., Levesque, J., and Bourgouin, P. (2001). Neural correlates of conscious self-regulation of emotion. *Journal of Neuroscience, 21*(18), RC165.

Bechara, A. and Damasio, A. R. (2005). The somatic marker hypothesis: A neural theory of economic decision. *Games and Economic Behavior, 52*(2), 336–72.

Bechara, A., Damasio, H., and Damasio, A. R. (2000). Emotion, decision making and the orbitofrontal cortex. *Cerebral Cortex, 10*(3), 295–307.

Blair, K. S., Smith, B. W., Mitchell, D. G., Morton, J., Vythilingam, M., Pessoa, L. et al. (2007). Modulation of emotion by cognition and cognition by emotion. *Neuroimage, 35*(1), 430–40.

Breiter, H. C., Gollub, R. L., Weisskoff, R. M., Kennedy, D. N., Makris, N., Berke, J. D. et al. (1997). Acute effects of cocaine on human brain activity and emotion. *Neuron, 19*(3), 591–611.

Cardinal, R. N., Parkinson, J. A., Hall, J., and Everitt, B. J. (2002). Emotion and motivation: the role of the amygdala, ventral striatum, and prefrontal cortex. *Neuroscience Biobehavioral Reviews, 26*(3), 321–52.

Critchley, H. D. (2002). Electrodermal responses: what happens in the brain. *Neuroscientist, 8*(2), 132–42.

Crowne, D. P. and Marlowe, D. (1960). A new scale of social desirability independent of psychopathology. *Journal of Consulting Psychology, 24*, 349–54.

Delgado, M. R. (2007). Reward-related responses in the human striatum. *Annals of the New York Academy of Sciences, 1104*, 70–88.

Delgado, M. R., Olsson, A., and Phelps, E. A. (2006). Extending animal models of fear conditioning to humans. *Biological Psychology, 73*(1), 39–48.

Delgado, M. R., Gillis, M. M., and Phelps, E. A. (2008a). Regulating the expectation of reward via cognitive strategies. *Nature Neuroscience, 11*(8), 880–81.

Delgado, M. R., Nearing, K. I., LeDoux, J. E., and Phelps, E. A. (2008b). Neural circuitry underlying the regulation of conditioned fear and its relation to extinction. *Neuron, 59*(5), 829–38.

Dillon, D. G. and LaBar, K. S. (2005). Startle Modulation During Conscious Emotion Regulation Is Arousal-Dependent. *Behavioral Neuroscience, 119*(4), 1118–24.

Ekman, P. and Friesen, W. V. (1971). Constants across cultures in the face and emotion. *Journal of Personality and Social Psychology, 17*(2), 124–29.

Foti, D. and Hajcak, G. (2008). Deconstructing reappraisal: descriptions preceding arousing pictures modulate the subsequent neural response. *Journal of Cognitive Neuroscience, 20*(6), 977–88.

Ghashghaei, H. T. and Barbas, H. (2002). Pathways for emotion: interactions of prefrontal and anterior temporal pathways in the amygdala of the rhesus monkey. *Neuroscience, 115*(4), 1261–79.

Giuliani, N. R., McRae, K., and Gross, J. J. (2008). The up- and down-regulation of amusement: Experiential, behavioral, and autonomic consequences. *Emotion, 8*(5), 714–719.

Goldin, P. R., McRae, K., Ramel, W., and Gross, J. J. (2008). The neural bases of emotion regulation: Reappraisal and suppression of negative emotion. *Biological Psychiatry, 63*(6), 577–86.

Gray, J. R. (2004). Integration of emotion and cognitive control. *Current Directions in Psychological Science, 13*(2), 46–48.

Green, M. J. and Malhi, G. S. (2006). Neural mechanisms of the cognitive control of emotion. *Acta Neuropsychiatrica, 18*(3-4), 144–53.

Gross, J. J. (1998a). Antecedent- and response-focused emotion regulation: divergent consequences for experience, expression, and physiology. *Journal of Personality and Social Psychology, 74*(1), 224–37.

Gross, J. J. (1998b). The emerging field of emotion regulation: an integrative review. *Review of General Psychology, 2*(3), 271–99.

Gross, J. J. (2002). Emotion regulation: affective, cognitive, and social consequences. *Psychophysiology, 39*(3), 281–91.

Gross, J. J. and John, O. P. (2003). Individual differences in two emotion-regulation processes: implications for affect, relationships, and well-being. *Journal of Personality and Social Psychology, 85*(2), 348–62.

Hamann, S. and Canli, T. (2004). Individual differences in emotion processing. *Current Opinion in Neurobiology, 14*(2), 233–38.

Hare, T. A., Camerer, C. F., and Rangel, A. (2009). Self-control in decision making involves modulation of the vmPFC valuation system. *Science, 324*(5927), 646–48.

Harenski, C. L. and Hamann, S. (2006). Neural correlates of regulating negative emotions related to moral violations. *Neuroimage, 30*(1), 313–24.

Hariri, A. R., Bookheimer, S. Y., and Mazziotta, J. C. (2000). Modulating emotional responses: Effects of a neocortical network on the limbic system. *Neuroreport: For Rapid Communication of Neuroscience Research, 11*(1), 43–48.

James, W. (1894). The physical basis of emotion. *Psychological Review, 101*, 205–210.

Johnstone, T., van Reekum, C. M., Urry, H. L., Kalin, N. H., and Davidson, R. J. (2007). Failure to regulate: counterproductive recruitment of top-down prefrontal-subcortical circuitry in major depression. *Journal of Neuroscience, 27*(33), 8877–84.

Kalisch, R., Wiech, K., Critchley, H. D., Seymour, B., O'Doherty, J. P., Oakley, D. A. et al. (2005). Anxiety reduction through detachment: subjective, physiological, and neural effects. *Journal of Cognitive Neuroscience, 17*(6), 874–83.

Kalisch, R., Wiech, K., Herrmann, K., and Dolan, R. J. (2006). Neural correlates of self-distraction from anxiety and a process model of cognitive emotion regulation. *Journal of Cognitive Neuroscience, 18*(8), 1266–76.

Kim, S. H. and Hamann, S. (2007). Neural correlates of positive and negative emotion regulation. *Journal of Cognitive Neuroscience,* **19**(5), 776–98.

Knutson, B. and Cooper, J. C. (2005). Functional magnetic resonance imaging of reward prediction. *Current Opinion in Neurology,* **18**(4), 411–417.

Kober, H., Barrett, L. F., Joseph, J., Bliss-Moreau, E., Lindquist, K., and Wager, T. D. (2008). Functional grouping and cortical-subcortical interactions in emotion: a meta-analysis of neuroimaging studies. *Neuroimage,* **42**(2), 998–1031.

Kober, H., Kross, E. F., Mende-Siedlecki, P., and Ochsner, K. N. (2009). Regulating craving for cigarettes and food: an fMRI study of cigarette smokers. *Annual Meeting of the Cognitive Neuroscience Society, San Francisco, CA.*

Kober, H., Kross, E. F., Mischel, W., Hart, C. L., and Ochsner, K. N. (2010). Regulation of craving by cognitive strategies in cigarette smokers. *Drug and Alcohol Dependence,* **106**(1), 52–5.

Kring, A. M. and Gordon, A. H. (1998). Sex differences in emotion: expression, experience, and physiology. *Journal of Personality and Social Psychology,* **74**(3), 686–703.

Lang, P. J., Greenwald, M. K., Bradley, M. M., and Hamm, A. O. (1993). Looking at pictures: affective, facial, visceral, and behavioral reactions. *Psychophysiology,* **30**(3), 261–73.

Lerner, J. S., Small, D. A., and Loewenstein, G. (2004). Heart strings and purse strings: carryover effects of emotions on economic decisions. *Psychological Science,* **15**(5), 337–41.

Levesque, J., Fanny, E., Joanette, Y., Paquette, V., Mensour, B., Beaudoin, G. et al. (2003). Neural circuitry underlying voluntary suppression of sadness. *Biological Psychiatry,* **53**(6), 502–510.

Lieberman, M. D., Eisenberger, N. I., Crockett, M. J., Tom, S. M., Pfeifer, J. H., and Way, B. M. (2007). Putting feelings into words: Affect labeling disrupts amygdala activity in response to affective stimuli. *Psychological Science,* **18**(5), 421–28.

Martin, L. N., Fareri, D. S., and Delgado, M. R. (2007). The influence of emotion-regulation strategies on risky decision making. *Annual Meeting of the Society for Neuroeconomics, Hull, MA.*

McRae, K., Ochsner, K. N., Mauss, I. B., Gabrieli, J. J. D., and Gross, J. J. (2008). Gender differences in emotion regulation: an fMRI study of cognitive reappraisal. *Group Processes and Intergroup Relations,* **11**(2), 143–62.

Milad, M. R. and Quirk, G. J. (2002). Neurons in medial prefrontal cortex signal memory for fear extinction. *Nature,* **420**(6911), 70–74.

Miller, E. K. and Cohen, J. D. (2001). An integrative theory of prefrontal cortex function. *Annual Review of Neuroscience,* **24** , 167–202.

O'Doherty, J. P. (2004). Reward representations and reward-related learning in the human brain: insights from neuroimaging. *Current Opinion in Neurobiology,* **14**(6), 769–76.

Ochsner, K. N. and Gross, J. J. (2008). Cognitive emotion regulation: Insights from social cognitive and affective neuroscience. *Current Directions in Psychological Science,* **17**(2), 153–58.

Ochsner, K. N., Bunge, S. A., Gross, J. J., and Gabrieli, J. D. E. (2002). Rethinking feelings: an fMRI study of the cognitive regulation of emotion. *Journal of Cognitive Neuroscience,* **14**(8), 1215–29.

Ochsner, K. N., Ray, R. D., Cooper, J. C., Robertson, E. R., Chopra, S., Gabrieli, J. D. et al. (2004). For better or for worse: neural systems supporting the cognitive down- and up-regulation of negative emotion. *Neuroimage,* **23**(2), 483–99.

Panksepp, J. (1998). *Affective neuroscience: the foundations of human and animal emotions. Series in affective science,* xii. New York, NY: Oxford University Press.

Patil, P. G., Apfelbaum, J. L., and Zacny, J. P. (1995). Effects of a cold-water stressor on psychomotor and cognitive functioning in humans. *Physiology and Behavior,* **58**(6), 1281–86.

Phan, K. L., Fitzgerald, D. A., Nathan, P. J., Moore, G. J., Uhde, T. W., and Tancer, M. E. (2005). Neural substrates for voluntary suppression of negative affect: a functional magnetic resonance imaging study. *Biological Psychiatry,* **57**(3), 210–219.

Phelps, E. A. and LeDoux, J. E. (2005). Contributions of the amygdala to emotion processing: from animal models to human behavior. *Neuron, 48*(2), 175–87.

Phelps, E. A., Delgado, M. R., Nearing, K. I., and LeDoux, J. E. (2004). Extinction learning in humans: role of the amygdala and vmPFC. *Neuron, 43*(6), 897–905.

Porcelli, A. J. and Delgado, M. R. (2009). Acute stress modulates risk taking in financial decision making. *Psychological Science, 20*(3), 278–83.

Potenza, M. N. and Winters, K. C. (2003). The neurobiology of pathological gambling: Translating research findings into clinical advances. *Journal of Gambling Studies, 19*(1), 7–10.

Quirk, G. J. and Beer, J. S. (2006). Prefrontal involvement in the regulation of emotion: convergence of rat and human studies. *Current Opinion in Neurobiology, 16*(6), 723–27.

Ray, R. D., Ochsner, K. N., Cooper, J. C., Robertson, E. R., Gabrieli, J. D., and Gross, J. J. (2005). Individual differences in trait rumination and the neural systems supporting cognitive reappraisal. *Cognitive, Affective and Behavioral Neuroscience, 5*(2), 156–68.

Richards, J. M. and Gross, J. J. (2000). Emotion regulation and memory: The cognitive costs of keeping one's cool. Year of Publication 2000. *Journal of Personality and Social Psychology, 79*(3), 410–24.

Schaefer, S. M., Jackson, D. C., Davidson, R. J., Aguirre, G. K., Kimberg, D. Y., and Thompson-Schill, S. L. (2002). Modulation of amygdalar activity by the conscious regulation of negative emotion. *Journal of Cognitive Neuroscience, 14*(6), 913–21.

Siegle, G. J., Thompson, W., Carter, C. S., Steinhauer, S. R., and Thase, M. E. (2007). Increased amygdala and decreased dorsolateral prefrontal BOLD responses in unipolar depression: related and independent features. *Biological Psychiatry, 61*(2), 198–209.

Sinha, R. (2007). The role of stress in addiction relapse. *Current Psychiatry Reports, 9*(5), 388–95.

Sinha, R., Lacadie, C., Skudlarski, P., Fulbright, R. K., Rounsaville, B. J., Kosten, T. R. . (2005). Neural activity associated with stress-induced cocaine craving: et ala functional magnetic resonance imaging study. *Psychopharmacology (Berl), 183*(2), 171–80.

Sokol-Hessner, P., Hsu, M., Curley, N. G., Delgado, M. R., Camerer, C. F., and Phelps, E. A. (2009). Thinking like a trader selectively reduces individuals' loss aversion. *Proceedings of the National Academy of Sciences, U.S.A., 106*(13), 5035–40.

Staudinger, M. R., Erk, S., Abler, B., and Walter, H. (2009). Cognitive reappraisal modulates expected value and prediction error encoding in the ventral striatum. *Neuroimage, 47*(2), 713–21.

Urry, H. L., van Reekum, C. M., Johnstone, T., Kalin, N. H., Thurow, M. E., Schaefer, H. S. et al. (2006). Amygdala and ventromedial prefrontal cortex are inversely coupled during regulation of negative affect and predict the diurnal pattern of cortisol secretion among older adults. *Journal of Neuroscience, 26*(16), 4415–25.

Van Boven, L., White, K., and Huber, M. (2009). Immediacy bias in emotion perception: current emotions seem more intense than previous emotions. *Journal of Experimental Psychology: General, 138*(3), 368–82.

Vohs, K. D. and Faber, R. J. (2007). Spent Resources: Self-Regulatory Resource Availability Affects Impulse Buying. *Journal of Consumer Research, 33*(4), 537–47.

Wager, T. D., Davidson, M. L., Hughes, B. L., Lindquist, M. A., and Ochsner, K. N. (2008). Prefrontal-subcortical pathways mediating successful emotion regulation. *Neuron, 59*(6), 1037–50.

Winkielman, P., Berridge, K. C., and Wilbarger, J. L. (2005). Unconscious affective reactions to masked happy versus angry faces influence consumption behavior and judgments of value. *Personality and Social Psychology Bulletin, 31*(1), 121–35.

Chapter 15

Reward processing and conscious awareness

Mathias Pessiglione, Liane Schmidt,
Stefano Palminteri, and Chris D. Frith

Abstract

Can our behavior be motivated by environmental signals that we are not aware of? In this chapter we cast light on this question, with a series of experiments investigating whether the human brain can deal with the reward-predicting properties of visual stimuli that subjects cannot consciously perceive. The experimental paradigms designed for this purpose bring together procedures that have been used for decades in separate scientific fields: subliminal perception on one side and incentive motivation on the other. We first sketch a short history of methods and concepts used in these two fields, and then we present psychophysics studies combining the two approaches to explore subliminal motivation in humans. Specifically, our previous studies have shown that the human brain is able to translate higher subliminal incentives into higher physical effort, and to use subliminal cues that predict gambles outcomes to make profitable decisions. We present here several novel variants of the original paradigms, to further explore the roles of top-down attention, strategic control and associative learning in conscious and subconscious incentive motivation.

15.1 Introduction—a brief history of concepts

15.1.1 Subliminal perception

The empirical quest for a "*limen,*" or threshold, below which perception is unconscious but still affects behavior, is as old as experimental psychology. Pioneering studies showed that some capacity for discrimination can persist in the absence of consciousness. In these early days, conscious awareness was probed by introspection, with the subjects sometimes being the experimenters themselves (as in Pierce and Jastrow, 1884). In one of these experiments, for instance, characters were presented at a distance, such that subjects reported seeing only a blurred spot. When forced to guess whether the characters were digits or letters, their performance was nonetheless better than chance (Sidis, 1898). Several demonstrations of this kind, showing above chance discrimination with no subjective awareness, were published during the first half of the twentieth century (for a review, see: Adams, 1957), until introspection was criticized as a valid method for assessing conscious awareness (Eriksen, 1960). To properly demonstrate an absence of awareness, experimenters were instead required to show that an objective measure, such as discrimination performance, was at chance level. The ironic implication is that the same observation, above chance discrimination, which was first interpreted as evidence for unconscious perception, was now taken as an indicator of conscious awareness.

The dilemma is still unresolved: should we go for subjective or objective measures if we want to separate subconscious from conscious processes? Ideally we would prefer our demonstration not to depend on dubious reports about the subjective feeling of being conscious. As Eriksen (1960) pointed out, the same percept may be considered as conscious by some subjects but unconscious by other subjects, or by the same subjects under different instructions. In other words, introspective measures make consciousness dependent on a volatile confidence criterion. By contrast, an objective measure, such as the percentage of correct discriminations, seems much more reliable. The problem with stringent objective criteria is that they are likely to kill the very phenomenon, subconscious processing, that we intend to study. For example, with an objective criterion, one would dismiss such an interesting phenomenon as blindsight. This syndrome is commonly observed after damage to the primary visual cortex and characterized by patients claiming they cannot see anything, yet showing impressive accuracy at discriminating between elementary visual patterns (Weiskrantz, 1999). On one side, authors attached to objective criteria would conclude that blindsight patients have a conscious visual percept, even if they fail to report it. On the other side, authors trusting subjective reports would draw the opposite conclusion: that discrimination performance has nothing to do with consciousness, since the two can be dissociated (Lau, 2008). From a methodological viewpoint, subjective reports can be used to classify each stimulation as consciously perceived or not, and hence to monitor conscious awareness on a trial-by-trial basis (Baars, 1988). On the contrary, discrimination performance is a statistical measure, which can only be assessed over a large number of trials, among which some occasional conscious perception may be missed. Indeed, demonstrating chance level discrimination raises the formal issue of accepting a null hypothesis, which remains problematic because a negative test can mistake insufficient statistical power for an absence of effect (Cheesman and Merikle, 1986).

In search for "*absolute subliminality*," some authors have formalized a dissociation procedure, which consists in showing that information about stimuli can be inaccessible for the conscious mind, as evidenced by a direct discrimination measure, but still available for some unconscious process indexed by an indirect measure (Reingold and Merikle, 1988). This procedure has been largely implemented in masked priming studies, in which processing of a visible target is influenced by the prior presentation of a related invisible prime. For example, after being exposed to a masked word, say "salt," subjects were unable to state whether the word was present or not, but favored semantically related words, like "pepper," in a subsequent forced choice (Marcel, 1983). These studies have been subjected to ferocious criticisms, however, such that subliminal semantic processing has been cyclically acclaimed and rejected, resulting at the end in substantial methodological improvement (see Kouider and Dehaene, 2007). Among further methodological requirements, one is that an equal number of subliminal stimulations, in the same visual conditions, should be used for direct and indirect measures (Holender, 1986). Another is that responses cannot be prepared in advance, to avoid direct motor specification, which might occur when using a small set of known stimuli (Abrams and Greenwald, 2000; Damian, 2001).

However, obtaining above chance indirect measures simultaneously with chance level direct measures does not necessarily equate to an effective subconscious processing in the absence of awareness. It would be the case if measures were both exclusive and exhaustive, meaning that the direct measure accounts for all and only conscious processing, and the indirect measure all and only unconscious processing. These assumptions are hard to implement in practice, so it may be argued that the two measures are likely to represent a mix of conscious and unconscious processes. This is why some authors suggested that the only convincing evidence for subconscious processing is a qualitatively different behavioral effect, compared to that obtained with conscious processing (Cheesman and Merikle, 1986). For instance, the mere exposure effect involves subjects being flashed subliminal stimuli and then tested on both recognition and preference. Typically, in the recognition test, subjects are unable to state which stimuli were previously presented, but in the preference judgment test, they favor the previously presented stimuli (Kunst-Wilson and Zajonc, 1980). Crucially, the effects are reversed when stimuli are explicitly and not subliminally presented, with above chance recognition of old stimuli and preference for novel stimuli. A qualitative difference could, in principle, be found as well in neuroimaging data, if conscious and subconscious processing recruit different brain circuits. Unfortunately, most brain-imaging studies have reported a quantitative difference, with the same regions being more activated when processing becomes conscious (see Marzi et al., 2004).

Nowadays, after a half century of intense controversy, subliminal perception can no longer be denied, whatever the criterion; but what representations exactly can be formed subconsciously is still a debated issue. An influential theory is that perception has two stages, with subconscious processing first, for lower-level information, and then conscious processing for higher level representation (Baars, 1988; Greenwald, 1992; Dehaene and Naccache, 2001). Although the frontier between lower and higher levels may still fluctuate, these authors agree that a large variety of short-lived information-processing stages can remain subconscious, including those involved in semantic representations. Some other stages may, however, need to be conscious, notably the strategic processing that would develop under volitional control and apply to longer time scales. Curiously, there was little investigation on whether and how the brain can process the reward-predicting properties of subliminal stimuli before our own publications (Pessiglione et al., 2007, 2008). One earlier attempt to motivate people with subliminal message was the famous "eat pop-corn" flashed on a movie screen of the US West Coast in 1957. The authors first claimed that the subliminal manipulation had boosted their sales but later admitted this was a fake (for a review, see: Pratkanis, 1992). Despite the fact that no well-controlled study could prove any effect on consumer behavior, the idea that you cannot defend yourself against subliminal advertising, because it directly targets your unconscious, became highly popular. Our aim was to revisit the concept of subliminal motivation, by applying a visual masking technique to paradigms developed for conditioning studies in animals. The general plan was to degrade the visibility of reward-predicting stimuli and look for dissociations between direct indicators, both objective and subjective, of conscious awareness, and indirect measures of incentive motivation.

15.1.2 Incentive motivation

Motivation is not an easy concept to investigate empirically, because it belongs to common language and accepts vague and various meanings. Several operational definitions of motivation were proposed in the course of the last century (for an extended review, see: Berridge, 2004). During the behaviorist era, motivation was first seen as a useless concept, as stimulus–response relationships were believed to exhaustively describe the observations. There is, indeed, a threat of circularity with motivational explanation: when an animal executes an action, it adds nothing to say that the animal had a motivation to execute the action. Later on, motivation was employed as a convenient intervening variable between experimental manipulation and behavioral observation (see Miller, 1971). The issue was that various manipulations can produce a same spectrum of observations; for instance, water deprivation and heat dehydration may result in more water drunk or more work for a sip. Instead of making all possible stimulus–response links, which would rapidly lead to a combinatorial explosion, it is parsimonious to link the above cited manipulations to thirst and then thirst to the behavioral observations. At this period (until 1960s), motivation was equated with homeostatic drive, assuming that behavior results from the need to keep some internal variables, such as glucose plasma level, at given set points. Drives like thirst or hunger would then develop from an error signal and trigger compensatory behavior in order to minimize the error. Thus, motivational explanations were formulated in terms of drive reduction, which may have reasonable face validity for food- or water-directed behavior, but much less for sex or dominance. Research on the biological correlates of motivation has nonetheless been long focused on identifying set points and error signals that would trigger drive-reduction behavior.

Several difficulties lead most authors to abandon the drive-reduction account of motivation. It was first argued that a transiently stable balance between opposing forces can give the illusion of homeostatic regulation. For instance, body weight may have no set point at all, but only fluctuating levels resulting from a balance between opponent systems. According to Bolles (1980), the fact that obesity rates have recently risen does not reflect a change in internal set-points, but in external availability and palability of food, which would have favored eating behavior. Thus, as other authors would put it, hedonic aspects of rewards may not be negligible in explaining behavior (Pfaffmann, 1960; Young, 1966; Cabanac, 1992). Further evidence was drawn from a patient whose esophagus was permanently damaged and who was fed through gastric fistula. Surprisingly, the patient insisted on chewing food at meals, before placing it in his stomach (Wolf and Wolff, 1943). This situation was reproduced in animals to show that satisfying appetite is not merely a matter of drive reduction (Miller and Kessen, 1952). Another line of evidence came from self-stimulation studies in animals with implanted electrodes. If the drive reduction theory was true, stimulation of a brain site that triggers eating behavior should be aversive, meaning that rats would want to stop it. The prediction turned out to be false: when given the possibility, the rats pressed levers to prolong the stimulation, just as they pressed levers to obtain food, such that eating electrodes were also reward electrodes (Valenstein, 1976).

The concept of incentive motivation was built on earlier reflections about the necessary features of a truly motivated behavior. It was first noted that all motivated behavior could be divided into appetitive and consummatory phases (Sherrington, 1906). The appetitive phase involves flexible approach behavior directed toward a goal, whereas the consummatory phase consists in stereotyped behavioral patterns elicited when the goal is within reach, such as chewing food, aggressive biting, or sexual copulation. Teitelbaum (1966) pointed to the flexibility of the appetitive phase as an essential feature of motivated behavior, including the possibility of learning a new, operant response or inferring a new strategy to obtain the goal. Epstein (1982) added two criteria, goal expectation and affective reaction, that are supposed to distinguish between truly motivated behavior and that of machine-learning algorithms. The most basic reinforcement learning algorithm would be something like "increase response frequency when you get a reward." Such an algorithm cannot account for some behavioral markers of motivation, such as autoshaping or incentive contrast (Crespi, 1942; Williams and Williams, 1969; Jenkins and Moore, 1973). These effects are obtained when the reward used to reinforce an operant response is suddenly increased: certain behavioral measures that are irrelevant to obtaining the reward, such as the speed of approach response or the rate of anticipatory licking, will change on the very next trial before any reinforcement can take place. These effects are usually explained by the fact that animals are expecting a reward, and not just activating context–action associations. Also, by contrast with learning machines, the affective manifestations (including somatic, autonomic, or hormonal markers) of the appetitive phase indicate that behavior is really motivated towards hedonic goals. Furthermore, Balleine and Dickinson (1998) underlined that not only the expected reward has to be represented during the appetitive phase, but also the contingency linking the behavior to the reward. This can be tested in extinction paradigms following devaluation of the reward, by satiation for instance. If the behavior is reduced, then it can be qualified as goal-directed, meaning dependent on updated reward expectation. Otherwise, it would be called a habit, which is mere activation of context–action links, without any goal representation.

Thus, contrary to the drive reduction theory where everything starts with homeostasis, incentive motivation theory makes things start with the hedonic experience of rewards. In the latter view, what motivates people is learned expectation of hedonic rewards (Bolles, 1972). This definition fits well with common intuition: when we question the motivation, or the motive, for an action, we basically wonder what expected reward the action is aimed at. More specifically, it has been assumed that the value of hedonic reward experience is transferred through associative learning to contingent cues, which thereby acquire motivational properties (Bindra, 1974). Of course, the tenants of incentive motivation theory would not claim that physiological states, such as hunger and satiation, play no role in motivating behavior. They propose instead that physiological states could magnify or attenuate the incentive/hedonic value of reward predictive cues (Toates, 1986). According to Berridge and Robinson (1998), the predictive cues become both liked and wanted, forming a gradient along which animals may move, from the most distal to the most proximal, up to reaching the reward. In their terminology, "liking" is an affective state reflecting the hedonic properties of the cue, whereas "wanting," also called "incentive salience," reflects the motivational value of the cue, which may attract attention and behavior. In normal situations "liking" and "wanting" usually go together, but they can be dissociated following certain brain modifications; for instance, drug addicts may still want to take substances that they do not particularly like anymore.

Associative learning is thus central to incentive motivation theory, which can be seen as a cognitive interpretation of the animal-conditioning literature that had been constituted during the behaviorist era, when cognitive representations were banished. In classical or Pavlovian conditioning, an arbitrary cue (say a bell ring) is repeatedly followed by a rewarding outcome (say a sausage), until it shows the capacity to elicit a vegetative manifestation (say salivation) that is normally observed in response to the reward (Pavlov, 1927). In operant or instrumental conditioning, access to reward (say a food pellet) is dependent on a behavioral response (say lever press), the frequency of which increases across trials according to the law of effect (Thorndike, 1911). Thus, Pavlovian learning involves building cue–outcome associations, and instrumental learning cue–response–outcome associations. Both types of learning depend on two main factors: contiguity (short delays between reward and cue or response) and contingency (more reward following specific cue or response). It is generally accepted that, in both cases, the learning rate is commensurate to a reward-prediction error, which is the difference between actual and predicted reward (Rescorla and Wagner, 1972). Basically this rule says that surprise may serve as a teaching signal: the more surprised you are, the more you learn about your environment. Note that the surprise has a sign: a positive prediction error (more reward than expected) will reinforce the associations between cues, responses, and outcomes; whereas negative ones (less reward than expected), will weaken these associations. The crucial role of prediction errors is well illustrated in blocking paradigms, where a reward that is already fully predicted by a first cue fails to be associated with other cues (Kamin, 1969). The Rescorla–Wagner learning rule has been developed and implemented in various models, providing a computational account of the incentive salience concept, which would reflect reward prediction for a given cue (Schultz et al., 1997; McClure et al., 2003). If we imagine a sequential chain of cues leading to reward, the incentive salience gradient would be learned from a teaching signal, equivalent to the difference of reward prediction between two successive cues, or two time-points (the so-called "temporal difference error").

Beyond the acquisition of incentive salience, we were interested in its effects on behavior, i.e., in the motivational processes occurring during the appetitive phase of goal-directed action. Outside the learning context, motivational effects can be divided into two types: energizing and directing behavior. Energizing behavior can be assessed as the amount of effort, for instance the number of lever presses, exerted by an animal to obtain a given reward (Walton et al., 2006). Directing behavior can be assessed as the alternative favored by the animal in choice situations, for instance in discounting paradigms where a small reward is compared to a larger reward associated with higher effort, longer delay, or lower probability (Cardinal, 2006). Working with humans, we chose to use monetary rewards, which offer several advantages: they are easy to quantify, they are not prone to satiation, and they provide a natural counterpart, losing money as opposed to winning money, to contrast punishment avoidance with reward seeking. The paradigms detailed below were originally designed for neuroimaging studies, in which we analyzed the BOLD signal to identify key brain areas and the skin conductance response, as an index of affective reactions (Pessiglione et al., 2007, 2008). Here, we focus on behavioral measures, and develop variants of the original designs in order to further investigate the relationships between motivational processes and conscious awareness.

15.2 Experimental part 1: energizing behavior

15.2.1 Original experiments: a case for subliminal motivation

A first series of experiments was designed to examine whether monetary incentives can subconsciously influence motor activation. To this aim we manipulated both the visibility and the amount of money presented in the different trials: subjects were flashed various coin images between two visual masks, with various durations (see Fig. 15.1A). In a visual-discrimination task, subjects were asked to report which incentive has been flashed, and whether they saw it or they had just been guessing. We thus observed two direct indicators of stimulus awareness: percentage of correct responses (objective measure) and percentage of seen responses (subjective measure). In the incentive-force task, subjects were asked to squeeze a handgrip, and explained that they would be allowed to keep a fraction of the monetary incentive, proportional to the force produced. Handgrip force was thus taken as an indirect measure reflecting incentive motivation. Subjects were given online visual feedback on the force exerted, visualized as a cursor moving up and down, and a cumulative total of the money won at the end of every trial. We used two criteria to select sessions where subjects were not consciously aware of the monetary incentive: objective measure at chance level and subjective measure at zero. In both cases, subjects still exerted more force for higher incentives (Pessiglione et al., 2007). This effect of incentive motivation was specifically underpinned by bilateral activation of a basal forebrain region known to be involved in reward processing (Robbins and Everitt, 1996; Pecina et al., 2006). The same region was activated, regardless of stimulus visibility, such that conscious awareness made no qualitative difference (no separate circuits for conscious and subconscious motivation), but a quantitative difference (more activation when

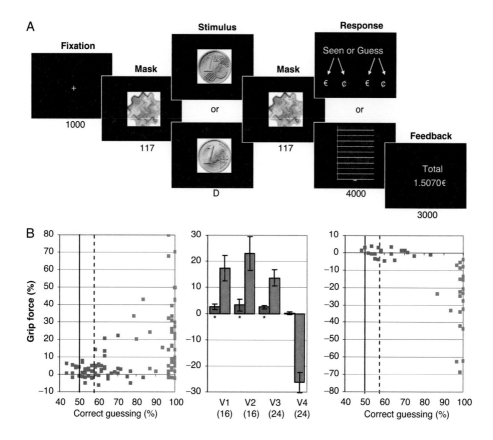

Fig. 15.1 Subliminal incentive motivation. (A) The tasks. Successive screenshots displayed in a single trial are shown from left to right, with durations in milliseconds. Subjects were first flashed a masked coin image (1¢ or 1€), representing the amount of money at stake. The duration D of cue display was varied between 33 and 117 ms to manipulate conscious awareness. Then they had to respond either by selecting a button press (visual-discrimination task) or by squeezing a handgrip (incentive-force task). In the perceptual-decision task, they had to report which coin was on the screen, and whether they saw it or just guessed. In the incentive-force task, they had to win the largest fraction possible of the money at stake. This fraction was proportional to the height reached by the cursor, which indicated the force exerted on the hand grip. The top of the graduated scale was adjusted to twice the subject's maximal force, and corresponded to a full monetary reward (1¢ or 1€). Finally, subjects were given feedback on the money won, including all previous trials. (B) The results. Middle: histograms represent differential grip force (1€−1¢) averaged across subjects (number in brackets) for the different variants of the paradigm (see text for details). Error bars are ± SEM. Dots represent subjects plotted on a diagram showing differential grip force against rate of correct guessing. Left: results of V1 to V3, where incentives have their normal meaning. Right: V4, where meanings were reversed (see explanations in text). Green = 33 ms; Red = 117 ms. Continuous vertical lines indicate chance level (50%) and dotted ones the threshold for significant above chance guessing at individual level (χ^2 test, $P<0.05$).

motivation becomes conscious). The energizing effect of monetary incentives was accompanied by an increase in skin conductance response, suggesting an emotional participation in addition to physical effort. The two measures, skin conductance and grip force, might respectively reflect the liking and wanting components of incentive motivation defined by Berridge and Robinson (2003). Using a similar task, but with supraliminal stimuli only, we showed that the two components can be dissociated following bilateral lesions of the basal ganglia (Schmidt et al., 2008): in these patients the skin conductance is still responsive to the amount of money at stake (liking is intact), but the grip force is no longer adapted (wanting is impaired).

15.2.2 **Novel experiments: testing effects of attention and training**

We constructed four variants of the original paradigm, and tested a total of 56 young healthy subjects. In contrast to the original neuroimaging experiment, subjects were not playing for real money. They were, nonetheless, assigned the goal to win as much virtual money as possible. We chose to compare a negligible incentive to a more appealing one (1¢ vs 1€), and a near threshold display to a visible one (33 vs 117 ms). Following presentation of mask/coin/mask sequence, there were two possible tasks: in the visual-discrimination task, subjects chose between four responses (seen 1€, seen 1¢, guess 1€, guess 1¢), whereas in the incentive-force task, they squeezed the handgrip in order to win as much as possible of the money at stake. The first variant, V1, was tested on 16 subjects to replicate the findings of the original experiment. The four cells (two incentives times two durations) of the design were randomly distributed over trials within each block. The two tasks were conducted in separate blocks, with the incentive-force task first (60 trials) and then the visual-discrimination task (120 trials). One potential caveat of this design is that subjects may be less motivated during the visual-discrimination task, because there is no money at stake, and hence pay less attention to the subliminal stimuli. Thus, even if visual discrimination is at chance, subjects could nonetheless see some stimuli during the incentive-force task, because they would pay more attention. To test out this possibility, we had 16 other subjects performing a second variant, V2, in which we mixed the two tasks, such that when they are flashed the incentives, subjects would not know whether they will subsequently have to answer the forced choice (with the left hand) or to squeeze the grip (with the right hand). In other words, we now had eight cells (two incentives times two durations times two tasks) randomly distributed over the 120 trials. With this design, subjects had to be equally attentive to the stimuli, whatever the task. Another potential criticism is that subliminal stimuli do not really trigger motivational processes, but just some degraded form of the motor response that is trained with supraliminal stimuli. To answer this critique, we tested 24 other subjects in a third variant, V3, in which the two durations were applied to different blocks, including 20 trials of 33/117/33 ms, successively. With this design, we were able to assess whether subliminal motivation can work before any conscious training of stimulus–response links can occur (with the first 33 ms block), and whether this training increases or not the effects of subliminal stimuli (with the comparison between the two 33 ms blocks).

We found no difference between the three variants of the task (Fig. 15.1B, middle diagram). All yielded a significant motivational effect at 33 ms (paired t-test, $P<0.05$), with more force produced for Euros compared to cents ($+2.5\pm1.0$, $+3.3\pm2.2$, and $+2.5\pm0.7\%$ for V1, V2, and V3, respectively). At this duration, percentage of correct choices in the three variants was 58.7 ± 2.5, 56.8 ± 1.9, and $59.8\pm1.7\%$, with a similar proportion of subjects whose performance did not differ from chance level (chi-2 test, $P>0.05$): 8/16, 8/16, and 13/24, respectively. Data from the three variants were pooled, increasing the sample size to 56 subjects, and to 29 the number of subjects with visual discrimination at chance level. The differential effect of incentives on force production was still significant in these last 29 subjects ($+1.9\pm0.6\%$ for Euros compared to cents, $P<0.01$), who appear on the left of the dotted line (Fig. 15.1B, left diagram). In fact, the paired t-test assessing motivational effect was still significant for subjects below chance level ($\leq 50\%$, objective criterion), or for subjects who reported seeing absolutely nothing of the 120 subliminal stimulations (subjective criterion).

These results rule out some interpretations of our original findings. A first interpretation would be that, because subjects are more motivated in the incentive-force task, they discriminate better the stimuli, and then apply more force when they guess that the money at stake is worthy. This would be plausible, since motivation has been shown to improve perceptual discrimination (Visser and Merikle, 1999). It would ruin the novelty of the result (and the concept of subliminal motivation) as the effect would be explained in terms of better decision making (and not of more energization). Subjects would decide whether the incentive is a cent or a Euro, and consequently decide to exert more or less force on the handgrip. Such an interpretation is no longer defendable, however, since the effect holds in a situation where subjects do not know which task they will have to do when they must pay attention to the stimuli. They were still at chance when asked to make a decision, but made a difference when asked to exert an effort. Thus, motor energization appeared to be more sensitive to subliminal incentives than perceptual decisions. A second interpretation would be that the effect of subliminal stimulation is due to motor training rather than incentive stimuli. This training would occur during supraliminal stimulation, where a certain degree of force could be progressively associated with each incentive. However, subjects who started with a block of subliminal stimuli also showed a differential effect on grip force ($+1.6\pm0.8\%$, $P<0.05$), before being administrated the block of supraliminal stimuli. After the supraliminal block, the effect of subliminal stimuli tended to increase (to $+3.3\pm1.1\%$), but not significantly so. It is unclear whether this non-significant increase was due to conscious training of incentive-force associations or just to more fatigue, which repeatedly enhanced the differential impact of incentives on grip force in all our experiments. However, it could be argued that, even if it works in the absence of training, the effect could still rely on subjects preparing in advance a mental set, where two levels of force must be applied to the two possible incentives, without any true motivational effect of subliminal incentives. This seems unlikely because such direct motor specification could equally be applied to the visual-discrimination task, and thus should have resulted in above-chance guessing. Indeed, two discrete motor responses, like button presses, seem easier to pre-link to the two incentives than two force levels on a continuum. We nonetheless designed a fourth variant, V4, of our paradigm to deal with the direct motor specification issue.

15.2.3 Novel experiments: testing effects of strategic control

In V4, the meaning of the coin images was reversed. Subjects were told that, whenever they are flashed a cent, the real stake would be one Euro, and vice versa. Thus, they could prepare in advance to exert a high level of force following cents presentation, and a low level following Euros. We tested the same 24 subjects who also performed V3, with the same design, where durations are assigned to different blocks (33/117/33 ms successively). The differential effect of subliminal incentives was null in both 33-ms blocks: -0.3 ± 0.9 and $+0.5 \pm 0.8\%$ (Fig. 15.1B, left diagram). Subjects were, in contrast, perfectly able to reverse their effort, squeezing harder for cents than for Euros, when the incentives were consciously visible (at 117 ms, with a differential effect of $-26.3 \pm 3.9\%$, $P<0.001$). This clearly suggests that the effects of subliminal incentives cannot be reduced to perceptual decision making, to motor training during conscious block, or to pre-configuring associations between monetary incentives and force levels. In other words, we obtained a qualitative dissociation, incentive motivation being reversible when conscious but not when subliminal. Note, however, that the instructions did have an impact, the effect of subliminal incentives being abolished when their meaning was reversed, as shown by the significant difference between V3 and V4 ($+2.5 \pm 0.7$ vs $+0.1 \pm 0.5\%$, $P<0.05$). This indicates that subliminal motivation is not out of control, since higher incentives did not automatically trigger higher force in a situation where it would not have been desirable. Such distinction is important to point out, as notions of unconscious and automatic are often confounded.

Taken together, the new behavioral results confirm our interpretation in terms of subliminal motivation: invisible stimuli predicting more reward have the capacity to energize behavior. This motivational interpretation was also supported by the other measures recorded during the original neuroimaging experiment, notably the specific activation of limbic circuits (and not motor or associative circuits) in the contrast between incentives, and the higher skin conductance response for higher incentives, revealing involvement of affective processes in addition to putative cold decision making and motor execution. The concept of subliminal motivation received further empirical support in a publication reporting that subliminal words expressing effort-related concepts can increase force production (Aarts et al., 2008). However, subliminal motivation effects were observed here with coin images, when they had their habitual meaning, the reward properties of which being well established. In the next section we address the issue of whether neutral subliminal stimuli can acquire reward properties so as to influence choices.

15.3 Experimental part 2: directing behavior

15.3.1 Original experiments: a case for subliminal instrumental conditioning

A second series of experiments was designed to assess whether instrumental learning can occur subconsciously. Initial steps had already been taken towards this demonstration, notably with the so-called implicit learning concept, meaning that behavioral responses can be adapted to the statistical structure of stimuli that fails to be reported explicitly (Knowlton et al., 1996; Destrebecqz and Cleeremans, 2001; Bayley et al., 2005). In implicit learning tasks using artificial grammar, serial reaction time, or probabilistic classification, authors have claimed that subjects can achieve good acquisition without explicit knowledge of the task structure. However, methods for assessing awareness of statistical contingencies have been criticized, principally on the issue that failure to answer retrospective questions about task structure does not prove any absence of awareness at the time of performing the task. In other words, questions were very demanding in terms of memory and subjects may have simply forgotten what they had been aware of (Wilkinson and Shanks, 2004; Lagnado et al., 2006). Thus, to formally test whether instrumental conditioning can occur without awareness, we took a more stringent approach: masking the cues, so that they remained unperceived. Subliminal conditioning studies in humans had so far been restricted to Pavlovian paradigms, such as fear conditioning (Clark and Squire, 1998; Knight et al., 2003; Olsson and Phelps, 2004), where subliminal stimuli (like unseen faces) are paired with unpleasant events (like white noise) to increase autonomic responses (like skin conductance). To our knowledge, subliminal instrumental conditioning, where decision making would be biased by unperceived cues predicting rewards or punishments, had never been demonstrated.

We used the same abstract cues, which were letters taken from a medieval font, and the same masking procedure to set up our visual-discrimination and instrumental-conditioning tasks (see Fig. 15.2A). In the visual-discrimination task, two masked cues were successively displayed on the screen, and subjects had to report whether or not they perceived a difference between the two stimulations. We reasoned that if subjects are unable to correctly discriminate between the masked cues, then they are also unable to build conscious representations of cue–outcome associations. We chose not to use a recognition test because identifying the cues would not be necessary to build conscious associations with the outcomes, discriminating them would indeed be sufficient. The procedure has also the advantage of not showing the cues unmasked, so that, by the end of the experiment, subjects had no idea what the cues look like. In the instrumental-conditioning task, subjects had to decide whether or not to make a risky response, which could be pressing or not pressing a button. Feedback about the response was displayed on the screen: "Go!" if they pressed the button, "No!" if they did not. Then they observed the outcome, which was neutral following a safe response, and either rewarding (monetary gain), neutral, or punishing (monetary loss) in the event of a risky response. Subjects were told that a subliminal cue, predicting the outcome of the risky response, was hidden

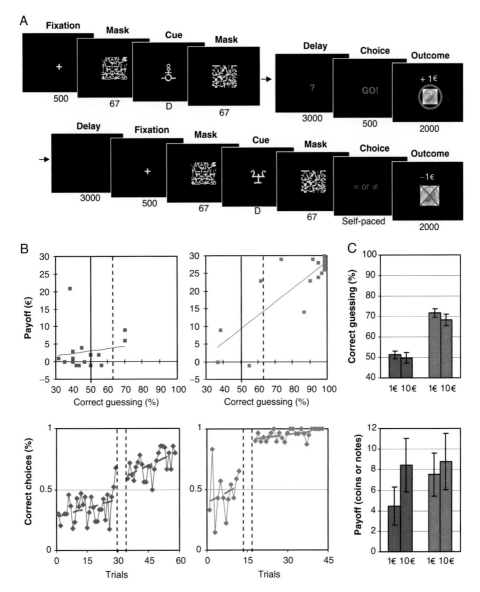

Fig. 15.2 Subliminal instrumental learning. (A) The tasks. Successive screenshots displayed in a single trial are shown from left to right, with durations in milliseconds. The duration D of cue display was varied from 33 to 83 ms to manipulate conscious awareness. The first four screens consisted in flashing a masked cue following a fixation cross, and were common to the instrumental-learning and visual-discrimination tasks. In the instrumental-learning task (top series), subjects chose to press or not press a response button, and subsequently observed the outcome. In the illustrated example, "Go" appeared on the screen because the subject had pressed the button, following the cue associated with a rewarding outcome (winning 1€). In the visual-discrimination task, a second masked cue was flashed, and subjects reported, by selecting one of two response buttons, whether or not they saw a difference. In variant V2 (see text), subjects could be given a monetary feedback about whether their response was correct or

not. **Fig. 15.2** (*contd.*) In the illustrated example, a punishing feedback (losing 1€) was given because the subject pressed the "=" button while the cues were different. (B) Results of variant V1. Top: dots represent subjects plotted on a diagram showing differential monetary payoff against percentage of correct guessing. Continuous vertical lines indicate chance level (50%) and dotted ones the threshold for significant above chance guessing at individual level (chi-2 test, $P<0.05$). Oblique lines represent the best fit using a linear regression. Bottom: learning curves represent percentage of correct responses across trials. The removed trials between vertical dotted lines correspond to the transition (an error followed by four consecutive correct responses). Periods before and after the transition have both been fitted using linear regression (oblique dotted lines). Green = 33 ms; Red = 83 ms. (C) Results of variant V2. Top: histograms represent percentage of correct guessing with feedbacks of ±1€ (left) and ±10€ (right). Bottom: histograms represent the number of coins won for the 1€ condition (left), and the number of notes won for the 10€ condition (right). Green: group average for subjects who were at chance level in the visual-discrimination task. Red: group average for subjects who were significantly above chance level (χ^2 test, $P<0.05$). Error bars are ± SEM.

between the mask images. As they would not see the cues, we encouraged them to follow their intuition, choosing the risky response if they had a feeling they were in a winning trial, and choosing a safe response if they felt it was a losing trial. Note that if subjects always made the same response, or if they performed at chance, their final payoff would be zero. On the contrary, subjects won money in this task, despite being at chance in the visual-discrimination task (Pessiglione et al., 2008). In other words, without the relevant feedback, subjects stayed at chance, but with the help of rewards and punishments, they learned to differentiate their responses to the various masked cues.

To model instrumental conditioning, we implemented a standard Q-learning algorithm, with inputs from individual histories of cues, choices, and outcomes. On every trial, the model estimates the likelihood of the risky response from the value of the displayed cue. If the risky response was actually taken, the model updates the value of the displayed cue in proportion to the prediction error, according to the Rescorla and Wagner rule. The parameters of the model were optimized such that likelihoods of risky responses provided the best fit of subjects' actual responses across conditioning sessions. The theoretical values of subliminal cues generated by this optimized algorithm were then used as regressors for analysis of brain-imaging data. Cue value correlated with activity in the ventral striatum, a component of limbic basal forebrain circuits. The same region was activated in a previous study using supraliminal cues (Pessiglione et al., 2006), such that again, conscious awareness made no qualitative difference in the brain circuits recruited to perform the task. Interestingly, the striatum has been involved as a major player in implicit/procedural (but not explicit/declarative) learning (Hikosaka et al., 1999; Packard and Knowlton, 2002; Graybiel, 2005). In our case, there was no correlation between ventral striatum activity and behavioral performance, indicating that this brain region equally learned the cue–outcome associations in all subjects, although not all subjects managed to bias their choices appropriately. The implication is that some learning occurred at the neuronal level, even in subjects who were playing at chance in the instrumental-conditioning task.

15.3.2 Novel experiments: testing for Q-learning properties (reward-sensitive deceleration)

The fact that neuronal activity followed a negatively accelerated, gradually increasing (for reward cues) or decreasing (for punishment cues) learning curve, is far from being trivial. Indeed, gradual learning curves have been criticized as an artifact of group averaging (Gallistel et al., 2004). Individual learning curves might be closer to step function, but due to the transition occurring at different latencies across subjects, the group average looks like a log function. Gallistel and colleagues acknowledge, however, that underlying associative learning might be gradual, but in this case would give rise to transitions when reaching a threshold. Following up this suggestion, we made the assumption that masking the cues would open a window to see gradual learning reflected in behavioral performance, whereas unmasking would allow conscious processing to generate abrupt transitions. Note that the analytical tools provided by Gallistel and colleagues are hard to implement with our paradigm, as responses were all or nothing decisions and learning sessions quite short (30 trials), which makes any increase in performance necessarily abrupt. We nonetheless tracked transitions as occurring between the last error and a plateau of successive correct trials. To examine whether transitions relate to conscious awareness, we progressively unmasked the cues, increasing their duration of display from 33 to 83 ms.

In a first variant, V1, of the subliminal conditioning paradigm, 16 subjects performed four learning sessions of step-by-step increasing durations (33/50/66/83 ms), each with three novel cues, presented 30 times in a random order, and associated with reward (+1€), neutral (0€) and punishment (−1€) outcomes. As with incentive-force tasks, subjects were not playing for real money but were nevertheless assigned the goal to win as much virtual money as possible. Then they were administered four sessions of the visual-discrimination task with the same range of durations (33/50/66/83 ms), each using another set of three novel cues presented in pairs for a same/different judgment. Each cue was presented the same number of times as in the conditioning task, to assess whether, by virtue of perceptual learning alone (without rewards and punishments), subjects could discriminate them better than chance level. In total, we used 24 cues, which were randomly assigned across subjects to the two tasks (instrumental learning/visual discrimination), four durations (33/50/66/83 ms), and three outcomes (+1€/0€/−1€).

Percentage of correct guessing in the visual-discrimination task was not significantly different from chance level at 33 ms (47.2±2.9%), but significantly above chance at the longer durations (respectively, 60.3±4.1, 70.4±4.9, and 82.0±5.5% for 50, 67, and 83 ms; paired t-test, all $P<0.05$). Subjects significantly won money at all durations (respectively, 2.8±1.4, 5.6±2.6, 12.6±3.2, and 21.4±2.6 € for 33, 50, 67, and 83 ms; paired t-test, all $P<0.05$), thus demonstrating an instrumental learning effect, even when unable to discriminate between the cues. Monetary payoff was significantly correlated with visual-discrimination performance at all durations. Linear regression crossed chance level (50%) at 3.2, 3.0, 5.5, and 9.0 € in the 33, 50, 67, and 83 ms sessions, respectively (Fig. 15.2B, top). These results, therefore, replicate the demonstration of subliminal instrumental conditioning reported in our original publication (Pessiglione et al., 2008), and show, in addition, that learning effects gradually increase as cues become more visible. To detect transitions in learning curves, we applied an a priori criterion of four consecutive correct trials. To compensate for between-subjects' differences in the latency of reaching the plateau, and hence to avoid averaging artifacts, we aligned individual curves at the transition (Fig. 15.2B, bottom). We next examined whether transitions could explain learning by comparing percentage of correct responses between the last trial before and the first trial after. These comparisons were not significant at 33 (67.9 to 59.1%) and 50 ms (72.0 to 77.3%), but significant at 67 (46.2 to 87.5%, $P<0.01$) and 83 ms (65.0 to 90.0%, $P<0.05$). This result suggests that, for shorter durations, sequences of consecutive correct trials occurred by chance and did not reflect learning, which occurred by gradual increments. For longer durations, in contrast, transitions largely explained learning effects, and presumably corresponded to the conscious realization of cue–outcome contingencies. Interestingly, residual gradual learning was observed before transitions at all durations, as if the putative conscious insights were preceded by incremental reinforcement episodes. Such speculations must be considered with caution, however, since we cannot know for sure whether the transitions detected with our arbitrary criterion correspond or not to conscious insight.

We tested 16 other subjects in a second variant of our paradigm (V2), to further assess the hypothesis that subliminal learning corresponds to gradual increments, whereas supraliminal learning corresponds to sudden insight leading to a step change in performance. We reasoned that the first type of learning should be dependent on the magnitude of reinforcement, which directly affects the size of prediction errors and hence of value updates. In contrast, conscious associations between cues and outcomes should not be faster to build up if we increase the reinforcement magnitude. We, therefore, decided to compare learning between two reward levels: 1 and 10€. We conducted three learning sessions, each including four novel cues presented 30 times each and associated with four different outcomes: +1€, −1€, +10€, and −10€. We also introduced the same feedback in the visual-discrimination task, to reward the correct responses and punish the others. The two reward levels were employed in two different sessions of 60 trials each. Assignment of the different cues to the tasks, sessions and outcomes was again randomized.

Introduction of monetary feedback into the visual-discrimination task was necessary to answer the critique that chance-level performance may be due to poor motivation, as seen with the incentive-force task. Feedback also encouraged subjects to try guessing whether the cues were identical or not, rather than just signaling when they pick up differences. We observed no significant effect of motivation in this task, as percentage of correct guessing was similar for 1 and 10€ (61.6±3.3 and 59.1±3.6%). The 16 subjects were then split into two halves, one being at chance level (51.3±2.5 for 1€ and 49.8±2.3 for 10€), the other significantly above chance (71.9±3.4 for 1€ and 68.3±5.4 for 10€). Interestingly, better-than-chance subjects learned to associate the cues with low (1€) and high (10€) outcomes (winning 7.5±2.1 low and 8.8±2.7 high) at an equal rate, whereas chance-level subjects seem to learn less with 1€ than with 10€ (4.5±1.9 low and 8.4±2.6 high). This difference was only marginally significant ($P<0.1$), however, probably due to the small number of subjects. If it is confirmed, this result would corroborate the link between conscious awareness and learning dynamics (abrupt versus gradual). More generally, it would support the existence of two learning systems: one incrementing values on the basis of reward-prediction errors, and one explicitly representing the associations between cues and outcomes.

15.4 **Conclusion**

Applying the standard masking procedures used in subliminal perception studies, we rendered stimuli inaccessible to the conscious mind. Following the definition of Dehaene et al. (2006), these stimuli can be called subliminal because they were attended but not reportable. When asked a direct question about the stimuli, subjects reported not seeing anything (subjective criterion) and their discrimination performance was at chance level (objective criterion). Adapting to humans some paradigms borrowed from animal-conditioning literature, we contrasted these direct measures with indirect measures indexing motivational effects: first, the amount of effort expended to win a subliminal incentive; and, second, the propensity to take a risky response after a subliminal abstract cue. Although subjects were unable to discriminate the relevant dimensions of subliminal stimuli, they nonetheless exhibited motivational effects. Namely, subliminal stimuli had the capacity to energize behavior, to acquire rewarding values through associations with outcomes, and to bias choices towards advantageous risk-taking. Compared with subliminal stimuli, consciously visible ones always yielded quantitatively greater effects, and occasionally some qualitative differences, such as the immediate adaptation to reversal of cue meanings, and the presence of abrupt transitions in learning curves.

Although it has not been demonstrated empirically before, that motivation can be subconscious may not be surprising for the general public. In particular, Freudian theory and subliminal advertising have both popularized the view that we can be motivated against our conscious will. It is worth pointing out some differences from the concept of subliminal incentive motivation that we have evidenced here. A notable difference is that motivational impulses in Freudian theory come from the inside, not from the environment. Also, subliminal stimuli never influenced behavior in a way that would not be desirable for the subjects. In other words, had they been aware of the stimuli, subjects would have behaved in a similar, and even amplified, way. Thus, there seems to be no value for advertisers in masking their messages, they would just reduce their impact on consumer behavior. It is unknown how long the effects of subliminal advertising would last. In our original study (Pessiglione et al., 2008), we showed that subliminal instrumental conditioning could bias the preferences, even after unmasking the cues. Subjects preferred the cues that had been paired with rewards, compared to those associated with punishments. However, this preference judgment test was done about 10 minutes after the conditioning sessions, and nobody knows whether or not the effect would survive an hour.

In conclusion, we have gathered a set of empirical evidence suggesting that incentive motivation can be triggered by stimuli that cannot be reported. If perception appeared to be subconscious, it is unclear whether or not subjects could have access to the information that they were being motivated. For instance, we might speculate that what we refer to as our instinct, or our intuition, relates to a conscious feeling elicited by unseen signals present in the environment. When we consider a choice, and get the intuition that alternative A is better than B, it could come from an environmental feature that we do not consciously perceive, but which has been associated in the past with A being successful. Further research will be needed to explore whether we can have access to, or learn to access, the feeling of being motivated by environmental signals that we do not perceive otherwise.

References

Aarts H, Custers R, and Marien H. Preparing and motivating behavior outside of awareness. *Science,* 2008; **319**: 1639.

Abrams RL and Greenwald AG. Parts outweigh the whole (word) in unconscious analysis of meaning. *Psychol Sci,* 2000; **11**: 118–24.

Adams JK. Laboratory studies of behavior without awareness. *Psychol Bull,* 1957; **54**: 383–405.

Baars BJ. A cognitive theory of consciousness. New York: Cambridge University Press, 1988.

Balleine BW and Dickinson A. Goal-directed instrumental action: contingency and incentive learning and their cortical substrates. *Neuropharmacology,* 1998; **37**: 407–19.

Bayley PJ, Frascino JC, and Squire LR. Robust habit learning in the absence of awareness and independent of the medial temporal lobe. *Nature,* 2005; **436**: 550–3.

Berridge KC. Motivation concepts in behavioral neuroscience. *Physiol Behav,* 2004; **81**: 179–209.

Berridge KC and Robinson TE. What is the role of dopamine in reward: hedonic impact, reward learning, or incentive salience? *Brain Res Brain Res Rev,* 1998; **28**: 309–69.

Berridge KC and Robinson TE. Parsing reward. *Trends Neurosci,* 2003; **26**: 507–13.

Bindra D. A motivational view of learning, performance, and behavior modification. *Psychol Rev,* 1974; **81**: 199–213.

Bolles RC. Reinforcement, expectancy, and learning. *Psychol Rev,* 1972; **79**: 394–409.

Bolles RW. Some functionalistic thoughts about regulation. In: Toates TW and Halliday T.W. (eds). *Analysis of motivational processes.* New York: Academic Press, 1980: 63–75.

Cabanac M. Pleasure: the common currency. *J Theor Biol,* 1992; **155**: 173–200.

Cardinal RN. Neural systems implicated in delayed and probabilistic reinforcement. *Neural Netw,* 2006; **19**: 1277–301.

Cheesman J and Merikle PM. Distinguishing conscious from unconscious perceptual processes. *Can J Psychol,* 1986; **40**: 343–67.

Clark RE and Squire LR. Classical conditioning and brain systems: the role of awareness. *Science,* 1998; **280**: 77–81.

Crespi LP. Quantitative variation of incentive and performance in the white rat. *Am J Psychol,* 1942; **55**: 467–517.

Damian MF. Congruity effects evoked by subliminally presented primes: automaticity rather than semantic processing. *J Exp Psychol Hum Percept Perform,* 2001; **27**: 154–65.

Dehaene S, Changeux JP, Naccache L, Sackur J, and Sergent C. Conscious, preconscious, and subliminal processing: a testable taxonomy. *Trends Cogn Sci,* 2006; **10**: 204–11.

Dehaene S and Naccache L. Towards a cognitive neuroscience of consciousness: basic evidence and a workspace framework. *Cognition,* 2001; **79**: 1–37.

Destrebecqz A and Cleeremans A. Can sequence learning be implicit? New evidence with the process dissociation procedure. *Psychon Bull Rev,* 2001; **8**: 343–50.

Epstein AN. The physiology of thirst. In: Pfaff DW (ed.). Physiological mechanisms of motivation. New York: Springer-Verlag, 1982: 25–55.

Eriksen CW. Discrimination and learning without awareness: a methodological survey and evaluation. *Psychol Rev*, 1960; **67**: 279–300.

Gallistel CR, Fairhurst S, and Balsam P. The learning curve: implications of a quantitative analysis. *Proc Natl Acad Sci U S A*, 2004; **101**: 13124–31.

Graybiel AM. The basal ganglia: learning new tricks and loving it. *Curr Opin Neurobiol*, 2005; **15**: 638–44.

Greenwald AG. New look 3. Unconscious cognition reclaimed. *Am Psychol* 1992; **47**: 766–79.

Hikosaka O, Nakahara H, Rand MK, Sakai K, Lu X, Nakamura K et al. Parallel neural networks for learning sequential procedures. *Trends Neurosci*, 1999; **22**: 464–71.

Holender D. Semantic activation without conscious identification in dichotic listening, parafoveal vision, and visual masking: a survey and appraisal. *Behav Brain Sci*, 1986; **9**: 1–23.

Jenkins HM and Moore BR. The form of the auto-shaped response with food or water reinforcers. *J Exp Anal Behav*, 1973; **20**: 163–81.

Kamin LJ. Selective association and conditioning. In: Mackintosh NJ and Honig WK (eds). *Fundamental issues in instrumental learning*. Halifax: Dalhousie University Press, 1969: 42–64.

Knight DC, Nguyen HT, and Bandettini PA. Expression of conditional fear with and without awareness. *Proc Natl Acad Sci U S A*, 2003; **100**: 15280–3.

Knowlton BJ, Mangels JA, and Squire LR. A neostriatal habit learning system in humans. *Science*, 1996; **273**: 1399–402.

Kouider S and Dehaene S. Levels of processing during non-conscious perception: a critical review of visual masking. *Philos Trans R Soc Lond B Biol Sci*, 2007; **362**: 857–75.

Kunst-Wilson WR and Zajonc RB. Affective discrimination of stimuli that cannot be recognized. *Science*, 1980; **207**: 557–8.

Lagnado DA, Newell BR, Kahan S, and Shanks DR. Insight and strategy in multiple-cue learning. *J Exp Psychol Gen*, 2006; **135**: 162–83.

Lau HC. A higher order Bayesian decision theory of consciousness. *Prog Brain Res*, 2008; **168**: 35–48.

Marcel AJ. Conscious and unconscious perception: experiments on visual masking and word recognition. *Cognit Psychol*, 1983; **15**: 197–237.

Marzi CA, Minelli A, and Savazzi S. Is blindsight in normals akin to blindsight following brain damage? *Prog Brain Res*, 2004; **144**: 295–303.

McClure SM, Daw ND, and Montague PR. A computational substrate for incentive salience. *Trends Neurosci*, 2003; **26**: 423–8.

Miller NE and Neal E. *Miller: selected papers*. Chicago: Aldine Atherton, 1971.

Miller NE and Kessen ML. Reward effects of food via stomach fistula compared with those of food via mouth. *J Comp Physiol Psychol*, 1952; **45**: 555–64.

Olsson A and Phelps EA. Learned fear of "unseen" faces after Pavlovian, observational, and instructed fear. *Psychol Sci*, 2004; **15**: 822–8.

Packard MG and Knowlton BJ. Learning and memory functions of the Basal Ganglia. *Annu Rev Neurosci*, 2002; **25**: 563–93.

Pavlov PI. *Conditioned reflexes*. London: Oxford University Press, 1927.

Pecina S, Smith KS, and Berridge KC. Hedonic hot spots in the brain. *Neuroscientist*, 2006; **12**: 500–11.

Pessiglione M, Petrovic P, Daunizeau J, Palminteri S, Dolan RJ, and Frith CD. Subliminal instrumental conditioning demonstrated in the human brain. *Neuron*, 2008; **59**: 561–7.

Pessiglione M, Schmidt L, Draganski B, Kalisch R, Lau H, Dolan RJ et al. How the brain translates money into force: a neuroimaging study of subliminal motivation. *Science*, 2007; **316**: 904–6.

Pessiglione M, Seymour B, Flandin G, Dolan RJ, and Frith CD. Dopamine-dependent prediction errors underpin reward-seeking behaviour in humans. *Nature*, 2006; **442**(7106): 1042–5.

Pfaffmann C. The pleasures of sensation. *Psychol Rev,* 1960; **67**: 253–68.

Pierce CS and Jastrow J. On small differences in sensation. *Mem Natl Acad Sci,* 1884; **3**: 75–83.

Pratkanis AR. The cargo-cult science of subliminal persuasion. *Skept Inq,* 1992; **16**: 260–72.

Reingold EM and Merikle PM. Using direct and indirect measures to study perception without awareness. *Percept Psychophys,* 1988; **44**: 563–75.

Rescorla RA and Wagner AR. A theory of Pavlovian conditioning: variations in the effectiveness of reinforcement and nonreinforcement. In: Black AH and Prokasy WF (eds). *Classical conditioning II: Current research and theory.* New York: Appleton-Century-Crofts, 1972: 64–99.

Robbins TW and Everitt BJ. Neurobehavioral mechanisms of reward and motivation. *Curr Opin Neurobiol,* 1996; **6**: 228–36.

Schmidt L, d'Arc BF, Lafargue G, Galanaud D, Czernecki V, Grabli D et al. Disconnecting force from money: effects of basal ganglia damage on incentive motivation. *Brain,* 2008; **131**: 1303–10.

Schultz W, Dayan P, and Montague PR. A neural substrate of prediction and reward. *Science,* 1997; **275**: 1593–9.

Sherrington CS. *The integrative action of the nervous system.* New York: C. Scribner's Sons, 1906.

Sidis B. *The psychology of suggestion.* New York: Appleton, 1898.

Teitelbaum P. The use of operant methods in the assessment and control of motivational states. In: Honig WK (ed.). *Operant behavior: areas of research and application.* New York: Appleton-Century-Crofts, 1966: 565–608.

Thorndike EL. *Animal intelligence: experimental studies.* New York: Macmillan, 1911.

Toates F. *Motivational systems.* Cambridge: Cambridge University Press, 1986.

Valenstein ES. The interpretation of behavior evoked by brain stimulation. In: Wauquier A and Rolls ET (eds). *Brain-stimulation reward.* New York: Elsevier, 1976: 557–75.

Visser TA, Merikle PM. Conscious and unconscious processes: the effects of motivation. *Conscious Cogn,* 1999; **8**: 94–113.

Walton ME, Kennerley SW, Bannerman DM, Phillips PE, and Rushworth MF. Weighing up the benefits of work: behavioral and neural analyses of effort-related decision-making. *Neural Netw,* 2006; **19**: 1302–14.

Weiskrantz L. *Consciousness lost and found.* Oxford: Oxford University Press, 1999.

Wilkinson L and Shanks DR. Intentional control and implicit sequence learning. *J Exp Psychol Learn Mem Cogn,* 2004; **30**: 354–69.

Williams DR and Williams H. Auto-maintenance in the pigeon: sustained pecking despite contingent non-reinforcement. *J Exp Anal Behav,* 1969; **12**: 511–20.

Wolf S and Wolff HG. *Human gastric function, an experimental study of a man and his stomach.* London: Oxford University Press, 1943.

Young PT. Hedonic organization and regulation of behavior. *Psychol Rev,* 1966; **73**: 59–86.

Chapter 16

Role of striatal dopamine in the fast adaption of outcome-based decisions

Roshan Cools

Abstract

The prefrontal cortex interacts with a set of deep brain subcortical structures, including in particular the striatum, to bias flexible decision making. The output of these fronto-striatal circuits is sensitive to modulation by brain dopamine. However, the relationship between dopamine and flexible decision making is complex and the effects of dopaminergic drugs are both baseline-dependent and outcome-specific. Specifically, opposite effects are observed on reward- and punishment-based reversal learning and in subjects with high and low baseline dopamine function. The reviewed results suggest that the striatum might mediate these opposite effects on reversal learning, even when it requires only the fast (single trial) adaptation of predictions based on explicit cues.

16.1 Introduction

Brain dopamine has been implicated in a wide variety of cognitive processes. Best known are its contributions to reinforcement (and habit) learning (Hollerman and Schultz, 1998; Dayan, 2008), as well as working memory (Goldman-Rakic, 1992). The data reviewed in this chapter suggest that dopamine is important not only for incremental reinforcement or habit learning and working memory, but also for the ability to rapidly adjust predictions based on explicit cues.

This high-level cognitive control of flexible behavior has been associated most commonly with the prefrontal cortex (PFC). Indeed, dopamine might act at the level of the PFC to affect high-level cognitive control. However, we also know that this region does not act in isolation, but rather interacts with a set of deep-brain subcortical structures, including the striatum. Furthermore, dopamine receptors are most abundant in the striatum. Consistent with this arrangement, we here elaborate on the working hypothesis that it is indeed the striatum that mediates the dopaminergic modulation of high-level flexible decision making, even when it implicates only the rapid single-trial adjustment of predictions based on explicit (outcome) cues.

16.1.1 Measuring flexible decision making

The experimental model that has been used most frequently to study the neurobiological mechanisms of flexible outcome-based decision making is the reversal learning paradigm. In standard probabilistic reversal learning paradigms, contingencies are instrumental and probabilistic, so that subjects choose a stimulus that is usually rewarded and avoid a stimulus that is usually punished. Specifically, on each trial, subjects are presented with two visual patterns (e.g. rectangles of colored stripes; Fig. 16.1). The task typically consists of an initial simple probabilistic visual discrimination, in which subjects have to learn to choose between the two patterns: one, for instance, with an 80:20 ratio of positive:negative feedback, and another with an 20:80 ratio of positive:negative feedback. Optimal performance maximizes reward and depends on consistent choices of the 80:20 pattern. This choice strategy should be maintained despite the so-called "probabilistic errors." After having completed this initial discrimination, the task proceeds to the second, reversal stage in which contingencies are reversed, without warning, so that the previously "incorrect" pattern is now usually rewarded and vice versa for the previously "correct" pattern. Upon reversal, the previously rewarded stimulus becomes punished and subjects must learn to select the other (previously punished) stimulus. Subjects typically perseverate and continue to respond to the previously rewarded pattern before eventually reversing their choice, after the so-called "final reversal error," to the newly rewarded pattern.

Flexible behavior on such tasks requires, among other things, the anticipation of biologically relevant events by learning signals of their occurrence, i.e., prediction. Models of reinforcement learning use a temporal difference prediction error signal, representing the difference between expected and obtained events, to update their predictions based on states of the environment (Sutton and Barto, 1998). A putative neuronal mechanism of the temporal prediction error signal for future reward is the fast phasic firing of dopamine cells in the ventral tegmental area (Montague et al., 1996; Schultz et al., 1997). According to this proposal, positive prediction error of reward, i.e., unexpected reward, produces a burst in the firing of dopamine neurons, whereas negative prediction error of reward, i.e., unexpected omission of reward, produces a pause in the firing of dopamine neurons. As such, the hypothesis that flexible decision making depends on dopamine is generally consistent with neurophysiological and computational evidence from the domain of reinforcement learning (Montague et al., 1996; Schultz et al., 1997; Frank, 2005).

Although demands for reinforcement learning are high in reversal learning paradigms, it should be recognized that reversal learning constitutes a special case of reinforcement learning. Adequate performance also depends on other processes, including prepotent response inhibition and stimulus-switching, when contingencies are reversed. Furthermore, simple reinforcement learning models do not encompass all aspects of reversal learning. For example, Hampton et al. (2006) have compared models to explain behavioral performance and neural activity (in the ventromedial prefrontal cortex) during a probabilistic reversal learning task. One model simulated knowledge of the abstract task structure, by which reversal is accompanied not only by value updating of the previously rewarded (chosen) stimulus, but also by value updating of the previously punished (unchosen)

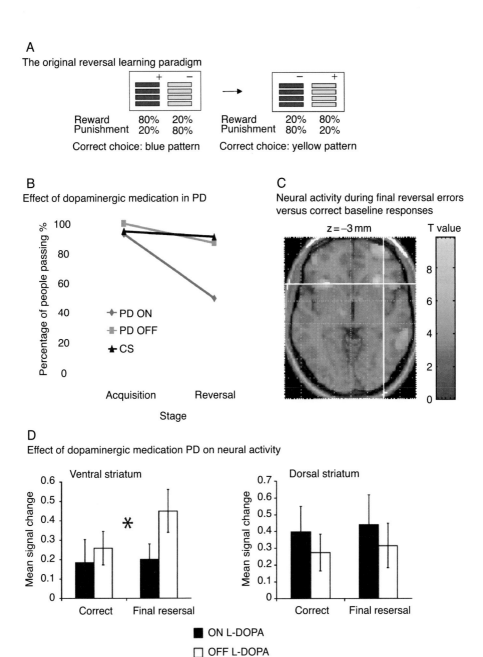

Fig. 16.1 (A) The probabilistic reversal learning paradigm. On each trial, subjects are presented two visual patterns (location randomized); one associated with an 80:20 ratio of positive:negative feedback and another with an 20:80 ratio of positive:negative feedback. Subjects choose between the two patterns. After a number of correct choices of the usually rewarded pattern, the contingencies reverse. Upon reversal, subjects shift to choosing the pattern that was previously usually punished and avoid the pattern that was previously usually rewarded. R. Cools, et al., Enhanced or Impaired Cognitive Function in Parkinson's Disease as a Function of Dopaminergic Medication and Task Demands, *Cerebral Cortex*, 2001 11(12) by permission of Oxford University Press. (B) Effect of dopaminergic medication in Parkinson's disease (PD) on probabilistic reversal learning (Cools et al., 2001). Significantly more patients ON their medication failed to obtain learning criterion at the reversal stage of the task than patients

Fig. 16.1 (*Contd.*) OFF their medication and age- and education-matched controls. There was no effect of group on the initial acquisition stage of the task. (C) Neural activity in healthy young volunteers during probabilistic reversal learning Reprinted from *Journal of Neuroscience*, 2002, R.Cools, L.Clark, A.M.Owen, and T.W.Robbins, Copyright 2002, with permission from Society of Neuroscience. Neural activity was increased in the ventral striatum, ventrolateral prefrontal cortex, dorsomedial prefrontal cortex and posterior parietal cortex during the final reversal error relative to baseline correct responses. (D) Effect of dopaminergic medication in PD on neural activity during probabilistic reversal learning Reprinted by permission from Macmillan Publishers Ltd: *Neuropsychopharmacology*, 32(1) R.Cools, S.J.G.Lewis, L.Clark, R.A.Barker, and T.W.Robbins, L-DOPA Disrupts Activity in the Nucleus Accumbers during Reversal Learning in Parkinson's Disease, Copyright 2007. PD patients exhibited increased activity in the ventral striatum (and other areas) during the final reversal error relative to baseline correct responses. This reversal-related activity in the ventral striatum (but not in other brain areas) was abolished when the same patients were scanned ON medication.

stimulus. The other model simulated simple reinforcement learning that did not incorporate such higher order knowledge. Performance and neural activity was fit better by the model that also simulated knowledge of the abstract task structure, i.e., knowledge about interdependencies between actions. Thus probabilistic reversal learning depends not necessarily only on implicit reinforcement learning, but might also implicate explicit higher order knowledge leading to the adoption of explicit decision strategies.

Probabilistic reversal learning paradigms with such a higher order abstract structure provide a unique opportunity to assess separately the neurobiological mechanisms of, on the one hand, outcome-induced adjustment based on explicit decision strategy, and, on the other hand, those of outcome-induced adjustment based on implicit decision strategy (i.e., reinforcement learning). For example, a recent electroencephalography study with healthy volunteers revealed that the negative deflection in electrical activity observed during punishment over the medial frontal cortex (also referred to as the feedback-related negativity; FRN), correlated significantly and positively with a (reinforcement learning model-derived) reward prediction error signal during a probabilistic reversal learning task (Chase et al., in press). Interestingly, the FRN (and the prediction error signal) was greatest during the probabilistic (misleading) errors that did not lead to immediate behavioral adjustment and was absent during the final reversal error that was followed directly by immediate behavioral adjustment. By contrast, a positive deflection was observed, corresponding to the P3, which was larger during the final reversal error than during probabilistic errors (Chase et al., in press). This finding suggests that the FRN signals implicit decisions based on reinforcement learning, while the P3 signals more explicit decision strategies based on higher order knowledge of the abstract task structure.

16.1.2 Investigating the role of dopamine in flexible decision making

One way to study the role of dopamine in human decision making is by assessing the effects of dopaminergic drugs; for example, in patients with Parkinson's disease (PD). Accumulating evidence indicates that there is large variability in the effects of dopaminergic drugs, which may either enhance or impair flexible decision making. The identification of factors that contribute to this large variability in drug efficacy has already helped to elucidate the complex relationship between dopamine and flexible decision making. Two of these factors will be highlighted in the present review.

First, drug effects depend on task demands and associated neural systems, so that, within the same people, the same drug improves some forms of flexible decision making, while simultaneously impairing other forms of flexible decision making. This point is illustrated by the observation that the same dopamine-enhancing drugs can improve the rapid switching between two well-learnt tasks, and simultaneously impair outcome-based reversal learning in mild PD patients (Cools et al., 2001). Furthermore, dopamine-enhancing drugs can even have opposite effects within one and the same paradigm of reversal learning, depending on the valence of the unexpected outcome that signals the reversal (see below). Second, drug effects depend on baseline dopamine levels, so that suboptimal dopamine levels are remedied, while already optimized dopamine levels are detrimentally overdosed by the same drug (Williams and Goldman-Rakic, 1995; Zahrt et al., 1997; Arnsten, 1998). Indeed stratification of drug effects by individual differences in baseline dopamine function has helped to isolate some important effects of dopamine (see below).

16.2 Flexible decision making in Parkinson's disease

Mild PD provides a particularly good model for investigating these task- and baseline-dependent effects of dopamine-enhancing drugs on flexible decision making for the following three reasons. First, the primary abnormality in the earliest stages of the disease is dopamine depletion in the striatum. The striatum is well known to be critical for flexible decision making as evidenced, for instance, by animal research demonstrating that lesions of the striatum impair reversal learning (Divac et al., 1967; Taghzouti et al., 1985; Annett et al., 1989; Stern and Passingham, 1995; Clarke et al., 2008). This is further supported by neuroimaging research in humans, which demonstrates an increased blood oxygenation level-dependent response in the striatum during the punishment events that signal the need for reversal (Cools et al., 2002). Second, PD is characterized by a spatiotemporal progression of dopamine depletion so that, at least in the early stages of the disease, there is an imbalance of dopamine with the most severe depletion occurring in the dorsal parts of the striatum, but with relatively preserved dopamine levels in the ventral striatum (Kish et al., 1988). Thus, PD is accompanied by naturally occurring variation in baseline dopamine levels within brain regions critically implicated in flexible decision making. A final reason for studying medication effects in PD is the known paradoxical effects of medication on cognitive function in these patients. Specifically, some PD patients exhibit compulsive medication intake, pathological gambling, or other forms of impulse control failure. It is thought that the common dopamine-enhancing medication, known to remedy the motor symptoms of the disease, might contribute to the development of this harmful pattern of severe decision-making abnormalities. How can the same medication improve some functions in PD, while impairing other functions?

Based on evidence from studies with experimental animals, indicating that too much dopamine can be as bad for cognitive performance as can too little dopamine (Williams and Goldman-Rakic, 1995; Zahrt et al., 1997; Arnsten, 1998), we and others have proposed the medication overdose hypothesis to account for the contrasting medication effects in PD (Gotham et al., 1988; Swainson et al., 2000; Cools et al., 2001). This hypothesis states that medication doses necessary to remedy the dopamine lack in the dorsal striatum may detrimentally "overdose" any area where dopamine levels are relatively intact, such as, for example, in the ventral striatum. To test this hypothesis, performance of a group of patients ON their normal dopaminergic medication was compared with that of a group of patients after they had abstained from their dopaminergic medication for about 18 h prior to the assessment (Cools et al., 2001, 2003). We assessed performance on a series of tasks associated with distinct fronto-striatal circuits. According to the medication overdose hypothesis, a beneficial effect of medication was predicted on tasks associated with the depleted dorsal striatum, but a detrimental overdose effect was predicted on tasks associated with relatively intact ventral fronto-striatal circuitry. First, our patients completed a paradigm of rapid task-switching (Rogers and Monsell, 1995), well-known to activate dorsolateral cortical brain areas, such as the lateral PFC and the posterior parietal cortex. Both these regions are strongly connected with the, in PD, severely depleted dorsal striatum. Dopaminergic medication was predicted to remediate an impairment on this task. The same patients also performed a task of probabilistic reversal learning, which implicates the ventral striatum, as well as the strongly connected ventral prefrontal cortex (Divac et al., 1967; Dias et al., 1996; Cools et al., 2002; Fellows and Farah, 2003; Clarke et al., 2008). This ventral circuit is relatively intact in PD and, accordingly, detrimental overdose effects of medication were predicted on reversal learning, i.e., impairment in patients ON medication relative to patients OFF medication. The results were consistent with the medication overdose hypothesis. On the one hand, dopaminergic medication remediated a task-switching deficit, associated with the severely depleted brain regions. By contrast, the same dopaminergic medication impaired reversal learning, associated with the relatively intact ventral striatum (Cools et al., 2001). These data suggest that dopaminergic medication in mild PD improves some cognitive functions by restoring dopamine levels in severely depleted brain areas like the dorsal striatum, while impairing other cognitive functions by detrimentally overdosing dopamine levels in relatively intact brain areas, like the ventral striatum.

To test this medication overdose hypothesis more directly, we subsequently investigated neural activity in PD with functional magnetic resonance imaging (fMRI). Specifically, a pharmacological fMRI experiment was designed to assess whether the behavioral effect of medication on probabilistic reversal learning was accompanied by a neural effect of medication during reversal learning on the ventral but not the dorsal striatum. A group of eight mild PD patients was scanned on two occasions: once ON their normal dopaminergic medication and once OFF their dopaminergic medication. In the scanner, subjects performed a probabilistic reversal learning task that was identical to the task used in the earlier neuropsychological study, apart from the fact that the fMRI task required multiple serial reversals (Cools et al., 2002). Again, subjects were presented with two abstract visual patterns; they had to choose the one that was usually correct. The contingencies were probabilistic, so that a correct response would occasionally lead to spurious negative feedback. Contingencies reversed following on average 12 correct trials. Following reversal, subjects would typically perseverate, that is, stick to the previously relevant pattern for a few trials, before eventually reversing to the newly relevant pattern. The critical event of interest was the final reversal error, which was by definition followed by the subjects switching their responding. Consistent with the overdose hypothesis, dopaminergic medication in PD modulated activity during this critical final reversal error in the relatively intact ventral striatum, but not in the severely depleted dorsal striatum (or the PFC). Patients OFF medication exhibited significant reversal-related activity centered on the nucleus accumbens (Cools et al., 2007), similar to that seen in healthy volunteers in an earlier study (Cools et al., 2002). Critically, this reversal-related activity was abolished when the same patients were scanned ON their medication. These neural effects were not confounded by differences between medication sessions in terms of performance, because medication did not induce an impairment on this well-practiced version of the task, in which reversals occurred over and over again.

The effect of dopamine-enhancing drugs on reversal-related activity in the ventral striatum is not restricted to PD patients, but extends to healthy volunteers whose dopamine neurons are intact, as predicted by the overdose hypothesis (Dodds et al., 2008; Clark et al., in preparation). In a study by Clark et al., healthy elderly volunteers were scanned during the exact same probabilistic reversal learning task with fMRI on two occasions: once after intake of an oral dose of levodopa (Sinemet 275 consisting of 250 mg levodopa and 25 mg carbidopa), and once after placebo. They found that, like dopaminergic medication in PD patients (Cools et al., 2007), levodopa in healthy elderly volunteers abolished reversal-related activity in the ventral striatum selectively during the punishment events that led to behavioral reversal. In another study by Dodds et al. (Dodds et al., 2008), young, healthy subjects were scanned on two occasions: once after intake of an oral dose of the catecholamine-enhancer methylphenidate (40mg) (which increases dopamine and noradrenaline), and once after placebo, again using the same reversal task. Methylphenidate abolished neural activity in the ventral striatum during punishment events that led to behavioral adjustment. Conversely, no such effects were seen during punishment events that did not lead to behavioral adjustment. The effects of levodopa and methylphenidate during the final reversal errors were selective to the ventral striatum and did not extend to other brain regions. Although the precise neural locus of the effects of levodopa and methylphenidate in healthy volunteers, i.e., the ventrolateral putamen, differed somewhat from that of medication in PD, i.e., centered on the nucleus accumbens, the similarity of these three patterns is remarkable. The discrepancy in the precise localization might reflect a genuine difference between dopaminergic modulation in healthy subjects versus PD patients. Alternatively, the discrepancy in precise localization within the ventral striatum might reflect the limits of fMRI localization due to low-level movement artifacts or suboptimal normalization procedures.

The selective effect of dopaminergic medication in PD on activity in the ventral striatum might well underlie the drug-induced impairment on reversal learning seen in the earlier neuropsychological study with PD patients (Cools et al., 2001). Furthermore, this drug-induced reversal deficit might contribute to the very severe decision-making abnormalities, such as pathological gambling and compulsive drug-use, seen in some PD patients. Indeed, PD patients with such severe decision-making abnormalities have been shown to exhibit excessive dopamine release in the ventral but not the dorsal striatum (Evans et al., 2006).

The overdose hypothesis could be further substantiated in future pharmacological fMRI studies with mild PD patients and matched controls. Specifically, dopaminergic drug effects should be assessed using tasks that activate both the dorsal and the ventral striatum. This approach will pave the way for a double dissociation within the same mild PD patients, with medication normalizing dorsal striatal activity, while disrupting ventral striatal activity. Conversely, in controls, medication should disrupt activity in both the ventral and the dorsal striatum, where dopamine levels should still be intact.

16.3 Parsing flexible decision making into punishment and reward components

The above-reviewed studies demonstrated not only that dopamine-enhancing drugs in mild PD can impair reversal learning, but also that they might do so by modulating processing in the relatively intact ventral striatum. What these studies did not demonstrate, however, was the exact neurocognitive mechanism by which dopamine impairs reversal learning. One major problem with the original (instrumental) reversal learning paradigm is that adequate reversal depends on multiple processes. Contingencies in this paradigm are instrumental; subjects are required to choose a rewarded stimulus and to avoid a punished stimulus, and thus have control over their outcomes. Upon reversal, the previously rewarded stimulus becomes punished and subjects must learn to select the other (previously punished) stimulus. Therefore, at the time of reversal (signaled by punishment; Cools et al., 2002; O'Doherty et al., 2003a; Remijnse et al., 2005; Hampton and O'Doherty J, 2007) subjects have to learn to both avoid the newly punished stimulus and to choose the newly rewarded stimulus. The critical punishment event signaling a reversal in these previous studies confounds, at least: (1) the need to establish a new association between the previously relevant stimulus and punishment; (2) the need to establish a new association between the newly relevant stimulus and reward; (3) the need to stop responding to the previously rewarded, but newly punished stimulus (i.e., response inhibition); and (4) the need to facilitate responding to the previously punished, but newly rewarded stimulus. The reversal deficit obtained in our previous study with PD patients might reflect any of these processes.

To better understand the role of dopamine in reversal learning, we recently conducted another medication withdrawal study in PD patients, for which we designed a novel reversal paradigm that allowed the separate assessment of its subcomponent processes. Specifically, based on recent work by Frank and colleagues (Frank et al., 2004), we were

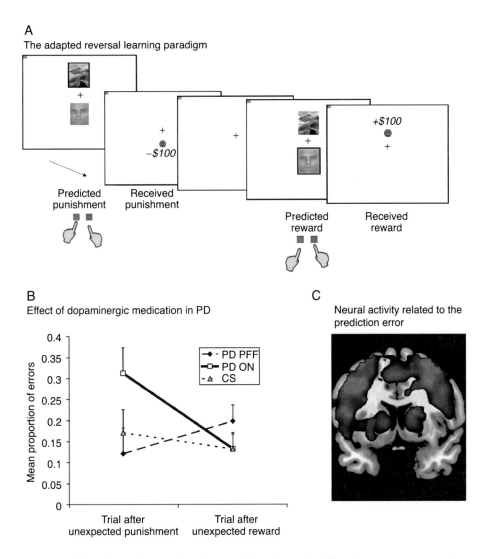

Fig. 16.2 (A) The adapted reversal learning paradigm. On each trial, subjects were presented two visual patterns, one associated with reward, the other associated with punishment. One of the two patterns was highlighted with a thick black border. Subjects predicted whether this highlighted stimulus would lead to reward or punishment. After their prediction (indicated by a left or right response on a red or green button), the outcome was presented, which depended on the highlighted stimulus and not on the response. Contingencies reversed repeatedly. Such reversals were signaled, either by an unexpected punishment (presented after a previously reward pattern was highlighted) or by an unexpected reward (presented after a previously punished pattern was highlighted). (B) Effect of dopaminergic medication in PD patients on reversal based on unexpected reward and reversal based on unexpected punishment (Cools et al., 2006). The mean proportion of errors on trials after the unexpected reward and the unexpected punishment are presented separately. Patients ON medication made more errors on trials after unexpected punishment than on trials after unexpected reward. This bias was reversed in patients OFF medication. (C) Neural activity related to the prediction error in young

Fig. 16.2 (*contd.*) healthy volunteers (Robinson et al., 2010). Activity related to the valence-independent absolute prediction error is displayed in red (all T-values > 2.5). Activity related to the valence-dependent, signed prediction error is displayed in blue (all t-values > 2.5).

interested to disentangle the new learning, upon reversal, of reward contingencies from the new learning, upon reversal, of punishment contingencies. In this novel paradigm (Fig. 16.2A), we presented two visual patterns (a face and a scene), one of which was associated with reward (a green, smiley face and a "+$100" sign), and one of which was associated with punishment (a red, sad face and a "–$100" sign). In the traditional reversal task, subjects had to choose between the stimuli in order to maximize reward. This was not the case in the novel paradigm. Instead, in the novel task the computer selected one of the stimuli by highlighting it with a thick black box. The subject then simply had to predict whether this highlighted stimulus would lead to reward or punishment; i.e., they had no control over these outcomes. Their prediction (indicated by a right or left button press) was followed by the actual outcome (either reward or punishment; Fig. 16.2A). Subjects were not provided with direct performance feedback but simply had to match their prediction with the outcome. For example, on a correct punishment prediction trial, subjects would both predict punishment and receive punishment. In other words, it was not the *response* of the subject that elicited reward or punishment, but rather the stimulus preceding the response; contingencies were no longer instrumental. Outcomes were deterministic and contingencies reversed after a variable criterion of 4, 5, or 6 correct responses.

The task consisted of two conditions. In one condition, reversals were signaled by unexpected punishment (after a previously rewarded stimulus was highlighted), while in the other, reversals were signaled by unexpected reward (after a previously punished stimulus was highlighted). On reversal trials of the unexpected reward condition, for instance, the previously punished stimulus was highlighted and followed unexpectedly by reward (Cools et al., 2006). The critical measure of interest was accuracy on the trial immediately after the unexpected outcome, which thus indexed fast single-trial adjustment of predictions based on relatively explicit (outcome) cues. Accuracy on these reversal trials measured how sensitive subjects were to unexpected reward versus unexpected punishment. A further advantage of the novel task was that it minimized demands for prepotent response inhibition, whilst matching response requirements between conditions. Both unexpected reward and unexpected punishment required a reversal of the prediction response, i.e., inhibition of the previous response and activation of the novel response. A deficit restricted to either of these two conditions could not be accounted for by a process that was not specific to the outcome-type, like response inhibition or response activation. Therefore, this new design enabled, for the first time, the separate measurement of fast single-trial reversal of predictions based on punishment and fast single-trial reversal of predictions based on reward.

Results revealed that there was no difference between the reward and punishment conditions in the healthy control subjects. However, dopaminergic medication in PD patients altered the balance between fast reversal based on unexpected reward and fast reversal based on unexpected punishment, so that patients ON medication had difficulty with punishment-based reversal, not with reward-based reversal (Cools et al., 2006). Conversely, patients OFF medication, if anything, had greater difficulty with reversal in the reward than in the punishment condition. Thus dopaminergic medication in PD induced a shift away from punishment-based reversal learning toward reward-based reversal learning. These results are remarkably consistent with those obtained using an entirely different probabilistic instrumental learning task by Frank et al. (Frank et al., 2004). Specifically, Frank et al. asked PD patients to choose between stimuli, some of which were rewarded more often than others. In this paradigm, outcomes depended on the subjects' choices, so subjects had control over their outcomes. At a subsequent test stage, subjects were presented novel combinations of these same stimuli, but this time no feedback was provided. PD patients were better at choosing the stimulus associated during the initial instrumental learning task with the highest reward probability than at avoiding the stimulus associated with the highest punishment probability. However, this was only the case when they were ON their medication. Withdrawal of medication reversed this bias, improving the avoidance of the punished stimulus relative to the approach of the rewarded stimulus. Subsequent studies have further strengthened these effects by revealing that parallel changes in reward–punishment biases are obtained in the response time domain. Medication facilitated response time speeding for reward maximization, but impaired response time slowing for punishment avoidance (Moustafa et al., 2008). Our study extends this work by showing that similar effects are seen also on fast single-trial reversal tasks, which do not require "implicit" incremental reinforcement learning but rather the rapid adaptation of predictions based on explicit (outcome) cues. Furthermore, the data from the novel prediction-based reversal task showed that the dopamine-induced bias towards reward and away from punishment is also observed when demands for response inhibition or activation are matched between conditions. Thus our study showed that the effects of dopamine on reinforcement learning tasks might reflect effects on the instantaneous formation of Pavlovian contingencies, rather than on the slow formation of instrumental actions or habits. An altered bias in the balance between fast updating of reward- and punishment-predictions might well underlie the dopamine-related deficit on the original probabilistic reversal learning task (Cools et al., 2001), as well as altered performance on other learning tasks, including the probabilistic selection task (Frank et al., 2004) and category learning tasks (Shohamy et al., 2006; 2008). In all these tasks, performance will be affected by changes in the ability to rapidly update reward and punishment predictions. Furthermore, poor punishment prediction might also underlie abnormal behavior on gambling tasks (Cools et al., 2003), e.g. by leading to reduced loss aversion (Moustafa et al., 2008).

16.4 Role of the striatum in flexible outcome-based decision making

So far, we have learned that (1) dopamine-enhancing drugs can impair probabilistic reversal learning; (2) dopamine-enhancing drugs abolish neural activity in the ventral striatum during probabilistic reversal learning. Specifically, they disrupt activity during the punishment event that leads to behavioral adjustment, but not during punishment that does not lead to behavioral adjustment. Finally (3) a dopamine-induced deficit on reversal learning is not restricted to incremental instrumental tasks, which require subjects to update actions and/or habits based on the integration of punishment and reward across a series of trials, but extends to fast single-trial Pavlovian learning tasks, which require subjects to rapidly adjust their predictions of punishment relative to those of reward.

Although these independent studies are consistent with each other and also with data obtained using different paradigms in different laboratories (Frank et al., 2004; Moustafa et al., 2008), they do raise an important question: what exactly is the role of the striatum in reversal learning and, more specifically, in the deficit caused by dopamine-enhancing drugs? The punishment-related activity in the striatum (observed in healthy volunteers and PD patients, who are OFF, but not ON dopamine-enhancing medication) during the original reversal paradigm is in apparent contrast to the robust finding that the striatum is active during reward processing. Activity in the striatum is seen during reward receipt (Schultz, 2002; O'Doherty et al., 2004; Yacubian et al., 2006) and/or during reward antic-ipation (Yacubian et al., 2006; Hare et al., 2008). Conversely, activity in the striatum is less consistently found during punishment. In fact, activity in the striatum is sometimes reduced below baseline during punishment (or reward omission) (McClure et al., 2003; O'Doherty et al., 2003b; Pessiglione et al., 2006; Yacubian et al., 2006; Tom et al., 2007; but see: Seymour et al., 2004, 2005, 2007; Jensen et al., 2007; Delgado et al., 2008). Yet, in our reversal studies, striatal activity is found (and abolished by dopamine-enhancing drugs) during the receipt of punishment, albeit only when this punishment signals behav-ioral adjustment. An important unresolved question, therefore, is whether we can recon-cile the generally accepted role of the striatum in reward processing with its role in reversal learning. One possibility is that the activity in the striatum during probabilistic reversal learning simply reflects the salience of the critical punishment event leading to behavioral adjustment (Zink et al., 2003). However, as noted above, the critical punishment event signaling reversals in the original paradigm confounds multiple processes and is accompanied not only by the processing of the salient punishment event, but also by prepotent response inhibition, new (Pavlovian) reward predictions and new (Pavlovian) punishment predictions. Our novel reversal learning paradigm, in which reversals are signaled by unexpected reward or unexpected punishment (Fig. 16.2A) provided a good model for disentangling these different possibilities. Salience and demands for response inhibition are matched between the reward and punishment conditions of this new task, as evidenced by the finding that accuracy on trials after unexpected rewards did not differ from that on trials after unexpected punishment in control subjects. Thus, if striatal activ-ity during reversal learning reflects salience-coding or response inhibition, then the unexpected reward and punishment events would activate the same region of the stria-tum to the same degree. Conversely, if striatal activity during reversal learning reflects valence-dependent coding, e.g. the aversive prediction error or the appetitive prediction error, then the unexpected reward and punishment events would activate (different parts of) the striatum to different degrees. Preliminary fMRI data from 16 young healthy volunteers (Robinson et al., in preparation) revealed that the answer to this question is: both; that is, distinct parts of the striatum exhibited valence-independent coding and valence-dependent coding of unexpected outcomes. To assess which brain regions conformed to valence-independent coding, for example, reflecting salience or response inhibition, we looked at activity associated with the absolute prediction error, derived from fitting a standard reinforcement learning model (see Cools et al., 2009, supplement for details). This analysis demonstrated highly significant valence-independent activity extending into the ventromedial striatum, as well as the dorsal anterior cingulate cortex, the ventrolateral PFC, and the orbitofrontal cortex. Conversely, to assess which brain regions conformed to valence-dependent coding, we looked at activity associated with the signed (appetitive) prediction error. Like the valence-independent analysis, this analysis also revealed activity in the striatum and the orbitofrontal cortex, albeit at a lower statistical threshold. However, this valence-dependent activity was located in different fronto-striatal regions, specifically, in more dorsal and lateral regions of the striatum, i.e., the putamen and the dorsal caudate nucleus, and in orbitofrontal regions just posterior to those seen in the valence-independent analysis (Fig. 16.2C). No increases in activity were found for the reverse contrast, i.e., the signed aversive prediction error.

The interpretation of the valence-independent activity remains somewhat ambiguous. It might represent (overlapping or adjacent) co-representation of distinct appetitive and aversive prediction errors in the striatum, as has been shown previously in the context of Pavlovian learning (Seymour et al., 2004; 2005; 2007; Jensen et al., 2007). Alternatively, it might reflect processing that is present in both our unexpected reward and punishment conditions, such as salience or response inhibition. The response inhibition account of the valence-nonspecific activity in the striatum, which was centered on the caudate nucleus, is plausible in the context of disrupted reversal learning after lesions in the caudate nucleus of monkeys (Divac et al., 1967; Clarke et al., 2008). These monkeys with lesions in the caudate nucleus displayed perseveration or disinhibition of responding when they encountered unexpected outcomes. However, we cannot exclude the possibility that the valence-independent activity seen in our study simply reflects the salience of the unexpected outcome. Indeed the finding of distinct valence-independent and valence-dependent patterns of activity in the striatum is also remarkable in the context of recent electrophysiological data from Matsumoto and Hikosaka (2009). These researchers recorded single-neuron activity in the midbrain of monkeys who performed a Pavlovian learning paradigm. The data revealed that different deeper and more superficial populations of midbrain dopamine neurons exhibit different responses to unexpected reward and unexpected punishment. Specifically, some populations of dopamine neurons exhibited valence-coding (increased firing for reward, decreased firing for punishment) and other neurons exhibited salience-coding of outcomes (increased firing for both reward and punishment). Future pharmacological fMRI studies will demonstrate whether the opposite effects of dopaminergic drugs (see above and below) are accompanied by distinct modulation of this valence-independent activity and/or valence-dependent activity in the striatum during unexpected reward and unexpected punishment.

16.5 Dopaminergic modulation of fast flexible outcome-based decision making in healthy volunteers

The reviewed studies in PD patients have revealed a key role for dopamine in regulating the balance between (reversal) learning from reward and (reversal) learning from punishment. This role is not specific to one particular task context but extends across different task domains (Frank et al., 2004; Cools et al., 2006; Moustafa et al., 2008). Thus dopamine-enhancing medication in mild PD improves both slow and fast learning based on reward, and impairs both slow and fast learning based on punishment. This shift in valence-specific processing might well underlie the severe impulse control disorder or other more subtle decision-making abnormalities seen in these patients. A critical question is whether this effect of enhancing dopamine on the balance between reward and punishment is also seen in healthy volunteers, as would be predicted from the overdose hypothesis outlined above. Alternatively, the potentiation of reward at the expense of punishment might be restricted to PD, thus reflecting some disease characteristic, like striatal dopamine depletion. To investigate this issue we have assessed the effects of dopamine receptor stimulation in healthy volunteers as a function of their baseline levels of dopamine function (Cools et al., 2009). It turns out that dopaminergic drug effects can be predicted not only from the type of task under study, but also from individual differences in baseline dopamine function. In this study we measured baseline dopamine synthesis capacity using positron emission tomography with the tracer 6-[^{18}F]fluoro-L-m-tyrosine (FMT). FMT is comparable to the more widely used [^{18}F]fluorodopa and indexes presynaptic dopamine synthesis capacity in striatal terminals of midbrain dopamine neurons. Because signal is unreliable in other brain regions of interest, such as the orbitofrontal cortex, we focused only on data from the striatum. There was large individual variability in baseline dopamine function, even in the healthy population, with some individuals having low dopamine synthesis capacity and others having high synthesis capacity. Results revealed that these individual differences in synthesis capacity were associated with individual differences in the effects of our dopaminergic drug. We employed bromocriptine, a dopamine receptor agonist with particular affinity for the D2 receptor family, and used to treat PD. Eleven young, healthy subjects were tested on two occasions: once after intake of a placebo pill, and once after intake of 1.25 mg bromocriptine. They performed the novel, fast-outcome prediction paradigm, enabling the separate investigation of the fast adaptation of reward- and punishment-predictions. As expected, we found a highly significant correlation between fast single-trial updating of reward predictions and baseline dopamine synthesis capacity in the striatum, so that subjects with low dopamine made more errors after unexpected reward than did subjects with high dopamine synthesis capacity. This is consistent with electrophysiological data from monkeys (Hollerman and Schultz, 1998) and shows that individual differences in the fast updating of reward-predictions reflect quantitative variation in baseline dopamine synthesis capacity (Schönberg et al., 2007). Intriguingly, the effect of the dopamine receptor agonist also depended on baseline dopamine synthesis capacity, so that bromocriptine improved the fast updating of reward-predictions to a greater extent in the low-dopamine subjects. In fact, in the high-dopamine subjects, it impaired fast updating of reward-predictions.

Such negative correlations were observed between the effect of bromocriptine and synthesis capacity in both the putamen and the caudate nucleus. This finding is consistent with an inverted U-shaped relationship between dopamine and cognitive performance, by which both insufficient, as well as excessive, dopamine receptor stimulation is associated with impairment (Arnsten, 1998). Until now, evidence for such a relationship was available only for D1 receptor stimulation in the PFC. The present study suggests that similar mechanisms underlie effects of D2 receptor stimulation in the striatum and the updating of outcome-predictions. This conclusion is further substantiated by the recent observation that effects of the nonspecific catecholamine enhancer methylphenidate on probabilistic reversal learning, correlated with drug effects on D2 receptor availability, as measured with $[^{11}C]$-raclopride radioligand positron emission tomography (Clatworthy et al., 2009). In the FMT study, the strongest positive correlation was obtained between synthesis capacity and relative scores, calculated by subtracting accuracy on punishment-predictions from accuracy on reward-predictions. In fact, in the low-dopamine subjects, bromocriptine improved the updating of reward-predictions but actually impaired the updating of punishment-predictions. This bias was reversed in the high-dopamine subjects. Thus, dopamine-enhancing drugs have contrasting effects on the fast updating of reward- and punishment-predictions not only in PD patients, but also in healthy volunteers. Specifically, such drugs benefit the updating of reward- but impair the updating of punishment-predictions in subjects with low dopamine baseline levels, as well as in PD patients. Conversely, they impair the updating of reward-predictions but improve the updating of punishment-predictions in subjects with already optimized or supra-optimal levels of dopamine. It might be noted that variability in dopamine synthesis capacity was measured only in the striatum. It is well possible that individual variability in striatal synthesis capacity correlates with individual variability in synthesis capacity in other brain regions. Therefore, we cannot draw strong conclusions about the regional specificity of the reported associations.

In conclusion, our data highlight two factors that may contribute to the large variability of dopaminergic drug effects on human cognition in general and on the fast adaptation of outcome-predictions in particular. First, different effects are seen depending on the particular task demands under study and the associated neural mechanism, as illustrated by the contrasting effect of dopamine-enhancing drugs on the updating of reward- and punishment-predictions in PD as well as in healthy volunteers. Second, drug effects depend on baseline levels of dopamine, as illustrated by our positron emission tomography study where drugs had opposite effects in low- and high-dopamine subjects. Finally, this work with human volunteers and patients demonstrates that striatal dopamine is likely implicated not only in incremental reinforcemental (or habit) learning and the slow updating of actions and habits, but also in the instantaneous updating of already established behavior based on changes in explicit outcome predictions, generally consistent with decades of work with experimental animals (Cools, 1980; Taylor and Robbins, 1984).

Acknowledgments

Some of the work reviewed in this chapter was conducted in the lab of Trevor Robbins within the University of Cambridge Behavioural and Clinical Neuroscience Institute

(BCNI) funded by a joint award from the Medical Research Council and the Wellcome Trust. Other work was conducted in the labs of Mark D'Esposito and William Jagust within the Helen Wills Neuroscience Institute at UC Berkeley and supported by NIH grants DA02060. Thanks to Luke Clark, Marieke van der Schaaf, Esther Aarts and Martine van Schouwenburg for helpful comments on earlier drafts of this paper.

References

Annett, L., McGregor, A., and Robbins, T. (1989). The effects of ibutenic acid lesions of the nucleus accumbens on spatial learning and extinction in the rat. *Behav Brain Res*, 31, 231–42.

Arnsten, A.F.T. (1998). Catecholamine modulation of prefrontal cortical cognitive function. *Trends Cogn Sci*, 2, 436–46.

Chase, H., Swainson, R., Drurham, L., and Benham, L., Cools, R. (in press (2010)) Feedback-related negativity codes prediction error, but not behavioural adjustment during probabilistic reversal learning *J Cogn Neurosci*, Feb 10, [Epub ahead of print].

Clark, L., Nawijn, L., Muller, U., Patsalos, P., Ratnaraj, N., Williams-Gray, C. et al. (In preparation) The effects of L-DOPA on brain responses during reversal learning in healthy older adults.

Clarke, H., Robbins, T., and Roberts, A. (2008). Lesions of the medial striatum in monkeys produce perseverative impairments during reversal learning similar to those produced by lesions of the orbitofrontal cortex. *J Neurosci*, 28, 10972–82.

Clatworthy, P.L., Lewis, S.J., Brichard, L., Hong, Y.T., Izquierdo, D., Clark, L. et al. (2009). Dopamine release in dissociable striatal subregions predicts the different effects of oral methylphenidate on reversal learning and spatial working memory. *J Neurosci*, 29, 4690–96.

Cools, A.R. (1980). Role of the neostriatal dopaminergic activity in sequencing and selecting behavioural strategies: facilitation of processes involved in selecting the best strategy in a stressful situation. *Behav Brain Res*, 1, 361–78.

Cools, R., Barker, R.A., Sahakian, B.J., and Robbins, T.W. (2001). Enhanced or impaired cognitive function in Parkinson's disease as a function of dopaminergic medication and task demands. *Cereb Cortex*, 11, 1136–43.

Cools, R., Clark, L., Owen, A.M., and Robbins, T.W. (2002). Defining the neural mechanisms of probabilistic reversal learning using event-related functional Magnetic Resonance Imaging. *J Neurosci*, 22, 4563–67.

Cools, R., Barker, R.A., Sahakian, B.J., and Robbins, T.W. (2003). L-Dopa medication remediates cognitive inflexibility, but increases impulsivity in patients with Parkinson's disease. *Neuropsychologia*, 41, 1431–41.

Cools, R., Altamirano, L., and D'Esposito, M. (2006). Reversal learning in Parkinson's disease depends on medication status and outcome valence. *Neuropsychologia*, 44, 1663–73.

Cools, R., Lewis, S., Clark, L., Barker, R., and Robbins, T.W. (2007). L-DOPA disrupts activity in the nucleus accumbens during reversal learning in Parkinson's disease. *Neuropsychopharmacology*, 32,180–89.

Cools, R., Frank, M., Gibbs, S., Miyakawa, A., Jagust, W., and D'Esposito, M. (2009). Striatal dopamine predicts outcome-specific reversal learning and its sensitivity to dopaminergic drug administration. *J Neurosci*, 29, 1538–43.

Dayan, P. (2008). The role of value systems in decision making. In: Strungmann Forum Report: better than conscious? *Decision making, the human mind, and implications for institutions* (Engel C and Singer W, eds), pp 51–70. Frankfurt, Germany: MIT Press.

Delgado, M.R., Li, J., Schiller, D., and Phelps, E.A. (2008). The role of the striatum in aversive learning and aversive prediction errors. *Philos Trans R Soc Lond B Biol Sci*, 363, 3787–800.

Dias, R., Robbins, T.W., and Roberts, A.C. (1996). Dissociation in prefrontal cortex of affective and attentional shifts. *Nature*, 380, 69–72.

Divac, I., Rosvold, H.E., and Szwarcbart, M.K. (1967). Behavioral effects of selective ablation of the caudate nucleus. *J Comp Physiol Psychol*, 63, 184–90.

Dodds, C.M., Muller, U., Clark, L., van Loon, A., Cools, R., and Robbins, T.W. (2008). Methylphenidate has differential effects on blood oxygenation level-dependent signal related to cognitive subprocesses of reversal learning. *J Neurosci*, 28, 5976–82.

Evans, A.H., Pavese, N., Lawrence, A.D., Tai, Y.F., Appel, S., Doder, M. et al. (2006). Compulsive drug use linked to sensitized ventral striatal dopamine transmission. *Ann Neurol*, 59, 852–58.

Fellows, L., and Farah, M. (2003). Ventromedial frontal cortex mediates affective shifting in humans: evidence from a reversal learning paradigm. *Brain*, 126, 1830–37.

Frank, M.J. (2005). Dynamic dopamine modulation in the basal ganglia: a neurocomputational account of cognitive deficits in medicated and nonmedicated Parkinsonism. *J Cogn Neurosci*, 17, 51–72.

Frank, M.J., Seeberger, L.C., and O'Reilly, R. C. (2004). By carrot or by stick: cognitive reinforcement learning in parkinsonism. *Science*, 306, 1940–43.

Goldman-Rakic, P. (1992). Dopamine-mediated mechanisms of the prefrontal cortex. *Semin Neurosci*, 4, 109–118.

Gotham, A.M., Brown, R.G., and Marsden, C.D. (1988) 'Frontal' cognitive function in patients with Parkinson's disease 'on' and 'off' levodopa. *Brain*, 111, 299–321.

Hampton, A.N., and O'Doherty, J. P. (2007). Decoding the neural substrates of reward-related decision making with functional MRI. *Proc Natl Acad Sci USA*, 104, 1377–82.

Hampton, A.N., Bossaerts, P., and O'Doherty, J.P. (2006). The role of the ventromedial prefrontal cortex in abstract state-based inference during decision making in humans. *J Neurosci*, 26, 8360–67.

Hare, T., O'Doherty, J., Camerer, C., Schultz, W., and Rangel, A. (2008). Dissociating the role of the orbitofrontal cortex and the striatum in the computation of goal values and prediction errors. *J Neurosci*, 28, 5623–30.

Hollerman, J.R., and Schultz, W. (1998). Dopamine neurons report an error in the temporal prediction of reward during learning. *Nat Neurosci*, 1, 304–9.

Jensen, J., Smith, A., Willeit, M., Crawley, A., Mikulis, D., Vitcu, I., and Kapur, S. (2007). Separate brain regions code for salience vs valence during reward prediction in humans. *Human Brain Mapping*, 28, 294–302.

Kish, S.J., Shannak, K., and Hornykiewicz, O. (1988). Uneven patterns of dopamine loss in the striatum of patients with idiopathic Parkinson's disease. *New Eng J Med*, 318, 876–80.

McClure, S., Berns, G., and Montague, P. (2003). Temporal prediction errors in a passive learning task activate human striatum. *Neuron*, 38, 339–46.

Matsumoto, M., and Hikosaka, O. (2009). Two types of dopamine neuron distinctly convey positive and negative motivational signals. *Nature*, 459, 837–41.

Montague, P.R., Dayan, P., and Sejnowski, T.J. (1996). A framework for mesercephalic dopamine systems based on predictive Hebbian learning. *J Neurosci*, 16, 1936–47.

Moustafa, A., Cohen, M., Sherman, S., and Frank, M. (2008). A role for dopamine in temporal decision making and reward maximization in parkinsonism. *J Neurosci*, 28, 12294–304.

O'Doherty, J., Critchley, H., Deichmann, R., and Dolan, R.J. (2003a). Dissociating valence of outcome from behavioral control in human orbital and ventral prefrontal cortices. *J Neurosci*, 23, 7931–39.

O'Doherty, J., Dayan, P., Friston, K., Critchley, H., and Dolan, R. (2003b). Temporal difference models and reward-related learning in the human brain. *Neuron*, 38, 329–37.

O'Doherty, J., Dayan, P., Schultz, J., Deichmann, R., Friston, K., and Dolan, R. (2004). Dissociable role of ventral and dorsal striatum in instrumental conditioning. *Science*, 304, 452–54.

Pessiglione, M., Seymour, B., Flandin, G., Dolan, R.J., and Frith, C.D. (2006). Dopamine-dependent prediction errors underpin reward-seeking behaviour in humans. *Nature*, **442**, 1042–45.

Remijnse, P.L., Nielen, M.M., Uylings, H.B., and Veltman, D.J. (2005). Neural correlates of a reversal learning task with an affectively neutral baseline: an event-related fMRI study. *Neuroimage*, **26**, 609–618.

Robinson, O.J., Frank, M.J., Sahakian, B.J., and Cools, R. (2010). Dissociable responses to punishment in distinct striatal regions during reversal learning. *Neuroimage*, **51**(4), 1459–67.

Rogers, R.D., and Monsell, S. (1995). Costs of a predictable switch between simple cognitive tasks. *J Exp Psychol*, **124**, 207–31.

Schönberg, T., Daw, N., Joel, D., and O'Doherty, J. (2007). Reinforcement learning signals in the human striatum distinguish learners from nonlearners during reward-based decision making. *J Neurosci*, **27**, 12860–67.

Schultz, W. (2002). Getting formal with dopamine and reward. *Neuron*, **36**, 241–63.

Schultz, W., Dayan, P., and Montague, P.R. (1997). A neural substrate of prediction and reward. *Science*, **275**, 1593–99.

Seymour, B., O'Doherty, J.P., Dayan, P., Koltzenburg, M., Jones, A.K., Dolan, R.J., Friston, K.J., and Frackowiak, R.S. (2004). Temporal difference models describe higher order learning in humans. *Nature*, **429**, 664–67.

Seymour, B., O'Doherty, J.P., Koltzenburg, M., Wiech, K., Frackowiak, R., Friston, K., and Dolan, R. (2005). Opponent appetitive-aversive neural processes underlie predictive learning of pain relief. *Nat Neurosci*, **8**, 1234–40.

Seymour, B., Daw, N., Dayan, P., Singer, T., and Dolan, R. (2007). Differential encoding of losses and gains in the human striatum. *J Neurosci*, **27**, 4826–31.

Stern, C., and Passingham, R. (1995). The nucleus accumbens in monkeys (Macaca fascicularis). *Exp Brain Res*, **106**, 239–47.

Sutton, R., and Barto, A.G. (1998). *Reinforcement learning*. Cambridge, MA: MIT Press.

Swainson, R., Rogers, R.D., Sahakian, B.J., Summers, B.A., Polkey, C.E., and Robbins, T.W. (2000). Probabilistic learning and reversal deficits in patients with Parkinson's disease or frontal or temporal lobe lesions: possible adverse effects of dopaminergic medication. *Neuropsychologia*, **38**, 596–612.

Taghzouti, K., Louilot, A., Herman, J., Le Moal, M., and Simon, H. (1985). Alternation behaviour, spatial discrimination, and reversal disturbances following 6-hydroxydopamine lesions in the nucleus accumbens of the rat. *Behav Neural Biol*, **44**, 354–63.

Taylor, J. and Robbins, T. (1984). Enhanced behavioural control by conditioned reinforcers following microinjections of d-amphetamine into the nucleus accumbens. *Psychopharmacology*, **84**, 405–12.

Tom, S., Fox, C., Trepel, C., and Poldrack, R. (2007). The neural basis of loss aversion in decision-making under risk. *Science*, **315**, 515–518.

Williams, G.V., and Goldman-Rakic, P.S. (1995). Modulation of memory fields by dopamine D1 receptors in prefrontal cortex. *Nature*, **376**, 572–75.

Yacubian J, Gläscher J, Schroeder K, Sommer T, Braus D, and Büchel C (2006) Dissociable systems for gain- and loss-related value predictions and errors of prediction in the human brain. *J Neurosci*, **26**, 9530–37.

Zahrt J, Taylor JR, Mathew RG, and Arnsten AFT (1997) Supranormal stimulation of D1 dopamine receptors in the rodent prefrontal cortex impairs spatial working memory performance. *J Neurosci*, **17**, 8528–35.

Zink CF, Pagnoni G, Martin ME, Dhamala M, and Berns GS (2003) Human striatal response to salient nonrewarding stimuli. *J Neurosci*, **23**, 8092–97.

Chapter 17

Investigating the role of the noradrenergic system in human cognition

Sander Nieuwenhuis and Marieke Jepma

Abstract

Animal research and computational modeling have indicated an important role for the noradrenergic system in the regulation of attention and behavior. According to a recent theory, the noradrenergic system is critical for the optimization of behavioral performance—by facilitating responses to motivationally significant stimuli and regulating the tradeoff between exploitative and exploratory behaviors (Aston-Jones and Cohen, 2005). However, until recently, crucial empirical tests of this theory in human subjects have been lacking. This is not so surprising since the study of neuromodulation in humans poses considerable methodological challenges. In this chapter we will discuss recent progress made in the development and validation of non-invasive measures and methods for investigating noradrenergic function in humans. This methodological progress has opened up new opportunities for testing predictions and further development of theories of noradrenergic function.

17.1 Introduction

As their name suggests, neuromodulators such as dopamine, acetylcholine, and norepinephrine (NE) modify the effects of neurotransmitters—the molecules that enable communication between neurons. Neuromodulatory systems are involved in almost every mental function, including attention, learning, and emotion (Robbins, 1997), and they are disturbed in many neurological and psychiatric disorders, such as attention-deficit/hyperactivity disorder (ADHD), post-traumatic stress disorder, and schizophrenia.

For a long time researchers have associated neuromodulators with basic, nonspecific functions such as signaling reward (dopamine) and regulating arousal (NE). But recent research has shown that neuromodulators have more specific functions in learning and decision making. This progress is especially apparent in cognitive neuroscience, in which neurophysiological data from animal studies have been used to develop highly sophisticated theories about the role of neuromodulatory systems in human cognition (Frank and Claus, 2006; Holroyd and Coles, 2002; Usher et al., 1999). This chapter focuses specifically on the role of the noradrenergic system in optimizing task performance, with a strong emphasis on the question of how we can investigate the function of this system in human subjects.

The locus coeruleus (LC) is the brainstem neuromodulatory nucleus responsible for most of the NE released in the brain. It has widespread projections throughout the neocortex. The LC-mediated noradrenergic innervation increases the responsivity of efferent target neurons (Berridge and Waterhouse, 2003), which can be modeled as a change in the gain (steepness) of the neurons' activation function (Servan-Schreiber et al., 1990). Although cell recordings in non-human primates have yielded a wealth of information regarding the dynamics of the noradrenergic system, to date there has been very little empirical research on the activation dynamics and function of this system in humans. This is not so surprising since the study of the noradrenergic system in humans poses considerable methodological challenges. First, the LC is a very small nucleus and lies deep within the brainstem, necessitating the use of refined non-invasive imaging techniques to record its activity. And second, it is not possible to directly measure the neurophysiological effects of NE in the human brain. The study of these effects requires the development of indirect measures, or the measurement of changes in behavior and brain activity brought about by pharmacological manipulations of the noradrenergic system. Nevertheless, if we want to achieve a thorough understanding of the functions of the human noradrenergic system, we need to confront these challenges.

In this chapter we will discuss recent progress made in the development and validation of non-invasive measures and methods for investigating noradrenergic function in humans. The discussed methods include functional imaging, scalp electrophysiology, the application of computational models of the monkey noradrenergic system to the study of human attention phenomena, pupillometry, and psychopharmacology. As we will show, this methodological progress has opened up new opportunities for testing predictions and further development of theories of noradrenergic function.

17.2 The function of phasic LC responses

When an animal is actively engaged in performing a task, LC neurons exhibit a rapid, phasic increase in discharge rate to task-relevant and otherwise motivationally salient stimuli. For example, such *LC phasic responses* are observed for target stimuli in a simple target-detection task in which monkeys are required to respond to rare target stimuli presented at random intervals embedded in a train of distractor stimuli. Provided that the animal is engaged in the task, these target stimuli cause a phasic increase in LC firing rate that peaks at approximately 100–150 ms post-target and approximately 200 ms prior to the response (Fig. 17.1; e.g., Aston-Jones et al., 1994; Clayton et al., 2004). Importantly, the LC does not exhibit this type of phasic response to distractor stimuli, nor is the phasic response associated with any other task-related events once training is complete

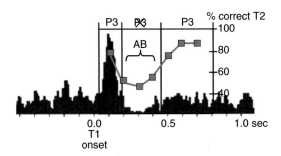

Fig. 17.1 Peristimulus time histogram of activity from a typical monkey locus coeruleus (LC) neuron during target trials in a target-detection task. Following the target (T1) LC activity exhibits a sharp phasic response, followed by a refractory period, followed by a return back to baseline. The plotted curve indicates typical results in a human attentional-blink (AB) experiment: accuracy for a second target (T2) is critically dependent on the time interval between the two targets. If T2 is presented 200–450 ms following T1, T2 accuracy is dramatically impaired and T2 does not elicit a second P3. Note the similarity in the timing of the LC refractory period, the attentional blink, and P3 occurrence.

(reward delivery, fixation point, response movements, etc.). However, similar phasic responses are elicited by unexpected, intense, threatening, or otherwise salient stimuli that demand effective processing and action (Aston-Jones et al., 1999).

The ensuing release of NE in cortical areas temporarily increases the responsivity of these areas to their afferent input (Berridge and Waterhouse, 2003), selectively potentiating any activity present concurrent with LC activation. It has been shown that, when applied in a temporally strategic manner (e.g., when driven by the identification and evaluation of motivationally relevant stimuli), increases in responsivity produce an increase in the signal-to-noise ratio of subsequent processing and a concomitant improvement in the efficiency and reliability of behavioral responses (Servan-Schreiber et al., 1990). Accordingly, it has been found that LC phasic activation reliably precedes, and is temporally linked to, behavioral responses to task-relevant stimuli (Bouret and Sara, 2004; Clayton et al., 2004). In addition, studies have reported a direct relation between the strength of LC activity and response accuracy in choice-reaction time tasks (Rajkowski et al., 2004). Together, these findings suggest that phasic noradrenergic signals play an important role in optimizing responses to motivationally significant stimuli (for an elaborate discussion of this topic, see Aston-Jones and Cohen, 2005).

17.3 Functional imaging of the LC

Functional magnetic resonance imaging (fMRI) would be a suitable and highly convenient method for measuring phasic LC signals in human subjects. But unfortunately, imaging of the LC with fMRI is far from straightforward, due to the LC's small size (~ 1 cm in length in humans) and its location deep down in the brainstem. Previous fMRI studies of the noradrenergic system have therefore either focused on LC projection areas (e.g., Strange and Dolan, 2007) or have been forced to note that their conclusions regarding activation in the LC region must remain tentative (e.g., Raizada and Poldrack, 2008; Sterpenich et al., 2006).

A relatively simple methodological requirement for LC imaging concerns immobilizing the subject's head to prevent motion of the LC from one voxel to the next, and investigating the data from individual subjects rather than the grand-average to prevent spatial "smearing." An alternative solution for the averaging problem is the use of a brainstem normalization algorithm to improve overlap of the brainstem across subjects for group analysis (Napadow et al., 2006). Another requirement is the use of high-resolution scan sequences designed to image small brain structures. This is needed to minimize the effects of partial volume averaging. A final challenge concerns the fact that the LC lies immediately adjacent to the fourth ventricle, resulting in movement artifacts caused by pulsatile flow of the cerebrospinal fluid. To remedy this problem one can use "cardiac gating" (Guimaraes et al., 1998). This means that the heart beat is used as a trigger for the fMRI image acquisition, so that each slice image is always acquired during the same moment of a heart-beat cycle. This maximizes the chance that the same brain tissue falls into a particular voxel every time it is measured.

A recent study has demonstrated that the above-described set of methods allows the effective measurement of blood oxygen-level dependent (BOLD) signals in dopaminergic midbrain nuclei (D'Ardenne et al., 2008). The authors suggest that, using these methods, it should also be possible to investigate other neuromodulatory nuclei such as the LC. Our group is currently making significant progress in this direction, but until this work begins to bear fruit, we will consider alternative approaches for localizing the LC. One such approach is the triangulation method (Komisaruk et al., 2002): the LC is closely surrounded by multiple nuclei with elementary sensory or motor functions (e.g, swallowing, detecting subtle facial stimulation). These regions can be functionally mapped with fMRI in a short period, thus generating for each individual a functional reference map for localizing the approximate location of the LC. Another approach is to use a noradrenergic drug agent and examine with fMRI whether the main effect of drug versus placebo activates a voxel cluster consistent with the estimated location of the LC. This voxel cluster can then be used as a region-of-interest for investigating task effects on LC activity (Minzenberg et al., 2008). Finally, neurochemists have recently developed a noradrenergic tracer (for use in humans); a radioactive molecule that has high affinity for the NE transporter and that can be imaged with positron emision tomography (Takano et al., 2008). This is likely to be an effective method for localizing the LC, which has a high density of NE transporters. Similar tracers have been successfully used in imaging other neuromodulatory systems in humans (e.g., dopamine; Cools et al., 2002).

17.4 The P3 component of the event-related potential

While relatively direct measurement of LC phasic activity using fMRI has not yet been realized, it seems possible to obtain non-invasive measures of the distant, post-synaptic effects of such phasic activity. In particular, it has recently been proposed that the modulatory effect of phasic NE release in the neocortex can be measured in human subjects by recording the P3(00) component of the scalp-recorded event-related potential (Nieuwenhuis et al., 2005a).

The P3 is a prominent, positive large-amplitude potential with a broad, midline scalp distribution, and a typical peak latency between 300 and 400 ms following presentation of stimuli in any sensory modality (for a review see Polich, 2007). First reported in 1965 (Sutton et al., 1965), the P3 has undoubtedly been the single most studied component of the event-related potential. Yet, until recently, psychologists and neuroscientists have failed to come up with a precise, mechanistic account that elucidates the functional role in information processing of the process underlying the P3, as well as its neural basis. Strong evidence for subcortical involvement in P3 generation has come from a study showing largely intact P3 components to unilaterally presented visual stimuli in the unstimulated hemisphere of a split-brain patient (Kutas et al., 1990). Given that in split-brain patients, interhemispheric transfer of information is not possible at the cortical level, this finding indicates that critical input and/or output signals of the P3 process must have passed through one of the intact subcortical commissures. The hypothesis that the P3 reflects the LC-mediated phasic enhancement of neural responsivity in the cortex is supported by a wealth of data from intracranial recordings, lesion studies, psychopharmacology, functional imaging, and other methods, as summarized below (for an extensive review see Nieuwenhuis et al., 2005a).

First, the antecedent conditions for the P3 are similar to those reported for the LC phasic response. In general, P3 amplitude is more closely related to the overall motivational significance and/or arousing nature of a given stimulus than to the affective valence of the stimulus. Important factors affecting the amplitude of the P3 are the subjective probability of the eliciting stimulus, its task-relevance, and its salience (e.g., intensity, novelty). Like the LC phasic response, the P3 is also enlarged for stimuli with intrinsic significance such as emotionally valent stimuli, whether experienced as positive or negative.

Second, the distribution and timing of intracranial and scalp-recorded P3 activity are consistent with the anatomical and physiological properties of the noradrenergic system. For example, functional imaging studies, intracranial recordings, and lesion studies have indicated that brain areas showing or contributing to P3 activity are scattered across the brain (Soltani and Knight, 2000), consistent with the widespread projections from the LC to cortical and subcortical areas. In addition, the pattern of P3 generators shows a spatial specificity that mirrors the projection density of the LC. Furthermore, P3 onset latency in simple two-alternative forced choice tasks is consistent with the latency of LC phasic activity (~150–200 ms), if one takes into account the relatively slow conduction velocity of LC fibers. Additionally, the relatively early timing of P3 activity in frontal and subcortical areas (e.g., thalamus; Klostermann et al., 2006) is consistent with the trajectory of LC fibers, which first reach these areas and only then veer backwards to innervate posterior cortical areas.

Third, several studies have reported direct evidence for an LC generator of the P3. These include psychopharmacological studies, which have shown that P3 amplitude is modulated in a systematic fashion by noradrenergic agents such as clonidine (Swick et al., 1994), and entirely abolished following drug-induced NE depletion (Glover et al., 1988).

Also, a recent study has found that individual differences in the noradrenergic gene that affects the activity of the alpha-2a receptor are a key determinant of P3 amplitude (Liu et al., 2009). In addition, lesion studies have demonstrated a selective effect on P3 amplitude of LC lesions (Pineda et al., 1989). Finally, larger and faster P3s are associated with more accurate and faster behavioral responses, a pattern that mirrors the relation between LC phasic activity and task performance, and that is consistent with the functional role ascribed to the noradrenergic system.

In the past, some authors have argued that the P3 peaks too late to influence behavioral responses, thereby challenging the LC–P3 theory. However, several counter-arguments are worth noting. First, even if the peak of the P3 sometimes occurs after the registration of the response, the *onset* of the P3 generally occurs before the response. Second, the potentiating influence of the noradrenergic system on behavioral responding is likely to be modest in typical laboratory tasks, which use simple stimuli and discrete button-press responses. These tasks are performed so quickly that the noradrenergic modulation of the relevant cortical areas (as reflected in the P3) may sometimes occur too late to facilitate the response. It is plausible that the facilitatory influence of the noradrenergic system is more prominent in real-life situations, which are characterized by multimodal, crowded sensory environments and a range of potential, often time-consuming response options. Finally, the LC-P3 theory does not claim that the P3 process is *necessary* for responding; of course, subjects can decide to respond before their perceptual system has fully analyzed the stimulus. The hypothesis claims that *if* the P3 occurs before the response, then the response will be facilitated and more efficient.

The LC–P3 theory offers a theoretical framework that allows the separate research literatures on the noradrenergic system and P3 each to inspire new predictions and research within the other domain. Because empirical knowledge about P3 function in humans by far exceeds that of the LC, it may prove fruitful for our understanding of LC function to identify and test cross-domain predictions inspired by the P3 literature.

17.5 Projections to the LC and the link with the orienting response

An important question is how the LC—this tiny brainstem nucleus—knows whether a stimulus is motivationally significant. To date, the best available answer is that some of the most prominent descending cortical projections to the LC come from two frontal brain structures that are thought to play a critical role in evaluating costs and rewards: the anterior cingulate cortex and the orbitofrontal cortex (Fig. 17.2; Arnsten and Goldman-Rakic, 1984; Aston-Jones and Cohen, 2005; Lee et al., 2005).

A growing body of work implicates the anterior cingulate cortex in action monitoring and reinforcement-guided decision making (Ridderinkhof et al., 2004; Rushworth et al., 2007). Activation of the anterior cingulate may provide a neural signal that greater control is required to successfully meet internal goals or external demands (Botvinick et al., 2004). As we have discussed, the LC is in a unique position neurophysiologically to provide such an augmentation in control by globally affecting system responsivity. There is also strong evidence that the orbitofrontal cortex plays an important role in reinforcement-guided decision making. For example, neurons in orbitofrontal cortex respond to the reward value of stimuli in varying modalities, and the magnitude of the neural response reflects the relative reward value of the corresponding stimuli (Rolls, 2004). Recent studies that have compared the distinctive contributions of the anterior cingulate and orbitofrontal cortex suggest that the former represents action–reward contingencies, whereas the latter represents stimulus–reward contingencies (Rushworth et al., 2007). Taken together, these findings suggest that the anterior cingulate and orbitofrontal cortex may jointly provide the LC with ongoing evaluations of task utility (see Section 17.7; Aston-Jones and Cohen, 2005).

In addition to these direct projections from frontal structures, many other cortical and limbic structures, including the amygdala and hypothalamus, have indirect connections with the LC. Interestingly, most of these cortical and limbic signals are relayed by the rostral part of the ventrolateral medulla, the area that provides the largest input to the LC (Fig. 17.2; Aston-Jones et al., 1986). Importantly, this same area of the medulla is also a key region for the regulation of the symphathetic branch of the autonomic nervous system. Neurons in this area are involved in controlling sympathetic activation of the pupil, sweat glands, the heart, and other autonomic organs. Indeed, LC firing rate and sympathetic nervous system activity have a strong temporal correlation (cf. Aston-Jones et al., 1996). Anatomical considerations suggest that this correlation reflects parallel downstream influences of a common afferent source in the medulla.

There is also ample evidence for a tight link between the psychophysiological manifestations of noradrenergic and sympathetic nervous system activity: the P3 and the *orienting response*, a collection of autonomic nervous system reflexes that includes pupillary dilation, a drop in skin resistance, and a momentary change in heart rate (Sokolov, 1963). In the 1970s, psychophysiologists were intrigued by the idea that the P3 might reflect a neural

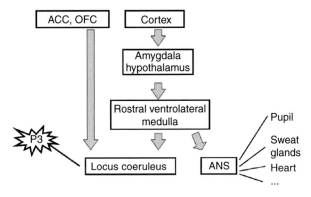

Fig. 17.2 Schematic outline of descending projections to the locus coeruleus and autonomic nervous system (ANS). Although there is substantial evidence that autonomic (mainly cardiovascular) responses have a direct influence on LC activity (Berntson et al., 1998), this anatomical route is too slow to explain the rapid, phasic LC responses to motivationally significant stimuli. ACC = anterior cingulate cortex; OFC = orbitofrontal cortex.

correlate of the orienting response. Like the P3, the orienting response is elicited by novel, intense, and otherwise motivationally significant stimuli. Moreover, both the P3 and the orienting response are well known to rapidly habituate to initially novel, task-irrelevant stimuli. In the 1980s, empirical and theoretical comparisons between the P3 and orienting response reached an impasse, in part because a neurobiological basis for these comparisons was lacking (Donchin et al., 1984). Our recent analysis suggests that the close link between these two phenomena reflects the co-activation of the noradrenergic and sympathetic systems by a common afferent pathway (Nieuwenhuis et al., in press).

17.6 The attentional blink as a marker of LC dynamics

Above, we have discussed that task-relevant stimuli in choice reaction-time tasks typically elicit a large P3 and that this may reflect the large LC phasic response to such stimuli. Nieuwenhuis and colleagues explored the question of what happens if we present a second task-relevant stimulus soon after the LC response to the first (Nieuwenhuis et al., 2005b). This question was inspired by the observation that the LC phasic response to task-relevant stimuli is typically followed by a brief period during which the LC is essentially inactive and unperturbable (due to local auto-inhibition; Aston-Jones et al., 1994). This so-called refractory period starts between 200 and 250 ms after the eliciting stimulus, and usually lasts until about 400–450 ms post-stimulus (Fig. 17.1). Importantly, human ERP experiments have shown that, if a second target stimulus is presented during roughly this interval, the target elicits no P3, consistent with the notion that the LC is refractory (Fig. 17.1; Vogel et al., 1998; Woods et al., 1980). In contrast, if the second target is presented a little later (>500 ms), when LC baseline activity is back up to normal, the target elicits a normal-sized P3.

Nieuwenhuis et al. (2005b) noted that the LC refractory period also coincides with the timing of a psychophysical phenomenon, the *attentional blink*: the transient impairment in perceiving the second of two targets presented in close temporal proximity in a rapid stream of distractors (Fig. 17.1; Shapiro et al., 1997). This observation led to the hypothesis that the attentional blink may be mediated by the momentary unavailability of noradrenergic potentiation during the refractory period associated with the first target. Because of the unavailability of NE, subsequent target stimuli that are presented during the refractory period do not receive the benefit of LC-mediated facilitation and, therefore, suffer a deficit in processing. To test this hypothesis, Nieuwenhuis and colleagues extended an existing computational model of monkey LC dynamics and its impact on target-detection performance (Gilzenrat et al., 2002). Computer simulations indicated that the model, when presented with an attentional-blink task, produced a pattern of deficit in its target-detection performance that was very similar to that associated with the attentional blink observed in empirical studies.

Aside from its occurrence and timing, the LC model explains various other properties of the attentional blink. For example, if the second target follows the first without intervening distractors, performance for the second target is often (partially) spared ("lag-1 sparing"; Shapiro et al., 1997). The LC model reproduces this phenomenon because the residuum of NE release associated with the first target benefits processing of the second target, allowing it to escape the disrupting effect of LC refractoriness. Another property of the attentional blink concerns the role of the distractor immediately following the first target (i.e., the T1+1 distractor). Many early studies have found that the attentional blink occurs only if the T1+1 distractor is presented, not if it is omitted, and therefore most models explain the attentional blink as the result of a process triggered by the presentation of the T1+1 distractor (Shapiro et al., 1997). In contrast, the core mechanism in the LC model produces an attentional blink regardless of the presence of the T1+1 distractor, because the occurrence of a LC phasic response is independent of this distractor item. Although this was initially regarded as a limitation of the LC model, recent empirical work has demonstrated that, provided that the probe task for second-target accuracy is sensitive enough, a substantial attentional blink can be observed even when the two targets are separated by a blank screen (Nieuwenstein et al., 2009).

Although fundamentally different from the LC model, two recent computational models of the attentional blink incorporate a crucial architectural component that produces target-evoked, transient, nonspecific attentional responses that facilitate the conscious identification of briefly presented, masked targets (the "blaster" in Bowman and Wyble, 2007; the "boost" function in Olivers and Meeter, 2008). The proponents of these models have explicitly recognized the similarity between the properties of these attentional mechanisms and properties of the LC (Bowman et al. 2007; Olivers, 2007), indicating a striking correspondence between computational and neurophysiological models of the attentional blink.

Finally, a couple of studies have provided indirect support for the involvement of the noradrenergic system in the attentional blink. First, functional imaging studies have suggested that target processing in the attentional blink task is mediated by a widespread cortical network including parietal cortex, anterior cingulate cortex, and lateral frontal cortex, which are some of the cortical areas with the densest noradrenergic innervation (cf. Nieuwenhuis et al., 2005b). Second, split-brain patients show a typical attentional blink even when the two targets are presented to two different hemispheres (Giesbrecht and Kingstone, 2004), suggesting a subcortical basis for the attentional blink. And third, a psychopharmacological study has found that changes in noradrenergic tone modulate the attentional blink (De Martino et al., 2008). This study found that beta-adrenergic blockade with propranolol impaired attentional-blink performance, whereas NE reuptake inhibition with reboxetine improved attentional-blink performance, at least for emotional target stimuli. However, another study found no reliable effect of the alpha-2 receptor agonist clonidine on the attentional blink (Nieuwenhuis et al., 2007). This is remarkable because the LC refractory period, proposed to be responsible for the attentional blink, is possibly caused by the activation of alpha-2 inhibitory autoreceptors in the LC (Aghajanian et al., 1977). It is unclear whether this discrepancy between model and data is due to insufficient sensitivity of the empirical study (e.g., dose too low; use of a between-subject design; see Nieuwenhuis et al., 2007, for an extensive discussion) or presents a falsification of the LC model of the attentional blink.

17.7 **Phasic versus tonic LC firing mode and corresponding control states**

Above, we have discussed that phasic LC responses facilitate responding to the motivationally significant stimuli that tend to elicit these responses. Here we discuss the function of tonic (baseline) changes in LC activity (i.e., changes happening over the course of multiple seconds or minutes). Levels of LC tonic activity vary systematically in relation to measures of task performance (Fig. 17.3). Aston-Jones and colleagues (1994) recorded LC activity in monkeys during performance of a target-detection task. Periods of intermediate tonic LC activity were accompanied by large LC phasic responses to target stimuli, and rapid and accurate responding. In contrast, periods of elevated tonic LC activity were consistently accompanied by relatively poor task performance, and distractible, restless behavior. Such phases were also consistently associated with a diminuition or absence of the target-evoked LC phasic responses observed during periods of good performance. These findings have led to the proposal that in the waking state there are two distinguishable modes of LC activity (Aston-Jones et al., 1999; Fig. 17.3): in the *phasic mode*, bursts of LC activity are observed in association with the outcome of task-related decision processes, and are closely associated with goal-directed behavior; in the *tonic mode*, LC baseline activity is elevated but phasic bursts of activity are absent and behavior is more distractible.

According to the recently proposed adaptive gain theory (Aston-Jones and Cohen, 2005; Cohen et al., 2004), the different modes of LC activity serve to regulate a fundamental tradeoff between two control states: exploitation versus exploration. The LC phasic

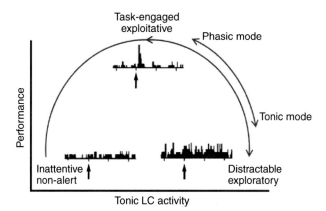

Fig. 17.3 Inverted-U relationship between tonic LC activity and performance on tasks that require focused attention. Moderate LC tonic activity is associated with optimal performance and prominent phasic LC activation following task-relevant stimuli (phasic LC mode). High levels of tonic LC activity are associated with poor performance and the absence of phasic LC activity (tonic LC mode). According to Aston-Jones and Cohen (2005), shifts along the continuum between the phasic and tonic LC modes drive corresponding changes in the exploitation-exploration tradeoff. Reprinted from Annual Review of Neuroscience 2005, 403–450, Aston-Jones, G. and Cohen, J., Copyright 2005, with permission from Annual Reviews.

mode promotes exploitative behavior by facilitating processing of task-relevant information (via the phasic response), while filtering out irrelevant stimuli (through low tonic responsivity). By increasing the phasic character of LC firing, the cognitive system is better able to engage in the task at hand, and maximize rewards harvested from this task. In contrast, the LC tonic mode promotes behavioral disengagement by producing a more enduring and less discriminative increase in responsivity. Although this degrades performance within the current task, it facilitates the disengagement of attention from this task, thus allowing potentially new and more rewarding behaviors to be emitted. Thus, the transition between the two LC modes can serve to optimize the tradeoff between exploitation and exploration of opportunities for reward, and thereby maximizes overall utility.

The adaptive gain theory further holds that the transition between phasic and tonic LC firing modes and the corresponding control states are driven by online assessments of utility by the frontal structures that provide a major input to the LC, the anterior cingulate and the orbitofrontal cortex (see Section 17.5). According to the theory, the utility signals in these brain areas are integrated over different timescales and then used to regulate LC mode (Aston-Jones and Cohen, 2005). Brief lapses in performance, in the context of otherwise high utility, augment the LC phasic mode, resulting in improved task performance. In contrast, enduring decreases in utility drive transitions to the LC tonic mode, promoting disengagement from the current task and facilitating exploration of behavioral alternatives.

17.8 Pupillometry can reveal LC-mediated control state

Most of the evidence for the hypothesized link between low utility, tonic LC firing mode, and a control state favoring exploratory behavior comes from animal studies, but even that evidence is sparse. Therefore, in order to generalize and further develop the adaptive gain theory (Aston-Jones and Cohen, 2005), it would be desirable to have at our disposal a non-invasive correlate measure of both tonic and phasic LC activity in humans. In recent work, Gilzenrat et al. (2010) have proposed that pupil diameter might provide such a measure.

In follow-up analyses of the target-detection task data discussed in Sections 17.2 and 17.7 (Aston-Jones et al., 1994), Rajkowski et al. (1993; see also Aston-Jones and Cohen, 2005) found that the monkey pupil diameter, which was recorded throughout the experiment, closely followed the LC tonic firing rate. Rajkowski and colleagues concluded that baseline pupil diameter varies with LC mode, such that the LC tonic mode is marked by a relatively large pupil diameter and the LC phasic mode is marked by a relatively small pupil diameter. Furthermore, a large number of studies with human subjects have shown that task processing is accompanied by rapid and large pupil dilations, consistent with the occurrence of an LC phasic response to task-relevant events (Kahneman, 1973). Typically, the size and duration of these dilations are positively correlated with task difficulty. Taken together, these previous human and animal studies show that task-related, effortful processing is associated with tonic constrictions (in the monkey) and phasic dilations (in the human) of the pupil. This tonic–phasic pupil interaction mirrors the negative correlation between tonic and phasic LC activity, suggesting that pupillary responses track LC firing rate, reflecting both its tonic and phasic character. This hypothesis is consistent with the close link between LC activity and autonomic nervous system activity discussed in Section 17.6.

Gilzenrat et al. (2010) conducted three experiments with young adults to investigate the value of pupil diameter as a marker of LC activity in humans. In Experiment 1 they examined the relationship between pupil diameter and task performance, using an auditory version of the target-detection task previously used in monkey LC studies. The results were consistent with the predictions of adaptive gain theory: trials with larger baseline pupil diameters were associated with poorer task performance, indicative of lapses of engagement mediated by spontaneous drift into LC tonic mode. Conversely, smaller baseline pupil diameters were associated with better performance, indicative of task engagement mediated by the LC phasic mode. In addition, larger baseline diameters were associated with smaller post-target dilations, and vice versa, consistent with the negative correlation between phasic and tonic LC activity.

In Experiment 2 the authors attempted to manipulate LC mode, and hence control state, by regulating the experienced processing conflict (~costs) and reward (which jointly determined task utility) across blocks of trials in a pitch-discrimination task (Kahneman and Beatty, 1967). The pupil exhibited smaller baseline diameters and larger dilations when both the amount of conflict and reward value were high, and likewise when both the amount of conflict and reward value were low. These results were predicted by the adaptive gain theory: both conditions encouraged the LC phasic mode as both signaled a need for recruitment of control (either due to high conflict, or negative feedback) in circumstances in which the required additional effort appeared to pay off (either in the form of positive feedback, or through a reduction in conflict). Conversely, the block with high, protracted conflict and low reward was associated with larger baseline pupil diameters and smaller dilations. This block promotes the LC tonic mode and hence an adaptive breakdown in the recruitment of control, as conflict remains high and feedback remains negative despite effortful performance.

Finally, in Experiment 3 the authors focused on the effect of dynamic changes in task utility on pupil diameter, and at the relationship between pupil diameter and a measure of task disengagement, using a novel diminishing-utility task. Subjects performed a series of tone discriminations of progressively increasing difficulty with rewards for correct performance that increased in value with increasing task difficulty. Initially, the increases in reward value outpaced increases in difficulty (and associated increases in errors), so that subjects remained engaged in the task. However, after several trials, the increases in difficulty led to sufficient numbers of errors as to reduce reward rate, even in the face of the increasing value of correct responses. At the beginning of every trial, subjects were allowed to press a reset button (an overt disengage behavior), which would start a new series of discriminations, beginning again with low difficulty and low reward value. Subjects behaved optimally on average, choosing to reset when the success (expected utility) of the discriminations began to decline. Early in each trial series there were large phasic pupil dilations for each discrimination. As would be predicted for LC phasic responses, these dilations declined in amplitude, and baseline (tonic) pupil diameter rose as the task became more difficult and expected utility began to decline. Baseline pupil diameter was greatest at the point at which subjects chose to abandon the current series, consistent with the hypothesis that this was mediated by an increase in LC tonic activity.

To summarize, in all three experiments the pupillometry and behavioral results showed a highly specific pattern that the adaptive gain theory would predict if pupil diameter indeed indexes LC activity: tonic and phasic pupil diameters (which were negatively correlated) were highly sensitive to dynamic changes in utility and highly predictive of task (dis)engagement. Thus, the confirmation of the theoretical predictions reaped a double reward: it served to validate the method, showing that pupillometry can reveal LC-mediated changes along the exploitation–exploration tradeoff; and it helped validate the adaptive gain theory, since the predicted pupil dynamics were dictated by an assumption of close correspondence with observed LC firing patterns.

However, although the diminishing-utility task used in Experiment 3 allowed subjects to disengage from the task, a limitation of this experiment was that there were no opportunities to actually explore other options. We have recently addressed this issue in a pupillometry study using an n-armed bandit task (Sutton and Barto, 1998). In this task subjects repeatedly chose one of four slot machines. The pay-offs of the four slots changed over time, such that the current pay-offs could only be learned through active sampling of the slots (i.e., exploration). Each choice made by the participants could be classified as exploitative or exploratory, by means of a model-based calculation of the expected value of the chosen slot relative to the other slots. The results confirmed our critical predictions that baseline pupil diameter was larger preceding exploratory versus exploitative choices, and that changes in baseline pupil diameter surrounding the transition between exploratory and exploitative control states were correlated with changes in task-related utility (Jepma and Nieuwenhuis, in press).

17.9 Pharmacological manipulations of LC-mediated control state

Pharmacological manipulations of the noradrenergic system provide a powerful means to study the functional role of this system in humans. The functional significance of the alpha-adrenergic and beta-adrenergic receptor systems are reviewed in detail elsewhere (Chamberlain et al., 2006a; Coull, 1994). Here we focus on the selective NE reuptake inhibitors atomoxetine, reboxetine, and desipramine, because administration of these drugs (at a clinically relevant dose) increases synaptic concentrations of norepinephrine, thus mimicking the effects of elevated NE release that characterize the tonic LC mode. Atomoxetine is a common treatment for ADHD and reboxetine and desipramine are antidepressant drugs used in the treatment of clinical depression. Acute administration of NE reuptake inhibitors has opposing effects: in the LC it leads to a reduction of firing activity through the increased activation of inhibitory autoreceptors within the LC; while in the forebrain it results in increased extracellular NE levels due to the reuptake blockade.

Importantly, the net effect of these two actions is still an increase in NE levels, and this effect is enhanced by chronic treatment (reviewed in Invernizzi and Garattini, 2004).

To date, no human or animal studies have directly investigated the effect of NE reuptake inhibitors on exploitative versus exploratory behaviors. However, there are several indications that these drugs promote behavioral disengagement and increase cognitive flexibility—other indications of the enduring and largely nonspecific increase in responsivity associated with the LC tonic mode. For example, acute and chronic treatment with desipramine has been found to improve rats' attentional set-shifting, a measure of cognitive flexibility (Lapiz et al., 2007). Furthermore, atomoxetine and desipramine have been reported to lead to improved reversal learning in discrimination tasks in which rats were trained to either reverse or retain a position-reward association learned in the previous session (Seu et al., 2009). In contrast, reboxetine did not improve performance during the retention phases, suggesting a specific improvement in cognitive flexibility, not in overall task performance. Interestingly, a similar facilitation in attentional set-shifting and reversal learning has been obtained with the alpha-2 receptor antagonists idazoxan and guanfacine, which also activate the NE system but are less suitable for use in humans (Devauges and Sara, 1990; Steere and Arnsten, 1997). Another consistent finding is that atomoxetine improves human subjects' ability to stop an ongoing motor response when cued to do so (Chamberlain et al., 2006b). Presumably the drug-related increase in cognitive flexibility facilitates disengaging from one task (responding) and switching to a new task (stopping the response). Remarkably, the same study found that atomoxetine did not improve reversal learning. Finally, reboxetine has been found to enhance social flexibility, as indicated by increased social engagement and cooperation and a reduction in self-focus in a stranger-dyadic social interaction paradigm (Tse and Bond, 2002).

We are currently conducting a study designed to provide a direct test of the effects of reboxetine on behavioral indices of task-(dis)engagement and the tradeoff between exploration and exploitation (Jepma et al., in press). One group of subjects receives reboxetine (4 mg single dose), a second group receives citalopram (30 mg; positive control), a selective serotonin reuptake inhibitor with comparable alerting effects and pharmacokinetic properties as reboxetine, and a third group receives a placebo. Subjects perform two tasks described in Section 17.8: the diminishing-utility task and the n-armed bandit task. For the diminishing-utility task our prediction is that subjects in the reboxetine group will reset (disengage) more often than subjects in the other two groups, because this type of behavior is indicative of the tonic LC mode. For the n-armed bandit task our prediction is that the reboxetine group will make more exploratory choices than the other two groups. Confirmation of these predictions will provide important support for the adaptive gain theory.

17.10 Concluding remarks

Much of the research reviewed in this chapter is exemplary for a research approach that has recently flourished: developing and validating measures and methods for studying a human neuromodulatory system (here: the noradrenergic system), and using these methodological advances to enhance our understanding of the role of this system in human cognition. In general, the work reviewed here is consistent with the adaptive gain theory, which posits a critical role for the noradrenergic system in the optimization of behavioral performance (Aston-Jones and Cohen, 2005). It seems probable that further research using the discussed methods will continue to unravel the function of this neuromodulatory system.

There are many similarities between the noradrenergic and dopaminergic systems. NE and dopamine are both neuromodulatory transmitters and have similar physiological effects on target systems (e.g., modulation of gain; Servan-Schreiber et al. 1990); like LC neurons, some midbrain dopamine neurons are responsive to both postitive and negative motivationally salient events (Matsumoto and Hikosaka, 2009); and like the noradrenergic system, the dopamine system has been implicated in the regulation of the exploration-exploitation tradeoff (sometimes referred to as the flexibility-stability tradeoff; Dreisbach et al., 2005; Frank et al., 2009). Despite these similarities, the relationships between these systems and how they interact has remained unclear. This is in part due to the fact that neuromodulatory systems are generally studied in isolation (but see Briand et al., 2007). A future challenge for empirical research will be to uncover how the noradrenergic and dopaminergic (and other modulatory) systems work in parallel to dictate cognitive function. An intriguing account of the interaction between dopamine and NE has been proposed by McClure et al. (2005; Aston-Jones and Cohen, 2005). This proposal builds on the hypothesis that phasic activity of (valence-sensitive) dopamine neurons reflects reward prediction errors for reinforcement learning (Schultz et al., 1997). Dopamine-guided reinforcement learning requires an annealing procedure, favoring exploration during learning in new (or changing) environments and promoting exploitation when reliable sources of reward have been discovered. The adaptive gain theory proposes that the noradrenergic system serves this function, implementing an annealing mechanism that is adaptive to ongoing estimates of utility.

Acknowledgements

The authors thank Mark Gilzenrat, Jonathan Cohen, and Gary Aston-Jones for the important contributions they have made to the research reviewed in this chapter. This research was supported by a VIDI-grant from the Netherlands Organization for Scientific Research.

References

Aghajanian, G.K., Cedarbaum, J.M., and Wang, R.Y. (1977). Evidence for norepinephrine-mediated collateral inhibition of locus coeruleus neurons. *Brain Research,* **136,** 570–77.

Arnsten, A.F. and Goldman-Rakic, P.S. (1984). Selective prefrontal cortical projections to the region of the locus coeruleus and raphe nuclei in the rhesus monkey. *Brain Research,* **306,** 9–18.

Aston-Jones, G. and Cohen, J.D. (2005). An integrative theory of locus coeruleus-norepinephrine function: adaptive gain and optimal performance. *Annual Review of Neuroscience,* **28,** 403–50.

Aston-Jones, G., Ennis, M., Pieribone, V.A., Nickell, W.T., and Shipley, M.T. (1986). The brain nucleus locus coeruleus: restricted afferent control of a broad efferent network. *Science,* **234,** 734–37.

Aston-Jones, G., Rajkowski, J., Kubiak, P., and Alexinsky, T. (1994). Locus coeruleus neurons in monkey are selectively activated by attended cues in a vigilance task. *Journal of Neuroscience,* **14,** 4467–80.

Aston-Jones, G., Rajkowski, J., Kubiak, P., Valentino, R. J., and Shipley, M. T. (1996). Role of the locus coeruleus in emotional activation. *Progress in Brain Research*, **107**, 379–402.

Aston-Jones, G., Rajkowski, J., and Cohen, J. (1999). Role of locus coeruleus in attention and behavioral flexibility. *Biological Psychiatry*, **46**, 1309–20.

Berridge C.W., and Waterhouse, B.D. (2003). The locus coeruleus-noradrenergic system: modulation of behavioral state and state-dependent cognitive processes. *Brain Research Reviews*, **42**, 33–84.

Botvinick, M.M., Cohen, J.D., and Carter, C.S. (2004). Conflict monitoring and anterior cingulate cortex: an update. *Trends in Cognitive Sciences*, **8**, 539–46.

Bouret, S. and Sara, S. J. (2004). Reward expectation, orientation of attention and locus coeruleus–medial frontal cortex interplay during learning. *European Journal of Neuroscience*, **20**, 791–802.

Bowman, H. and Wyble, B. (2007). The simultaneous type, serial token model of temporal attention and working memory. *Psychological Review*, **114**, 38–70.

Bowman, H., Wyble, B., Chennu, S., and Craston, P. (2007). A reciprocal relationship between bottom-up trace strength and the attentional blink bottleneck: relating the LC-NE and ST(2) models. *Brain Research*, **1202**, 25–42.

Briand, L.A., Gritton, H., Howe, W.M., Young, D.A., and Sarter, M. (2007). Modulators in concert for cognition: modulator interactions in the prefrontal cortex. *Progress in Neurobiology*, **83**, 69–91.

Chamberlain, S. R., Müller, U., Blackwell, A. D., Robbins, T. W., and Sahakian, B. J. (2006a). Noradrenergic modulation of working memory and emotional memory in humans. *Psychopharmacology*, **188**, 397–407.

Chamberlain, S.R., Müller, U., Blackwell, A. D., Clark, L., Robbins, T. W., Sahakian, B. J. (2006b). Neurochemical modulation of response inhibition and probabilistic learning in humans. *Science*, **311**, 861–63.

Clayton, E.C., Rajkowski, J., Cohen, J.D., and Aston-Jones, G. (2004). Phasic activation of monkey locus coeruleus neurons by simple decisions in a forced choice task. *Journal of Neuroscience*, **24**, 9914–20.

Cohen, J.D., Aston-Jones, G., and Gilzenrat, M.S. (2004). A systems level theory on attention and cognitive control. In M.I. Posner (ed.), *Cognitive neuroscience of attention* (pp. 71–90). New York, NY: Guilford Press.

Cools, R., Stefanova, E., Barker, R.A., Robbins, T.W., and Owen, A.M. (2002). Dopaminergic modulation of high-level cognition in Parkinson's disease: the role of the prefrontal cortex revealed by PET. *Brain*, **125**, 584–94.

Coull, J. T. (1994). Pharmacological manipulations of the alpha 2-noradrenergic system. *Effects on cognition. Drugs and Aging*, **5**, 116–26.

D'Ardenne, K., McClure, S.M., Nystrom, L.E., and Cohen, J.D. (2008). BOLD responses reflecting dopaminergic signals in the human ventral tegmental area. *Science*, **319**, 1264–67.

De Martino, B., Strange, B.A., and Dolan, R.J. (2008). Noradrenergic neuromodulation of human attention for emotional and neutral stimuli. *Psychopharmacology*, **197**, 127–36.

Devauges, V. and Sara, S.J. (1990). Activation of the noradrenergic system facilitates an attentional shift in the rat. *Behavioural Brain Research*, **39**, 19–28.

Donchin, E., Heffley, E., Hillyard, S.A., Loveless, N., Maltzman, I., Ohman, A., Rosler, F., Ruchkin, D., and Siddle, D. (1984). Cognition and event-related potentials. *II. The Orienting Reflex and P300. Annals of the New York Academy of Sciences*, **425**, 39–57.

Dreisbach, G., Müller, J., Goschke, T., Strobel, A., Schulze, K., Lesch, K.P., and Brocke, B. (2005). Dopamine and cognitive control: the influence of spontaneous eyeblink rate and dopamine gene polymorphisms on perseveration and distractibility. *Behavioral Neuroscience*, **119**, 483–90.

Frank, M.J. and Claus, E.D. (2006). Anatomy of a decision: striato-orbitofrontal interactions in reinforcement learning, decision making, and reversal. *Psychological Review*, **113**, 300–26.

Frank, M.J., Doll, B.B., Oas-Terpstra, J., and Moreno, F. (2009). Prefrontal and striatal dopaminergic genes predict individual differences in exploration and exploitation. *Nature Neuroscience*.

Giesbrecht, B. and Kingstone, A. (2004). Right hemisphere involvement in the attentional blink: evidence from a split-brain patient. *Brain and Cognition,* 55, 303–306.

Gilzenrat, M.S., Holmes, B.D., Rajkowski, J., Aston-Jones, G., and Cohen, J.D. (2002). Simplified dynamics in a model of noradrenergic modulation of cognitive performance. *Neural Networks,* 15, 647–63.

Gilzenrat, M.S., Nieuwenhuis S., Jepma, M., and Cohen, J.D. (2010). Pupil diameter tracks changes in control state predicted by the adaptive gain theory of locus coeruleus function. *Cognitive, Affective, and Behavioral Neuroscience,* 10, 252–69.

Glover, A., Ghilardi, M.F., Bodis-Wollner, I., and Onofrj, M. (1988). Alterations in event-related potentials (ERPs) of MPTP-treated monkeys. *Electroencephalography and Clinical Neurophysiology,* 71, 461–68.

Guimaraes, A.R., Melcher, J.R., Talavage, T.M., Baker, J.R., Ledden, P., Rosen, B.R., Kiang, N.Y., Fullerton, B.C., and Weisskoff, R.M. (1998). Imaging subcortical auditory activity in humans. *Human Brain Mapping,* 6, 33–41.

Holroyd, C.B. and Coles, M.G. (2002). The neural basis of human error processing: reinforcement learning, dopamine, and the error-related negativity. *Psychological Review,* 109, 679–709.

Invernizzi, R.W. and Garattini, S. (2004). Role of presynaptic alpha2-adrenoceptors in antidepressant action: recent findings from microdialysis studies. *Progress in Neuropsychopharmacology and Biological Psychiatry,* 28, 819–27.

Jepma, M. and Nieuwenhuis, S. (2010). Pupil diameter predicts changes in the exploration-exploitation tradeoff: Evidence for the adaptive gain theory of locus coeruleus function. *Journal of Cognitive Neuroscience* 28 July [Epub ahead of print].

Jepma, M., te Beek, E.T., Wagenmakers, E.-J., van Gerven, J.M.A., and Nieuwenhuis, S. (2010). The role of the noradrenergic system in the exploration-exploitation trade-off: A psychopharmalogical study. *Frontiers in Human Neuroscience,* 4, 170.

Kahneman, D. (1973). *Attention and effort.* Englewood Cliffs, NJ: Prentice-Hall.

Kahneman, D. and Beatty, J. (1967). Pupillary responses in a pitch-discrimination task. *Perception and Psychophysics,* 2, 101–105.

Klostermann, F., Wahl, M., Marzinzik, F., Schneider, G.H., Kupsch, A., and Curio, G. (2006). Mental chronometry of target detection: human thalamus leads cortex. *Brain,* 129, 923–31.

Komisaruk, B.R., Mosier, K.M., Liu, W.C., Criminale, C., Zaborszky, L., Whipple, B., and Kalnin, A. (2002). Functional localization of brainstem and cervical spinal cord nuclei in humans with fMRI. *American Journal of Neuroradiology,* 23, 609–617.

Kutas, M., Hillyard, S.A., Volpe, B.T., and Gazzaniga, M.S. (1990). Late positive event-related potentials after commissural section in humans. *Journal of Cognitive Neuroscience,* 2, 258–71.

Lapiz, M.D., Bondi, C.O., and Morilak, D.A. (2007). Chronic treatment with desipramine improves cognitive performance of rats in an attentional set-shifting test. *Neuropsychopharmacology,* 32, 1000–1010.

Lee, H.S., Kim, M.A., and Waterhouse, B.D. (2005). Retrograde double-labeling study of common afferent projections to the dorsal raphe and the nuclear core of the locus coeruleus in the rat. *Journal of Comparative Neurology,* 481, 179–93.

Liu, J., Kiehl, K.A., Pearlson, G., Perrone-Bizzozero, N.I., Eichele, T., and Calhoun, V.D. (2009). Genetic determinants of target and novelty-related event-related potentials in the auditory oddball response. *Neuroimage,* 46, 809–816.

Matsumoto, M. and Hikosaka, O. (2009). Two types of dopamine neuron distinctly convey positive and negative motivational signals. *Nature,* 459, 837–41.

McClure S.M., Gilzenrat M.S., Cohen J.D. (2005). An exploration-exploitation model based on norepinephrine and dopamine activity. In Weiss Y., Schölkopf B., Platt J. (Eds.), *Advances in neural information processing systems* 18 (pp. 867–74). Cambridge, MA: MIT Press.

Minzenberg, M.J., Watrous, A.J., Yoon, .J.H., Ursu, S., and Carter, C.S. (2008). Modafinil shifts human locus coeruleus to low-tonic, high-phasic activity during functional MRI. *Science*, 322, 1700–2.

Napadow, V., Dhond, R., Kennedy, D., Hui, K. K., and Makris, N. (2006). Automated brainstem co-registration (ABC) for MRI. *Neuroimage*, 32, 1113–1119.

Nieuwenhuis, S., Aston-Jones, G., and Cohen, J. D. (2005a). Decision making, the P3, and the locus coeruleus-norepinephrine system. *Psychological Bulletin*, 131, 510–32.

Nieuwenhuis, S., Gilzenrat, M. S., Holmes, B. D., and Cohen, J. D. (2005b). The role of the locus coeruleus in mediating the attentional blink: a neurocomputational theory. *Journal of Experimental Psychology General*, 134, 291–307.

Nieuwenhuis, S., van Nieuwpoort, I.C., Veltman, D.J., and Drent, M.L. (2007). Effects of the noradrenergic agonist clonidine on temporal and spatial attention. *Psychopharmacology*, 193, 261–69.

Nieuwenstein, M. R., Potter, M. C., and Theeuwes, J. (2009). Unmasking the attentional blink. *Journal of Experimental Psychology: Human Perception and Performance*, 35, 159–69.

Nieuwenhuis, S., de Geus, E.J., and Aston-Jones, G. (in press). The anatomical and functional relationship between the P3 and autonomic components of the orienting response. *Psychophysiology*.

Olivers, C. N. (2007). The time course of attention: It's better than we thought. *Current Directions in Psychological Science*, 16, 11–15.

Olivers, C.N., and Meeter, M. (2008). A boost and bounce theory of temporal attention. *Psychological Review*, 115, 836–63.

Pineda, J.A., Foote, S.L., and Neville, H.J. (1989). Effects of locus coeruleus lesions on auditory, long-latency, event-related potentials in monkey. *Journal of Neuroscience*, 9, 81–93.

Polich, J. (2007). Updating P300: an integrative theory of P3a and P3b. *Clinical Neurophysiology*, 118, 2128–48.

Raizada, R.D.S. and Poldrack, R.A. (2008). Challenge-driven attention: interacting frontal and brainstem systems. *Frontiers in Human Neuroscience*, 1:3.

Rajkowski, J., Kubiak, P., and Aston-Jones, G. (1993). Correlations between locus coeruleus (LC) neural activity, pupil diameter and behavior in monkey support a role of LC in attention. *Society for Neuroscience Abstracts*, 19, 974.

Rajkowski, J., Majczynski, H., Clayton, E., and Aston-Jones, G. (2004). Activation of monkey locus coeruleus neurons varies with difficulty and performance in a target detection task. *Journal of Neurophysiology*, 92, 361–71.

Ridderinkhof, K.R., Ullsperger, M., Crone, E.A., and Nieuwenhuis, S. (2004). The role of the medial frontal cortex in cognitive control. *Science*, 306, 443–47.

Robbins, T. W. (1997). Arousal systems and attentional processes. *Biological Psychology*, 45, 57–71.

Rolls, E. T. (2004). The functions of the orbitofrontal cortex. *Brain and Cognition*, 55, 11–29.

Rushworth, M.F., Behrens, T., Rudebeck, P., and Walton, M.E. (2007). Contrasting roles for cingulate and orbitofrontal cortex in decisions and social behaviour. *Trends in Cognitive Sciences*, 11, 168–76.

Schultz, W., Dayan, P., and Montague, P. R. (1997). A neural substrate of prediction and reward. *Science*, 275, 1593–99.

Servan-Schreiber, D., Printz, H., and Cohen, J. D. (1990). A network model of catecholamine effects: gain, signal-to-noise ratio, and behavior. *Science*, 249, 892–95.

Seu, E., Lang, A., Rivera, R.J., and Jentsch, J.D. (2009). Inhibition of the norepinephrine transporter improves behavioral flexibility in rats and monkeys. *Psychopharmacology*, 202, 505–519.

Shapiro, K.L., Arnell, K.A., and Raymond, J.E. (1997). The attentional blink: a view on attention and a glimpse on consciousness. *Trends in Cognitive Sciences*, 1, 291–96.

Sokolov, E. N. (1963). *Perception and the conditioned reflex*. Oxford: Pergamon Press.

Soltani, M. and Knight, R.T. (2000). Neural origins of the P300. *Critical Reviews in Neurobiology*, 14, 199–224.

Steere, J.C. and Arnsten, A.F. (1997). The alpha-2A noradrenergic receptor agonist guanfacine improves visual object discrimination reversal performance in aged rhesus monkeys. *Behavioral Neuroscience*, 111, 883–91.

Sterpenich, V., D'Argembeau, A., Desseilles, M., Balteau, E., Albouy, G., Vandewalle, G., Degueldre, C., Luxen, A., Collette, F., and Maquet, P. (2006). The locus ceruleus is involved in the successful retrieval of emotional memories in humans. *Journal of Neuroscience*, 26, 7416–23.

Strange, B.A. and Dolan, R.J. (2007). Beta-adrenergic modulation of oddball responses in humans. *Behavioral and Brain Functions*, 3:29.

Sutton, R. S. and Barto, A. G. (1998). *Reinforcement learning: an introduction.* MIT Press, Cambridge MA.

Sutton, S., Braren, M., Zubin, J., and John, E. R. (1965). Evoked-potential correlates of stimulus uncertainty. *Science*, 150, 1187–88.

Swick, D., Pineda, J.A., and Foote, S.L. (1994). Effects of systemic clonidine on auditory event-related potentials in squirrel monkeys. *Brain Research Bulletin*, 33, 79–86.

Takano, A., Varrone, A., Gulyás, B., Karlsson, P., Tauscher, J., and Halldin, C. (2008). Mapping of the norepinephrine transporter in the human brain using PET with (S,S)-[18F]FMeNER-D2. *Neuroimage*, 42, 474–82.

Tse, W.S. and Bond, A.J. (2002). Difference in serotonergic and noradrenergic regulation of human social behaviours. *Psychopharmacology*, 159, 216–21.

Usher, M., Cohen, J.D., Servan-Schreiber, D., Rajkowski, J., and Aston-Jones, G. (1999). The role of locus coeruleus in the regulation of cognitive performance. *Science*, 283, 549–54.

Vogel, E.K., Luck, S.J., and Shapiro, K.L. (1998). Electrophysiological evidence for a postperceptual locus of suppression during the attentional blink. *Journal of Experimental Psychology. Human Perception and Performance*, 24, 1656–74.

Woods, D.L., Hillyard, S.A., Courchesne. E., and Galambos, R. (1980). Electrophysiological signs of split-second decision making. *Science*, 207, 655–57.

Chapter 18

Interoception and decision making

Martin P. Paulus

Abstract

Three constructs are reviewed that have important contributions to risky decision making. First, interoception and its neural substrates are reviewed, the characteristics of interoceptive processing as they relate to decision making are discussed, and the relationship between interoception and reward is outlined. Second, the notion of alliesthesia is introduced and the connection to interoception is provided, together with the presumed underlying neural substrates. Third, we propose a heuristic homeostatic decision-making model, which is based on existing mathematical formulations of prospect theory augmented by a variable that indicates the internal state of the individual. Based on this extension, it can be shown that individuals undergo preference reversals in decision-making situations. It is argued that these three approaches can be used to better quantify and understand decision-making dysfunctions in individuals with psychiatric disorders.

18.1 Interoception

Interoception is (a) sensing the physiological condition of the body (Craig, 2002), (b) representing—possibly conscqiously—the internal state (Craig, 2009) within the context of ongoing activities, and (c) initiating motivated action to homeostatically regulate the internal state (Craig, 2007). Receptors that are involved in interoception can be divided, based on the type of stimulus they respond to as: mechanoreceptors, chemoreceptors, thermoreceptors, and osmoreceptors. As a consequence, interoception includes a range of sensations such as pain (LaMotte et al., 1982), temperature (Craig and Bushnell, 1994), itch (Schmelz et al., 1997), tickle (Lahuerta et al., 1990), sensual touch (Vallbo et al., 1995; Olausson et al., 2002), muscle tension (Light and Perl, 2003), air hunger (Banzett et al., 2000), stomach pH (Feinle, 1998), and intestinal tension (Robinson et al., 2005), which together provide an integrated sense of the body's physiological condition (Craig, 2002). These sensations travel via small-diameter primary afferent fibers, which are thought to comprise a cohesive system for homeostatic afferent activity that parallels the efferent sympathetic nervous system (Craig, 2007), and terminate on projection neurons in the most superficial layer of the spinal dorsal horn. The modality-selective lamina I spinothalamic neurons project to a specific thalamo-cortical relay nucleus, which in turn projects to a discrete portion of dorsal posterior insular cortex. The posterior insula provides topographic and modality-specific interoceptive signals to the anterior insular cortex for integration (Craig, 2003). These topographically organized and modality-specific pathways that carry interoceptive signals are integrated in the anterior insula cortex (Craig, 2003), which is integrally connected with subcortical (Chikama et al., 1997), limbic (Reynolds and Zahm, 2005), and executive control brain systems (Jasmin et al., 2004). An organism's interoceptive state and hedonic state are integrated via reciprocal connections of the anterior insular cortex to corticolimbic and striatal reward circuit components such as: (a) anterior cingulate (Augustine, 1996), which is important for error processing (Carter et al., 1998; Critchley et al., 2005) and evaluation of action selection (Goldstein et al., 2007; Rushworth and Behrens, 2008), to (b) amygdala (Augustine, 1985; Jasmin et al., 2003, 2004; Reynolds et al., 2005), which is critical for processing stimulus salience (Paton et al., 2006), (c) nucleus accumbens (Reynolds et al., 2005), which processes the incentive motivational aspects of rewarding stimuli (Robinson and Berridge, 2008), and (d) orbitofrontal cortex (Ongur and Price, 2000), which has been implicated in context-dependent evaluation of environmental stimuli (Bechara et al., 2000; O'Doherty et al., 2001; Schoenbaum et al., 2003; Rolls, 2004a, 2004b; Kringelbach, 2005; Schoenbaum et al., 2006; Rolls and Grabenhorst, 2008). Thus, the anterior insula has access to a multidimensional representation and integration of the current and possibly anticipated feeling state (Paulus and Stein, 2006) and is important for the capacity to be aware (Craig, 2002; Critchley et al., 2004) of oneself, others, and the environment (Craig, 2009). The columnar organization of the insular cortex shows a highly organized anterior–inferior to posterior–superior gradient (for example, see: Mesulam and Mufson, 1982), similar to other parts of the brain where cortical representations are based on modulatory or selective feedback circuits (Shipp, 2005). Therefore, it is not surprising that insular cortex is involved in a wide range of processes, including pain (Tracey et al., 2000), interoceptive (Critchley et al., 2004), emotion-related (Phan et al., 2002), cognitive (Huettel et al., 2004), and social functions (Eisenberger et al., 2003). In summary, the insular cortex is important for subjective feeling states (Craig, 2002; Critchley et al., 2004), and takes part in modulatory control of decision making by interacting with other limbic, and cortical areas (Garavan et al., 1999)

However, the relationship between interoception and subjective awareness is complex. For example, individuals with anxiety disorders, such as panic attacks, report more cardiac sensations and report more frequently aversive interoceptive events than healthy control subjects. However, they also had a marked tendency to underestimate their level of physical exertion (Vaitl, 1996). Subjects with high emotional reactivity showed a higher degree of interoceptive awareness based on the heart-beat detection task and higher trait anxiety, which has been taken to suggest that a chronically increased sympathetic outflow might be one variable contributing to the establishment of high interoceptive awareness (Pollatos et al., 2007a). Further analyses showed that the relationship between emotional arousal and trait anxiety was mediated by differences in interoceptive awareness (Pollatos et al., 2007b). Thus, there is some evidence that anxious individuals show increased interoceptive sensitivity, which may be associated with reduced interoceptive accuracy. Moreover, the degree to which interoceptive modulation is consciously reported varies with the type of interoceptive stimuli used.

18.1.1 Aversive probe: non-hypercapnic inspiratory breathing restriction

Respiratory sensations motivate humans to behaviorally modulate their breathing and are the sensory urge component of the respiratory motivation-to-action neural system (Davenport and Vovk, 2008). Respiratory sensations are the result of subcortical and cortical processes: (1) discriminative processing—awareness of the spatial, temporal, and intensity components of the respiratory input (i.e., what is sensed); and (2) affective processing—evaluative and emotional components of the respiratory input (i.e., how it feels). Humans can easily detect mechanical loads added to inspiration (Davenport et al., 2007), i.e., inspiratory resistive (R) loads. In contrast to expiratory breathing restriction, which affects CO_2 (Lopata et al., 1977), inspiratory breathing restriction results in stable, unchanged CO_2 levels (Lofaso et al., 1992), which is consistent with the finding that CO_2 levels have no regulatory effect on inspiratory breathing effort (Clague et al., 1990). The standard protocol requires the subject to inspire against the load at the beginning of the inspiratory effort and continue to breathe against the load throughout the inspiration. The detection of an R load is associated with a respiratory-related evoked potential, which has several peaks that indicate the transition from an early sensory component to a later cognitive aspect (Davenport et al., 1986, 2007; Revelette and Davenport, 1990; Knafelc and Davenport, 1999). Several studies have shown that breathing restriction affects processing of both pleasant and unpleasant stimuli (Ritz and Thons, 2002; Gomez et al., 2004, 2005). Thus, non-hypercapnic inspiratory breathing restriction is a powerful experimental tool to induce an aversive interoceptive state.

18.1.2 Pleasant probe: mechano-receptive C-fiber stimulation via slow stroke

The mechanic stimulation of the skin is mediated by several skin receptors, which have been associated traditionally only with discriminative stimulus processing but whose molecular mechanisms are only beginning to be understood (Frings, 2008). Within the skin, mechano-receptive CT (C tactile) afferents are a distinct type of unmyelinated, low-threshold units, which have been found abundantly in the hairy skin but have not been found in glabrous skin of humans and other mammals (Vallbo et al., 1993). These CT fibers are poor in encoding discriminative aspects of touch (Vallbo et al., 1995), but well-suited to encoding slow, gentle touch (Vallbo et al., 1999). Some investigators have proposed that these fibers in hairy skin may be part of a system for processing pleasant and socially relevant aspects of touch (Vallbo, 1999; McGlone et al., 2007). Moreover, these fibers may also have a role in pain inhibition (Olausson et al., 2010). Although the subjective effects of mechanic stimulation of the skin is mostly due to first-order sensory fibers (Harrington and Merzenich, 1970) or slow habituation A-β discriminative fibers(Olausson et al., 2000), CT afferents may have a particular potential to elicit pleasant subjective experience alongside behavioral, hormonal, and autonomic responses during gentle touch between individuals (Olausson et al., 2008). Subjectively, selective stimulation of these fibers gives rise to an inconsistent perception of weak or pleasant touch and can elicit a sympathetic skin response (Olausson et al., 2008). Prior imaging studies have shown that positively affective touch and temperature are represented in parts of the orbitofrontal and pregenual cingulate cortex, as well as ventral striatum (Rolls, 2010). Subjective pleasantness and richness to touch stimulation are modulated by parietal cortex, the insula, and ventral striatum, and touch to the forearm compared with touch to the glabrous skin of the hand revealed activation in the mid-orbitofrontal cortex (McCabe et al., 2008). Thus, mechano-receptive C-fiber stimulation provides another experimental tool to induce a pleasant interoceptive state.

18.2 Reward, urges, and cravings

Reward is a complex construct (Robinson et al., 2008) that can be defined operationally as an object or stimulus that increases the frequency of a behavior (Skinner, 1981), or experientially as an incident that induces a feeling of pleasure and an action towards obtaining it, i.e., it includes hedonic and incentive motivational aspects (Robinson et al., 2008). Typically, the feeling is described as "pleasurable" or "positive" and the individual acts to approach the object associated with reward. In contrast, objects associated with, or predicting, the lack of reward result in an "aversive" experience and an avoidance action. Some investigators have proposed that the internal state is an important factor for the relative desirability of different stimuli (Loewenstein, 1996). Consistent with this idea, a neuroimaging study has shown that the repeated administration of an initially pleasantly valued stimulus resulted in increased satiety-related aversion, which was accompanied by increased insula activation (Small et al., 2001), demonstrating a role of the insula in modifying the degree of reward experience.

Reward processing is not restricted to the positive experience. Negative affective states (i.e., aversion, dysphoria, or pain) are as important an aspect of hedonic processing as positive affective states of pleasure/euphoria (Baker et al., 1986). As argued by Craig (2002, 2009), both feeling and action are intimately linked with the internal homeostatic state of the individual. The notion of feeling and action as critically dependent on the homeostatic state of the individual, within the context of drug-related urges, is well illustrated by the notion of "affective contrast," as postulated by Solomon (1980) some 30 years ago.

Craving has been described as an intense affect associated with a strong urge to act (Singleton and Gorelick, 1998). Several craving models (see: Tiffany, 1999) have been put forth to explain the psychological processes underlying the expression of craving. Regardless of the model one might favor, it is not difficult to see how the dynamic valuation and strong incentive properties of interoceptive stimuli make them essential elements to the craving experience, i.e., the hedonic component of the body state associated with the incentive to act is an important characteristic of craving. For example, an interoceptive response to conditioned cues may result in a strong craving sensation with the urge to act to receive the cue-predictive stimulus, e.g. a drug.

Urges can be conceptualized as strong incentives to act. The processes underlying urges are complex. Some have suggested a stage approach that involves a motivation-to-action system (Baker et al., 1986). Initially, a stimulus triggers a neural cascade underlying the urge, i.e., the physical need to respond to the stimulus, which is then translated into a targeted goal. Next, actions are deployed to satisfy the urge-desire, and evidence is collected by neural systems to examine success of urge-related action. Finally, the sensory system determines whether the urge was satisfied (Davenport, 2008). Urge-related processes are closely related to the incentive motivational aspects of reward because both focus on approach or avoidance behaviors that are initiated in response to a stimulus. The degree of urge is an integral component of the current interoceptive state (Davenport, 2008), as evidenced by several studies. In chronic smokers, situational pain increases urge ratings and produces shorter latencies to smoke, which may be related in part to pain-induced negative affect (Ditre and Brandon, 2008). Exercise reduces alcohol urges, which re-emerge afterwards (Ussher et al., 2004). Taken together, the degree of urge is influenced by the factors that are clearly affected by the internal state of the individual and may reflect the interplay between limbic sensory cortex (insula) and limbic motor cortex (anterior cingulate).

18.3 Alliesthesia

Alliesthesia is a physiological construct introduced in 1973 to connect the stimulations that come from the "milieu exterieur" and affect the "milieu interieur" (Cabanac, 1971). Alliesthesia critically links reward, which is typically ascribed to external stimuli, to the internal state of the individual, as a result of interoception. Cabanac proposed that a given external stimulus can be perceived either as pleasant or unpleasant, depending upon interoceptive signals (Cabanac, 1971). In particular, negative alliesthesia refers to the notion that repeated administration of a stimulus will affect the internal milieu in such a way that the rewarding aspects of the stimulus are attenuated, e.g., the second or third piece of chocolate does not feel as good as the first. In contrast, positive alliesthesia is observed if the repeated administration of a stimulus changes the internal milieu in such a way as to increase its reward aspects. For example, fasting can enhance the subjective pleasantness of food images (Stoeckel et al., 2007). These phenomena can also be observed in animals. Specifically, pre-feeding has been associated with negative alliesthesia (Zhao and Cabanac, 1994), whereas food restriction was found to increase the sensory reward derived from alcohol, which is an example of positive alliesthesia (Soderpalm and Hansen, 1999).

Based on the alliesthesia construct, some investigators proposed a dynamic, homeostatic hypothesis of pleasure regulation (Cabanac et al., 2002; Ramirez and Cabanac, 2003). This hypothesis proposes that (1) we experience the intensity of a reward based on the evaluation of the stimulus relative to our internal state (Cabanac, 1992), and (2) we engage regulatory mechanisms to maximize the hedonic aspect of the internal state. The alliesthesia construct can be applied to both rewarding and aversive stimuli, but, additionally, the alliesthesia concept provides an explicit connection between the internal state (i.e., interoception) and rewarding or aversive stimuli in the environment. In particular, the reference to an internal state identifies additional circuitry, e.g., insular cortex and its connectivity to frontal cortical and extended amygdala circuits, which can be empirically tested for its role in processing appetitive or aversive stimuli.

Interoception is strongly related to reward, urge, and craving, as detailed above, and alliesthesia emphasizes that these aspects are dependent on the pre-existing internal state of the individual, which may undergo positive/negative alliesthetic changes. Thus, three components appear critical for decision-making processes involving the degree to which an individual favors one option over another: (1) the internal or homeostatic state as signaled via C-fiber afferents converging to the insular cortex; (2) the cognitive state of the individual, which includes a "contextualized" representation of the interoceptive state (Shipp, 2005); and (3) the learned associations of the external stimulus with previous outcomes including predicted internal states.

18.4 **Decision making**

Decision making consists of the process of transforming options into actions according to the individual's preference, which may result in experiencing an outcome that leads to a different psychological and physiological state of the decision maker. In particular, emotional states have powerful effects on how individuals process chance events or evaluate outcomes (Loewenstein, 1996). Moreover, because the brain must not only evaluate what is occurring now, but also what may occur in the future (Montague et al., 2006), anticipated feeling states are important modulators of decision-making behavior. Traditional decision-making psychology has sought to establish rules and quantitative theories about how individuals establish preferences among uncertain options. These theories have been based on the concept of utility (Von Neumann and Morgenstern, 1947; Luce and Raiffa, 1957), a measure of human value, which is related to the degree of preference for an option in a decision-making situation. The probability and magnitude of a reward or punishment associated with an option are critical elements in the complex function that is used to compute the individual's utility. In particular, the magnitude of the utility is then thought to represent a quantitative value of a preference of an option in a decision-making situation. Traditional approaches to understanding decision making are based on economic theory (Von Neumann et al., 1947) and mathematical choice psychology (Kahneman and Tversky, 1979).

More recently, several investigators have augmented this approach to include affective or visceral factors (Slovic, 1995; Loewenstein, 1996; Rottenstreich and Hsee, 2001), which profoundly changes the preference structure of available options. For example, individuals often under-appreciate, hardly remember, and have difficulty explaining the influence of these factors on their decision making (Loewenstein, 1996). These insights are consistent with systems neuroscience approaches (Platt and Glimcher, 1999; Breiter et al., 2001;

Knutson et al., 2005) and neurobiologically informed theories (Gold and Shadlen, 2001; Schultz, 2006) that have been proposed to delineate where and how the brain computes decisions.

The inclusion of visceral factors (Loewenstein, 1996) and affect heuristics (Slovic, 1995), i.e., the notion that the assessment of risk is primarily driven by associative emotional processes, as part of decision making has moved this process from a rational selection of options based on preference structures into the realm of homeostatic maintenance behaviors. Therefore, decision making can be considered a homeostatic process. Homeostasis in this context can be defined as a dynamic physiological, cognitive, and affective steady state (Craig, 2002), which results from the integration of multiple bottom-up sensory afferents, which are integrated with top-down cognitive and affective control processes to be dynamically stable, i.e., resistant to internal and external perturbations.

Decisions maintain or bring individuals into a new homeostatic state. Temporally, decision making can be divided into three stages (Ernst and Paulus, 2005): (1) the assessment and formation of preferences among possible options; (2) the selection and execution of an action (and inhibition of inappropriate actions); and (3) the experience or evaluation of an outcome. During the first stage, a value or utility is assigned to each available option (Kahneman and Tversky, 1984), which determines the preference structure of the decision-making situation. However, the brain must not only evaluate what is occurring now, but also what may or may not occur in the future (Montague et al., 2006). The current state of the individual, time to experience an outcome, the degree to which the outcome is advantageous, and the likelihood that an outcome will be observed are important variables that determine the preference structure. The decision maker incorporates outcome-related information, action-related information, and contextual or situational information to select an action.

18.5 Conceptual and heuristic model of homeostatic decision making

As reviewed above, interoceptive processing is highly related to both hedonic and incentive motivational processing, alliesthesia emphasizes that these aspects are dependent on the pre-existing internal state of the individual, and these processes are plastic via various learning processes. The connection between interoception, alliesthesia, and decision making is important because it provides a conceptual and potentially quantitative approach to examine how individuals change their preferences when choosing among several available options. Specifically, one can begin to apply these constructs to individuals who choose to use drugs even in the presence of obvious adverse consequences. It is argued here that the altered interoceptive state of an individual using drugs changes the value of the available option due to alliesthesia, i.e., due to the increased positive contrast and attenuated negative contrast of the projected outcomes associated with drug-taking.

One approach to quantify the effect of an internal state change of the individual is to begin with the standard prospect theory model (Kahneman et al., 1984). In this approach, individuals subjectively transform probabilities into decision weights and outcomes into values, relative to a reference point, which in turn depends on the individual's expectation, aspiration, and situation. The critical element of prospect theory (Kahneman et al., 1979) is the fact that probabilities, p, in decision-making situations are transformed non-linearly into weights $w(p)$. Tversky and Kahneman used a one-parameter function, which transforms probabilities into weights and has the property of being regressive, asymmetric, and s-shaped:

$$w(p) = \frac{p^\delta}{\left(p^\delta + (1-p)^\delta\right)^{1/\delta}}$$

Typically, value functions are expressed as power functions, i.e., the value of a certain amount, x, is given by:

$$v(x) = x^{\sigma+}$$

The, σ^+ symbol indicates that the power law differs for positive and negative values.

Cumulative prospect theory states that the valuation of the probability, p, that an individual will gain \$x is given by $w(p)*v(x)$. Moreover, this valuation is different for gains than for losses, thus $w^+(p)$ or $v^+(p)$ is not the same as $w^-(p)$ or $v^-(p)$.

Prelec (1998) derived an alternative formulation based on an axiomatic approach, which assures that the probability weight is not proportional across the entire probabilistic scale, that most weights are smaller than the actual probabilities, and is based on the axiom of compound invariance, which states that the equivalence of two gambles is preserved when these gambles are repeated n times with adjusted gains:

$$w(p) = \exp\left\{-\beta^+(-\ln(p)^\alpha\right\}$$

This function has the advantage that it can be easily estimated using standardized certainty equivalent techniques, $(c) \sim (x, p)$, i.e., what is the value c that makes the gamble equal to the probability p of gaining x?

Therefore, in order to examine the effect of an internal reference point explicitly, an internal state variable was added to the value function prior to obtain homeostatic values. Thus, in combination, the formula for a positively valued outcome reads:

$$SubjectiveValue(x)^+ = \exp\{-\beta^+(-\ln(p)^\alpha\}*(x-s)^{\sigma+}$$

Or, for negatively valued outcomes due to the steeper value function:

$$SubjectiveValue(x)^- = \exp\{-\beta^+(-\ln(p)^\alpha\}*(x-s)^{\sigma-}$$

It is important to note, however, that the positive and negative subjective value function is with respect to the difference between the gain (or loss) and the current internal state. The critical question is whether the introduction of an internal state enables one to observe preference reversals. The existence of such reversals would provide the proof of principle that the explicit reference to an internal state can alter decision making in such a way that presumably sub-optimal decisions are selected because they function to serve the internal needs of the individual better than the mathematically predicted optimal choice.

To determine whether possible preference reversals exist, two gambles were chosen with arbitrary money units. The first choice consisted of selecting an option that would always result in a gain of 0.2 money units. The second choice resulted in a variable outcome with 50% possibility of gaining 1 unit or 50% gaining nothing. As shown in Fig. 18.1, the subjective value curves show clearly that at $s = 0$ and $s = 0.2$ the greater subjective value reverses from the risky option to the safe option and then again from the safe option to the risky option. Thus, subjective value as calculated by an extended prospect theory model enables one to observe preference reversal from risk-taking to risk-averse and vice versa.

Clearly, there are several limitations to this approach. First, this analysis is merely a semi-quantitative proof of principle to determine whether internal states can be incorporated into a model to explain differences in risky decision making. Second, the quantification of the internal state per se may pose some significant experimental problems. In particular, in the current formulation, we assume that the value function is determined by the difference between a quantified scalar that is called the internal state and the reward magnitude; however, one could construct other functions that take into account different value attributes. Third, the functional form of the current approach is based on the specific implementation of the probability weighing function as suggested by Prelec (1998), the extension to other weighing functions would help to determine whether this

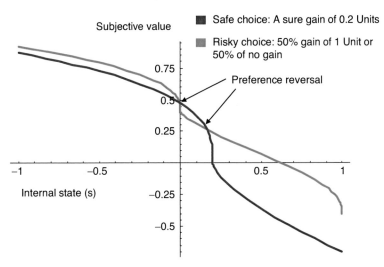

Fig. 18.1 Result of a simulation of the extended prospect theory model incorporating an internal state into the model. The subjective values of two choice options are shown as a function of varying internal state. The safe choice (selecting a sure gain of 0.2 units) is shown in blue and the risky choice (selecting an option with an uncertain outcome with 50% gaining 1 unit or 50% gaining nothing) is shown in red. There are two clear preference reversals at s = 0 and s = 0.2.

reversal is more generic, i.e., holds for a series of weight functions. Similarly, it was presumed that the primary effect of the internal state is to alter the value function and would not directly affect the probability weight function. It would be important to examine experimentally, whether this is indeed the case. Finally, the extension of this approach to temporal choice was not discussed here but is straight-forward. Preliminary analyses show preference reversals in time as they occur in variably distributed outcomes for risky versus safe choices.

The combination of interoception and alliesthesia to models of decision making adds several specific experimental approaches and predictions to the current conceptualization of dysfunction of risky decision making. First, alliesthesia necessitates a better delineation of the individual's internal state by experimental means. One approach is to determine the reactivity of the interoceptive system using a number of different interoceptive stimulations. Alternatively, one may begin to examine physiological correlates of internal states as covariates of cognitive and affective stimulation paradigms. Second, the insula is clearly a key neural substrate for interoceptive processing, yet the neuroanatomical characteristics of the insula support the idea that different processes occur in different parts of the insular cortex. Moreover, the insula is strongly integrated in various cortical and subcortical neural systems. Therefore, we need to better delineate which aspect of insular function is altered and in what direction, as well as which other brain areas are important contributors to this altered functioning. Third, modulating the internal state clearly contributes to the incentive motivational aspects of interoceptive processing. For example, a thirsty individual will perceive cues predicting water with greater "urgency" than a non-thirsty individual. However, we know precious little how to modify the internal state to attenuate the incentive motivational properties of drug-related cues.

Taken together, risky decision making cannot be viewed in isolation from the internal state of the individual. Several important processes need to be investigated using both neuroimaging and other technologies to clearly explicate the role of the internal state of the individual. It is proposed here that the internal state is processed via ascending C-fiber afferent, leading to a global representation of the internal milieu in the anterior insular cortex, which has profound effects on the valuation of available options in risky decision making situations. This approach also necessitates the development of behavioral paradigms to probe different aspects of decision making and to provide converging validity of some of the proposed decision-making constructs. Decision making will need to be examined within the homeostatic context of the individual. It is not clear yet whether dysfunctional decision making in individuals with psychiatric disorders is a consequence of altered assessment, execution, or evaluation stages of decision making or whether it is adequate decision making in the context of an altered homeostatic balance.

Acknowledgments

During the preparation of this article, the author was supported by NIH grants DA13186, DA016663 and Dept of Veterans Affairs Clinical.

References

Augustine, J.R. (1985). The insular lobe in primates including humans. *Neurol Res,* 7, 2–10.

Augustine, J.R. (1996). Circuitry and functional aspects of the insular lobe in primates including humans. *Brain Res Brain Res Rev,* 22, 229–44.

Baker, T.B., Morse, E., and Sherman, J.E. (1986). The motivation to use drugs: a psychobiological analysis of urges. *Nebr Symp Motiv,* 34, 257–323.

Banzett, R.B., Mulnier, H.E., Murphy, K., Rosen, S.D., Wise, R.J., and Adams, L. (2000). Breathlessness in humans activates insular cortex. *Neuroreport,* 11, 2117–20.

Bechara, A., Damasio, H., and Damasio, A.R. (2000). Emotion, decision making and the orbitofrontal cortex. *Cereb Cortex,* 10, 295–307.

Breiter, H.C., Aharon, I., Kahneman, D., Dale, A., and Shizgal, P. (2001). Functional imaging of neural responses to expectancy and experience of monetary gains and losses. *Neuron,* 30, 619–39.

Cabanac, M. (1971). Physiological role of pleasure. *Science,* 173, 1103–7.

Cabanac, M. (1992). Pleasure: the common currency. *J Theor Biol,* 155, 173–200.

Cabanac, M., Guillaume, J., Balasko, M., and Fleury, A. (2002). Pleasure in decision making situations. *BMC Psychiatry,* 2, 7.

Carter, C.S., Braver, T.S., Barch, D.M., Botvinick, M.M., Noll, D., and Cohen, J.D. (1998). Anterior cingulate cortex, error detection, and the online monitoring of performance. *Science,* 280, 747–9.

Chikama, M., McFarland, N.R., Amaral, D.G., and Haber, S.N. (1997). Insular cortical projections to functional regions of the striatum correlate with cortical cytoarchitectonic organization in the primate. *J Neurosci,* 17, 9686–705.

Clague, J.E., Carter, J., Pearson, M.G., and Calverley, P.M. (1990). Relationship between inspiratory drive and perceived inspiratory effort in normal man. *Clin Sci (Lond),* 78, 493–96.

Craig, A.D. (2002). How do you feel? Interoception: the sense of the physiological condition of the body. *Nat Rev Neurosci,* 3, 655–66.

Craig, A.D. (2003). Interoception: the sense of the physiological condition of the body. *Curr Opin Neurobiol,* 13, 500–5.

Craig, A.D. (2007). Interoception and emotion: a neuroanatomical perspective. In: M. Lewis, J. M. Haviland-Jones, and L. Feldman Barrett (eds), Handbook of emotions, 3rd edn, pp. 272–90. New York: Guilford Press.

Craig, A.D. (2009). How do you feel now? The anterior insula and human awareness. *Nat Rev Neurosci,* 10, 59–70.

Craig, A.D. and Bushnell, M.C. (1994). The thermal grill illusion: unmasking the burn of cold pain. *Science,* 265, 252–5.

Critchley, H.D., Wiens, S., Rotshtein, P., Ohman, A., and Dolan, R.J. (2004). Neural systems supporting interoceptive awareness. *Nat Neurosci,* 7, 189–95.

Critchley, H.D., Tang, J., Glaser, D., Butterworth, B., and Dolan, R.J. (2005). Anterior cingulate activity during error and autonomic response. *Neuroimage,* 27, 885–95.

Davenport, P. W. (2008). Urge-to-cough: what can it teach us about cough? *Lung,* 186, Suppl 1, S107–S111.

Davenport, P.W. and Vovk, A. (2009). Cortical and subcortical central neural pathways in respiratory sensations. *Respir Physiol Neurobiol,* 167, 72–86.

Davenport, P.W., Friedman, W.A., Thompson, F.J., and Franzen, O. (1986). Respiratory-related cortical potentials evoked by inspiratory occlusion in humans. *J Appl Physiol,* 60, 1843–8.

Davenport, P.W., Chan, P.Y., Zhang, W., and Chou, Y.L. (2007). Detection threshold for inspiratory resistive loads and respiratory-related evoked potentials. *J Appl Physiol,* 102, 276–85.

Ditre, J.W. and Brandon, T.H. (2008). Pain as a motivator of smoking: effects of pain induction on smoking urge and behavior. *J Abnorm Psychol*, **117**, 467–72.

Eisenberger, N.I., Lieberman, M.D., and Williams, K.D. (2003). Does rejection hurt? An FMRI study of social exclusion. *Science*, **302**, 290–2.

Ernst, M. and Paulus, M.P. (2005). Neurobiology of decision making: a selective review from a neuro-cognitive and clinical perspective. *Biol. Psychiatry*, **58**, 596–604.

Feinle, C. (1998). Role of intestinal chemoreception in the induction of gastrointestinal sensations. *Dtsch Tierarztl Wochenschr*, **105**, 441–4.

Frings, S. (2008). Primary processes in sensory cells: current advances. *J Comp Physiol A Neuroethol. Sens Neural Behav Physiol.*

Garavan, H., Ross, T.J., and Stein, E.A. (1999). Right hemispheric dominance of inhibitory control: an event-related functional MRI study. *Proc Natl Acad Sci USA*, **96**, 8301–6.

Gold, J.I. and Shadlen, M.N. (2001). Neural computations that underlie decisions about sensory stimuli. *Trends Cogn Sci*, **5**, 10–16.

Goldstein, R.Z., Tomasi, D., Rajaram, S., Cottone, L.A., Zhang, L., Maloney, T. et al. (2007). Role of the anterior cingulate and medial orbitofrontal cortex in processing drug cues in cocaine addiction. *Neuroscience*, **144**, 1153–9.

Gomez, P., Stahel, W.A., and Danuser, B. (2004). Respiratory responses during affective picture viewing. *Biol Psychol*, **67**, 359–73.

Gomez, P., Zimmermann, P., Guttormsen-Schar, S., and Danuser, B. (2005). Respiratory responses associated with affective processing of film stimuli. *Biol Psychol*, **68**, 223–35.

Harrington, T. and Merzenich, M.M. (1970). Neural coding in the sense of touch: human sensations of skin indentation compared with the responses of slowly adapting mechanoreceptive afferents innervating the hairy skin of monkeys. *Exp Brain Res*, **10**, 251–64.

Huettel, S.A., Misiurek, J., Jurkowski, A.J., and McCarthy, G. (2004). Dynamic and strategic aspects of executive processing. *Brain Res*, **1000**, 78–84.

Jasmin, L., Rabkin, S.D., Granato, A., Boudah, A., and Ohara, P.T. (2003). Analgesia and hyperalgesia from GABA-mediated modulation of the cerebral cortex. *Nature*, **424**, 316–20.

Jasmin, L., Burkey, A.R., Granato, A., and Ohara, P.T. (2004). Rostral agranular insular cortex and pain areas of the central nervous system: a tract-tracing study in the rat. *J Comp Neurol*, **468**, 425–40.

Kahneman, D. and Tversky, A. (1979). Prospect theory: An analysis of decision under risk. *Econometrica*, **47**, 263–91.

Kahneman, D. and Tversky, A. (1984). Choices, values, and frames. *Am Psychol*, **39**, 341–50.

Knafelc, M. and Davenport, P.W. (1999). Relationship between magnitude estimation of resistive loads, inspiratory pressures, and the RREP P(1) peak. *J Appl Physiol*, **87**, 516–22.

Knutson, B., Taylor, J., Kaufman, M., Peterson, R., and Glover, G. (2005). Distributed neural representation of expected value. *J Neurosci*, **25**, 4806–12.

Kringelbach, M.L. (2005). The human orbitofrontal cortex: linking reward to hedonic experience. *Nat Rev Neurosci.*, **6**, 691–702.

Lahuerta, J., Bowsher, D., Campbell, J., and Lipton, S. (1990). Clinical and instrumental evaluation of sensory function before and after percutaneous anterolateral cordotomy at cervical level in man. *Pain*, **42**, 23–30.

LaMotte, R.H., Thalhammer, J.G., Torebjork, H.E., and Robinson, C.J. (1982). Peripheral neural mechanisms of cutaneous hyperalgesia following mild injury by heat. *J Neurosci*, **2**, 765–81.

Light, A.R. and Perl, E.R. (2003). Unmyelinated afferent fibers are not only for pain anymore. *J Comp Neurol*, **461**, 137–9.

Loewenstein, G. (1996). Out of control: visceral influences on behavior. *Organizational Behavior and Human Decision Processes,* **65**, 272–92.

Lofaso, F., Isabey, D., Lorino, H., Harf, A., and Scheid, P. (1992). Respiratory response to positive and negative inspiratory pressure in humans. *Respir Physiol,* **89**, 75–88.

Lopata, M., La Fata, J., Evanich, M.J., and Lourenco, R.V. (1977). Effects of flow-resistive loading on mouth occlusion pressure during CO_2 rebreathing. *Am Rev Respir Dis,* **115**, 73–81.

Luce, R. D. and Raiffa, H. (1957). *Games and decisions.* New York: Wiley.

McCabe, C., Rolls, E.T., Bilderbeck, A., and McGlone, F. (2008). Cognitive influences on the affective representation of touch and the sight of touch in the human brain. *Soc Cogn Affect Neurosci,* **3**, 97–108.

McGlone, F., Vallbo, A.B., Olausson, H., Loken, L., and Wessberg, J. (2007). Discriminative touch and emotional touch. *Can J Exp Psychol,* **61**, 173–83.

Mesulam, M.M. and Mufson, E.J. (1982). Insula of the old world monkey. *III: Efferent cortical output and comments on function. J Comp Neurol.,* **212**, 38–52.

Montague, P.R., King-Casas, B., and Cohen, J.D. (2006). Imaging valuation models in human choice. *Annu Rev Neurosci,* **29**, 417–48.

O'Doherty, J., Kringelbach, M.L., Hornak, J., Andrews, C., and Rolls, E.T. (2001). Abstract reward and punishment representations in the human orbitofrontal cortex. *Nat Neurosci,* **4**, 95–102.

Olausson, H., Wessberg, J., and Kakuda, N. (2000). Tactile directional sensibility: peripheral neural mechanisms in man. *Brain Res,* **866**, 178–87.

Olausson, H., Lamarre, Y., Backlund, H., Morin, C., Wallin, B.G., Starck, G. et al. (2002). Unmyelinated tactile afferents signal touch and project to insular cortex. *Nat Neurosci,* **5**, 900–4.

Olausson, H., Cole, J., Rylander, K., McGlone, F., Lamarre, Y., Wallin, B.G. et al. (2008). Functional role of unmyelinated tactile afferents in human hairy skin: sympathetic response and perceptual localization. *Exp Brain Res,* **184**, 135–40.

Olausson, H., Wessberg, J., Morrison, I., McGlone, F., and Vallbo, A. (2010). The neurophysiology of unmyelinated tactile afferents. *Neurosci Biobehav Rev* **34**, 185–91.

Ongur, D. and Price, J.L. (2000). The organization of networks within the orbital and medial prefrontal cortex of rats, monkeys and humans. *Cereb Cortex,* **10**, 206–19.

Paton, J.J., Belova, M.A., Morrison, S.E., and Salzman, C.D. (2006). The primate amygdala represents the positive and negative value of visual stimuli during learning. *Nature,* **439**, 865–70.

Paulus, M.P. and Stein, M.B. (2006). An insular view of anxiety. *Biol Psychiat,* **60**, 383–7.

Phan, K.L., Wager, T., Taylor, S.F., and Liberzon, I. (2002). Functional neuroanatomy of emotion: a meta-analysis of emotion activation studies in PET and fMRI. *Neuroimage.,* **16**, 331–48.

Platt, M.L. and Glimcher, P.W. (1999). Neural correlates of decision variables in parietal cortex. *Nature,* **400**, 233–8.

Pollatos, O., Herbert, B.M., Kaufmann, C., Auer, D.P., and Schandry, R. (2007a). Interoceptive awareness, anxiety and cardiovascular reactivity to isometric exercise. *Int J Psychophysiol,* **65**, 167–73.

Pollatos, O., Traut-Mattausch, E., Schroeder, H., and Schandry, R. (2007b). Interoceptive awareness mediates the relationship between anxiety and the intensity of unpleasant feelings. *J Anxiety Disord,* **21**, 931–43.

Prelec, D. (1998). The probability weigthing function. *Econometrica,* **66**, 497–527.

Ramirez, J.M. and Cabanac, M. (2003). Pleasure, the common currency of emotions. *Ann NY Acad Sci,* **1000**, 293–95.

Revelette, W.R. and Davenport, P.W. (1990). Effects of timing of inspiratory occlusion on cerebral evoked potentials in humans. *J Appl Physiol,* **68**, 282–88.

Reynolds, S.M. and Zahm, D.S. (2005). Specificity in the projections of prefrontal and insular cortex to ventral striatopallidum and the extended amygdala. *J Neurosci,* **25**, 11757–67.

Ritz, T. and Thons, M. (2002). Airway response of healthy individuals to affective picture series. *Int J Psychophysiol,* **46,** 67–75.

Robinson, T.E. and Berridge, K.C. (2008). Review. *The incentive sensitization theory of addiction: some current issues. Philos Trans R Soc Lond B Biol Sci,* **363,** 3137–46.

Robinson, S.K., Viirre, E.S., Bailey, K.A., Gerke, M.A., Harris, J.P., and Stein, M.B. (2005). Randomized placebo-controlled trial of a selective serotonin reuptake inhibitor in the treatment of nondepressed tinnitus subjects. *Psychosom Med,* **67,** 981–8.

Rolls, E.T. (2004). Convergence of sensory systems in the orbitofrontal cortex in primates and brain design for emotion. *Anat Rec A Discov Mol Cell Evol Biol,* **281,** 1212–25.

Rolls, E.T. (2004). The functions of the orbitofrontal cortex. *Brain Cogn,* **55,** 11–29.

Rolls, E.T. and Grabenhorst, F. (2008). The orbitofrontal cortex and beyond: from affect to decision making. *Prog Neurobiol,* **86,** 216–44.

Rolls, E.T. (2010). The affective and cognitive processing of touch, oral texture, and temperature in the brain. *Neurosci Biobehav Rev.*

Rottenstreich, Y. and Hsee, C.K. (2001). Money, kisses, and electric shocks: on the affective psychology of risk. *Psychol. Sci.,* **12,** 185–90.

Rushworth, M.F. and Behrens, T.E. (2008). Choice, uncertainty and value in prefrontal and cingulate cortex. *Nat Neurosci,* **11,** 389–97.

Schmelz, M., Schmidt, R., Bickel, A., Handwerker, H.O., and Torebjork, H.E. (1997). Specific C-receptors for itch in human skin. *J Neurosci,* **17,** 8003–8.

Schoenbaum, G., Setlow, B., Saddoris, M.P., and Gallagher, M. (2003). Encoding predicted outcome and acquired value in orbitofrontal cortex during cue sampling depends upon input from basolateral amygdala. *Neuron,* **39,** 855–67.

Schoenbaum, G., Roesch, M.R., and Stalnaker, T.A. (2006). Orbitofrontal cortex, decision making and drug addiction. *Trends Neurosci,* **29,** 116–24.

Schultz, W. (2006). Behavioral theories and the neurophysiology of reward. *Annu Rev Psychol,* **57,** 87–115.

Shipp, S. (2005). The importance of being agranular: a comparative account of visual and motor cortex. *Philos Trans R Soc Lond B Biol Sci,* **360,** 797–814.

Singleton, E.G. and Gorelick, D.A. (1998). Mechanisms of alcohol craving and their clinical implications. *Recent Dev Alcohol,* **14,** 177–95.

Skinner, B.F. (1981). Selection by consequences. *Science,* **213,** 501–4.

Slovic, P. (1995). The construction of preference. *Am Psychol,* **50,** 364–71.

Small, D.M., Zatorre, R.J., Dagher, A., Evans, A.C., and Jones-Gotman, M. (2001). Changes in brain activity related to eating chocolate: From pleasure to aversion. *Brain,* **124,** 1720–33.

Soderpalm, A.H. and Hansen, S. (1999). Alcohol alliesthesia: food restriction increases the palatability of alcohol through a corticosterone-dependent mechanism. *Physiol Behav,* **67,** 409–15.

Solomon, R.L. (1980). The opponent-process theory of acquired motivation: the costs of pleasure and the benefits of pain. *Am Psychol,* **35,** 691–712.

Stoeckel, L.E., Cox, J.E., Cook, E.W., III, and Weller, R.E. (2007). Motivational state modulates the hedonic value of food images differently in men and women. *Appetite,* **48,** 139–44.

Tiffany, S.T. (1999). Cognitive concepts of craving. *Alcohol Res Health,* **23,** 215–24.

Tracey, I., Becerra, L., Chang, I., Breiter, H., Jenkins, L., Borsook, D. et al. (2000). Noxious hot and cold stimulation produce common patterns of brain activation in humans: a functional magnetic resonance imaging study. *Neurosci Lett,* **288,** 159–62.

Ussher, M., Sampuran, A.K., Doshi, R., West, R., and Drummond, D.C. (2004). Acute effect of a brief bout of exercise on alcohol urges. *Addiction,* **99,** 1542–7.

Vaitl, D. (1996). Interoception. *Biol Psychol,* **42,** 1–27.

Vallbo, A.B. (1999). Bridging sensory signals in the monkey and percepts in the human mind. *Brain Res Bull,* **50,** 319–20.

Vallbo, A., Olausson, H., Wessberg, J., and Norrsell, U. (1993). A system of unmyelinated afferents for innocuous mechanoreception in the human skin. *Brain Res,* **628,** 301–4.

Vallbo, A.B., Olausson, H., Wessberg, J., and Kakuda, N. (1995). Receptive field characteristics of tactile units with myelinated afferents in hairy skin of human subjects. *J Physiol,* **483,** 783–95.

Vallbo, A.B., Olausson, H., and Wessberg, J. (1999). Unmyelinated afferents constitute a second system coding tactile stimuli of the human hairy skin. *J Neurophysiol,* **81,** 2753–63.

Von Neumann, J. and Morgenstern, O. (1947). *Theory of games and economic behavior,* 2nd edn. Princeton: Princeton University Press.

Zhao, C. and Cabanac, M. (1994). Experimental study of the internal signal of alliesthesia induced by sweet molecules in rats. *Physiol Behav,* **55,** 169–73.

Neurodevelopmental and clinical aspects

Chapter 19

A neural systems model of decision making in adolescents

Monique Ernst

Abstract

This chapter focuses on a heuristic neural systems model of motivated behavior. This model provides hypotheses for mechanisms underlying changes in behavior across development and psychopathology. The fractal triadic model (FTM) posits that goal-directed behavior results from the interaction among three nodes of behavioral control These three functional nodes are centered on the amygdala, striatum, and medial prefrontal cortex, which contribute to avoidance, approach, and modulation, respectively. They feed two distinct neural circuits: one that is modulated primarily by appetitive stimuli and serves approach behavior, and one that is modulated primarily by aversive stimuli and serves avoidance behavior. The behavioral output results from the integration of the information that is processed by these two neural circuits and is submitted to the control of the supervisory node. Such organization of three functional nodes subserving two neural circuits relies on the well-described structural and functional heterogeneity of these nodes. In addition, asynchrony in the maturational trajectories not only among the nodes, but also among the subunits of these nodes, is the central principle that underlies the typical behavioral changes seen in adolescence. Functional neuroimaging research is beginning to examine ontogenic changes in neural responses to reward-related processes that can further inform this heuristic model. The present chapter will address the major points mentioned above and will end with selected questions proposed as priority for future research.

19.1 Introduction

Adolescence is a life stage during which young people are beginning to experience highly charged feelings (e.g., romantic passion) and ideas (e.g., idealistic convictions) about their world. Strong emotions about both self and others are common and it is widely recognized that such emotions are the prime motivators of adolescent behavior. This review will examine this broad theme from a neuroscience perspective, and "deconstruct" adolescent-motivated behavior into components that can be used in a mechanistic, explanatory theory, the fractal triadic model.

Much has been written on typical adolescent behavior (see reviews: Arnett, 1999; Crews et al., 2007; Dahl, 2004; Ernst et al., 2006, 2008; Gardner and Steinberg, 2005; Steinberg, 2004). Three main aspects of adolescent behavior prevail: (1) novelty-seeking with attend-ant risk-taking and sensation-seeking; (2) peer social pre-eminence; and (3) magnifica-tion of emotions. These characteristics form the landscape of "motivated behavior" or "decision making" in adolescence. Each has been queried separately by studies ranging from behavioral observations to molecular or genetic investigations across species. The theme being addressed here is how these behavioral features systematically come together at a critical point in time to produce the stereotypical behavioral pattern of adolescence.

Neurobiological theories of behaviors are multiple (see review: Ernst and Fudge, 2009), and they have arisen from a variety of disciplines, each providing a unique perspective. For example, reinforcement research proposes conditioning mechanisms as the basis of behavior and accordingly promotes the role of amygdala and ventral striatum as prime candidates of modulators of behavior (e.g., Martin-Soelch et al., 2007; Robbins et al., 1989). Functional neuroimaging research uses a tool that provides images of activation patterns across the whole brain and thus favors theories operating at the neural-network level (e.g., Casey et al., 2008; Ernst et al., 2006). Electrophysiological research analyzes cellular activity and advances theories implicating electrical signal as conveyor of infor-mation, which is translated into action (e.g., Schultz, 2006). Lesion studies examine how essential a given brain structure is to a specific behavior or function. This type of research also fosters neural systems theories (e.g., Bechara et al., 1994; Damasio, 1996). Finally, neurochemical work manipulates chemical components known to affect behavior, like neurotransmitters or hormones, and lends itself to neurochemical models of behavior (e.g., the dopamine-reward hypothesis, Gardner, 1999; for review, see: Ernst et al., 2008). The key point is that behavioral theories are only partial, as they are shaped within the boundaries of the research tools that were employed to formulate them. However, they all model an aspect of behavioral regulation that is of great consequence for the ultimate goal of neuroscience: to advance our understanding of the mechanisms underlying behaviors and to provide strategies to normalize impaired behavior. Finally, non-biological fields, such as mathematics, engineering, physics, and computer science, are bound to play a critical role in formalizing models and integrating the extreme complexities of motivated behavior (e.g., Chambers et al., 2007; Dayan et al., 2000; Deco and Rolls, 2005; Frank, 2006; Gold and Shadlen, 2001; Schultz et al., 1997). While highly appealing, these math-ematical (computational) models are difficult to understand, which hampers their use among the neuroscience and clinical community.

With particular reference to adolescence and neural development, and based on func-tional neuroimaging research, a consistent theme has emerged. This theme describes the combination of immature cognitive control processes, subserved by prefrontal cortical regions, with more active emotion processes mediated by subcortical structures. Whereas the protracted development of cognitive function is clear, both from behavioral and neural perspectives, the nature of the development of affective function has not been as systematically studied, probably because the field of affective neuroscience has lagged behind that of cognitive neuroscience, and the study of emotion confronts specific challenges that make it more difficult to investigate. Nonetheless, the framework proposed by a number of authors (e.g., Forbes and Dahl, 2005; Hare and Casey, 2005; Yurgelun-Todd, 2007) that rests on marked developmental changes in cognitive (e.g., Bunge and Wright, 2007; Casey et al., 2005; Luna et al., 2004; Rubia et al., 2006) and in emotion neural substrates (e.g., Guyer et al., 2008; Monk et al., 2003; Van den Bos and Güroglu, 2009) across childhood and adolescence is being fully captured in the model presented here. The goal of the present work is to integrate works from basic, cognitive, and affective neuroscience into a more detailed heuristic model, the fractal triadic model, that can be tested in future research.

19.2 **The fractal triadic model (FTM)**

19.2.1 **Background**

Three lines of research have inspired the formulation of the fractal triadic model (FTM). First, temperament research has recognized that motivated behavior operates along a dimensional continuum extending between two poles, i.e., one extreme dominated by approach behavior and the other extreme dominated by avoidance behavior (e.g., Kagan and Sidman, 2004). Second, these behavioral extremes have been mapped onto specific neural substrates that share roles, but are characterized by a dominant contribution to these roles (see next section). For example, neuroscience research recognizes the amygdala as playing a dominant role in avoidance (Davis, 2006; LeDoux, 2000) and the nucleus accumbens/ventral striatum in approach (Di Chiara, 2002; Di Chiara and Bassareo, 2007; Wise, 2004). In addition, neuroscience research has assigned to the prefrontal cortex higher order cognitive function, such as inhibition, working memory, planning, and rule formation (e.g., Miller and Cohen, 2001). Third, experts in clinical research on adolescence have posited an imbalance between affective maturation and cognitive maturation, leading to a lag in emotional maturity relative to cognitive maturity (Dahl, 2004; Steinberg, 2005). The triadic model integrates these concepts by proposing a three systems equilibrium that modulates motivated behavior.

19.2.2 **Description**

The FTM is based on the principle that motivated behavior results from the regulation of a balance between approach to, and avoidance of, stimuli or situations. Accordingly, three (triadic) functional nodes make up the model, each underlying regulatory, approach and avoidance functions, that can be schematized as a large triangle (see Fig. 19.1).

Each node is assigned a representative structure that has been shown to have a dominant role corresponding to the function of this node. The concept of functional dominance assumes that each structure subserves a diversity of roles, among which one predominates, as seen from the behavioral consequences of lesion studies. The amygdala heads the avoidance network, the ventral striatum heads the approach network, and the prefrontal cortex heads the regulatory network (see Fig. 19.1). However, as will be

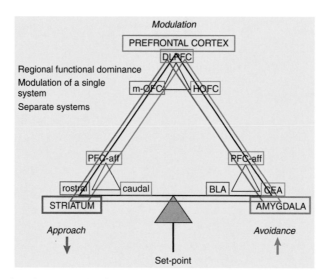

Fig. 19.1 Fractal triadic model. The fractal triadic model (FMT) is a heuristic neural systems model of motivated behavior that is based on a tripartite organization. The guiding principle posits that these three systems achieve a balance that determines a threshold for approach vs. avoidance response. This balance corresponds to a set-point that is biologically determined and varies as a function of age or psychopathology (e.g., substance use disorder). The three FTM nodes include: (1) circuits associated with approach behavior and dominated by striatal function, (2) circuits associated with avoidance behavior and dominated by amygdala function, and (3) circuits associated with regulatory processing and dominated by prefrontal cortical function. Each node participates in all three functions (fractal organization), but possesses a privileged role as noted above. Subunits showing specialized contribution to each function are proposed, based on literature in animals (see: Ernst and Fudge, 2009). In adolescence, the set-point is determined by the unique maturation pattern of these nodes and their subunits (see text). Finally, how these three nodes govern motivated behavior remains in question. Is there one single system (black triangle) or two interacting valence-related systems (red and blue triangles)?
DLPFC = dorsolateral prefrontal cortex, m-OFC = medial orbital frontal cortex, l-OFC = lateral orbital frontal cortex, PFC-aff = prefrontal cortical afferents, Ant = anterior striatum, Post = posterior striatum, BLA = basolateral amygdala, CEA = central amygdala.

discussed later, each of these structures has also been shown to contribute in various degrees to all three avoidance, approach, and modulation functions. Thus, we can assign a local triadic circuit to each structure. These are schematized in Fig. 19.1: Modulation (prefrontal cortex): DLPFC—m-OFC—l-OFC; Approach (striatum): rostral striatum—caudal striatum—PFC-aff; Avoidance (amygdala): CEA—BLA—PFC-aff. This neural systems model can thus be schematized as a fractal organization, whereby a shape can be subdivided into components, each being a small copy of the whole (Fig. 19.1).

The critical question concerns the nature of the mechanisms under which this fractal system operates. Mainly, how many separate functional networks can be identified? We can constrain answers to two main schemes, although other alternatives are conceivable: (1) a hierarchical organization based on a single network, or (2) a parallel organization based on two distinct, but interactive networks, one that monitors approach and one that monitors avoidance (Fig. 19.1). To facilitate discussion of these alternatives, a scenario of how incoming information from the environment (input) can be processed and translated into an adapted behavioral response (output) is presented in Fig. 19.2.

19.2.3 General modus operandi of a motivated behavior

We present a generic, highly simplified, schematic scenario of how environmental stimuli can generate a behavioral response (Fig. 19.2). This scenario is organized along the classical framework of "input–process–output" information-processing model. It is a graphic representation of the flow of information from detection, perception, interpretation, integration into goal, action preparation, and finally action execution. Therefore, it starts with the detection of a signal and ends up with the completion of an action.

This scenario also adopts the principle of a default mode for responding to stimuli. This default mode favors approach behavior, since approach (e.g., feeding and reproduction) is a sine qua non of survival.

19.2.3.1 Somatosensory signal

First captured by sensory organs, information about external stimuli is sent to, and processed by, primary somatosensory cortical areas. The somatosensory signal is then transmitted to "affective interpreters," the amygdala and the ventral striatum.

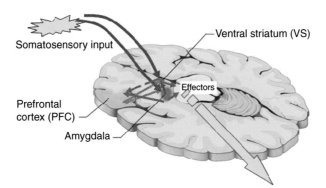

Fig. 19.2 Depiction of the path of information originating from a stimulus on a transaxial plane passing through the amygdala and striatum. The blue arrows refer to the somatosensory signal projected to subcortical areas from primary and secondary somatosensory cortical areas. The amygdala (red arrows) processes this signal and conveys it back to (1) brainstem effector centers, which generate an immediate freeze/flight response if the signal denotes acute threat, (2) back to prefrontal cortex (particularly BA25, 14), which makes the processed signal available to higher order function, and (3) to the ventral striatum, which, through communication with the prefrontal cortex, generates a motor action. The ventral striatum (purple arrows) can also project the signal back to brainstem effectors, but this route consists of relatively few striatal efferents. Most of the information is sent back to the prefrontal cortex indirectly, passing through ventral pallidum and thalamus. Finally, the prefrontal cortex (brown arrows), particularly its "limbic part" (BA 25, orbitofrontal region), sends projections directly back to the ventral striatum and amygdala, where it further modulates the processed signal.

19.2.3.2 Amygdala

The amygdala processes an affective value, which is relayed to three stations, brainstem nuclei, ventral striatum, and prefrontal cortex, using three different routes. If interpreted as an imminent threat, the amygdala signal is dispatched to the brainstem nuclei, which generate an immediate freeze or flight response. Another route is through projections to the ventral striatum. If interpreted as negative but not of survival value, the signal is transmitted to the ventral striatum and moderates the default mode of approach response. The third route proceeds through the prefrontal cortex. The amygdala sends its processed signal to cortical regions, particularly the orbital frontal cortex, which, in turn, generates an affective representation of the stimulus. Other cortical areas also use this signal to update higher order functions, including working memory, inhibition, planning, or rule formation, which are part of the cognitive construct of executive function.

19.2.3.3 Ventral striatum

The ventral striatum spurs the processing of the signal across striato-pallido-thalamo-cortical-striatal loops that ultimately generate a behavioral scheme. The behavioral scheme is actualized through the extra-pyramidal motor output pathway. The striatal system is most active in response to behavioral reinforcement, i.e., positive, such as lure of a reward, or negative, such as avoidance of a punishment. Therefore, the more affectively loaded is the incoming information, the more active is the striatal system.

In summary, both amygdala and ventral striatum, so-called "interpreters," provide their "interpreted" or processed information about the environmental stimuli directly or indirectly to the prefrontal cortex.

19.2.3.4 Prefrontal cortex

The prefrontal cortex is the site of higher order cognitive processing (e.g., Miller et al., 2001). This is where the information is stored and manipulated for higher purposes, such as behavioral organization or metacognition. Phylogenetically, the anterior medial prefrontal cortex appears to be the most evolved brain region, serving self- and other-referential cognitive processes. In this regard, the privileged anatomical and functional relations between the amygdala/ventral striatum and the anterior medial prefrontal cortex suggest a path for the communication of affective tags of environmental stimuli to higher order cognitive processes for use in complex behavioral responses, such as reflective decision making. Furthermore, these cortical–subcortical links are reciprocal, permitting prefrontal cortex to modulate the coding of affective information.

19.3 Structural and functional heterogeneity of the FTM nodes

The FTM is based on both specialization and diverseness of regional function. Such organization lends itself to redundancy but refinement and better control of information.

This heterogeneity is epitomized in two recent works with rats on the nucleus accumbens function (Faure et al., 2008; Reynolds and Berridge, 2008). These studies examined the behavioral outputs, both appetitive and aversive responses, after selective and very discretely localized inactivation of parts of the nucleus accumbens. These inactivations were performed by microinjections of an inhibitor (DNQX) of the excitatory glutamate (GLU) receptors. These studies examined whether these GLU-related behavioral effects were modulated by dopamine (Faure et al., 2008) and by environmental context (Reynolds et al., 2008). These studies reported two key observations: (1) manipulations of excitatory GLU receptors influenced appetitive and defensive behavior as a function of the site of GLU antagonist injection within the nucleus accumbens, and (2) manipulations of the environment (familiar vs. stressful), in which these manipulations occurred, significantly altered the injection-related behavioral effects. These investigators provided the metaphor of a keyboard, in which the DNQX microinjections are the fingers hitting the keys. Each note of the keyboard corresponds to a motivation, but the lower notes might be away from threat and the higher notes towards reward. The environment in which the keyboard is played changes the overall tonality of the keyboard: a stressful environment lowers the tonality and generates mainly fearful responses, and a pleasant environment raises the tonality and generates mainly appetitive responses. However, some keys become mixed and generate both appetitive and fearful responses in the stressful context. This suggests that these keys can modulate separate neural circuits, one that controls fearful behavior and another that controls appetitive behavior. Context would influence the ability of the keys to respond to either positive or negative stimuli or would influence the type of information coming to these keys (reducing the appetitive or aversive incoming signals).

19.3.1 Amygdala

Each node of the FTM, including amygdala, striatum, and medial prefrontal cortex, is composed of subregions (for review: Ernst et al., 2009). The amygdala comprises multiple nuclei, including the cortical-like nuclei or the basolateral nuclear group (BLNG: lateral, basal, and accessory basal nuclei) and the striatal-like medial and central nuclei (CEA), which are part of the medial and central extended amygdalae.

Schematically, the BLNG is the receiving port and is composed predominantly of excitatory GLU neurons, and the medial and central nuclei are the output ports and are composed predominantly of inhibitory GABA neurons (for review: Ernst and Fudge, 2009; Stefanacci and Amaral, 2000). Although their function is certainly more complex, the medial extended amygdala is involved in social information processing (social threat and maternal behavior), and the central extended amygdala determines motor and autonomic responses, such as freezing and startle to fear stimuli.

Whereas the amygdala as a whole is notably known for its role in fear (e.g., LeDoux, 2000), its role in reward is also well established (e.g., Baxter and Murray, 2002). In a review of the literature of Pavlovian conditioning studies, Everitt and colleagues (Everitt et al., 2003) proposed a double dissociation of function between the BLNG and the CEA, suggesting that these subsystems mediate different kinds of associative representation formed during Pavlovian conditioning. They proposed that the BLNG is required for coding current affective value, whereas the CEA mediates stimulus–response representations and motivational influences on behavior.

These influences on behavior would be mediated by the modulation of the nucleus accumbens indirectly via CEA projections to the dopamine nuclei in the ventral tegmentum and substantia nigra, or directly via the BLNG. This organization for processing appetitive stimuli parallels that reported for the processing of aversive stimuli, in which affective tagging is assigned to the BLNG and encoding stimulus–response Pavlovian associations, is assigned to the CEA. However, the information about aversive stimuli is processed in a serial manner from BLNG to CEA to brainstem nuclei without implicating the ventral striatum.

This partial and highly simplified summary of the anatomical and functional heterogeneity of the amygdala needs to be further qualified by the notion of dominant function. Such dominant function is defined by the behavioral consequences of the inactivation of the amygdala. Convergent evidence across species supports the reduction of fear responses in animals with lesioned amygdala, whereas consequences on appetitive behavior have not yet been systematically reported.

19.3.2 Ventral striatum

This region of the striatum is mostly involved in affective-related processes. It is referred to as the "limbic striatum" and receives projections from the amygdala and those cortical regions most influenced by the amygdala (e.g., subgenual medial prefrontal area). The ventral striatum comprises the shell and the core of the nucleus accumbens, as well as the ventromedial areas of the caudate nucleus and the putamen.

As mentioned above, the shell of the nucleus accumbens contributes to the processing of motivated behavior in response to both positive and negative stimuli along a rostrocaudal gradient, and these accumbens responses are modulated by the context in which these stimuli occur (Faure et al., 2008; Reynolds et al., 2008). A similar functional gradient seems to be more generalized along the entire rostrocaudal extent of the striatum (Fudge and Haber, 2002; Fudge et al., 2004;Selemon and Goldman-Rakic, 1985).

Other functional dissociations of the core and the shell of the nucleus accumbens have been delineated (e.g., Parkinson et al., 1999; Pecina, 2008). For example, Parkinson and colleagues (Parkinson et al., 1999) have proposed that the shell is critical for the behavioral effect of stimulants, whereas the core was implicated in mechanisms underlying the expression of conditioned stimulus–unconditioned stimulus (CS–US) associations, similar to the tagging of an affective value. This organization is reminiscent of the amygdala for which the BLNG specializes in affective tagging and the CEA in the behavioral responses to stimuli.

Similar to the amygdala, this functional heterogeneity of the ventral striatum needs to be moderated by the notion of dominant function. When the ventral striatum is inactivated, the most consistent consequence is a reduction of approach behavior (e.g., Adam et al., 2008).

19.3.3 Medial prefrontal cortex (mPFC)

This region comprises the anterior cingulate cortex, including the dorsal, anterior, and subgenual sections. Surrounding the anterior cingulate cortex, and following a caudal–rostral direction, are the supplementary motor area, Brodmann area (BA) 10, and medial orbital frontal cortex (BA 11). The mPFC, particularly the subgenual cingulate cortex (BA 25 and 14), is the cortical region most tightly connected with the amygdala and ventral striatum.

The mPFC, as a whole, has been implicated in a number of functions, including conflict detection, planning, rule formation, social processing, self-reflection, inhibition, representation of affective values, but also responses to reward and punishment (e.g., Bush et al., 2000; Carter and van Veen, 2007; Dehaene and Changeux, 2000; Rushworth et al., 2004; Schall et al., 2002; van den Bos and Güroglu, 2009). However, overall, less is known about the exact role of these regions because their functions may be unique to the human species and not accessible to study in lower animals.

The mPFC role in reward or punishment/threat is not straightforward. However, it is clear that appetitive/aversive information about environmental stimuli is used in higher level processes. In addition, mPFC plays an important role in monitoring and controlling amygdala and striatum activity, based on the direct and indirect reciprocal connections between these structures (for review: Ernst et al., 2009).

In summary, we provided a very coarse description of the heterogeneity of the three nodes of the FTM. However, the main point conveyed by this section is that each node contributes to all three functions of approach, avoidance, and regulation, in addition to carrying a dominant role defined by the most impaired behavior after inactivation. This architecture begs the question of functional organization. As already indicated, among a number of alternatives, two possible schemes can be entertained: a single network or two interactive networks (see Fig. 19.2). The FTM also provides a framework against which to study maturational changes.

19.4 **Further characterization of the FTM**

This section is twofold. First, it will provide support for separate networks that are modulated preferentially by appetitive or aversive stimuli. Second, it will examine how various maturation rates among each functional unit and subunit of the FTM can influence behavior.

19.4.1 **Two interactive networks in response to appetitive and aversive stimuli**

In studies of responses to reward or penalties, findings commonly report, on the one hand, activation of striatal regions and medial OFC in response to appetitive stimuli (e.g., monetary gain, beautiful faces) (e.g., Aharon et al., 2001; Breiter et al., 2001; Delgado et al., 2000; Ernst et al., 2005; Knutson et al., 2001, 2003; O'Doherty et al., 2004; Rogers et al., 2004), and, on the other hand, activation of amygdala, hippocampus, insula and lateral OFC in response to aversive stimuli (e.g., monetary losses, aversive pictures, or angry or fearful faces) (e.g., Becerra et al., 2001; Tom et al., 2007; Zald and Pardo, 1997). Although studies also report recruitment of structures from both sets of regions in either aversive or appetitive conditions (e.g., Becerra et al., 2001; Jensen et al., 2003; Seymour et al., 2007;

Zalla et al., 2000), the relative differential activation patterns to appetitive vs. aversive stimuli reflect the preferential regional sensitivity described above.

In support of this dual organization, we will briefly present two fMRI studies with adults from our laboratory. The first study (Hardin et al., 2007) contrasts neural responses to favorable vs. unfavorable monetary outcomes in a positive (gain vs. nogain) and a negative (loss vs. noloss) context. The second study (Nawa et al., 2008) contrasts performance on a monetary betting task in a social vs. nonsocial condition.

19.4.1.1 Monetary context

Hardin and colleagues (Hardin et al., 2007) used a monetary gambling paradigm that asked players to select one of two options provided by a wheel of fortune (Fig. 19.3a). Each option was defined by the probability of a $gain in the appetitive condition, or of a $loss in the aversive condition.

In the appetitive condition, the favorable outcome was a $gain ($0.50 to $7.00), and the unfavorable outcome was the absence of gain ($0.00). In the aversive condition, the favorable outcome was the avoidance of a $loss ($0.00), and the unfavorable outcome was a $loss ($0.50 to $7.00). These two appetitive and aversive conditions were presented in blocks, such that the dollar amount at stake was the same in either condition.

Findings showed that ventral striatum, medial OFC, and medial PFC were modulated preferentially by the outcomes of the appetitive context, and amygdala, hippocampus, and insula were modulated preferentially by the outcomes of the aversive context (Fig. 19.3b). No other regions were involved in these contrasts. These findings are eloquent support for a functional dichotomy in neural circuits underlying affective processes. Such relative segregation of function may give rise to different patterns of behavioral responses to positive or negative stimuli depending on their relative maturational state. The FTM introduce a third term to this appetitive–aversive balance in the form of a regulatory system that helps maintain a set-point for this balance.

19.4.1.2 Social context

The second study by Nawa and colleagues (Nawa et al., 2008) provides another example of how context can modulate the relative engagement of the appetitive and aversive network. In this study, a betting task performed in the mere presence of another unfamiliar player (social condition) was found to engage the amygdala and PFC more than when the task was performed by the participant alone; in contrast, when performed in the "alone" condition, the betting task engaged the ventral striatum more than when performed in the presence of another player. These findings suggest that the presence of another unfamiliar person would induce a state of alarm in the subjects, which would activate the threat system and moderate the engagement of the reward system during a betting task.

19.4.1.3 Summary

In summary, the key notion we wish to underline is that each node and its subunits has its own developmental trajectory pattern, and it is the coordination among these nodes at any given point in time that shapes motivated behavior. Much more needs to be learned

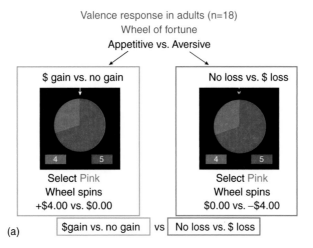

(a)

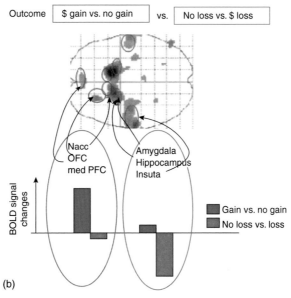

(b)

Fig. 19.3 Wheel of Fortune Paradigm (Ernst et al., 2004; Hardin et al., 2007) and evidence for a 2-valence-related network organization; (a) depicts the paradigm. The same wheel of fortune played in two blocks of two different conditions. In one block, participants can only win or not win (appetitive condition), and in the other block, participants can only lose or not lose (aversive condition). The contrast was how outcome was modulated by the context. (b) Presents the glass brain of the contrast. Findings showed a clear segregation of activation patterns: nucleus accumbens (Nacc), medial prefrontal cortex (medPFC), and orbitofrontal cortex (OFC) were sensitive to outcomes in the appetitive context (green lines), whereas the amygdala, hippocampus, and insula were sensitive to outcomes in the aversive context (red lines). The bar graph is a schematized rendition of the pattern seen in the study.

about these functional developmental patterns and how they interact with one another. This will be achieved through basic and human research advancing hand in hand in this quest. The FTM provides a framework that can help guide such systematic study. In the next section, we will provide a brief survey of work in humans. A review of adolescent developmental changes reported in the animal literature can be found in Ernst and Fudge (2009) and will not be addressed here.

19.4.2 Maturational trajectories of the FTM components affecting adolescent behavior

The notion of heterogeneity in regional maturational trajectories is well accepted (e.g., Casey et al., 2008; Ernst et al., 2006; Luna and Sweeney, 2004). The most prevalent theory posits a delay in the maturation of the regulatory control systems within the PFC, relative to the maturation of the processors of emotion, including amygdala and striatum. This dissociation in maturation was supported by findings from structural MRI showing ongoing changes in white matter (taken as an index of myelination) and volume (index of dendritization) in the prefrontal cortex extending through late adolescence (up to 25 years of age) (Giedd et al., 1999; Lu and Sowell, 2009). Subcortical structures did not show similar striking changes and were thus thought to be already mature, or close to mature, at adolescence.

This maturational imbalance between emotional and cognitive neural substrates was thought to at least partly explain adolescent behaviors, particularly the more intense and labile emotions, and the poor decision making in emotional contexts (poor inhibition or modulation of emotional responses). However, the high level of risk that adolescents take could not be explained by an indiscriminative imbalance between emotion and cognition. The direction of adolescent decision making, i.e., risk-taking with disregard for, or even attraction to, potential dangers and heightened lure of reward, suggests a bias in the function of the neural correlates of appetitive vs. aversive coding. Adolescent decision making would generically be characterized by a stronger system that favors approach to stimuli and typically responds to appetitive stimuli relative to a system that favors avoidance of stimuli and typically responds to aversive stimuli. The FTM modified the former dual cognitive/affective-system model by separating the appetitive and aversive aspects within the affective system.

The FTM proposes that during adolescence, the set-point for the balance of approach–avoidance behavior is displaced physiologically towards approach behavior in the context of decision making. This distinct set-point results from the functional (maturational) state of each of the regulatory, appetitive and aversive neural systems. This dynamic tripartite organization is quite flexible and provides latitude for adaptive behavior. For example, responses to threat may vary as a function of context. In a positive context (e.g., among familiar friendly peers), the adolescent response to threat may be reduced, whereas in a negative context (e.g., among unfamiliar unfriendly peers), this response may be exacerbated relative to adults. This model needs to be qualified by the huge interindividual variability in behavioral responses and the notion that this description is only generic. In addition, it suggests that all three components of the model undergo maturational changes. Indeed, functional alterations have been shown to also affect subcortical structures, including amygdala (changes in the density of amygdalocortical projections (Cunningham et al., 2002) and striatum (changes in dopamine activity; see review: Ernst et al., 2009), although in a more subtle way than those affecting PFC (see review: Ernst et al., 2009). At present, the few developmental studies comparing adolescents to adults on responses to rewards seem to support the FTM premises (see Table 19.1).

19.4.3 Developmental functional neuroimaging studies of reward-related processes

At present, the developmental neuroimaging work on reward-related processes is based solely on cross-over studies. The gold-standard for such work remains longitudinal studies, and efforts are being made to conduct this type of research.

Behaviorally, observational and clinical data seem to concur on enhanced risk-taking, enhanced sensitivity to reward, and reduced sensitivity to punishment in adolescence. An example of behavioral data supporting this framework is given in Fig. 19.4 (Ernst et al., 2005). In the context of a simple binary decision making, measures of sensitivity to punishment or to reward can be taken in three different stages of the decision-making process: (1) during the formation of a preference leading to the selection of one option, (2) during the anticipation of the reward or punishment, or (3) during the receipt of the reward or punishment (Ernst and Paulus, 2005). These different stages in reward processes have been examined in the few developmental studies published to date (see Table 19.1).

19.4.3.1 Formation of preference

As can be seen in Table 19.1, during the formation of a preference, the PFC (OFC/ACC) was found, in one study, to be less engaged in adolescents than in adults (Eshel et al., 2007). However, in another study, it was found to be more engaged in adolescents than in adults (van Leijenhorst et al., 2006). The paradigms used in these two studies significantly differ in the type of risk-taking, as well as the nature and manipulation of reward

Table 19.1 Summary of findings from developmental functional neuroimaging studies comparing adolescents to adults. Empty cells signify the absence of report of significant differences between adolescents and adults

	Risk selection		Gain anticipation		Ouctome: gain vs. nogain	
Ventral striatum			Decreased	Bjork et al., 2004	Increased	Ernst et al., 2005
						Galván et al., 2006
						Spicer et al., 2007
Amygdala					Decreased	Ernst et al., 2005
OFC	Increased	Van Leijenhorst et al., 2006			Increased	Spicer et al., 2007
	Decreased	Eshel et al. 2007				

magnitude. In the former study, there was no optimal choice: both reward magnitude and probability vary between options and participants could earn real money. In the latter study, there was an optimal choice, only probability was manipulated, and participants did not earn a specific money amount associated with their choice. Any of these differences could have accounted for the discrepancies in the result of these two studies. No age-related differences in striatal or amygdala activation were reported in either study.

19.4.3.2 Reward anticipation

Only one study specifically examined reward anticipation (Bjork et al., 2004). This study reported reduced ventral striatal activation in adolescents compared to adults. Interpretation of these findings can be twofold. The interpretation that was favored by the authors is that the lower activation indicates a reduced reward system response to the appetitive anticipation. Another possible, but opposite, account is that the reduced striatal activation indicates a more efficient reward response based on similar performance level between adults and adolescents. This question is still open. No significant activation differences between age groups were reported in the amygdala or PFC.

19.4.3.3 Reward receipt

Three independent studies reported greater ventral striatum activation in response to gains in adolescents compared to adults (Ernst et al., 2005; Galván et al., 2006; Spicer et al., 2007). One of these studies also found less amygdala modulation by outcomes in adolescent compared to adults (Ernst et al., 2005). Another study found greater OFC activation in adolescents compared to adults (Spicer et al., 2007).

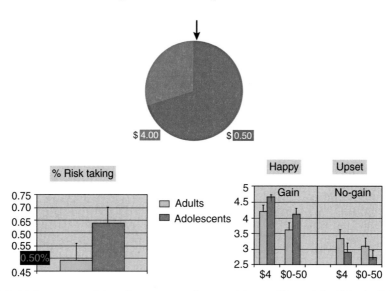

Fig. 19.4 Adolescent vs. adult performance on the appetitive condition of the Wheel of Fortune paradigm (Ernst et al., 2005). Adolescents take more risk, i.e., select more often the 30% chance of gain than the 70% chance of gain. During outcomes, they report being happier at receiving a gain than adults and less upset at missing a gain than adults.

In summary, these few studies are the very first indications, in humans, of age-related differences in the coding of incentives in the context of a decision-making or "go" paradigm. These age-related differences are presumably reflective of the ontogenic changes occurring in the underlying neural substrates of the processes under study. So far, findings from incentive-related studies in adolescents vs. adults seem to support greater responses of the neural system more closely associated with approach behavior (i.e., striatal structures), weaker engagement of both the neural systems more closely associated with avoidant behavior (i.e., amygdala), and the neural systems associated with supervisory function (i.e., PFC).

19.5 **Conclusion**

The fractal triadic model is proposed as a heuristic neural systems model of motivated behavior. It is based on a biological homeostatic balance established among three functional nodes whose set-point might also be programmed biologically, that is, determined in part by the genetic make-up and its interaction with the environment. This set-point varies as a function of neural maturation (and thus age), which is characterized by different trajectories among different regions and even subregions. This maturational asynchrony may be partially responsible for the unique set point of the balance of the triadic node, particularly during adolescence. Empirical evidence in humans is starting to emerge from functional neuroimaging studies. Many more studies are needed in order to prove or disprove this pattern of functional organization in the coding of reward-related behavior.

A critical aspect of this research is the complexity of the processes under scrutiny. For example, it will be critical to carefully parse out the various parameters of behavior that can contribute to age-group differences. One such parameter is the effect of self-agency. In other words, to what extent the group differences observed so far reflect the reward itself or the contingency of the reward on subjects' own actions (e.g., Bar-Haim et al., 2009; Zink et al., 2004). Another fundamental question is whether incentives differentially influence cognitive processes in adolescents and adults, based on ontogenic changes in neural systems. A third question concerns the effect of social context, which becomes so important during adolescence. In this regard, we can expect social context to modulate reward-related processes in unique ways during adolescence, not only quantitatively, but also qualitatively. Finally, it is critical to keep in mind that the set-point for reward-related behaviors in the context of decision making can be different in other contexts, including passive exposure to emotionally loaded stimuli, or cognitive demands, such as response inhibition. For example, whereas amygdala engagement seems to be weaker in adolescents compared to adults during reward-related decision making (Ernst et al., 2005), it is stronger in adolescents than in adults during exposure to negatively valenced facial expressions (Guyer et al., 2008).

In closing this chapter, we wish to acknowledge that the FTM could not have been formulated without the formidable work of so many basic and clinical scientists and theorists, who, unfortunately, could not all be included in this work.

Acknowledgments

This work was supported by the Intramural Research Program of the National Institute of Mental Health of the NIH.

References

Adam, J., Baulac, M., Hauw, J.J., Laplane, D., and Duyckaerts, C. (2008). Behavioral symptoms after pallido-nigral lesions: a clinico-pathological case. *Neurocase*, **14**(2), 125–30.

Aharon, I., Etcoff, N., Ariely, D., Chabris, C.F., O'Connor, E., and Breiter, H.C. (2001). Beautiful faces have variable reward value: fMRI and behavioral evidence. *Neuron*, **32**(3), 537–51.

Arnett, J.J. (1999). Adolescent storm and stress, reconsidered. *Am Psychol*, **54**(5), 317–26.

Bar-Haim, Y., Fox N.A., Benson, B., Guyer, A.E., Williams, A., Nelson E.E., et al. (2009). Neural correlates of reward processing in adolescents with a history of inhibited temperment. *Psychol Sci*, **20**(8), 1009–18.

Baxter, M.G. and Murray, E.A. (2002). The amygdala and reward. *Nat Rev Neurosci*, **3**(7), 563–73.

Becerra, L., Breiter, H.C., Wise, R., Gonzalez, R.G., and Borsook, D. (2001). Reward circuitry activation by noxious thermal stimuli. *Neuron*, **32**(5), 927–46.

Bechara, A., Damasio, A.R., Damasio, H., and Anderson, S.W. (1994). Insensitivity to future consequences following damage to human prefrontal cortex. *Cognition*, **50**(1–3), 7–15.

Bjork, J.M., Knutson, B., Fong, G.W., Caggiano, D.M., Bennett, S.M., and Hommer, D.W. (2004). Incentive-elicited brain activation in adolescents: similarities and differences from young adults. *J Neurosci*, **24**(8), 1793–802.

Breiter, H.C., Aharon, I., Kahneman, D., Dale, A., and Shizgal, P. (2001). Functional imaging of neural responses to expectancy and experience of monetary gains and losses. *Neuron*, **30**(2), 619–39.

Bunge, S.A. and Wright, S.B. (2007). Neurodevelopmental changes in working memory and cognitive control. *Curr Opin Neurobiol*, **17**(2), 243–50.

Bush, G., Luu, P., and Posner, M.I. (2000). Cognitive and emotional influences in anterior cingulate cortex. *Trends Cogn Sci*, **4**(6), 215–22.

Carter, C.S. and van Veer, V. (2007). Anterior cingulate cortex and conflict detection: an update of theory and data. *Cogn Affect Behav Neurosci*, **7**(4), 367–79.

Casey, B.J., Galván, A., and Hare, T.A. (2005). Changes in cerebral functional organization during cognitive development. *Curr Opin Neurobiol*, **15**(2), 239–44.

Casey, B.J., Getz, S., and Galván, A. (2008). The adolescent brain. *Dev Rev*, **28**(1), 62–77.

Chambers, R.A., Bickel, W.K., and Potenza, M.N. (2007). A scale-free systems theory of motivation and addiction. *Neurosci Biobehav Rev*, **31**(7), 1017–45.

Crews, F., He, J., and Hodge, C. (2007). Adolescent cortical development: a critical period of vulnerability for addiction. *Pharmacol Biochem Behav*, **86**(2), 189–99.

Cunningham, M.G., Bhattacharyya, S., and Benes, F.M. (2002). Amygdalo-cortical sprouting continues into early adulthood: implications for the development of normal and abnormal function during adolescence. *J Comp Neurol*, **453**(2), 116–30.

Dahl, R.E. (2004). Adolescent brain development: a period of vulnerabilities and opportunities. Keynote address. *Ann NY Acad Sci*, **1021**, 1–22.

Damasio, A.R. (1996). The somatic marker hypothesis and the possible functions of the prefrontal cortex. *Philos Trans R Soc Lond B Biol Sci*, **351**(1346), 1413–20.

Davis, M. (2006). Neural systems involved in fear and anxiety measured with fear-potentiated startle. *Am Psychol*, **61**(8), 741–56.

Dayan, P., Kakade, S., and Montague, P.R. (2000). Learning and selective attention. *Nat Neurosci*, 3 Suppl, 1218–23.

Deco, G. and Rolls, E.T. (2005). Attention, short-term memory, and action selection: a unifying theory. *Prog Neurobiol*, **76**(4), 236–56.

Dehaene, S. and Changeux, J.P. (2000). Reward-dependent learning in neuronal networks for planning and decision-making. *Prog Brain Res*, **126**, 217–29.

Delgado, M.R., Nystrom, L.E., Fissell, C., Noll, D.C., and Fiez, J.A. (2000). Tracking the hemodynamic responses to reward and punishment in the striatum. *J Neurophysiol*, **84**(6), 3072–77.

Di Chiara, G. (2002). Nucleus accumbens shell and core dopamine: differential role in behavior and addiction. *Behav Brain Res*, **137**(1–2), 75–114.

Di Chiara, G. and Bassareo, V. (2007). Reward system and addiction: what dopamine does and doesn't do. *Curr Opin Pharmacol*, **7**(1), 69–76.

Ernst, M. and Fudge, J.L. (2009). A developmental neurobiological model of motivated behavior: Anatomy, connectivity and ontogeny of the triadic nodes. *Neurosci Biobehav Rev*, **33**(3), 367–82.

Ernst, M. and Paulus, M.P. (2005). Neurobiology of Decision-making: A Selective Review from a Neurocognitive and Clinical Perspective. *Biol Psychiatry*, **58**(8), 597–604.

Ernst, M. and Spear, L.P. (2008). Development of reward systems in adolescence. In M. De Haan and M.R.Gunnar (eds), *Handbook of developmental social neuroscience*. New York City: Guilford Press.

Ernst, M., Nelson, E.E., McClure, E.B., Monk, C.S., Eshel, N., Zarahn, E. et al. (2004). Choice selection and reward anticipation: an fMRI study. *Neuropsychologia*, **42**, 1585–97.

Ernst, M., Nelson, E.E., Jazbec, S., McClure, E.B., Monk, C.S., Leibenluft, E. et al. (2005). Amygdala and nucleus accumbens in responses to receipt and omission of gains in adults and adolescents. *Neuroimage*, **25**(4), 1279–91.

Ernst, M., Pine, D.S., and Hardin, M. (2006). Triadic model of the neurobiology of motivated behavior in adolescence. *Psychol Med*, **36**(3), 299–312.

Ernst, M., Romeo, R., and Andersen, S.L. (2009). Neurobiology of the development of motivated behaviors in adolescence: A window into a neural systems model. *Pharmacol Biochem Behav*, **93**(3), 199–211.

Eshel, N., Nelson, E.E., Blair, R.J., Pine, D.S., and Ernst, M. (2007). Neural substrates of choice selection in adults and adolescents: development of the ventrolateral prefrontal and anterior cingulate cortices. *Neuropsychologia*, **45**(6), 1270–79.

Everitt, B.J., Cardinal, R.N., Parkinson, J.A., and Robbins, T.W. (2003). Appetitive behavior: impact of amygdala-dependent mechanisms of emotional learning. *Ann NY Acad Sci*, **985**, 233–50.

Faure, A., Reynolds, S.M., Richard, J.M., and Berridge, K.C. (2008). Mesolimbic dopamine in desire and dread: enabling motivation to be generated by localized glutamate disruptions in nucleus accumbens. *J Neurosci*, **28**(28), 7184–92.

Forbes, E.E. and Dahl, R.E. (2005). Neural systems of positive affect: relevance to understanding child and adolescent depression? *Dev Psychopathol*, **17**(3), 827–50.

Frank, M.J. (2006). Hold your horses: a dynamic computational role for the subthalamic nucleus in decision-making. *Neural Netw*, **19**(8), 1120–36.

Fudge, J.L., and Haber, S.N. (2002). Defining the caudal ventral striatum in primates: cellular and histochemical features. *J Neurosci*, **22**(23), 10078–82.

Fudge, J.L., Breitbart, M.A., and McClain, C. (2004). Amygdaloid inputs define a caudal component of the ventral striatum in primates. *J Comp Neurol*, **476**(4), 330–47.

Galván, A., Hare, T.A., Parra, C.E., Penn, J., Voss, H., Glover, G., and Casey, B.J. (2006). Earlier development of the accumbens relative to orbitofrontal cortex might underlie risk-taking behavior in adolescents. *J Neurosci*, **26**(25), 6885–92.

Gardner, E.L. (1999). The neurobiology and genetics of addiction: Implications of the reward deficiency syndrome for therapeutic strategies in chemical dependency. In J. Elster (ed.), Addiction:Entries and Exits. (pp. 57–119). New York: Russell Sage Foundation.

Gardner, M. and Steinberg, L. (2005). Peer influence on risk taking, risk preference, and risky decision-making in adolescence and adulthood: an experimental study. *Dev Psychol*, **41**(4), 625–35.

Giedd, J.N. et al. (1999). Brain development during childhood and adolescence: a longitudinal MRI study. *Nat Neurosci*, **2**(10), 861–63.

Gold, J.I. and Shadlen, M.N. (2001). Neural computations that underlie decisions about sensory stimuli. *Trends Cogn Sci.*, **5**(1), 10–16.

Guyer, A.E., Monk, C.S., McClure-Tone, E.B., Nelson, E.E., Roberson-Nay, R., Adler, A.D. et al. (2008). A Developmental Examination of Amygdala Response to Facial Expressions. *J Cogn Neurosci*, **20**(9), 1565–82.

Hardin, M., Pine, D.S., and Ernst, M. (2007). How money talks to the brain: The influence of contextual valence in processing decision outcomes [Abstract]. *The Society for Neuroeconomics Annual Conference*, 27–30.

Hare, T.A. and Casey, B.J. (2005). The neurobiology and development of cognitive and affective control. *Cog Brain, Behav*, **9**(3), 273–86.

Jensen, J., McIntosh, A.R., Crawley, A.P., Mikulis, D.J., Remington, G., and Kapur, S. (2003). Direct activation of the ventral striatum in anticipation of aversive stimuli. *Neuron*, **40**(6), 1251–57.

Kagan, J. and Sidman, N.C. (2004). *The long shadow of temperament*. Cambridge: Belknap Press of Harvard University Press.

Knutson, B., Fong, G.W., Adams, C.M., Varner, J.L., and Hommer, D. (2001). Dissociation of reward anticipation and outcome with event-related fMRI. *Neuroreport*, **12**(17), 3683–87.

Knutson, B., Fong, G.W., Bennett, S.M., Adams, C.M., and Hommer, D. (2003). A region of mesial prefrontal cortex tracks monetarily rewarding outcomes: characterization with rapid event-related fMRI. *J Comp Pysiol Psychol*, **47**, 419–27.

LeDoux, J.E. (2000). Emotion circuits in the brain. *Annu Rev Neurosci*, **23**, 155–84.

Lu, L.H. and Sowell, E.R. (2009). Morphological development of the brain: waht has imaging told us? In J.M. Rumsey and M. Ernst (eds), *Neuroimaging in developmental clinical neuroscience*. Cambridge, U.K.: Cambridge University.

Luna, B. and Sweeney, J.A. (2004). The emergence of collaborative brain function: FMRI studies of the development of response inhibition. *Ann NY Acad Sci*, 1021, 296–309.

Luna, B., Garver, K.E., Urban, T.A., Lazar, N.A., and Sweeney, J.A. (2004). Maturation of cognitive processes from late childhood to adulthood. *Child Dev.*, **75**(5), 1357–72.

Martin-Soelch, C., Linthicum, J., and Ernst, M. (2007). Appetitive conditioning: neural bases and implications for psychopathology. *Neurosci Biobehav Rev*, **31**(3), 426–40.

Miller, E.K. and Cohen, J.D. (2001). An integrative theory of prefrontal cortex function. *Annu Rev Neurosci*, **24**, 167–202.

Monk, C.S., McClure, E.B., Nelson, E.E., Zarahn, E., Bilder, R.M., Leibenluft, E. et al. (2003). Adolescent immaturity in attention-related brain engagement to emotional facial expressions. *Neuroimage*, **20**, 420–8.

Nawa, N.E., Nelson, E.E., Pine, D.S., and Ernst, M. (2008). Do you make a difference? Social context in a betting task. *Soc Cogn Affect Neurosci*, **3**(4), 367–76.

O'Doherty, J., Dayan, P., Schultz, J., Deichmann, R., Friston, K., and Dolan, R.J. (2004). Dissociable roles of ventral and dorsal striatum in instrumental conditioning. *Science*, **304**(5669), 452–4.

Parkinson, J.A., Olmstead, M.C., Burns, L.H., Robbins, T.W., and Everitt, B.J. (1999). Dissociation in effects of lesions of the nucleus accumbens core and shell on appetitive pavlovian approach behavior and the potentiation of conditioned reinforcement and locomotor activity by D-amphetamine. *J Neurosci*, **19**(6), 2401–11.

Pecina, S. (2008). Opioid reward "liking" and "wanting" in the nucleus accumbens. *Physiol Behav*, **94**(5), 675–80.

Reynolds, S.M. and Berridge, K.C. (2008). Emotional environments retune the valence of appetitive versus fearful functions in nucleus accumbens. *Nat Neurosci*, **11**(4), 423–5.

Robbins, T.W., Cador, M., Taylor, J.R., and Everitt, B.J. (1989). Limbic-striatal interactions in reward-related processes. *Neurosci Biobehav Rev*, **13**(2–3), 155–62.

Rogers, R.D., Ramnani, N., Mackay, C., Wilson, J.L., Jezzard, P., Carter, C.S., and Smith, S.M. (2004). Distinct portions of anterior cingulate cortex and medial prefrontal cortex are activated by reward processing in separable phases of decision-making cognition. *Biol Psychiatry*, **55**(6), 594–602.

Rubia, K., Smith, A.B., Woolley, J., Nosarti, C., Heyman, I., Taylor, E., and Brammer, M. (2006). Progressive increase of frontostriatal brain activation from childhood to adulthood during event-related tasks of cognitive control. *Hum Brain Mapp*, **27**(12), 973–93.

Rushworth, M.F., Walton, M.E., Kennerley, S.W., and Bannerman, D.M. (2004). Action sets and decisions in the medial frontal cortex. *Trends Cogn Sci*, **8**(9), 410–417.

Schall, J.D., Stuphorn, V., and Brown, J.W. (2002). Monitoring and control of action by the frontal lobes. *Neuron*, **36**(2), 309–22.

Schultz, W. (2006). Behavioral theories and the neurophysiology of reward. *Annu Rev Psychol*, **57**, 87–115.

Schultz, W., Dayan, P., and Montague, P.R. (1997). A neural substrate of prediction and reward. *Science*, **275**(5306), 1593–99.

Selemon, L.D. and Goldman-Rakic, P.S. (1985). Longitudinal topography and interdigitation of corticostriatal projections in the rhesus monkey. *J Neurosci*, **5**(3), 776–94.

Seymour, B., Daw, N., Dayan, P., Singer, T., and Dolan, R. (2007). Differential encoding of losses and gains in the human striatum. *J Neurosci*, **27**(18), 4826–31.

Spicer, J., Galván, A., Hare, T.A., Voss, H., Glover, G., and Casey, B. (2007). Sensitivity of the nucleus accumbens to violations in expectation of reward. *Neuroimage*, **34**(1), 455–61.

Stefanacci, L. and Amaral, D.G. (2000). Topographic organization of cortical inputs to the lateral nucleus of the macaque monkey amygdala: a retrograde tracing study 11557. *J Comp Neurol*, **421**(1), 52–79.

Steinberg, L. (2004). Risk taking in adolescence: what changes, and why?. *Ann NY Acad Sci*, **1021**, 51–58.

Steinberg, L. (2005). Cognitive and affective development in adolescence 569. *Trends Cogn Sci*, **9**(2), 69–74.

Tom, S.M., Fox, C.R., Trepel, C., and Poldrack, R.A. (2007). The neural basis of loss aversion in decision-making under risk. *Science*, **315**(5811), 515–518.

van Leijenhorst, L., Crone, E.A., and Bunge, S.A. (2006). Neural correlates of developmental differences in risk estimation and feedback processing. *Neuropsychologia*, **44**(11), 2158–70.

van Leijenhorst, L., Zanolie, K., Van Meel, C.S., Westenberg, P.M., Rombouts, S.A., and Crone, E.A. (2010). What motivates the adolescent? Brain regions mediating reward sensitivity across adolescence. *Cereb Cortex*, **20**(1), 61–9.

van den Bos, W., and Güroglu, B. (2009). The role of the ventral medial prefrontal cortex in social decision-making. *J Neurosci*, **29**(24), 7631–32.

Wise, R.A. (2004). Dopamine, learning and motivation. *Nat Rev Neurosci*, **5**(6), 483–94.

Yurgelun-Todd, D. (2007). Emotional and cognitive changes during adolescence. *Curr Opin Neurobiol*, **17**(2), 251–57.

Zald, D.H. and Pardo, J.V. (1997). Emotion, olfaction, and the human amygdala: amygdala activation during aversive olfactory stimulation. *Proc Natl Acad Sci USA*, **94**(8), 4119–24.

Zalla, T., Koechlin, E., Pietrini, P., Basso, G., Aquino, P., Sirigu, A., and Grafman, J. (2000). Differential amygdala responses to winning and losing: a functional magnetic resonance imaging study in humans. *Eur J Neurosci*, **12**(5), 1764–70.

Zinc, C.F., Pagnoni, G., Martin-Skursi, M.E., Chappelow, J.C., Berns, G.J. (2004). Human stratal responses to monetary reward depend on saliency. *Neuron*, **42**(3), 509–17.

Chapter 20

Risky and impulsive components of adolescent decision making

B.J. Casey, Todd A. Hare, and Adriana Galván

Abstract

Adolescence is a developmental period often characterized as a time of impulsive and risky choices leading to increased incidence of unintentional injuries and violence, alcohol and drug abuse, unintended pregnancy, and sexually transmitted diseases. Traditional neurobiological and cognitive explanations for such suboptimal decisions have failed to account for nonlinear changes in behavior observed during adolescence, relative to childhood and adulthood. This review provides a biologically plausible conceptualization of the neural mechanisms underlying these nonlinear changes in behavior, of a heightened sensitivity to incentives while impulse control is still relatively immature during this period. Recent human imaging and animal studies provide a biological basis for this view, suggesting differential development of limbic reward systems relative to top-down control systems during adolescence, relative to childhood and adulthood. Finally, a mathematical model is provided to further distinguish these constructs of impulsivity and risky choices to further characterize developmental and individual differences in suboptimal decisions during this period.

20.1 Introduction

Of the over 13,000 adolescent deaths recorded in the United States each year by The National Center for Health Statistics, the leading causes are all preventable motor vehicle crashes, unintentional injuries, homicide, and suicide (Eaton et al., 2006). Decisions teens make that increase their likelihood of a fatal outcome include deciding to drive a vehicle after drinking or without a seat belt, to carry a weapon, to use illegal substances, and to engage in unprotected sex resulting in unintended pregnancies and STDs, including HIV infection (2005 National Youth Risk Behavior Survey—YRBS). These statistics underscore the significance of understanding risky and impulsive decision making in adolescents.

A number of cognitive and neurobiological hypotheses have been postulated for why adolescents engage in suboptimal choice behavior. In a recent review of the literature on human adolescent brain development, Yurgelun-Todd (2007) suggests that cognitive development through the adolescent years is associated with progressively greater efficiency of cognitive control capacities. This efficiency is described as dependent on maturation of the prefrontal cortex as evidenced by increased activity within focal prefrontal regions (Rubia et al., 2000; Tamm et al., 2002) and diminished activity in irrelevant brain regions (Brown et al., 2005; Durston et al., 2006). Several groups have shown that changes in prefrontal development from adolescence to adulthood are associated with less suboptimal and risky choices (e.g., Eshel et al., 2006). While these studies assess the transition out of adolescence into adulthood, they fail to examine the transition into adolescence from childhood. As such, one can only speculate as to whether this pattern is specific to adolescence or a general phenomenon of development.

The general pattern of improved cognitive control with maturation of the prefrontal cortex (Crone et al 2007), suggests a linear increase in development from childhood to adulthood. Yet the consequences of suboptimal decisions observed during adolescence represent a nonlinear change in behavior that can be distinguished from childhood and adulthood, as evidenced by the National Center for Health Statistics on adolescent behavior and mortality.

If cognitive control and an immature prefrontal cortex were the basis for suboptimal choice behavior, then children should look remarkably similar, or even worse, than adolescents, given their less developed prefrontal cortex and cognitive abilities. Thus, immature prefrontal function alone, cannot account for adolescent choice behavior. The context in which decisions are made is an important consideration too, as children typically have less unsupervised social and sexual activities than adolescents.

An accurate conceptualization of cognitive and neurobiological changes during adolescence must treat adolescence as a transitional developmental period (Spear, 2000), rather than a single snapshot in time. In other words, to understand this developmental period, transitions into and out of adolescence are necessary for distinguishing distinct attributes of this period of development (Casey et al., 2005a, 2005b). Establishing developmental trajectories for cognitive and neural processes is essential in characterizing these transitions and constraining interpretations about changes in behavior during this period. On a cognitive or behavioral level, adolescents are characterized as impulsive (diminished cognitive control) and risk-taking (behavioral bias toward incentives), with these constructs used synonymously and without appreciation for distinct developmental trajectories for each. On a neurobiological level, human imaging and animal studies suggest distinct neurobiological bases and developmental trajectories for the neural systems that underlie these separate constructs of impulse control and risk-taking.

We have developed a testable neurobiological model of adolescent development within this framework that builds on rodent models (Laviola et al., 1999; Spear, 2000; Brenhouse et al., 2008) and recent imaging studies of adolescence (Ernst et al., 2005; Galván et al., 2006; Galván et al., 2007; Hare et al., 2008). Figure 20.1 depicts this model.

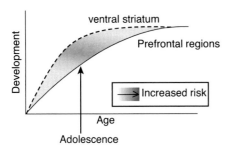

Fig. 20.1 Neurobiological model depicting later development of top-down prefrontal regions relative to subcortical limbic regions involved in desire and fear. This imbalance in development of these systems is suggested to be at the core of risky choice behavior in adolescents in contrast to the popular view of adolescent behavior being due to the protracted development of the prefrontal cortex alone. Adapted from Somerville et al., 2009.

This characterization of adolescence goes beyond exclusive association of risky behavior to the immaturity of the prefrontal cortex. Instead, the proposed neurobiological model illustrates how limbic subcortical and prefrontal top-down control regions must be considered together. The figure illustrates different developmental trajectories for these systems, with limbic systems developing earlier than prefrontal control regions. According to this model, the individual is biased more by functionally mature limbic regions during adolescence (i.e., imbalance of subcortical limbic relative to prefrontal cortical control), compared to children, for whom these systems (i.e., limbic and prefrontal) are both still developing; and compared to adults, for whom these systems are fully mature.

This perspective provides a basis for nonlinear shifts in behavior across development, due to earlier maturation of this limbic relative to less mature top-down prefrontal control region. With development and experience, the functional connectivity between these regions provides a mechanism for top-down control of this circuitry (Hare et al., 2008). Further, the model reconciles the contradiction of health statistics of risky behavior during adolescence, with the astute observation by Reyna and Farley (2006) that adolescents are quite capable of rational decisions and understand risks of behaviors in which they engage. However, in emotionally salient situations, the subcortical limbic system will win out over control systems, given its maturity relative to the prefrontal control system.

This model is similar in part to other recent models of adolescent development (Ernst et al., 2005; Nelson et al., 2005; Steinberg, 2008) suggesting heightened emotionality during adolescence due to less top-down regulation. However, the present model differs in that it emphasizes the dynamic interplay between subcortical and cortical brain systems across development that results in heightened sensitivity to both appetitive and aversive cues, and accounts for the nonlinearity of adolescent behavior change by integrating findings from children, adolescents and adult into the model.

Evidence from behavioral and human imaging studies to support this model will be provided in the context of actions in rewarding and emotional contexts (Galván et al., 2006, 2007; Hare et al., 2008, Cauffman et al., 2010; Figner et al., 2009). In addition, we speculate on why the brain may develop in this way and why some teenagers may be at greater risk for making suboptimal decisions leading to poorer long-term outcomes (Galván et al., 2007; Hare et al., 2008). Finally, we offer a mathematical model for formalizing these decision processes further.

20.2 **Development of decision making**

We review classic cognitive developmental studies in the context of cortically driven cognitive/impulse control and provide behavioral and neuranatomical evidence for its distinction from subcortical processes involved in detecting appetitive and aversive cues. A core component of optimal decision making is the ability to suppress inappropriate representations of choices in favor of goal-directed ones, especially in the presence of compelling incentives, typically referred to as cognitive or impulse control (Casey et al., 2000b, 2002, 2005). We review classic cognitive developmental literature in the context of changes in cortically driven cognitive/impulse control with age and provide behavioral and neuranatomical evidence for its distinction from risky related choices supported by subcortical systems.

A number of classic developmental studies have shown that this ability develops throughout childhood and adolescence (Flavell et al., 1966; Pascual-Leone, 1970; Case, 1972; Keating and Bobbitt, 1978). Several theorists have argued that this development is due to increases in processing speed and efficiency (e.g., Case, 1985; Bjorklund, 1985, 1987), but others have suggested "inhibitory" processes are the key factor (Harnishfeger and Bjorklund, 1993). According to this account, suboptimal decision making in childhood is due to greater susceptibility to interference from competing sources that must be suppressed (e.g., Diamond, 1985; Brainerd and Reyna, 1993 Dempster, 1993; Munakata and Yerys, 2001; Casey et al., 2002a). Thus optimal decision making requires the control of impulses and/or delay of immediate gratification for optimization of outcomes (Mischel et al., 1989) and this ability matures in a linear fashion across childhood and adolescence.

Adolescent decision making has been described as suboptimal in that it is characterized by impulsivity and sensation-seeking. These constructs are often used as if synonymous, yet they rely on different cognitive and neural processes that suggest distinct neural correlates and distinct developmental trajectories. Specifically, a review of the literature suggests that impulsivity diminishes with age across childhood and adolescence (Casey et al., 2002a, 2005b; Galván et al., 2007) and is associated with protracted development of the prefrontal cortex (Casey et al., 2005), although there are differences in the degree to which a given individual is impulsive or not, regardless of age (Eigsti et al., 2006).

In contrast, to impulse/cognitive control, sensation-seeking/risk-taking appears to show a curvilinear pattern, with an increase during adolescence relative to childhood and adulthood (Galván et al., 2007; Cauffman et al., 2010; Figner et al., 2009). Further, human imaging studies, suggest an increase in subcortical activation (e.g., ventral striatum) when making risky choices (Montague and Berns, 2002; Matthews et al., 2004; Kuhnen and Knutson, 2005) that is exaggerated in adolescents, relative to children and adults (Ernst et al., 2005; Galván et al., 2006, van Leijenhorst et al., 2009). These findings suggest distinct neural systems for the constructs of risky and impulsive behavior, as well as different trajectories, with earlier development of risk-taking systems relative to control systems, that show a protracted and linear developmental course, in terms of overriding inappropriate choices and actions in favor of goal-directed ones.

20.2.1 Evidence from neuroimaging studies of human brain development

Recent investigations of adolescent brain development have been based on advances in neuroimaging methodologies that can be easily used with developing human populations. These methods rely on magnetic resonance imaging (MRI) methods and include: structural MRI, which is used to measure the size and shape of structures; functional MRI, which is used to measure patterns of brain activity; and diffusion tensor imaging (DTI), which is used to index connectivity of white matter fiber tracts. Evidence for our developmental model of competition between cortical and subcortical regions is supported by immature structural and functional connectivity as measured by DTI and fMRI, respectively.

20.2.2 MRI studies of human brain development

Several studies have used structural MRI to map the anatomical course of normal brain development (Casey et al., 2005). Although total brain size is approximately 90% of its adult size by age 6 years, the gray and white matter subcomponents of the brain continue to undergo dynamic changes throughout adolescence. Data from recent longitudinal MRI studies indicate that gray matter volume has an inverted U-shape pattern, with greater regional variation than white matter (Giedd, 2004; Gogtay et al., 2004; Sowell et al., 2003, 2004). In general, regions subserving primary functions, such as motor and sensory systems, mature earliest; higher-order association areas, which integrate these primary functions, mature later (Gogtay et al., 2004; Sowell et al., 2004). For example, studies using MRI-based measures show that cortical gray matter loss occurs earliest in the primary sensorimotor areas and latest in the dorsolateral prefrontal and lateral temporal cortices (Gogtay et al., 2004). This pattern is consistent with nonhuman primate and human postmortem studies showing that the prefrontal cortex is one of the last brain regions to mature (Huttenlocher, 1979; Bourgeois et al., 1994), while subcortical and sensorimotor regions develop sooner. In contrast to gray matter, white matter volume increases in a roughly linear pattern, increasing throughout development, well into adulthood (Gogtay et al., 2004). These changes presumably reflect ongoing myelination of axons by oligodendrocytes enhancing neuronal conduction and communication of relevant connections.

Although less attention has been given to subcortical regions when examining structural changes, some of the largest changes in the brain across development are seen in these regions, particular in portions of the basal ganglia like the striatum (Sowell et al., 1999,) and especially in males (Giedd et al., 1996). Developmental changes in structural volume within basal ganglia and prefrontal regions are interesting in light of known developmental processes (e.g. dendritic arborization, cell death, synaptic pruning, myelination) that are occurring during childhood and adolescence. These processes allow for fine-tuning and strengthening of connections between prefrontal and subcortical regions with learning that may coincide with greater cognitive control (e.g., signaling of prefrontal control regions to adjust behavior (Casey et al., 2006 Casey and Durston, 2006).

It is unclear how structural changes relate to behavior changes, however. A number of studies are beginning to show indirect associations between these changes using MRI-based volume and cognitive function using neuropsychological measures (e.g., Casey et al., 1997; Sowell et al., 2003). Specifically, associations have been reported between MRI-based prefrontal cortical and basal ganglia regional volumes and measures of cognitive control that represent an optimal choice (i.e., ability to override an inappropriate choice/action in favor of another; Casey et al., 1997a, 1997b). These findings suggest that cognitive changes are reflected in structural changes in the brain and underscore the importance of subcortical (striatum), as well as cortical (e.g., prefrontal cortex) development.

20.2.3 DTI studies of human brain development

The MRI-based morphometry studies reviewed suggest that cortical connections are being fine-tuned with the elimination of an over-abundance of synapses and strengthening of relevant connections with development and experience. Recent advances in MRI technology, like DTI, provide a potential tool for examining the role of specific white matter tracts to the development of the brain and behavior with greater detail. Relevant to this paper are the neuroimaging studies that have linked the development of fiber tracts with improvements in cognitive ability. Specifically, associations between DTI-based measures of prefrontal white matter development and cognitive control in children have been shown. In one study, development of this capacity was positively correlated with prefrontal-parietal fiber tracts (Nagy et al., 2004) consistent with functional neuroimaging studies showing differential recruitment of these regions in children relative to adults.

Using a similar approach, Liston and colleagues (2005) have shown that white matter tracts in frontostriatal and frontoparietal circuits continue to develop across childhood into adulthood, but only those frontostriatal tracts that are correlated with impulse control, as measured by performance on a go/no-go task (Liston et al., 2006; Casey et al, 2007). The prefrontal fiber tracts were defined by regions of interest identified in a fMRI study using the same task (Durston et al., 2002, Epstein et al., 2007). Across these developmental DTI studies, fiber tract measures were correlated with development, but specificity of particular fiber tracts with cognitive performance were shown by dissociating the particular tract (Liston et al., 2005, Casey et al., 2007) or cognitive ability (Nagy et al., 2004). These findings underscore the importance of examining not only regional structural changes, but also circuitry related changes when making claims about age-dependent changes in neural substrates of cognitive development.

20.2.4 Functional MRI studies of behavioral and brain development

Although structural changes, as measured by MRI and DTI, have been associated with behavioral changes during development, a more direct approach for examining structure–function associations is to measure changes in the brain and behavior simultaneously, as with fMRI. The ability to measure functional changes in the developing brain with MRI has significant potential for the field of developmental science. In the context of the current chapter, fMRI provides a means for constraining interpretations of adolescent decision making. As stated previously, the development of the prefrontal cortex is believed to play an important role in the maturation of higher cognitive abilities, such as decision making and goal-oriented choice behavior (Casey et al., 1997a, 2002b). Many paradigms have been used, together with fMRI, to assess the neurobiological basis of these abilities, including go/no-go, flanker, stop signal, and anti-saccade tasks (Casey et al., 1997b, 2000a; Luna et al., 2001; Bunge et al., 2002; Durston et al., 2003). Collectively, these studies show that children recruit distinct but often larger, more diffuse prefrontal regions when performing these tasks than do adults. The pattern of activity within brain regions central to task performance (i.e., that correlate with cognitive performance) become more focal or fine-tuned with age, while regions not correlated with task performance diminish in activity with age. This pattern has been observed across both cross-sectional (Brown et al., 2005) and longitudinal studies (Durston et al., 2006) and across a variety of paradigms. Although neuroimaging studies cannot definitively characterize the mechanism of such developmental changes (e.g., dendritic arborization, synaptic pruning) the findings reflect development within, and refinement of, projections to and from, activated brain regions with maturation and suggest that these changes occur over a protracted period of time (Casey et al., 1997a, 2002a; Luna et al., 2001; Bunge et al., 2002; Moses et al., 2002; Schlaggar et al., 2002; Tamm et al., 2002; Turkletaub et al., 2003; Thomas et al., 2004; Brown et al., 2005; Crone et al., 2006).

How can this methodology inform us about whether adolescent decisions are indeed impulsive or are risky? Impulse control, as measured by tasks such as the go/no-go task, show a linear pattern of development across childhood and adolescence, as described above. However, recent neuroimaging studies have begun to examine reward-related processing specific to risk-taking in adolescents (Bjork et al., 2004; May et al., 2004; Ernst et al., 2005; Galván et al., 2005). These studies have focused primarily on the region of the ventral striatum, a region implicated in learning and predicting reward outcomes.

Overall, few studies have examined how the development of reward circuitry in subcortical regions changes in conjunction with development of cortical prefrontal regions. Moreover, how these neural changes coincide with reward-seeking, impulsivity, or risk-taking behaviors remains relatively unknown. Our neurobiological model proposes that the combination of heightened responsiveness to rewards and immaturity in behavioral control areas may bias adolescents to seek immediate, rather than long-term gains, perhaps explaining their increase in risky decision making. Tracking subcortical (e.g., ventral striatum) and cortical (e.g., prefrontal) development of decision making across childhood through adulthood, provides additional constraints on whether changes reported in adolescence are specific to this period of development, or reflect maturation that is steadily occurring in a somewhat linear pattern from childhood to adulthood.

Empirical evidence from a recent fMRI study helps to support our neurobiological model and takes a transitional approach to understanding adolescence by examining changes prior to, and following, adolescence. In this study, (Galván et al., 2006), we examined behavioral and neural responses to reward manipulations across development, focusing on brain regions implicated in reward-related learning and behavior in animal (Hikosaka and Watanabe, 2000; Pecina et al., 2003; Schultz, 2006) and adult imaging studies (e.g. Knutson et al., 2001; O'Doherty et al., 2004) and in studies of addiction (Hyman and Malenka, 2001; Volkow and Li, 2004). Based on rodent models (Laviola et al., 1999; Spear, 2000) and previous imaging work (Ernst et al., 2005), we hypothesized that, relative to children and adults, adolescents would show exaggerated activation of the ventral striatum in concert with less mature recruitment of top-down prefrontal control regions. Galván et al., (2006) provided findings in support of this hypothesis by showing that the extent of activity (volume of activity) in the ventral striatum to reward was similar to that observed in adults, whereas the extent of activity in prefrontal regions was more similar to children. Figure 20.2 shows the resulting elevated magnitude of activity (percent change in MR signal) in the ventral striatum in adolescents relative to children and adults in the ventral striatum. Recent work showing delayed functional connectivity between prefrontal and limbic subcortical regions in adolescence relative to adults, provides a mechanism for the lack of top-down control of regions related to desire and fear (Hare et al., 2008).

These findings are consistent with rodent models (Laviola et al., 2003) and previous imaging studies (Ernst et al., 2005) showing enhanced accumbens activity to rewards during adolescence. Indeed, relative to children and adults, adolescents showed an exaggerated accumbens response in anticipation of reward. However, both children and adolescents showed a less mature response in prefrontal control regions than adults. These findings suggest that different developmental trajectories for these regions may underlie the enhancement in accumbens activity, relative to children or adults, which may in turn relate to the increased impulsive and risky decisions observed during this period of development.

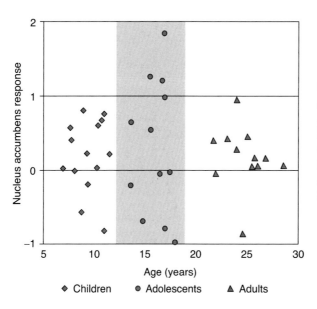

Fig. 20.2 Activity in the ventral striatum to anticipated reward as a function of age, for each individual subject, showing enhanced activity between roughly 13 to 18 years. Adapted from Galván et al, 2007.

Differential recruitment of prefrontal and subcortical regions have been reported across a number of developmental fMRI studies (Luna et al., 2001; Casey et al., 2002b; Monk et al., 2003; Thomas et al., 2004). Typically these findings have been interpreted in terms of immature prefrontal regions, rather than an imbalance between prefrontal and subcortical regional development. Given evidence of prefrontal regions in guiding appropriate actions in different contexts (Miller and Cohen, 2001), immature prefrontal activity might hinder appropriate estimation of future outcomes and appraisal of risky choices, and might thus be less influential on reward valuation than the accumbens. This pattern is consistent with previous research showing elevated subcortical, relative to cortical activity when decisions are biased by immediate over long-term gains (McClure et al., 2004). Further, accumbens activity has been shown, with fMRI, to positively correlate with subsequent risk-taking behaviors (Kuhnen and Knutson, 2005). During adolescence, relative to childhood or adulthood, immature ventral prefrontal cortex may not provide sufficient top-down control of robustly activated reward processing regions (e.g., accumbens), resulting in less influence of prefrontal systems (orbitofrontal cortex) relative to the accumbens in reward valuation.

Outside of the functional neuroimaging literature, there is evidence to suggest a differential relative maturity of subcortical limbic brain structures, as compared to prefrontal regions, which may be most pronounced during adolescence. Evidence for the continued pruning of prefrontal cortical synapses well into development has been established in both nonhuman primates and humans (Rakic et al., 1986; Huttenlocher, 1997), with greater regional differentiation suggested in the human brain (Huttenlocher, 1997), such that cortical sensory and subcortical areas undergo dynamic synaptic pruning earlier than higher order association areas. This conceptualization of cortical development is consistent with anatomical MRI work demonstrating protracted pruning of gray matter in higher order prefrontal areas that continue through adolescence (e.g., Giedd et al., 1999) relative to subcortical regions. For example, the ventral striatum and amygdala show neuroanatomical changes during this time of life, but to a lesser degree than association cortices. In an anatomical MRI experiment, subcortical measurements of the ventral striatum was not predicted by age, unlike prefrontal regions that were strongly negatively predicted by age (Sowell et al., 2002). In terms of amygdala maturation, the volumetric analyses of the human amygdala show a substantially reduced slope of change magnitude relative to cortical areas in 4–18-year-olds (Giedd et al., 1996). Taken together, these findings suggest a protracted developmental time course of the prefrontal cortex relative to these limbic subcortical regions.

20.3 Comparative and evolutionary perspectives on adolescence

A question that emerges from this imbalance model of adolescent brain development is: Why would the brain be programmed to develop in this way? This question may be addressed best by taking a step back, and defining adolescence. Adolescence is the transitional period between childhood and adulthood often co-occurring with puberty. Puberty marks the beginnings of sexual maturation (Graber and Brooks-Gunn, 1998) and can be defined by biological markers. Adolescence can be described as a progressive transition into adulthood with a nebulous ontogenetic time course (Spear, 2000). Evolutionarily speaking, adolescence is the period in which independence skills are acquired to increase success upon separation from the protection of the family, though increase chances for harmful circumstances (e.g., injury, depression, anxiety, drug use and addiction (Kelley et al., 2004). Independence-seeking behaviors are prevalent across species, such as increases in peer-directed social interactions and intensifications in novelty seeking and risk-taking behaviors. Psychosocial factors impact adolescent propensity for risky behavior. However, risky behavior may be defined as the product of a biologically driven imbalance between increased novelty and sensation seeking in conjunction with immature "self-regulatory competence" (Steinberg, 2004). Our neurobiological data suggest this occurs through differential development of these two systems (limbic and control).

Speculation would suggest that this developmental pattern is an evolutionary feature in that an individual needs to engage in high-risk behavior to leave a safe and familiar niche in order to find a mate and procreate. Thus, risk-taking appears to coincide with the time in which hormones drive adolescents to seek out sexual partners. In today's society—when adolescence may extend indefinitely—with children living with parents and having financial dependence and choosing mates later in life, this evolution may be deemed inappropriate.

There is evidence across species for heightened novelty-seeking and risk-taking during the adolescent years consistent with this view. Seeking out same-age peers and fighting with parents, which all help get the adolescent away from the home territory for mating, is seen in other species, including rodents, nonhuman primates, and some birds (Spear, 2000). Relative to adults, periadolescent rats show increased novelty-seeking behaviors in a free-choice novelty paradigm (Laviola et al, 1999). Neurochemical evidence indicates that the balance in the adolescent brain between cortical and subcortical dopamine systems, begins to shift toward greater cortical dopamine levels during adolescence (Spear, 2000; Brenhouse et al., 2008). Similarly, protracted dopaminergic enervation through adolescence into adulthood has been shown in the nonhuman primate prefrontal cortex as well (Rosenberg and Lewis, 1995). Thus this elevated apparent risk-taking appears to be across species and to have important adaptive purposes.

20.4 Maladaptive behavior: adolescents and risk factors

Individual differences in impulse control and taking risks has been recognized in psychology for some time (Benthin et al., 1993). Perhaps one of the classic examples of individual differences reported in these abilities in the social, cognitive, and developmental psychology literature, is delay of gratification (Mischel et al., 1989). Delay of gratification is typically assessed in 3 to 4-year-old toddlers. The toddler is asked whether they would prefer a small reward (one cookie) or a large reward (two cookies). The child is then told that the experimenter will leave the room in order to prepare for upcoming activities and explains to the child that if she remains in her seat and does not eat a cookie, she will receive the large reward. If the child does not or cannot wait, she should ring a bell to summon the experimenter and thereby receive the smaller reward. Once it is clear the child understands the task, she is seated at the table with the two rewards and the bell. Distractions in the room are minimized, with no toys, books, or pictures. The experimenter returns after 15 minutes or after the child has rung the bell, eaten the rewards, or shown any signs of distress. Mischel showed that children typically behave in one of two ways: (1) either they ring the bell almost immediately in order to have the cookie, which means they only get one; or (2) they wait and optimize their gains, and receive both cookies. This observation suggests that some individuals are better than others in their ability to control impulses in the face of highly salient incentives and this bias can be detected in early childhood (Mischel et al., 1989), and they appear to remain throughout adolescence and young adulthood (Eigsti et al, 2006).

What might explain individual differences in optimal decision making and behavior? Some theorists have postulated that dopaminergic mesolimbic circuitry, implicated in reward processing, underlies risky behavior (Blum et al., 2000). Individual differences in this circuitry, such as allelic variants in dopamine-related genes, resulting in too little or too much dopamine in subcortical regions, might relate to the propensity to engage in risky behavior (O'Doherty, 2004). The ventral striatum has been shown to increase in activity immediately prior to making risky choices on monetary-risk paradigms (Montague and Berns, 2002; Matthews et al., 2004; Kuhnen and Knutson, 2005) and as described previously, adolescents show exaggerated striatal activity to rewarding outcomes relative to children or adults (Ernst et al., 2005; Galván et al., 2006). Collectively, these data suggest that adolescents may be more prone to risky choices as a group (Gardner and Steinberg, 2005), but some adolescents will be more prone than others to engage in risky behaviors, putting them at potentially greater risk for negative outcomes. Therefore, it is important to consider individual variability when examining complex brain–behavior relationships related to risk-taking and reward processing in developmental populations.

To explore individual differences in risk-taking behavior, Galván and colleagues (2007) recently examined the association between activity in reward-related neural circuitry in anticipation of a large monetary reward with personality trait measures of risk-taking and impulsivity in adolescence. Functional magnetic resonance imaging and anonymous self-report rating scales of risky behavior, risk perception and impulsivity were acquired in individuals between the ages of 7 and 29 years. There was a positive association between ventral striatal activity and the likelihood of engaging in risky behavior across development. This activity varied as a function of individuals' ratings of anticipated positive or negative consequences of such behavior. The individuals who perceived risky behaviors as leading to dire consequences, activated the ventral striatum less to reward. This negative association was driven by the child participants, whereas a positive association was seen in the adults who rated the consequences of such behavior as positive.

In addition to linking risk-taking to reward circuitry, Galván also showed no association between activity of this circuitry and ratings of impulsivity, further distinguishing the constructs of impulsivity and risk-taking (Galván et al., 2007). These findings suggest that during adolescence, some individuals may be more prone to engage in risky behaviors due to developmental changes in concert with variability in a given individual's predisposition to engage in risky behavior, rather than to simple changes in impulsivity.

Collectively, these data suggest that although adolescents as a group are considered risk-takers (Gardner and Steinberg, 2005), some adolescents will be more prone than others to engage in risky behaviors, putting them at potentially greater risk for negative outcomes. These findings underscore the importance of considering individual variability when examining complex brain–behavior relationships related to risk-taking and reward processing in developmental populations. Further, these individual and developmental differences may help explain vulnerability in some individuals to risk-taking associated with substance use, and ultimately, addiction.

20.5 Drift diffusion model of adolescent decision making

Adolescent behavior has repeatedly been characterized as impulsive and risky (Steinberg, 2004, 2007), yet this review of the imaging and animal literature suggests different neurobiological substrates and different developmental trajectories for these behaviors. A model of decision making that may help to further characterize impulsive and risky choice behavior in adolescence is that of the drift diffusion model (DDM). Such a model has appeal, given the many studies that have applied the equivalent of the DDM to decision-making processes (Barnard, 1946; Wald, 1947; Stone, 1960; Laming, 1968; Ratcliff, 1978; Ratcliff et al., 1999, 2003, 2004).

The DDM provides a formal framework for making specific, testable predictions about the mechanisms underlying decisions. It is a continuous version of the random walk model, providing a mathematical description of the decision process involved in two alternative forced choices (e.g., engage in an act or not). The DDM assumes that the signal upon which a decision must be made is noisy, and thus at any single point in time there is uncertainly about which alternative is optimal or correct. Accordingly, it integrates the difference between information favoring one alternative vs. the other over time, as the accumulation of evidence builds (drift rate), and reaches a decision when the magnitude of this difference reaches a critical value (the threshold).

The mathematical description of this process is given by:

$$x' = A + c\eta,$$

where x is the evidence favoring one decision over the other, and x' denotes its rate of change over time. x' is determined by a drift term A, denoting the average increase in evidence for the correct choice per unit time, and $c\eta$ represents random fluctuations (noise) in this evidence. The decision process can be seen as analogous to the diffusion of a gas particle toward one of two boundaries (the decision thresholds); a signal (e.g., a stimulus) favoring one alternative produces a "drift," so that it is more likely to reach the corresponding boundary, though random fluctuations still may drive it toward the other. Key parameters of the DDM, in addition to the drift rate, are the starting point

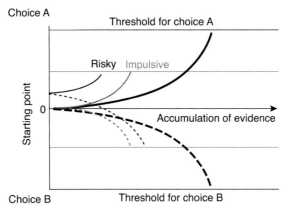

Fig. 20.3 Drift diffusion model incorporating psychological constructs of impulsivity in light gray and risk in dark gray, as separate parameters to explain changes in decision making with development, relative to mature decision making (shown in dark black). Impulsivity (in light gray) is defined by a change in threshold for making a decision. As thresholds get closer, the faster a response choice is made and the greater likelihood of an incorrect choice as observed in children. Risk-taking (in dark gray) is defined by a change in the starting point. A change in starting point would lead to favoring the choice closest to that point (riskier) as observed in adolescents' bias toward incentive-based actions.

(behavioral bias) and the decision threshold (sufficient evidence). Both the threshold and starting, which we suggest are key in understanding impulsive and risky choices during development, respectively, are driven largely by reinforcement learning mechanisms and subjects' history and/or traits, while drift rate is influenced by top-down mediated processes.

In the context of how this model may help characterize development of decision making, one can take the simple example of deciding to engage in an act or not (e.g., go/no-go laboratory task). Figure 20.3 illustrates the basic parameters of the DDM of a simple two-choice decision task without any developmental or individual biases implemented in black. In the case of the go/no-go task, we will assume that choice A is a go response and choice B is a no-go response. Now, if we alter the threshold in the DDM (see Fig. 20.3 in light gray), we can account for changes in impulsivity across development. Manipulation of the threshold parameter results in decisions being made with less time for sufficient accumulation of evidence and therefore more misses of the targets and more false alarms in detecting the nontarget. In other words, as thresholds are moved closer together, the process will reach them more quickly, but will be more likely to cross the wrong one because there will be less time to be influenced by the drift force (i.e., speed accuracy trade-off). This pattern of performance is similar to that reported on go/no-go tasks in children, as evidenced by lower d prime scores (Durston et al., 2006). D prime takes into account both hits and false alarms and provides a measure of sensitivity in the discrimination and detection of target stimuli relative to nontarget stimuli (note: a similar pattern could be observed by simply varying noise $c\eta$ linearly with age).

Since the behavioral and imaging literature suggests sensitivity to incentives is associated with increased risk-taking during adolescence (Ernst et al., 2005; Eshel et al., 2005;

Galván et al., 2006, 2007; Hare et al., 2008, Cauffman et al., 2010; Figner et al., 2009), we manipulate a second parameter to account for this construct. Specifically, to reflect this construct in the model, we manipulate the starting point (see Fig. 20.3 in dark gray). A change in starting point would lead to greater selection of the associated choice closest to that point (e.g., to engage in an act or go in laboratory task) and less selection of the alternative (not to engage in an act). In Fig. 20.3, this bias is shown as choosing choice A more than B. Thus, if choice A is a go response, then the likelihood of the response choice is higher and thus a higher rate of detecting targets, but likewise, a higher rate of incorrectly detecting a nontarget (false alarm). This pattern of performance differs from the previously described impulsivity manipulation of moving the thresholds closer, but captures changes in performance from childhood to adolescence. Specifically, adolescents make more false alarms than adults on go/no-go tasks, but fewer misses than children (Durston et al., 2006). The same pattern of performance can be seen when experimentally manipulating reinforcement or frequency of preceding events in adults (Montague et al., 1996, Casey et al., 2001; Durston et al., 2002), as that manipulation parallels an increased sensitivity to environmental cues that we observe during adolescence and is driven subcortically.

According the model, the starting point and the threshold will bias top-down processes related to the drift rate. As the threshold increases from childhood to adolescence, general performance will begin to improve, but then be biased by changes in the starting point (sensitivity to environmental cues) during adolescence. Clearly individual differences in impulsive and risky behavior will further bias these two parameters differentially and further influence the drift rate. Future efforts to incorporate temporal dynamics into the DDM over longer time periods (e.g., years) may help in the formal quantification of changes in decision processes over development.

20.6 **Discussion**

Human imaging studies show structural and functional changes in frontostriatal regions (Jernigan et al., 1991; Giedd 1996; Giedd et al., 1999; Sowell et al., 1999; for review, Casey et al., 2005b) that seem to parallel increases in cognitive control and self-regulation (Casey et al., 1997a; Rubia et al., 2000; Luna and Sweeney, 2001, 2004; Steinberg, 2004, 2008). These changes appear to show a shift in activation of prefrontal regions from diffuse to more focal recruitment over time (Casey et al., 1997a; Bunge et al., 2002; Moses et al., 2002; Brown et al., 2005; Durston et al., 2006) and elevated recruitment of subcortical regions during adolescence (Luna et al., 2001; Casey et al., 2002a; Durston et al., 2006). Although neuroimaging studies cannot definitively characterize the mechanism of such developmental changes, these changes in volume and structure may reflect development within, and refinement of, projections to and from these brain regions during maturation suggestive of fine-tuning of the system with development.

Taken together, the findings synthesized here indicate that increased risk-taking behavior in adolescence is associated with different developmental trajectories of subcortical pleasure and cortical control regions. However, this is not to say that adolescents are not capable of making rational decisions, rather that, in emotionally charged situations, the more mature limbic system may win over the prefrontal control system in deciding on a choice.

Although adolescence has been distinguished as a period characterized by reward-seeking and risk-taking behaviors (Spear, 2000; Gardner and Steinberg, 2005), individual differences in neural responses to reward, predispose some adolescents to take more risks than others, putting them at greater risk for negative outcomes. Mathematical models that incorporate these psychological constructs may lead to formalized tests of theoretical accounts of the development of decision making. These findings provide crucial groundwork by synthesizing the various findings related to impulsivity and risk-taking in adolescence and in understanding individual differences and developmental markers for propensities for suboptimal choices leading to negative consequences.

Acknowledgments

This work was supported in part by NIDA R01 DA018879, NIMH P50 MH62196, NSF 06-509, and NSF 0720932 to BJC, the Mortimer D. Sackler family, the Dewitt-Wallace fund, and by the Weill Cornell Medical College Citigroup Biomedical Imaging Center and Imaging Core.

References

Barnard, G.A. (1946). Sequential tests in industrial statistics. *Journal of Royal Statistical Society Supplement*, **8**, 1–26.

Bennett, C. M. and Baird, A. A. (2006). Anatomical changes in the emerging adult brain: a voxel-based morphometry study. *Human Brain Mapping*, **27**, 766–77.

Benthin, A., Slovic, P., and Severson H. (1993). A psychometric study of adolescent risk perception. *Journal of Adolescence*, **16**, 153–68.

Berridge, K. C. and Robinson T. E. (1998). What is the role of dopamine in reward: hedonic impact, reward learning, or incentive salience? *Brain Research Reviews*, **28**, 309–69.

Bjork, J. M., Knutson, B., Fong, G. W., Caggiano, D. M., Bennett, S. M., and Hommer, D. W. (2004). Incentive-elicited brain activation in adolescents: similarities and differences from young adults. *Journal of Neuroscience*, **24**, 1793–802.

Bjorkland, D. F. (1985). The role of conceptual knowledge in the development of organization in children's memory. In C. J. Brainerd and M. Pressley (eds) *Basic processes in memory development: progress in cognitive development research.* (pp. 103–42). New York: Springer-Verlag.

Bjorkland, D. F. (1987). How age changes in knowledge base contribute to the development of children's memory: an interpretive review. *Developmental Review*, **7**, 93–130.

Blum, K., Braverman, E., Holder, J., Lubar, J., Monastra, V. et al. (2000). Reward deficiency syndrome: a biogenetic model for the diagnosis and treatment of impulsive, addictive and compulsive behaviors. *Journal of Psychoactive Drugs*, **32** Suppl: i–iv, 1–112.

Brainerd, C. J. and Reyna, V. F. (1993). Memory independence and memory interference in cognitive development. *Psychological Review*, **100**, 42–67.

Brenhouse H.C., Sonntag K.C., Andersen S.L. (2008). Transient D1 dopamine receptor expression on prefrontal cortex projection neurons: relationship to enhanced motivational salience of drug cues in adolescence. *Journal of Neuroscience*, **28(10)**:2375–82.

Bourgeois, J. P., Goldman-Rakic, P. S., and Rakic, P. (1994). Synaptogenesis in the prefrontal cortex of rhesus monkeys. *Cerebral Cortex*, **4**, 78–96.

Brown, T. T., Lugar, H. M., Coalson, R. S., Miezin, F. M., Petersen, S. E., and Schlaggar, B. L. (2005). Developmental changes in human cerebral functional organization for word generation. *Cerebral Cortex*, 15, 275–90.

Bunge, S. A., Dudukovic, N. M., Thomason, M. E., Vaidya, C. J., and Gabrieli, J. D. (2002). Immature frontal lobe contributions to cognitive control in children: evidence from fMRI. *Neuron*, 33, 301–11.

Case, R. (1972). Validation of a neo-Piagetian capacity construct. *Journal of Experimental Child Psychology*, 14(2), 287–302.

Casey, B.J. and Durston, S. (2006). From behavior to cognition to the brain and back: what have we learned from functional imaging studies of ADHD. *American Journal of Psychiatry*, 163(6), 957–60.

Casey, B. J., Trainor, R. J., Orendi, J. L., Schubert, A. B., Nystrom, L. E., Giedd, J. N. et al. (1997a). A developmental functional MRI study of prefrontal activation during performance of a go-no-go task. *Journal of Cognitive Neuroscience*, 9, 835–47.

Casey, B. J., Castellanos, F. X., Giedd, J. N., Marsh, W. L., Hamburger, S. D., Schubert, A. B. et al. (1997b). Implication of right frontostriatal circuitry in response inhibition and attention-deficit/hyperactivity disorder. *Journal of the American Academy of Child and Adolescent Psychiatry*, 36, 374–83.

Casey, B. J., Giedd, J. N., and Thomas, K. M. (2000a). Structural and functional brain development and its relation to cognitive development. *Biological Psychology*, 54, 241–57.

Casey, B.J., Amso, D., and Davidson, M.C. (2006). Learning about learning and development with neuroimaging. In M. Johnsons and Y. Munakata (eds) *Attention and performance XXI: processes of change in brain and cognitive development*, pp.513–33. Cambridge, MA: MIT

Casey, B. J., Tottenham, N., Liston, C., and Durston, S. (2005a). Imaging the developing brain: what have we learned about cognitive development? *Trends in Cognitive Science*, 9, 104–110.

Casey, B. J., Galván, A., and Hare, T. A. (2005b). Changes in cerebral functional organization during cognitive development. *Current Opinion in Neurobiology*, 15, 239–44.

Casey, B. J., Thomas, K. M., Welsh, T. F., Badgaiyan, R. D., Eccard, C. H., Jennings, J. R. et al. (2000b). Dissociation of response conflict, attentional selection, and expectancy with functional magnetic resonance imaging. *Proceedings of the National Academy of Science*, 97, 8728–33.

Casey, B.J., Forman, S.D., Franzen, P., Berkowitz, A., Braver, T.S., Nystrom, L.E. et al. (2001) Sensitivity of prefrontal cortex to changes in target probability. *Human Brain Mapping*, 13–26–33.

Casey, B. J., Thomas, K. M., Davidson, M. C., Kunz, K., and Franzen, P. L. (2002a). Dissociating striatal and hippocampal function developmentally with a stimulus-response compatibility task. *Journal of Neuroscience*, 22, 8647–52.

Casey, B. J., Tottenham, N., and Fossella, J. (2002b). Clinical, imaging, lesion and genetic approaches toward a model of cognitive control. *Developmental Psychobiology*, 40, 237–54.

Cauffman, E., Shulman, E. P., Steinberg, L., Claus, E., Banich, M. T., Graham, S. J. et al. (2010). Age differences in affective decision making as indexed by performance on the Iowa Gambling Task. *Developmental Psychology*, 46(1), 193–207.

Crone, E.A. and van der Molen, M.W. (2007). Development of decision making in school-aged children and adolescents: evidence from heart rate and skin conductance analysis. *Child Dev.* 78(4), 1288–301.

Crone, E., Donohue, S., Honomichl, R., Wendelken, C., and Bunge, S. (2006). Brain regions mediating flexible rule use during development. *Journal of Neuroscience*, 26, 11239–47.

Dempster, F. N. (1993). Resistance to interference: developmental changes in a basic processing mechanism. In M. L. Howe and R. Pasnak (eds) *Emerging themes in cognitive development*, Vol. 1: *Foundations*, pp. 3–27. New York: Springer.

Diamond, A. (1985). Development of the ability to use recall to guide action, as indicated by infants' performance on AB. *Child Development*, 56, 868–83.

Durston, S., Hulshoff Pol, H. E., Casey, B. J., Giedd, J. N., Buitelaar, J. K., and van Engeland, H. (2001). Anatomical MRI of the developing human brain: what have we learned? *Journal of American Academy of Child Adolescent Psychiatry*, 40, 1012–20.

Durston, S., Thomas, K. M., Worden, M. S., Yang, Y., and Casey, B. J. (2002). The effect of preceding context on inhibition: an event-related fMRI study. *Neuroimage*, 16, 449–53.

Durston, S., Davidson, M. C., Thomas, K. M., Worden, M. S., Tottenham, N., Martinez, A. et al. (2003). Parametric manipulation of conflict and response competition using rapid mixed-trial event-related fMRI. *Neuroimage*, 20, 2135–41.

Durston, S., Davidson, M. C., Tottenham, N., Galván, A., Spicer, J., Fossella, J. et al. (2006). A shift from diffuse to focal cortical activity with development. *Developmental Science*, 1, 18–20.

Eaton, L. K., Kinchen, S., Ross, J., Hawkins, J., Harris, W. A., Lowry, R. et al. (2006). Youth Risk Behavior Surveillance United States, 2005, Surveillance Summaries. *Morbidity and Mortality Weekly Report*, 55, 1–108.

Eigsti, I. M., Zayas, V., Mischel, W., Shoda, Y., Ayduk, O., Dadlani, M. B. et al. (2006). Predicting cognitive control from preschool to late adolescence and young adulthood. *Psychological Science*, 17, 478–84.

Epstein, J. N., Casey, B. J., Tonev, S. T., Davidson, M., Reiss, A., Garrett, A. et al. (2007) ADHD- and medication-related brain activation effects in concordantly affected parent–child dyads with ADHD. *J Child Psychol Psychiatry*, 48(9), 899–913.

Ernst, M., Nelson, E. E., Jazbec, S., McClure, E. B., Monk, C. S., Leibenluft, E. et al. (2005). Amygdala and nucleus accumbens in responses to receipt and omission of gains in adults and adolescents. *Neuroimage*, 25, 1279–91.

Ernst M, Pine DS, and Hardin M. (2006). Triadic model of the neurobiology of motivated behavior in adolescence. *Psychol Med*, 36(3):299–312.

Eshel N, Nelson EE, Blair RJ, Pine DS, and Ernst M. (2007). Neural substrates of choice selection in adults and adolescents: development of the ventrolateral prefrontal and anterior cingulate cortices. *Neuropsychologia*, 45(6):1270–9.

Flavell, J. H., Feach, D. R., and Chinsky, J. M. (1966). Spontaneous verbal rehearsal in a memory task as a function of age. *Child Development*, 37, 283–99.

Figner, B., Mackinlay, R. J., Wilkening, F., and Weber, E. U. (2009). Risky choice in children, adolescents, and adults: affective versus deliberative processes and the role of executive functions. *Proceedings of the Society for Research in Child Development, Denver, CO, USA*.

Galván, A., Hare, T. A., Davidson, M., Spicer, J., Glover, G., and Casey, B. J. (2005). The role of ventral frontostriatal circuitry in reward-based learning in humans. *Journal of Neuroscience*, 25(38), 8650–56.

Galván, A., Hare, T. A., Parra, C. E., Penn, J., Voss, H., Glover, G. et al. (2006). Earlier development of the accumbens relative to orbitofrontal cortex might underlie risk-taking behavior in adolescents. *Journal of Neuroscience*, 26, 6885–92.

Galván, A., Hare, T., Voss, H., Glover, G., and Casey, B. J. (2007). Risk-taking and the adolescent brain: who is at risk? *Developmental Science*, 10, F8–F14.

Gardner, M. and Steinberg, L. (2005). Peer influence on risk-taking, risk preference, and risky decision making in adolescence and adulthood: an experimental study. *Developmental Psychology*, 41, 625–35.

Giedd, J. N. (2004). Structural magnetic resonance imaging of the adolescent brain. *Annals of the New York Academy of Sciences*, 1021, 77–85.

Giedd, J. N., Snell, J. W., Lange, N., Rajapakse, J. C., Casey, B. J., Kozuch, P. L. et al. (1996). Quantitative magnetic resonance imaging of human brain development: ages 4–18. *Cerebral Cortex*, 6, 551–60.

Giedd, J. N., Blumenthal, J., Jeffries, N. O., Castellanos, F. X., Liu, H., Zijdenbos, A. et al. (1999). Brain development during childhood and adolescence: a longitudinal MRI study. *Nature Neuroscience*, 2, 861–63.

Gogtay, N., Giedd, J. N., Lusk, L., Hayashi, K. M., Greenstein, D., Vaituzis, A. C. et al. (2004). Dynamic mapping of human cortical development during childhood through early adulthood. *Proceedings of the National Academy of Sciences of the United States of America*, 101, 8174–79.

Graber, J. A. and Brooks-Gunn, J. (1998). Puberty. In E. A. Blechman, and K. D. Brownell (eds) *Behavioral medicine and women a comprehensive handbook*, pp. 51–8. New York, NY: Guilford Press.

Hare, T. A., Tottenham, N., Galván, A., Voss, H. U., Glover, G. H., and Casey, B. J. (2008). Biological substrates of emotional reactivity and regulation in adolescence during an emotional go-no-go task. *Biol Psychiatry*, **63**(*10*), 927–34.

Harnishfeger, K. K. and Bjorkland, F. (1993). The ontogeny of inhibition mechanisms: a renewed approach to cognitive development. In **M. L. Howe and R. Pasnek** (eds) *Emerging themes in cognitive development*, Vol. *1*, pp. 28–49. New York: Springer-Verlag.

Hikosaka, K. and Watanabe, M. (2000). Delay activity of orbital and lateral prefrontal neurons of the monkey varying with different rewards. *Cerebral Cortex*, **10**, 263–71.

Huttenlocher, P. R. (1979). Synaptic density in human frontal cortex developmental changes and effects of aging. *Brain Research*, **163**, 195–205.

Huttenlocher, P. R. (1997). Regional differences in synaptogenesis in human cerebral cortex. *Journal of Comparative Neurology*, **387**, 167–78.

Hyman, S. E. and Malenka, R. C. (2001). Addiction and the brain: the neurobiology of compulsion and its persistence. *Nature Reviews Neuroscience*, **2**, 695–703.

Jernigan, T. L., Zisook, S., Heaton, R. K., Moranville, J. T., Hesselink, J. R., and Braff, D. L. (1991). Magnetic resonance imaging abnormalities in lenticular nuclei and cerebral cortex in schizophrenia. *Archives of General Psychiatry*, **48**, 811–23.

Keating, D. P. and Bobbitt, B. L. (1978). Individual and developmental differences in cognitive processing components of mental ability. *Child Development*, **49**, 155–67.

Kelley, A. E., Schochet, T., and Landry, C. (2004). *Annals of the New York Academy of Sciences*, **1021**, 27–32.

Knutson, B., Adams, C. M., Fong, G. W., and Hommer, D. (2001). Anticipation of increasing monetary reward selectively recruits nucleus accumbens. *Journal of Neuroscience*, **21**, RC159.

Kuhnen, C. M. and Knutson, B. (2005). The neural basis of financial risk-taking. *Neuron*, **47**, 763–70.

Laming, D. R. J. (1968). *Information theory of choice-reaction times*. New York: Academic Press.

Laviola, G., Adriani, W., Terranova, M. L., and Gerra, G. (1999). Psychobiological risk factors for vulnerability to psychostimulants in human adolescents and animal models. *Neuroscience and Biobehavioral Reviews*, **23**, 993–1010.

Laviola, G., Macri, S., Morley-Fletcher, S., and Adriani, W. (2003). Abstract risk-taking behavior in adolescent mice: psychobiological determinants and early epigenetic influence. *Neuroscience and Biobehavioral Reviews*, **27**, 19–31.

Liston, C., Watts, R., Tottenham, N., Davidson, M. C., Niogi, S., Ulug, A. M. et al. (2005). Frontostriatal microstructure modulates efficient recruitment of cognitive control. *Cerebral Cortex*, **16**, 553–60.

Liston, C., Watts, R., Tottenham, N., Davidson, M. C., Niogi, S., Ulug, A. M. et al. (2006). Frontostriatal microstructure modulates efficient recruitment of cognitive control. *Cerebral Cortex*, **16**(*4*), 553–60.

Luna, B. and Sweeney, J. A. (2004). The emergence of collaborative brain function: FMRI studies of the development of response inhibition. *Annals of the New York Academy of Sciences*, **1021**, 296–309.

Luna, B., Thulborn, K. R., Munoz, D. P., Merriam, E. P., Garver, K. E., Minshew, N. J. et al. (2001). Maturation of widely distributed brain function subserves cognitive development. *Neuroimage*, **13**, 786–93.

Matthews, S. C., Simmons, A.N., Lare, S.D., and Paulus, M.P. (2004). Selective activation of the nucleus accumbens during risk-taking decision making. *Neuroreport*, **15**, 2123–27.

May, J. C., Delgado, M. R., Dahl, R. E., Stenger, V. A., Ryan, N. D., Fiez, J. A. et al. (2004). Event-related functional magnetic resonance imaging of reward-related brain circuitry in children and adolescents. *Biological Psychiatry*, **55**, 359–66.

McClure, S. M., Laibson, D. I., Loewenstein, G., and Cohen, J. D. (2004). Separate neural systems value immediate monetary rewards. *Science*, **306**, 503–507.

Miller, E. K. and Cohen. J. D. (2001). An integrative theory of prefrontal cortex function. *Annual Review of Neuroscience*, 24, 167–202.

Monk, C. S., McClure, E. B., Nelson, E. E., Zarahn, E., Bilder, R. M., Leibenluft, E. et al. (2003). Adolescent immaturity in attention-related brain engagement to emotional facial expressions. *Neuroimage*, 20, 420–28.

Mischel, W., Shoda, Y., and Rodriguez, M. I. (1989). Delay of gratification in children. *Science*, 244, 933–38.

Montague, P. R. and Berns, G. S. (2002). Neural economics and the biological substrates of valuation. *Neuron*, 36, 265–84.

Montague, P.R., Dayan, P., and Sejnowski, T.J. (1996). A framework for mesencephalic dopamine systems based on predictive Hebbian learning. *J Neurosci,* 16, 1936–47.

Moses, P., Roe, K., Buxton, R. B., Wong, E. C., Frank, L. R., and Stiles J. (2002). Functional MRI of global and local processing in children. *Neuroimage*, 16, 415–24.

Munakata, Y. and Yerys, B. E. (2001). All together now: when dissociations between knowledge and action disappear. *Pscychological Science*, 12, 335–37.

Nagy, Z,. Westerberg, H., and Klingberg, T. (2004). Maturation of white matter is associated with the development of cognitive functions during childhood. *Journal of Cognitive Neuroscience*, 16, 1227–33.

Nelson, E. E., Leibenluft, E., McClure, E. B., and Pine, D. S. (2005). The social re-orientation of adolescence: A neuroscience perspective on the process and its relation to psychopathology. *Psychological Medicine*, 35, 163–74.

O'Doherty, J. P. (2004). Reward representations and reward-related learning in the human brain: Insights from neuroimaging. *Current Opinions in Neurobiology*, 14, 769–76.

Pascual-Leone, J. A. (1970). A mathematical model for transition in Piaget's developmental stages. *Acta Psychologica*, 32, 301–45.

Pecina, S., Cagniard, B., Berridge, K. C., Aldridge, J. W., and Zhuang X. (2003). Hyperdopaminergic mutant mice have higher "wanting" but not "liking" for sweet rewards. *Journal of Neuroscience*, 23, 9395–9402.

Rakic, P., Bourgeois, J. P., Eckenhoff, M. F., Zecevic, N., and Goldman-Rakic, P. S. (1986). Concurrent overproduction of synapses in diverse regions of the primate cerebral cortex. *Science*, 232, 232–35.

Rakic, P., Bourgeois, J-P., and Goldman-Rakic, P. S. (1994). *Synaptic development of the cerebral cortex: implications for learning, memory, and mental illness.* In **J. van Pelt, M. A. Corner, H. B. M. Uylings, and F. H. Lopes da Silva** (eds) *Progress in brain research, The self-organizing brain: from growth cones to functional networks*, Vol. *102*, pp. 227–43. Amsterdam: Elsevier.

Ratcliff, R. (1978). A theory of memory retrieval. *Psychological Review*, 85, 59–108.

Ratcliff, R. and Smith, P. L. (2004). A comparison of sequential sampling models for two-choice reaction time. *Psychological Review*, 111, 333–67.

Ratcliff, R., Van Zandt, T., and McKoon, G. (1999). Connectionist and diffusion models of reaction time. *Psychological Review*, 106, 261–300.

Ratcliff, R., Thapar, A., and McKoon, G. (2003). A diffusion model analysis of the effects of aging on brightness discrimination. *Perception and Psychophysics*, 65, 523–35.

Reyna, V. F. and Farley, F. (2006). Risk and rationality in adolescent decision making: Implications for theory, practice, and public policy. *Psychological Science in the Public Interest*, 7, 1–44.

Rosenberg, D. R. and Lewis, D. A. (1995). Postnatal maturation of the dopaminergic innervation of monkey prefrontal and motor cortices: a tyrosine hydroxylase immunohistochemical analysis. *The Journal of Comparative Neurology*, 358, 383–400.

Rubia, K., Overmeyer, S., Taylor, E, Brammer, M., Williams, S. C., Simmons, A. et al. (2000). Functional frontalisation with age: mapping neurodevelopmental trajectories with fMRI. *Neuroscience and Biobehavioral Reviews*, 24, 13–19.

Schlaggar, B. L., Brown, T. T., Lugar, H. M., Visscher, K. M., Miezin, F. M., and Petersen, S. E. (2002). Functional neuroanatomical differences between adults and school-age children in the processing of single words. *Science*, 296, 1476–79.

Schultz, W. (2006). Behavioral theories and the neurophysiology of reward. *Annual Reviews of Psychology*, 57, 87–115.

Somerville, L.H., Jones, R.M., and Casey, B.J. (2010). A time of change: Behavioral and neural correlates of adolescent sensitivity to appetitive and aversive environmental cues. *Brain and Cognition*, 72, 124–33.

Somerville, L. H., Fani, N., and McClure-Tone, E. B. (in press). Behavioral and neural representations of emotional facial expressions across the lifespan. *Developmental Neuropsychology*.

Sowell, E. R., Peterson, B. S., Thompson, P. M. Welcome, S. E., Henkenius, A. L., and Toga, A. W. (2003). Mapping cortical change across the human life span. *Nature Neuroscience*, 6, 309–315.

Sowell, E. R., Thompson, P. M., Holmes, C. J., Jernigan, T. L., and Toga, A. W. (1999). In vivo evidence for post-adolescent brain maturation in frontal and striatal regions. *Nature Neuroscience*, 2, 859–61.

Sowell, E. R., Thompson, P. M., and Toga, A. W. (2004). Mapping changes in the human cortex throughout the span of life. *Neuroscientist*, 10, 372–92.

Sowell, E. R., Trauner, D. A., Gamst, A., and Jernigan, T. L. (2002). Development of cortical and subcortical brain areas in childhood and adolescence: a structural MRI study. *Developmental Medicine and Child Neurology*, 44(1), 4–16.

Spear, L. P. (2000). The adolescent brain and age-related behavioral manifestations. *Neuroscience and Biobehavioral Reviews*, 24, 417–63.

Steinberg, L. (2004). Risk-taking in adolescence: what changes, and why? *Annals of the New York Academy of Sciences*, 1021, 51–8.

Steinberg, L. (2007). Risk-taking in adolescence: new perspectives from brain and behavioral science. *Current Directions in Psychological Science*, 16, 55–9.

Steinberg, L. (2008). A social neuroscience perspective on adolescent risk-taking. *Developmental Review*, 28, 78–106.

Steinberg, L., and Morris, A. S. (2001). Adolescent development. *Annual Review of Psychology*, 52, 83–110.

Stone, M. (1960). Models for choice reaction time. *Psychometrika*, 25, 251–60.

Tamm, L., Menon, V., and Reiss. A. L. (2002). Maturation of brain function associated with response inhibition. *Journal of the American Academy of Child and Adolescent Psychiatry*, 41, 1231–38.

Thomas, K. M., Hunt, R. H., Vizueta, N., Sommer, T., Durston, S., Yang, Y. et al. (2004). Evidence of developmental differences in implicit sequence learning: an FMRI study of children and adults. *Journal of Cognitive Neuroscience*, 16, 1339–51.

Turkeltaub, P.E., Gareau, L., Flowers, D.L., Zeffiro, T.A., and Eden, G.F. (2003). Development of neural mechanisms for reading. *Nature Neuroscience*, 6, 767–73.

Van Leijenhorst, L., Zanolie, K., Van Meel, C. S., Westenberg, P. M., Rombouts, S. A. R. B., and Crone, E. A. (2009). What motivates the adolescent? Brain regions mediating reward sensitivity across adolescence. *Cerebral Cortex* (on line)

Volkow, N. D. and Li, T. K. (2004). Drug addiction: the neurobiology of behaviour gone awry. *Nature Reviews Neuroscience*, 5, 963–70.

Wald, A. (1947). *Sequential Analysis*. New York: John Wiley & Sons, Inc.

Yurgelun-Todd, D. (2007). Emotional and cognitive changes during adolescence. *Current Opinion in Neurobiology*, 17, 251–57.

Zald, D. H., Boileau, I., El-Dearedy, W., Gunn, R., McGlone, F., Dichter, G. S., and Dagher, A. (2004). Dopamine transmission in the human striatum during monetary reward tasks. *Journal of Neuroscience*, 24, 4105–4112.

Chapter 21

Abnormalities in monetary and other non-drug reward processing in drug addiction*

Rita Z. Goldstein

Abstract

Adaptations of the reward circuit to intermittent and chronic supraphysiological stimulation by drugs increase reward thresholds. As a consequence, response to non-drug reinforcers in individuals with chronic drug use or addiction, may be decreased. Clinical symptoms include anhedonia and compulsive drug use, at the expense of the attainment of other rewarding experiences and despite detrimental consequences to the individual's functioning. While most addiction studies focus on the increased valuation of drug reward and drug-related cues, in this chapter we instead review the behavioral and neurobiological evidence for decreased valuation of non-drug reinforcers and cues. Future research should directly address the following question: is processing of drug reward enhanced at the expense of non drug-related reward (at least in certain subgroups of addicted individuals)? Or are these two processes independent?

21.1 The phenomenology and neurobiology of drug addiction

Addiction is a chronic disease characterized by repeated periods of drug craving, intoxication, bingeing, and withdrawal (American Psychiatric Association, 1994). This cycle culminates in the escalated preoccupation with the attainment and consumption of the substance. In particular, the compulsive consumption of the drug occurs at the expense of the attainment of other rewarding experiences and despite detrimental consequences

* Notice: This manuscript has been authored by Brookhaven Science Associates, LLC under Contract No. DE-AC02-98CHI-886 with the US Department of Energy. The United States Government retains, and the publisher, by accepting the article for publication, acknowledges, a world-wide license to publish or reproduce the published form of this manuscript, or allow others to do so, for the United States Government purposes.

to the individual's functioning (encompassing physical health and other personal, social, and occupational goals). This pattern continues despite attempts of the addicted individual to stop or curtail drug use and even when the rewarding experiences from the drug are markedly reduced (Goldstein and Volkow, 2002).

Animal and human studies show that drugs of abuse exert their reinforcing and addictive effects by activating, and ultimately co-opting, the brain's reward system, a phylogenetically ancient circuitry normally involved in the reward sensations that are essential to learning and survival. The hub of this system consists of the mesolimbic and mesocortical dopamine (DA) fibers, which originate in the ventral tegmental area and terminate in the ventral striatum (VStr, which encompasses the nucleus accumbens), ventral pallidum, amygdala, hippocampus, and prefrontal cortex (PFC). This circuit's drug-induced stimulation occurs directly by triggering DA action or indirectly, by modulating other neurotransmitters (e.g., glutamate, gamma aminobutyric acid, endogenous opioids, acetylcholine, cannabinoids, and serotonin). Specifically, all addictive substances increase DA in the mesolimbic brain regions (Volkow et al., 1997a) as directly associated with the reinforcing effects (self-reports of "high", "rush," and "euphoria") of the drugs (cocaine, methylphenidate, and amphetamine) (Laruelle et al., 1995; Volkow et al., 2002a). This is different from non-drug primary ("natural") reinforcers for which increases in DA appear to occur mostly for reward prediction rather than to the reward itself (Koob and Bloom, 1988; Pontieri et al., 1996, 1998; Schultz et al., 2000). Furthermore, natural reinforcers induce DA increases within the physiological range that habituate with repeated consumption or decrease with satiety. In contrast, drugs of abuse induce supraphysiological DA increases that do not habituate (Bassareo et al., 2002) and that encode for motivation to procure the drug irrespective of whether the drug is pleasurable or not (McClure et al., 2003). Thus, these DA responses imply that drugs are reinforcing not just because they are pleasurable, but because by increasing DA they are being processed as salient stimuli that will inherently motivate further procurement of more drug (regardless of whether the drug is consciously perceived as pleasurable or not) and will facilitate conditioned learning (Volkow et al., 2004a).

With chronic use, striatal DA D2 receptor availability is reduced (Nader and Czoty, 2005; Nader et al., 2006; Volkow et al., 1990, 1997a) as associated with altered function in dopaminergically innervated corticolimbic areas (encompassing the orbitofrontal cortex and anterior cingulate cortex) that mediate processing of reward salience and motivation (McClure et al., 2004b; Wolfram Schultz, 2006; Volkow et al., 1993). Given these long-lasting decreases in DA function, it has been proposed that addicted individuals may take the drug to compensate for the decreased stimulation of DA-regulated reward pathways by non-drug rewards (Volkow et al., 2004a). Indeed, enhanced processing of drug reward and drug-related cues has been frequently studied (Childress et al., 1999; Di Chiara and Imperato, 1988). However, it is still not clear whether this enhanced drug-reward processing is achieved at the expense of non-drug-reward processing in drug-addicted individuals or whether these are independent processes. Several theoretical accounts, mostly based on animal evidence, have been proposed to resolve this issue.

21.2 **An underlying change in the value of reward in drug addiction: theoretical accounts**

The reward-deficiency syndrome hypothesis posits that individuals prone to addiction have a deficit in recruiting DA motivational circuitry by non-drug rewards, such that abused drugs are uniquely able to normalize DA levels in the VStr to readily motivate drug-taking behavior (Blum et al., 2000). The allostatic hypothesis suggests a chronic deviation of the brain's reward "set-point" after repeated prolonged exposure to drugs of abuse, which are powerfully reinforcing owing to their potent ability to activate the brain's reward system. Specifically, it is proposed that the brain reward thresholds become chronically elevated and do not appear to return to baseline levels with abstinence (Koob and Le Moal, 1997). The incentive motivation model posits that, with repeated drug use, cues associated with drug-taking acquire incentive value through sensitization of the brain's reward system. As the number of paired cue-drug presentations increases, the incentive value of these cues intensifies, making them increasingly "wanted." With ongoing use, drug cue incentive salience becomes excessive, "wanting" transforms into drug craving, and drug cues become potent perpetuators of further excessive drug taking, despite awareness of associated adverse consequences (Robinson and Berridge, 1993, 2001, 2003). Similarly, a core symptom of our impaired response inhibition and salience attribution (I-RISA) model was postulated to encompass a disproportionate salience, or value, attribution to the drug of choice with a concomitant decrease in the value attributed to other primary and secondary reinforcers by drug-addicted individuals, together enhancing motivation to procure drugs at the expense of the drive to attain most other non-drug-related goals (Goldstein and Volkow, 2002).

Consistent with these models, animal research suggests that, after chronic drug administration, the value of a drug reward is increased (Ahmed and Koob, 1998; Ahmed et al., 2002), while that of a non-drug reward is decreased (Grigson and Twining, 2002). Similarly, human cocaine-addicted subjects, but not controls, showed reduced activation of corticolimbic brain areas when viewing an erotic (non-drug) video, than when exposed to a cocaine video (Garavan et al., 2000). In contrast, other human studies show blunted subjective responses to drug rewards (intravenous methylphenidate), suggesting reductions in the subjective value of drug reward in addicted individuals (Volkow et al., 1997b). Yet a third possibility is that of a generally drug-sensitized brain-reward circuit, where heightened drug motivation may "spillover" to non-drug rewards (Robinson and Berridge, 2003). Here, evidence from animal studies suggests that drug sensitization can increase the incentive value of other rewards, such as sucrose or other foods, a sexually receptive female (for male rats), and conditioned stimuli for such rewards (Fiorino and Phillips, 1999a, 1999b; Nocjar and Panksepp, 2002; Taylor and Horger, 1999; Wyvell and Berridge, 2001). Similarly, in human-addicted individuals, evidence suggests that some cocaine-addicted individuals are hypersexual (Washton and Stone-Washton, 1993) and some substance-dependent individuals may be hyper-responsive to money rewards (Bechara et al., 2002). To resolve these discrepancies, studies could target certain subgroups within addicted individuals, such that heterogeneity in the addicted population vis-à-vis sensitivity to reward is explicitly addressed. One such subgrouping could be based on recency of drug use that is associated with enhanced anhedonia but better cognitive functioning (Woicik et al., 2008) and prefrontal drug cue-reactivity (Wilson et al., 2004) in currently addicted individuals. Studies could also dissociate the subjective value of an expected reward (before reward is received) from reward perception at consumption (when reward is received/experienced). Other important dissociations have been suggested by the incentive motivation theory. Here, it is hypothesized that "wanting" drugs (e.g., how much an animal will work to acquire a drug) increases to pathological levels without a parallel increase in drug's hedonic properties or its "liking" (Robinson and Berridge, 1993, 2001, 2003). This specific hypersensitivity (i.e., sensitization) to the incentive motivational (i.e., "wanting" but not "liking") effects of drugs (and drug-related stimuli) is hypothesized to ultimately lead to increasingly compulsive patterns of drug-seeking and drug-taking behavior. Clearly, more experimental designs directly examining the value attributed to drug rewards specifically, as it compares with the value attributed to primary non-drug rewards, are needed to further the study of drug addiction.

21.3 Enhanced processing of drug cues at the expense of non-drug cues in human drug addiction?

In this section we review the behavioral evidence suggesting enhanced processing of drug vs. non-drug reward in human drug addiction.

21.3.1 Subjective reports

An impressive body of research has documented the subjective overpowering effects of drugs of abuse (Fox et al., 2005; Gawin, 1991; Lasagna et al., 1955; Leyton et al., 2005; Von Felsinger et al., 1955), suggesting that conditioned drug-related responses trigger an intense desire for the drug, possibly exceeding desire for all other non-drug reinforcers (Volkow et al., 2006b). We have recently developed a brief self-report measure (sensitivity to reinforcement of addictive and other primary rewards, STRAP-R) that dissociates "liking" from "wanting" of expected "drug" rewards as compared to "food" and "sex" while respondents report about three different situations ("current" lab situation, and hypothetical "in general," and "under drug influence") (Goldstein et al., 2008a). Results in 20 cocaine-addicted individuals revealed that the reinforcers' relative subjective value changed when reporting about the drug-related context ("under drug influence:" drug>food; otherwise: drug<food). This relative paling of other rewards in the environment was highest in the addicted individuals with the youngest age of cocaine-use onset, suggesting this subjective value shift may represent a cumulative (and not acute) effect of drug use or it may predispose individuals to more intense early drug experimentation and subsequent development of drug addiction.

21.3.2 Objective choice behavior

Although essential, because uniquely human, self-reports are limited due to their potential modulation by extraneous factors encompassing demand characteristics (and social desirability), as well as imperfect awareness of one's own mental processes, which may be all the more pronounced in drug addiction (Goldstein et al., in press). To overcome this limitation, experimental paradigms have directly tested choice behavior. Here, juxtaposing choice for drug against choice for competing reinforcers, studies have shown that previously drug-exposed animals choose cocaine over novelty (Reichel and Bevins, 2008), adequate maternal behavior (Mattson et al., 2001), and even food, a primary reinforcer needed for survival (Aigner and Balster, 1978; Woolverton and Anderson, 2006; Zombeck et al., 2008). Parallel human studies use the multiple-choice procedure that provides an index of the relative reinforcing value of a drug vs. alternative reinforcers (Griffiths et al., 1993, 1996). Here, studies show that drug-addicted individuals routinely choose their drug of choice over money (Donny et al., 2003; Hart et al., 2000; Martinez et al., 2007b). This effect is modulated by drug dose, as recently demonstrated: choice for immediate alcohol (vs. 1-week delayed monetary delivery) increased with alcohol dose (12, 24, or 36 ounces) in 27 young binge-drinkers (>5 drinks at one sitting twice a week) (Benson et al., 2009). Interestingly, at the highest alcohol dose, alcohol choice was enhanced even in the immediate monetary payment condition (Benson et al., 2009). This is important because, compared to controls, drug-addicted individuals show preference for immediate over delayed reward as associated with risky or disadvantageous decision making (reviewed below in S21.6). Whether such preference for immediate reward may be biased in the context of, and towards, the drug of choice (and away from other non drug rewards), remains to be tested.

We developed a picture-choice task to provide an opportunity for testing choice for drug-related, as compared to competing, reinforcers (pleasant and unpleasant pictures) outside of an acute drug-administration paradigm, therefore suitable for use even when direct drug administration is not feasible or ethical (e.g., in abstaining or treatment-seeking drug-addicted individuals) (Moeller et al., 2009). Results showed that 20 cocaine-addicted individuals selected more, and worked more for, cocaine pictures than matched healthy control subjects. Results also revealed modulation of the drug-picture choice by the alternative pictures, such that the drug-picture choice was equivalent to pleasant-picture choice but enhanced when compared to unpleasant-picture choice, possibly indicative of modulation of actual drug choice by other pleasant or aversive stimuli in drug-addicted individuals as consistent with both human and animal studies (Ahmed and Koob, 1997; Brown and Erb, 2007; Christensen et al., 2008; Higgins et al., 2004; Lenoir et al., 2007; Sinha et al., 2000, 2006; Stairs et al., 2006). Importantly, higher choice for viewing cocaine pictures, even when directly compared to selections of the other positively valued and reportedly more pleasant pictures, correlated with higher frequency of actual cocaine use (as possibly indicative of higher drug-addiction severity). It is, therefore, possible that such choice behavior would be differently expressed depending on an individual's phase within the addiction cycle (e.g., intoxication, craving, bingeing, withdrawal) and consequently remains to be studied longitudinally and in various subgroups within the heterogeneous-addicted population (e.g., those who are positive vs. negative for cocaine in urine, an objective measure of recency and frequency of use). Overall, such disadvantageously enhanced drug choice could provide a marker of the neurocognitive dysfunction that characterizes drug addiction.

21.3.3 Cognitive processes

Cognitive studies similarly demonstrate that drug-related cues elicit a unique pattern of reactions in drug-addicted individuals. For instance, exposure to drug-related stimuli (e.g., pictures, paraphernalia) in drug-addicted individuals impacts classical neuropsychological measures of cognitive interference (e.g., the Stroop effect) (Carter and Tiffany, 1999; Duka and Townshend, 2004; Franken et al., 2000; Hester et al., 2006; Mogg and Bradley, 2002) as indicative of attention bias and automatic cue reactivity. Similarly, tailoring other neuropsychological measures to specifically target drug addiction also shows promising results, e.g., drug-addicted as compared to control subjects name more drug-related words, while there are no group differences on the regular/neutral semantic fluency (naming animals or fruits/vegetables) (Goldstein et al. 2007c). Thereby, one could test the underlying mechanisms which, in addition to attention bias, may also include overlearning of drug-predictive cues (Redish, 2004), "fresher" memory traces of drug effects (Lee et al., 2006), and heightened arousal/autonomic reactions evidenced in addicted individuals in response to drug-related cues (Carter and Tiffany, 1999b; Ehrman et al. 1992; Glautier and Drummond, 1994; Margolin et al., 1994; Sinha et al., 2000). An open question in these studies is whether this bias to drug-related processing decreases efficiency of non-drug related processing, which would be evidenced by a cognitive compromise under a neutral context, as indeed suggested using classical neuropsychological studies in addiction (e.g., Woicik et al., 2008). We speculate that this cognitive compromise in addicted individuals is not fully driven by a neutral (i.e., not motivating) context, and that even under high levels of motivation, compromised neurocognitive functioning could be detected as suggested by results of neuroimaging studies, as reviewed next.

21.4 Neuroimaging studies utilizing monetary reward in drug-addicted individuals

Neuroimaging research has predominantly focused on responses to drug-related stimuli alone and rarely examined how these findings compare with the processing of non-drug reinforcers. We, therefore, next review the neuroimaging studies that used non-drug-related reward in addicted individuals. We start with reviewing the studies that utilized money as a reinforcer. The importance of using monetary reward lies in the conditioning between monetary availability and drug procurement. If processing of this secondary generalizable reinforcer is compromised in addicted individuals, it is possible that, for this population, only more immediate drug-related cues (e.g., pictures or a video; see: Garavan et al., 2000) or the drug itself, could activate this circuit at a comparable level with that induced by a non-drug-related reward in the non-drug-addicted individual. Such evidence would provide support for the possibility that processing of non-drug reward is compromised in drug addiction.

In a functional magnetic resonance imaging (fMRI) study, we examined responses to monetary reward received for correct performance on a sustained attention task in 16 cocaine-addicted (abstinence 1–90 days) as compared to 13 healthy control subjects

(Goldstein et al., 2007b). Sustained monetary reward was associated with a robust and complex neuronal activation pattern in the comparison subjects (Fig. 21.1): there was a trend for the left orbitofrontal (OFC) to respond in a graded fashion (45¢>1¢>0¢), the lateral and medial PFC (including anterior cingulate cortex) responded instead to the two conditions of monetary value equally (45¢ = 1¢>0¢), while the mesencephalon displayed a third pattern of sensitivity to the highest available reward only (45¢>1¢ = 0¢). In general, these results were consistent with role of the (a) OFC in relative reward processing in the primate (Tremblay and Schultz, 1999) and in healthy human subjects (Breiter et al., 2001; Elliott et al., 2003; Knutson et al., 2000; Kringelbach et al., 2003; O'Doherty et al., 2001); (b) PFC in the control of attention (Hornak et al., 2004), possibly irrespective of reward magnitude (Watanabe, 1989); and (c) mesencephalon in an all-or-nothing reward processing in the primate (Tobler et al., 2005) and in healthy human subjects (Elliott et al., 2003). The cocaine-addicted subjects did not display this complex pattern of activation to monetary reward, demonstrating either reduced regional fMRI signal in the between-group analyses, or less sensitivity to differences between the monetary conditions in the within-group analyses. A relative exception was the left cerebellum, where only the cocaine abusers displayed a significant monetary effect (45¢>0¢; note, however, that the between-group analysis still showed larger reward-related activations in the comparison subjects). This within-subjects result is consistent with reports of compensatory mechanisms in the cerebellum in psychopathology, e.g., over-reliance on the cerebellum by cocaine abusers during a working memory task (Hester and Garavan, 2004) and by Parkinson's patients during a rewarded task (Goerendt et al., 2004). Extending our prior study (Goldstein et al., 2007b), we recently reported that anterior cingulate hypoactivations in cocaine users cannot be attributed to task difficulty or disengagement but that, nevertheless, emotional salience modulates this region's responses in proportion to drug use severity (Goldstein et al., 2009a).

Interestingly, using a self-report measure adapted from studies in opiate addiction (Martin-Soelch et al., 2001), our results showed that, while most controls reported valuing higher amounts of money more than lower amounts, more than half of the cocaine-addicted individuals rated the value of all monetary amounts equally ($10 = $1000) (Goldstein et al., 2007a) (Fig. 21.2). Eighty-five percent of the variance in this constrained subjective sensitivity to monetary reward gradients in the cocaine abusers was attributed to lateral OFC, amygdala, and medial frontal gyrus responses to monetary reward. This finding may seem perplexing in light of the frequently used delay discounting and gambling reward paradigms, where time and reward contingencies are juxtaposed to examine the effects of the created conflict on decision-making/choice behavior (e.g., Bechara and Damasio, 2002; McClure et al., 2004a). In contrast, in our study, subjects did not choose between smaller immediate vs. larger delayed monetary rewards. Instead, we focused on the individual's subjective experience (evaluation of a non-drug reward). We interpreted these findings to suggest preserved reward sensitivity (illustrated by the small squares in Fig. 21.3A) that would allow the detection of differences between reinforcers in the healthy control subjects (monotonically positive function). In contrast, the low sensitivity

Fig. 21.1 Average fMRI signals in the left orbitofrontal cortex (A: OFC), prefrontal cortex (B: PFC, mean signal), right mesencephalon (C: MSN), and left cerebellum (D: CBL) as a function of monetary reward (white = 0¢; gray = 1¢; black = 45¢) and diagnostic group (left: 16 cocaine abusers; right: 12 comparison subjects, ss). Bar graphs represent mean % signal change from baseline ± SEM. ANOVA F results are presented on the right: df = 2, 25 (Money) or 1, 26 (Group). Results of significant t-tests are marked inside the figures: df = 11 (comparison subjects), 15 (cocaine), 26 (group differences); all significant t>|2.1|; *P<0.05; **P<0.01. Adapted with permission from: Goldstein et al., 2007b; figure #2.

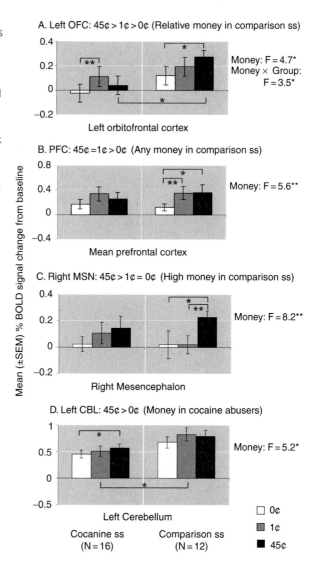

A. Left OFC: 45¢ > 1¢ > 0¢ (Relative money in comparison ss)

Left orbitofrontal cortex

Money: F = 4.7*
Money × Group: F = 3.5*

B. PFC: 45¢ = 1¢ > 0¢ (Any money in comparison ss)

Mean prefrontal cortex

Money: F = 5.6**

C. Right MSN: 45¢ > 1¢ = 0¢ (High money in comparison ss)

Right Mesencephalon

Money: F = 8.2**

D. Left CBL: 45¢ > 0¢ (Money in cocaine abusers)

Left Cerebellum

Money: F = 5.2*

Mean (±SEM) % BOLD signal change from baseline

Cocaine ss (N = 16)   Comparison ss (N = 12)

☐ 0¢
■ 1¢ (gray)
■ 45¢

in cocaine abusers (large squares in Fig. 21.3B) would not permit the distinction between stimuli of different gradations but rather allow an all-or-nothing identification only of the stimuli that reach the threshold required for perception of reinforcement (step function). Results of this self-reported data need to be confirmed with more objective measures of behavior, especially given the impairments in self-awareness in addiction, as we recently suggested (Goldstein et al., in press). It also remains to be determined whether different subgroups within the addicted population (e.g., urine positive vs. negative for the drug) would evidence differential subjective (or more objective) sensitivity to non-drug reward (as indeed suggested by our preliminary results, Fig. 21.2B).

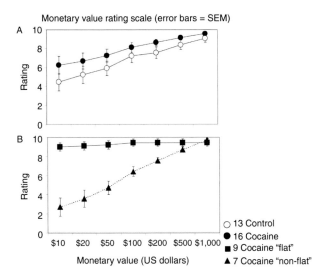

Monetary value rating scale (error bars = SEM)

Fig. 21.2 Money value rating scale. A: Subjective ratings in control subjects (N = 13, white) compared with cocaine abusers (N = 16, black). B: Data presented for two cocaine subgroups: subjects with flat ratings on the money rating scale (N = 9, black squares) vs. subjects with non-flat ratings (N = 7, black triangles). Error bars represent standard error.

Adapted with permission from: (Goldstein et al., 2007a; figure #2.

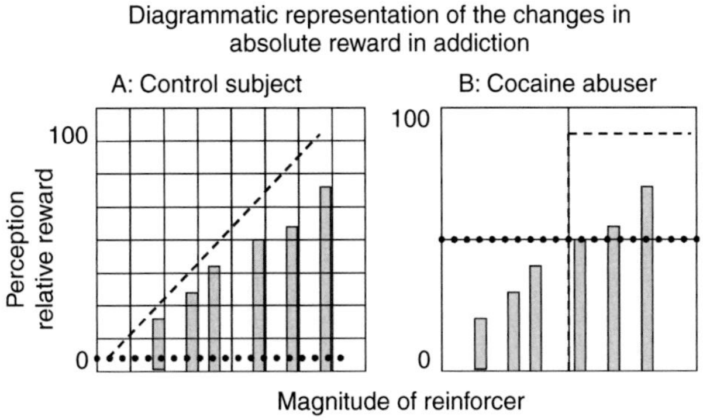

○ 13 Control
● 16 Cocaine
■ 9 Cocaine "flat"
▲ 7 Cocaine "non-flat"

Diagrammatic representation of the changes in absolute reward in addiction

A: Control subject   B: Cocaine abuser

Magnitude of reinforcer

Fig. 21.3 Diagrammatic representation of the changes in relative and absolute reward in addiction. Dotted lines reflect the threshold for a stimulus to be perceived as reinforcing: the threshold is lower in the non-addicted (A) and higher in the drug-addicted (B) individual. Dashed lines reflect the function that describes the perception of a stimulus as subjectively valuable. The high sensitivity to the reinforcers (small squares, A) allows the detection of small reinforcers and differences in magnitude between reinforcers in control subjects (*monotonically positive function*). The low sensitivity in cocaine abusers (large squares, B) does not permit the distinction between stimuli of different gradations but rather identify only those that reach the threshold required for the stimulus to be perceived as reinforcing (*step function*).

With permission from: Goldstein et al., 2007a; figure #4.

Using the same sustained-attention task and monetary reward quantities (45¢, 1¢ and 0¢), while recording event-related potentials (ERPs), we replicated the impact of monetary reward on neural responses (measured here with the P300 ERP component) in healthy young adults (Goldstein et al., 2006). This result was consistent with a large body of literature implicating the P300 in processing reward magnitude and valence (e.g., Yeung and Sanfey, 2004). Importantly, we subsequently replicated these results in 18 healthy individuals matched on age and other demographic factors to cocaine-addicted individuals (abstinence 0–4 days) (Goldstein et al., 2008b): while in the control subjects the amplitude of the P300 component was higher in the 45¢ condition than the 0¢ condition, a similar P300 response to money was not significant in the cocaine-addicted subjects. In parallel, only the control subjects reacted faster to the highest monetary condition (45¢) as compared to the neutral cue (0¢). Importantly, only in the control subjects, these P300 amplitude differentials directly intercorrelated with the respective behavioral adjustments to the monetary incentive (45¢>0¢ with accuracy and 1¢>0¢ with reaction time); in the cocaine-addicted subjects, the better the accuracy adjustment for the high monetary condition, the less frequent the cocaine use during the year preceding the study. Our most recent results suggest that such compromised P300 responses to money characterize both cocaine urine positive and cocaine urine negative currently addicted individuals (unpublished observation).

Overall, reduced sensitivity to non-drug reward (as objectively measured with fMRI and ERPs) may represent an additional symptom of the reward threshold elevations and reward sensitivity decreases characterizing chronic drug use (Ahmed and Koob, 1998; Ahmed et al., 2002), hypothesized to result from adaptations of the reward circuit to intermittent and chronic supraphysiological stimulation by drugs (Volkow and Fowler, 2000).

21.4.1 Neuroimaging studies focusing on the ventral striatum

Note that in our fMRI study, the VStr (or dorsal striatum) was not activated to money (Goldstein et al., 2007b), which could be attributed to technical factors (e.g., statistical threshold, signal loss) or the lack of incorporation into the task design of an anticipatory phase (reward contingencies were constant and predictable). Other fMRI studies of monetary reward anticipation showed the expected VStr activations in healthy control subjects (e.g., Knutson et al., 2005). Utilizing this same monetary incentive delay task, authors recently showed that, while the VStr was activated to both gain and loss (gain>loss) in healthy control subjects, these activations were significantly higher than in abstinent alcoholics (recruited from an inpatient detoxification treatment program, abstinence 5–37 days) (Wrase et al., 2007). Interestingly, the alcoholics with the highest VStr monetary gain activations had the lowest self-reported alcohol craving. Importantly, alcohol (vs. neutral) pictures elicited significant right VStr activation in the alcoholics and the higher this activation, the more the alcohol craving (Wrase et al., 2007). Consistent with the premise of the current review, the authors interpreted these findings to reflect the selective diversion of motivational resources away from conventional rewards and toward drug rewards in addicted individuals (these findings were not interpreted to reflect a global deficit of brain activation in alcoholics, e.g., due to hypoperfusion, or a selective blunting of the VStr). Although the direct comparison between the different classes of reinforcers (money vs. drug cues) remains to be accomplished, this study offers strong support for the hypothesis that the value of drug-related cues overpowers that of non-drug-related cues in addicted individuals. In a similar vein, we recently reported that even abstract cues, such as drug words (but not neutral words), activated the mesencephalon (the main source of dopamine release and projection to the VStr) in cocaine users but not demographically matched healthy control subjects; these increased drug-related mesencephalic responses were associated with enhanced verbal fluency specifically for drug (but not neutral) words in the addicted subjects (Goldstein et al., 2009b).

Opposite evidence has also been suggested. Here, a modified version of the monetary incentive delay fMRI task was used in 23 controls and 23 abstinent treatment-seeking alcoholics (scanned 6–26 days after abstinence) (Bjork et al., 2008b). While there were no differences between the groups during the anticipatory phase, the VStr (and insula and anterior cingulate cortex) showed higher responses in the alcoholics than controls to reward delivery ($5.0 or $.5) vs. no reward ($0.0); these regions were also deactivated by reward-outcome deferrals (i.e., frustration) in the alcoholics more than in the controls. The authors interpreted these results as indicative of a physiological signature of reward-centric bias in addiction, and of motivational and emotional instability/impulsivity/greater urgency to alleviate negative emotions (Bjork et al., 2008b). Because this task has been designed to emphasize the anticipatory and not consummatory phase, and given some inconsistencies in this study (e.g., although there were significant reaction time responses to reward in controls but not alcoholics, the controls did not show VStr responses to reward during the reward delivery phase), these results await replication and validation in other populations of addicted individuals. Of note here are also previous positron emission tomography (PET) studies that measured regional cerebral blood flow during processing of monetary reward in addicted (e.g., smokers, opiate users) and non-addicted individuals (Martin-Soelch et al., 2001, 2003); here too conclusive statements should be deferred due to lack of direct comparisons between the study groups.

21.5 Other non-monetary reward

Studies of neural responses to drug-related vs. non-drug-related cues (including potential reinforcers) in addicted vs. non-addicted individuals have generally utilized electrophysiological recordings, while subjects view drug-related, pleasant, unpleasant, and neutral pictures. Including non-drug emotional stimuli, in addition to the usual drug-related vs. neutral pictures, add to the fledgling emotional neuroscience literature in drug addiction (Aguilar de Arcos et al., 2005; Verdejo-Garcia et al., 2006). For example, we used an ERP component, the LPP, as a psychophysiological measure of automatic (Hajcak et al., 2007) or bottom-up (Ferrari et al., 2008) motivated attention bias elicited by drug-related stimuli in 20 active cocaine-addicted individuals (abstinence 0–14 days), as compared to matched controls (unpublished observation). Preliminary results showed that the LPPs elicited by cocaine pictures were similar to LPPs elicited by the other emotional pictures only in the addicted individuals; in the controls, LPPs elicited by the cocaine pictures were instead comparable to LPPs elicited by the neutral pictures, and both were significantly smaller than LPPs elicited by the other emotional pictures. These findings suggest that, for the cocaine-addicted subjects, but not controls, both cocaine and emotional stimuli automatically increase attention. A recent study in active heroin-addicted individuals (24-h abstinence) reported similar drug-related P300 enhancements (Lubman et al., 2009) as correlated with baseline craving (Lubman et al., 2008). The more recent study (Lubman et al., 2009) also showed lack of the typical P300 reward enhancement to pleasant vs. neutral or drug pictures, consistent with inhibited responding to non-drug reinforcers in addicted individuals. Compromised responsiveness to pleasant pictures in heroin-addicted individuals was similarly reported in a recent fMRI study, where the bilateral dorsolateral PFC was activated to pleasant pictures in 18 healthy controls but not in 16 abstinent (1–24 weeks), inpatient, male, heroin addicts (Zijlstra et al., 2009). Interestingly, in initially detoxified alcoholic subjects, VStr and thalamic response to pleasant vs. neutral stimuli predicted drinking days and alcohol intake within a 6-month follow-up period (Heinz et al., 2007). Taken together, the preserved responding to non-drug reinforcers may characterize individuals with less pronounced illness severity or reflect a protective factor in drug-addicted individuals. Indeed, offspring of alcoholics with higher DA D2 receptor availability may be protected against developing alcoholism through more adaptive recruitment of corticolimbic circuits (including the OFC) needed for positive emotion regulation (Volkow et al., 2006a).

A promising line of functional neuroimaging research has been using masked cues to study processing of stimuli outside of conscious awareness. In an event-related fMRI study in 21 cocaine patients, 33 ms "unseen" cocaine (and sexual) cues activated the subcortical reward circuitry (encompassing the VStr/pallidum, amygdala, insula, OFC, as characterized by prior studies in humans: Childress, 2002; McClure et al., 2004b) and in animals (Di Chiara and Imperato, 1988; Koob and Bloom, 1988; Wise, 2005) (Childress et al., 2008). Importantly, the "unseen" cocaine cue-induced ventral pallidum/amygdala activation predicted future positive affect to visible versions of these same cues (in an off-magnet affective-priming task, two days later). This correlation demonstrated the functional significance of the "unseen" cues, consistent with recent reports showing that appetitive signals (e.g., for money: Pessiglione et al., 2007; a tasty juice: McCabe et al., 2009b; or happy faces: Winkielman et al., 2005) outside of conscious attention can influence ongoing (e.g., grip force: Pessiglione et al., 2007) or subsequent (e.g., seat choice: McCabe et al., 2009b; or drinking of a novel beverage: Winkielman et al., 2005) motivated behavior.

21.6 Association with impulsivity in drug addiction

A modified value attributed to rewards in the environment may alter underlying stimulus-reinforcement association learning. This modified response to reinforcement in drug-addicted individuals may in turn contribute to cognitive-behavioral and emotional impairments that take the form of over-valuation or bias towards immediate reward and discounting of delayed rewards (Kirby and Petry, 2004; Monterosso et al., 2007) that together can lead to disadvantageous decision making (Bechara et al., 2002; Bolla et al., 2003) and impulsivity (Bjork et al., 2008a; Moeller et al., 2005). The impact of reward on tasks of decision making and other higher-order executive functions (e.g., set-shifting, concept formation, reversal learning) is further reviewed elsewhere in this volume (see Chapter 22).

In our fMRI monetary-reward task, we observed a significant correlation between the dorsolateral PFC response to monetary reward and trait self-reported inhibitory control (measured with Tellegen's Multidimensional Personality Questionnaire: Tellegen and Waller, 1997) in cocaine-addicted individuals (Fig. 21.4), suggesting that hyposensitivity to reward in the PFC is associated with the reduced self-control (impulsivity) reported by the cocaine abusers (Goldstein et al., 2007b). This result highlighted that the association between the PFC and control of behavior (Miller and Cohen, 2001) may be modulated by the PFC sensitivity to reinforcement. Subcortical regions may also be involved. For example, the higher the mesencephalic (ventral tegmental area/substantia nigra) response to money, the more the self-reported reward-dependence as possibly modulating less impulsivity (measured as exploratory excitability) in healthy individuals (Krebs et al., 2009). In contrast, VStr activation to monetary reward was associated with higher impulsivity, or the objectively measured preference for immediate over delayed rewards (Hariri et al., 2006). It remains to be determined whether these differences pertain to the brain region examined and underlying mechanisms (e.g., DA D2 receptor availability) or the measurement chosen (e.g., self-report vs. objective/behavioral measures of impulsivity).

21.7 Modulating factors

Thus, neural responses to reward seem to differ between addicted individuals and healthy control subjects, and these differences are behaviorally significant. However, the effect of the following factors needs to be considered when interpreting results of these studies; clearly more studies and the identification of additional factors is needed.

21.7.1 Perceived opportunity to consume drugs

A recent study showed attenuated dorsal striatal (caudate) responses to both monetary gains and losses (on a card-guessing task for which subjects could earn $1.00 or lose $.50) in 18 male habitual cigarette smokers, told that they would be able to smoke during the study, as compared to those who anticipated having to wait several hours before having the opportunity to smoke (Wilson et al., 2008). The authors concluded that monetary gains were processed as less rewarding and monetary losses as more punishing by individuals anticipating an opportunity to smoke soon, relative to those expecting a significant delay before having the chance to smoke, as modulated by the negative affect associated with imminent drug use further increasing the desire to engage in drug use (Wilson et al., 2008). This factor needs to be explicitly examined in other drug-addicted populations (e.g., cocaine urine positive vs. negative individuals, current users vs. abstinent or treatment-seeking individuals).

21.7.2 Sex differences

Recent evidence points to other modulating factors, such as hormones or gender. For example, during the midfollicular phase (days 4–8 after onset of menses, when estrogen

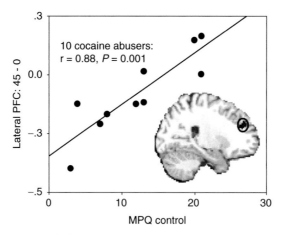

Fig. 21.4 Correlation between the lateral PFC and inhibitory control in 16 cocaine abusers. Scatterplot shows association between the fMRI signal change for monetary reward as compared to the neutral cue (45¢>0¢) in the lateral PFC with MPQ self-control (r = 0.88, P = 0.001); the inserted statistical map of brain activation depicts the cluster location corresponding to this correlation. Thresholded at P<0.05 uncorrected. Minimum cluster size 100 contiguous voxels, 2700 mm³. Adapted with permission from: Goldstein et al., 2007b; figure #3.

is unopposed by progesterone), women anticipating uncertain rewards activated the OFC and amygdala more than during the luteal phase (6–10 days after luteinizing hormone surge) (Dreher et al., 2007). Similar differences (follicular>luteal phase) were seen during reward delivery in the mesencephalon, striatum, and left fronto-polar cortex. Activity in the amygdalo-hippocampal complex was positively correlated with estradiol level, regardless of menstrual cycle phase. Also, men activated the ventral putamen more than women during anticipation of uncertain rewards, whereas women more strongly activated the anterior medial PFC at time of reward delivery (Dreher et al., 2007).

21.7.3 Age

Signal increases in the right VStr during anticipation of responding for large gains vs. non-gains positively correlated with age and, in a direct comparison, 12 adolescents (12–17 years of age) evidenced less recruitment of the right VStr and extended amygdala compared with 12 young adults (22–28 years) (Bjork et al., 2004). However, another study reported the opposite pattern, where exaggerated magnitude of VStr activity, relative to PFC activity, was observed in 13 adolescents (13–17 years), compared with 12 adults (23–29 years), and 16 children (7–11 years) (Galvan et al., 2006).

21.8 The underlying mechanism for a possible reward value shift in drug addiction

Dopamine is an essential neurotransmitter in processing reward and reward prediction errors (McClure et al., 2004b; Wolfram Schultz, 2006; Volkow et al., 1993) and in salience enhancement (Volkow et al., 2002b, 2004b). The abnormalities in reward processing in drug addiction are therefore not surprising and are consistent with similar compromises in other dopaminergically mediated psychopathologies. For example, monetary incentives do not modulate grip force in patients with bilateral striatal-pallidal damage (Schmidt et al., 2008) and Parkinson's disease patients are less proficient in learning the predictive value of monetary reward cues, displaying diminished functional connectivity of the mesencephalon and VStr (Schott et al., 2007). In healthy individuals, a preliminary pharmacological fMRI study suggested that a dopaminergic agent (0.25 mg/kg oral dopadextroamphetamine vs. placebo) modulated VStr responses during anticipation of gains, such that responses were blunted in peak amplitude but extended in duration (Knutson et al., 2004). However, the association between DA and reward processing is not linear. For example, higher baseline striatal DA synthesis is associated with better reward-learning but worse learning with further dopaminergic intervention (with bromocriptine) in healthy controls; in contrast, lower baseline striatal DA synthesis is associated with better punishment-learning and DA enhancement improves reward learning (Cools et al., 2009). It is, therefore, possible that improving baseline DA function in selected subgroups of drug-addicted individuals may improve their reward processing. In this context, preliminary results in our laboratory showed a direct correlation between baseline DA receptor availability (measured with C11 raclopride and PET), and thalamic and medial PFC response to money (measured with fMRI) in seven cocaine-addicted individuals (Asensio et al., accepted).

More direct evidence for the role of DA in the modified reward valuation in addicted individuals derives from another PET study, where blunted amphetamine-induced DA release in the VStr (and dorsal striatum) was predictive of actual choice for cocaine over money (and not of positive subjective drug effects) in 24 cocaine-addicted individuals (14 days abstinence), as compared to 24 controls (Martinez et al., 2007). These results were all the more compelling as subjects could choose to receive $5 or self-administer smoked cocaine (6 or 12 mg) with street value <$5. Although results of this study need to be validated using a more immediate monetary gain (the $5 gain was delayed, given as a merchandise voucher redeemable at local stores and paid upon discharge from the study), choice on this self-administration paradigm may model relapse (drug choice followed a priming dose/drug cue). In fact, the authors interpreted these results to indicate that the cocaine-addicted individuals who are most vulnerable to relapse are those with the lowest presynaptic DA function because their DA levels may be insufficient to provide the signal that could shift habitual behavior (drug choice, lesser reward) to a more advantageous behavior (monetary choice, greater reward).

21.9 **Summary and conclusions**

We reviewed evidence for a modified valuation of monetary and other non-drug-related reward in drug-addicted individuals. These abnormalities may contribute to the ascribed motivational impairments and deficits in controlling drug-taking behavior in drug-addicted individuals. For example, restricted range of subjective valuation of reward may play a mediating role in the ability to use internal cues and feedback from the environment to inhibit inappropriate (drug-escalated) behavior. Moreover, a "flattened" sensitivity to gradients in reward may predispose individuals to disadvantageous decisions (e.g., trading a car for a couple of cocaine hits). Without a relative context, drug use and its intense effects (craving and high) could become all the more overpowering.

21.10 Recommendations

Anhedonia (common during acute and long-term drug withdrawal) and difficulty to replace drug-taking behaviors with other, less harmful, activities are common symptoms in drug addiction. Targeting the neurobiology of reward processing in addiction may be beneficial in devising behavioral and pharmacological intervention strategies to alleviate these symptoms. For example, drug abusers who evidence a compromised sensitivity to non-drug reward could be identified for tailored interventions to improve associated cognitive-emotional skills (e.g., attention, response shifting, learning and memory, general value estimations). Because decreased DA striatal release may be associated with reduced activation in the OFC and anterior cingulate cortex to non-drug reward, and enhanced activation in these same regions in response to drug-related cues as correlated with drug craving (Volkow et al., 2004a), pharmacological enhancement or direct brain stimulation of these dopaminergically innervated corticolimbic brain regions may also be beneficial.

21.11 Future directions

Both positive (vouchers, privileges) and negative (incarceration) reinforcers are used in the management of the drug abuser. Therefore, future research needs to be expanded to include negative reinforcers. A particularly important question to be explored is how reward value could modulate choice behavior such that non-drug rewards would be chosen over drug use in addicted individuals. Here promising new approaches suggest that stimuli in a virtual environment (computer game) can acquire motivational properties that persist and modify behavior in the real world (McCabe et al., 2009).

Acknowledgment

Time dedicated to working on this chapter was supported by grants from the National Institute on Drug Abuse (1R01DA023579 and R21DA02062).

References

Aguilar de Arcos, F., Verdejo-Garcia, A., Peralta-Ramirez, M. I., Sanchez-Barrera, M., and Perez-Garcia, M. (2005). Experience of emotions in substance abusers exposed to images containing neutral, positive, and negative affective stimuli. *Drug and Alcohol Dependence,* 78, 159–67.

Ahmed, S.H. and Koob, G.F. (1997). Cocaine- but not food-seeking behavior is reinstated by stress after extinction. *Psychopharmacology,* 132(3), 289–95.

Ahmed, S.H. and Koob, G.F. (1998). Transition from moderate to excessive drug intake: change in hedonic set point. *Science,* 282(5387), 298–300.

Ahmed, S.H., Kenny, P.J., Koob, G.F., and Markou, A. (2002). Neurobiological evidence for hedonic allostasis associated with escalating cocaine use. *Nat Neurosci,* 5(7), 625–26.

Aigner, T.G. and Balster, R.L. (1978). Choice behavior in rhesus monkeys: cocaine versus food. *Science,* 201(4355), 534–35.

American Psychiatric Association. (1994). *Diagnostic and statistical manual of mental disorders,* 4th edn. Washington, DC: American Psychiatric Association.

Asensio, S., Romero, M.J., Romero, F.J., Wong, C., Alia-Klein, N., Tomasi, D. et al. (accepted). Dopamine D2 receptor availability predicts thalamic and medial prefrontal response to reward in cocaine addiction. *Synapse.*

Bassareo, V., De Luca, M.A., and Di Chiara, G. (2002). Differential expression of motivational stimulus properties by dopamine in nucleus accumbens shell versus core and prefrontal cortex. *J Neurosci,* 22(11), 4709–4719.

Bechara, A.B. and Damasio, H. (2002). Decision making and addiction (part I): impaired activation of somatic states in substance dependent individuals when pondering decisions with negative future consequences. *Neuropsychologia,* 40, 1675–89.

Bechara, A.B., Dolan, S., and Andrea, H. (2002). Decision making and addiction (part II): myopia for the future or hypersensitivity to reward. *Neuropsychologia,* 40, 1690–1705.

Benson, T.A., Little, C.S., Henslee, A.M., and Correia, C.J. (2009). Effects of reinforcer magnitude and alternative reinforcer delay on preference for alcohol during a multiple-choice procedure. *Drug Alcohol Depend,* 100(1–2), 161–63.

Bjork, J.M., Momenan, R., Smith, A.R., and Hommer, D.W. (2008a). Reduced posterior mesofrontal cortex activation by risky rewards in substance-dependent patients. *Drug Alcohol Depend,* 95(1–2), 115–28.

Bjork, J.M., Smith, A.R., and Hommer, D.W. (2008b). Striatal sensitivity to reward deliveries and omissions in substance dependent patients. *Neuroimage,* 42(4), 1609–21.

Blum, K., Braverman, E.R., Holder, J.M., Lubar, J.F., Monastra, V.J., Miller, D. et al. (2000). Reward deficiency syndrome: a biogenetic model for the diagnosis and treatment of impulsive, addictive, and compulsive behaviors. *J Psychoactive Drugs,* 32 Suppl: i–iv, 1–112.

Bolla, K. I., Eldreth, D. A., London, E. D., Kiehl, K. A., Mouratidis, M., Contoreggi, C. et al. (2003). Orbitofrontal cortex dysfunction in abstinent cocaine abusers performing a decision making task. *Neuroimage,* 19(3), 1085–94.

Breiter, H.C., Aharon, I., Kahneman, D., Dale, A., and Shizgal, P. (2001). Functional imaging of neural responses to expectancy and experience of monetary gains and losses. *Neuron,* 30(2), 619–39.

Brown, Z.J. and Erb, S. (2007). Footshock stress reinstates cocaine seeking in rats after extended post-stress delays. *Psychopharmacology,* 195(1), 61–70.

Carter, B.L. and Tiffany, S.T. (1999). Meta-analysis of cue-reactivity in addiction research. *Addiction,* 94(3), 327–40.

Childress, A.R., Mozley, P. D., McElgin, W., Fitzgerald, J., Reivich, M., and O'Brien, C. P. (1999). Limbic activation during cue-induced cocaine craving. *Am J Psychiatry,* 156(1), 11–18.

Childress, A.R., Franklin, T.R., Listerud, J., Acton, P.D., O'Brien, C.P. (2002). Neuroimaging of cocaine craving states: cessation, stimulant administration, and drug cue paradigms. In **K. L. Davis, Charney, D., Coyle, J.T., Nemeroff, C.** (Ed.), *Neuropsychopharmacology: The Fifth Generation of Progress* (pp. 1575–90).

Childress, A.R., Ehrman, R.N., Wang, Z., Li, Y., Sciortino, N., Hakun, J. et al. (2008). Prelude to passion: limbic activation by "unseen" drug and sexual cues. *PLoS ONE,* 3(1), e1506.

Christensen, C.J., Silberberg, A., Hursh, S.R., Huntsberry, M.E., and Riley, A.L. (2008). Essential value of cocaine and food in rats: Tests of the exponential model of demand. *Psychopharmacology,* 198(2), 221–29.

Cools, R., Frank, M.J., Gibbs, S.E., Miyakawa, A., Jagust, W., and D'Esposito, M. (2009). Striatal dopamine predicts outcome-specific reversal learning and its sensitivity to dopaminergic drug administration. *J Neurosci,* 29(5), 1538–43.

Di Chiara, G. and Imperato, A. (1988). Drugs abused by humans preferentially increase synaptic dopamine concentrations in the mesolimbic system of freely moving rats. *Proc Natl Acad Sci USA*, **85**(14), 5274–78.

Donny, E.C., Bigelow, G.E., and Walsh, S.L. (2003). Choosing to take cocaine in the human laboratory: Effects of cocaine dose, inter-choice interval, and magnitude of alternative reinforcement. *Drug and Alcohol Dependence*, **69**(3), 289–301.

Dreher, J.C., Schmidt, P.J., Kohn, P., Furman, D., Rubinow, D., and Berman, K.F. (2007). Menstrual cycle phase modulates reward-related neural function in women. *Proc Natl Acad Sci USA*, **104**(7), 2465–70.

Duka, T. and Townshend, J.M. (2004). The priming effect of alcohol pre-load on attentional bias to alcohol-related stimuli. *Psychopharmacology*, **176**, 353–61.

Ehrman, R., Robbins, S.J., Childress, A.R., and O'Brien, C.P. (1992). Conditioned responses to cocaine-related stimuli in cocaine abuse patients. *Psychopharmacology*, **107**(4), 523–29.

Elliott, R., Newman, J.L., Longe, O.A., and Deakin, J.F. (2003). Differential response patterns in the striatum and orbitofrontal cortex to financial reward in humans: a parametric functional magnetic resonance imaging study. *J Neurosci*, **23**(1), 303–307.

Ferrari, V., Codispoti, M., Cardinale, R., and Bradley, M.M. (2008). Directed and motivated attention during processing of natural scenes. *Journal of Cognitive Neuroscience*, **20**(10), 1753–61.

Fiorino, D.F. and Phillips, A.G. (1999a). Facilitation of sexual behavior and enhanced dopamine efflux in the nucleus accumbens of male rats after D-amphetamine-induced behavioral sensitization. *J Neurosci*, **19**(1), 456–63.

Fiorino, D.F. and Phillips, A.G. (1999b). Facilitation of sexual behavior in male rats following d-amphetamine-induced behavioral sensitization. *Psychopharmacology (Berl)*, **142**(2), 200–208.

Fox, H.C., Talih, M., Malison, R., Anderson, G.M., Kreek, M.J., and Sinha, R. (2005). Frequency of recent cocaine and alcohol use affects drug craving and associated responses to stress and drug-related cues. *Psychoneuroendocrinology*, **30**(9), 880–91.

Franken, I.H.A., Kroon, L.Y., Wiers, R.W., and Jansen, A. (2000). Selective cognitive processing of drug cues in heroin dependence. *Journal of Psychopharmacology*, **14**, 395–400.

Galvan, A., Hare, T.A., Parra, C.E., Penn, J., Voss, H., Glover, G. et al. (2006). Earlier development of the accumbens relative to orbitofrontal cortex might underlie risk-taking behavior in adolescents. *J Neurosci*, **26**(25), 6885–92.

Garavan, H., Pankiewicz, J., Bloom, A., Cho, J.K., Sperry, L., Ross, T.J. et al. (2000). Cue-induced cocaine craving: neuroanatomical specificity for drug users and drug stimuli. *Am J Psychiatry*, **157**(11), 1789–98.

Gawin, F.H. (1991). Cocaine addiction: psychology and neurophysiology. *Science*, **251**(5001), 1580–86.

Glautier, S. and Drummond, D.C. (1994). Alcohol dependence and cue reactivity. *J Stud Alcohol*, **55**(2), 224–29.

Goerendt, I.K., Lawrence, A.D., and Brooks, D.J. (2004). Reward processing in health and Parkinson's disease: neural organization and reorganization. *Cereb Cortex*, **14**(1), 73–80.

Goldstein, R.Z., and Volkow, N.D. (2002). Drug addiction and its underlying neurobiological basis: neuroimaging evidence for the involvement of the frontal cortex. *Am J Psychiatry*, **159**(10), 1642–52.

Goldstein, R.Z., Cottone, L.A., Jia, Z., Maloney, T., Volkow, N.D., and Squires, N.K. (2006). The effect of graded monetary reward on cognitive event-related potentials and behavior in young healthy adults. *International Journal of Psychophysiology*, **62**(2), 272–79.

Goldstein, R.Z., Tomasi, D., Alia-Klein, N., Cottone, L.A., Zhang, L., Telang, F. et al. (2007a). Subjective sensitivity to monetary gradients is associated with frontolimbic activation to reward in cocaine abusers. *Drug Alcohol Depend*, **87**(2–3), 233–40.

Goldstein, R.Z., Alia-Klein, N., Tomasi, D., Zhang, L., Cottone, L.A., Maloney, T. et al. (2007b). Is decreased prefrontal cortical sensitivity to monetary reward associated with impaired motivation and self-control in cocaine addiction? *Am J Psychiatry*, **164**(1), 43–51.

Goldstein, R.Z., Woicik, P.A., Lukasik, T., Maloney, T., and Volkow, N.D. (2007c). Drug fluency: a potential marker for cocaine use disorders. *Drug Alcohol Depend,* **89**(1), 97–101.

Goldstein, R., Woicik, P., Moeller, S., Telang, F., Jayne, M., Wong, C. et al. (2008a). Liking and wanting of drug and non-drug rewards in active cocaine users: the STRAP-R questionnaire. *J Psychopharmacol.*

Goldstein, R.Z., Parvaz, M. A., Maloney, T., Alia-Klein, N., Woicik, P. A., Telang, F. et al. (2008b). Compromised sensitivity to monetary reward in current cocaine users: an ERP study. *Psychophysiology,* **45**(5), 705–713.

Goldstein, R.Z., Alia-Klein, N., Tomasi, D., Carrillo, J.H., Maloney, T., Woicik, P.A. et al. (2009a). Anterior cingulate cortex hypoactivations to an emotionally salient task in cocaine addiction. *Proc Natl Acad Sci USA,* **106**(23), 9453–58.

Goldstein, R.Z., Tomasi, D., Alia-Klein, N., Carrillo, J.H., Maloney, T., Woicik, P.A. et al. (2009b). Dopaminergic response to drug words in cocaine addiction. *Journal of Neuroscience,* **29**(18), 6001–6006.

Goldstein, R.Z., Craig, A.D., Bechara, A., Garavan, H., Childress, A.R., Paulus, M.P. et al. (in press). The neurocircuitry of impaired insight in drug addiction. *Trends Cogn Sci.*

Goldstein, R.Z., Woicik, P.A., Maloney, T., Tomasi, D., Alia-Klein, N., Shan, J. et al. (2010). Oral methyphenidate normalizes cingulate activity in cocaine addiction during a salient cognitive task. *National Academy of Science USA,* Sep 21; **107**(38), 16667–77 [Epub ahead of print].

Giffiths, R.R., Troisi, J.R., Silverman, K., and Mumford, G.K. (1993). Multiple-choice procedure: An efficient approach for investigating drug reinforcement in humans. *Behavioural Pharmacology,* **4**, 3–13.

Griffiths, R.R., Rush, C.R., and Puhala, K.A. (1996). Validation of the multiple-choice procedure for investigating drug reinforcement in humans. *Experimental and Clinical Psychopharmacology,* **4**, 97–106.

Grigson, P.S. and Twining, R. C. (2002). Cocaine-induced suppression of saccharin intake: a model of drug-induced devaluation of natural rewards. *Behav Neurosci,* **116**(2), 321–33.

Hajcak, G., Dunning, J.P., and Foti, D. (2007). Neural response to emotional pictures in unaffected by concurrent task difficulty: an event-related potential study. *Behavioral Neuroscience,* **121**(6), 1156–62.

Hariri, A.R., Brown, S.M., Williamson, D.E., Flory, J.D., de Wit, H., and Manuck, S.B. (2006). Preference for immediate over delayed rewards is associated with magnitude of ventral striatal activity. *J Neurosci,* **26**(51), 13213–13217.

Hart, C.L., Haney, M., Foltin, R.W., and Fischman, M.W. (2000). Alternative reinforcers differentially modify cocaine self-administration by humans. *Behavioural Pharmacology,* **11**(1), 87–91.

Heinz, A., Wrase, J., Kahnt, T., Beck, A., Bromand, Z., Grusser, S.M. et al. (2007). Brain activation elicited by affectively positive stimuli is associated with a lower risk of relapse in detoxified alcoholic subjects. *Alcohol Clin Exp Res,* **31**(7), 1138–47.

Hester, R. and Garavan, H. (2004). Executive dysfunction in cocaine addiction: evidence for discordant frontal, cingulate, and cerebellar activity. *J Neurosci,* **24**(49), 11017–22.

Hester, R., Dixon, V., and Garavan, H. (2006). A consistent attentional bias for drug-related material in active cocaine users across word and picture versions of the emotional Stroop task. *Drug and Alcohol Dependence,* **81**, 251–57.

Higgins, S.T., Heil, S.H., and Lussier, J.P. (2004). Clinical implications of reinforcement as a determinant of substance use disorders. *Annual Review of Psychology,* **55**, 431–61.

Hornak, J., O'Doherty, J., Bramham, J., Rolls, E.T., Morris, R.G., Bullock, P.R. et al. (2004). Reward-related reversal learning after surgical excisions in orbito-frontal or dorsolateral prefrontal cortex in humans. *J Cogn Neurosci,* **16**(3), 463–78.

Kirby, K.N. and Petry, N.M. (2004). Heroin and cocaine abusers have higher discount rates for delayed rewards than alcoholics or non-drug-using controls. *Addiction,* **99**(4), 461–71.

Knutson, B., Westdorp, A., Kaiser, E., and Hommer, D. (2000). FMRI visualization of brain activity during a monetary incentive delay task. *Neuroimage,* **12**(1), 20–27.

Knutson, B., Bjork, J.M., Fong, G.W., Hommer, D., Mattay, V.S., and Weinberger, D.R. (2004). Amphetamine modulates human incentive processing. *Neuron,* **43**(2), 261–69.

Knutson, B., Taylor, J., Kaufman, M., Peterson, R., and Glover, G. (2005). Distributed neural representation of expected value. *J Neurosci,* **25**(19), 4806–4812.

Koob, G.F. and Bloom, F.E. (1988). Cellular and molecular mechanisms of drug dependence. *Science,* **242**(4879), 715–23.

Koob, G.F., and Le Moal, M. (1997). Drug abuse: hedonic homeostatic dysregulation. *Science,* **278**(5335), 52–58.

Krebs, R., Schott, B.H., and Duzel, E. (2009). Personality traits are differentially associated with patterns of reward and novelty processing in the human substantia nigra/ventral tegmental area. *Biol Psychiatry,* **65**(2), 103–110.

Kringelbach, M.L., O'Doherty, J., Rolls, E.T., and Andrews, C. (2003). Activation of the human orbitofrontal cortex to a liquid food stimulus is correlated with its subjective pleasantness. *Cereb Cortex,* **13**(10), 1064–71.

Laruelle, M., Abi-Dargham, A., van Dyck, C.H., Rosenblatt, W., Zea-Ponce, Y., Zoghbi, S.S. et al. (1995). SPECT imaging of striatal dopamine release after amphetamine challenge. *J Nucl Med,* **36**(7), 1182–90.

Lasagna, L., Von Felsinger, J.M., and Beecher, H.K. (1955). Drug-induced mood changes in man. I. Observations on healthy subjects, chronically ill patients, and postaddicts. *J Am Med Assoc,* **157**(12), 1006–20.

Lee, J.L., Milton, A.L., and Everitt, B.J. (2006). Cue-induced cocaine seeking and relapse are reduced by disruption of drug memory reconsolidation. *J Neurosci,* **26**(22), 5881–87.

Lenoir, M., Serre, F., Cantin, L., and Ahmed, S.H. (2007). Intense sweetness surpasses cocaine reward. *PLoS ONE, Aug 1;* **2**(1), e698.

Leyton, M., Casey, K.F., Delaney, J.S., Kolivakis, T., and Benkelfat, C. (2005). Cocaine craving, euphoria, and self-administration: a preliminary study of the effect of catecholamine precursor depletion. *Behav Neurosci,* **119**(6), 1619–27.

Lubman, D.I., Allen, N.B., Peters, L.A., and Deakin, J.F. (2008). Electrophysiological evidence that drug cues have greater salience than other affective stimuli in opiate addiction. *J Psychopharmacol,* **22**(8), 836–42.

Lubman, D.I., Yucel, M., Kettle, J.W., Scaffidi, A., Mackenzie, T., Simmons, J.G. et al. (2009). Responsiveness to drug cues and natural rewards in opiate addiction: associations with later heroin use. *Arch Gen Psychiatry,* **66**(2), 205–212.

Margolin, A., Avants, S.K., and Kosten, T.R. (1994). Cue-elicited cocaine craving and autogenic relaxation: Association with treatment outcome. *J Subst Abuse Treat,* **11**(6), 549–52.

Martin-Soelch, C., Chevalley, A.F., Kunig, G., Missimer, J., Magyar, S., Mino, A. et al. (2001). Changes in reward-induced brain activation in opiate addicts. *Eur J Neurosci,* **14**(8), 1360–68.

Martin-Soelch, C., Missimer, J., Leenders, K.L., and Schultz, W. (2003). Neural activity related to the processing of increasing monetary reward in smokers and nonsmokers. *Eur J Neurosci,* **18**(3), 680–88.

Martinez, D., Narendran, R., Foltin, R.W., Slifstein, M., Hwang, D.R., Broft, A. et al. (2007). Amphetamine-induced dopamine release: markedly blunted in cocaine dependence and predictive of the choice to self-administer cocaine. *Am J Psychiatry,* **164**(4), 622–29.

Mattson, B.J., Williams, S., Rosenblatt, J.S., and Morrell, J.I. (2001). Comparison of two positive reinforcing stimuli: Pups and cocaine throughout the postpartum period. *Behavioral Neuroscience,* **115**(3), 683–94.

McCabe, J.A., Tobler, P.N., Schultz, W., Dickinson, A., Lupson, V., and Fletcher, P.C. (2009). Appetitive and aversive taste conditioning in a computer game influences real-world decision making and subsequent activation in insular cortex. *J Neurosci*, **29**(4), 1046–51.

McClure, S.M., Daw, N.D., and Montague, P.R. (2003). A computational substrate for incentive salience. *Trends Neurosci*, **26**(8), 423–28.

McClure, S.M., Laibson, D.I., Loewenstein, G., and Cohen, J.D. (2004a). Separate neural systems value immediate and delayed monetary rewards. *Science*, **306**(5695), 503–507.

McClure, S.M., York, M.K., and Montague, P.R. (2004b). The neural substrates of reward processing in humans: the modern role of FMRI. *Neuroscientist*, **10**(3), 260–68.

Miller, E.K. and Cohen, J.D. (2001). An integrative theory of prefrontal cortex function. *Annu Rev Neurosci*, **24**, 167–202.

Moeller, F.G., Hasan, K.M., Steinberg, J.L., Kramer, L.A., Dougherty, D.M., Santos, R.M. et al. (2005). Reduced anterior corpus callosum white matter integrity is related to increased impulsivity and reduced discriminability in cocaine-dependent subjects: diffusion tensor imaging. *Neuropsychopharmacology*, **30**(3), 610–617.

Moeller, S.J., Maloney, T., Parvaz, M.A., Dunning, J.P., Alia-Klein, N., Woicik, P.A. et al. (2009). Enhanced choice for viewing cocaine pictures in cocaine addiction. *Biol Psychiatry*, **66**(2), 169–76.

Mogg, K. and Bradley, B.P. (2002). Selective processing of smoking-related cues in smokers: Manipulation of deprivation level and comparison of three measures of processing bias. *Journal of Psychopharmacology*, **16**, 385–92.

Monterosso, J.R., Ainslie, G., Xu, J., Cordova, X., Domier, C.P., and London, E.D. (2007). Frontoparietal cortical activity of methamphetamine-dependent and comparison subjects performing a delay discounting task. *Hum Brain Mapp*, **28**(5), 383–93.

Nader, M.A. and Czoty, P.W. (2005). PET imaging of dopamine d2 receptors in monkey models of cocaine abuse: genetic predisposition versus environmental modulation. *American Journal of Psychiatry*, **162**(8), 1473–82.

Nader, M.A., Morgan, D., Gage, H.D., Nader, S.H., Calhoun, T.L., Buchheimer, N. et al. (2006). PET imaging of dopamine D2 receptors during chronic cocaine self-administration in monkeys. *Nature Neuroscience*, **9**(8), 1050–56.

Nocjar, C. and Panksepp, J. (2002). Chronic intermittent amphetamine pretreatment enhances future appetitive behavior for drug- and natural-reward: interaction with environmental variables. *Behav Brain Res*, **128**(2), 189–203.

O'Doherty, J., Kringelbach, M.L., Rolls, E.T., Hornak, J., and Andrews, C. (2001). Abstract reward and punishment representations in the human orbitofrontal cortex. *Nat Neurosci*, **4**(1), 95–102.

Pessiglione, M., Schmidt, L., Draganski, B., Kalisch, R., Lau, H., Dolan, R.J. et al. (2007). How the brain translates money into force: a neuroimaging study of subliminal motivation. *Science*, **316**(5826), 904–906.

Pontieri, F.E., Tanda, G., Orzi, F., and Di Chiara, G. (1996). Effects of nicotine on the nucleus accumbens and similarity to those of addictive drugs. *Nature*, **382**(6588), 255–57.

Pontieri, F.E., Passarelli, F., Calo, L., and Caronti, B. (1998). Functional correlates of nicotine administration: similarity with drugs of abuse. *J Mol Med*, **76**(3-4), 193–201.

Redish, A.D. (2004). Addiction as a computational process gone awry. *Science*, **306**(5703), 1944–7.

Reichel, C. M. and Bevins, R. A. (2008). Competition between the conditioned rewarding effects of cocaine and novelty. *Behavioral Neuroscience*, **122**(1), 140–50.

Robinson, T.E. and Berridge, K.C. (1993). The neural basis of drug craving: an incentive-sensitization theory of addiction. *Brain Res Brain Res Rev*, **18**(3), 247–91.

Robinson, T.E. and Berridge, K.C. (2001). Incentive-sensitization and addiction. *Addiction*, **96**(1), 103–114.

Robinson, T.E. and Berridge, K.C. (2003). Addiction. *Annu Rev Psychol*, **54**, 25–53.

Schmidt, L., d'Arc, B.F., Lafargue, G., Galanaud, D., Czernecki, V., Grabli, D. et al. Disconnecting force from money: effects of basal ganglia damage on incentive motivation. *Brain*, **131**, 1303–10.

Schott, B.H., Niehaus, L., Wittmann, B.C., Schutze, H., Seidenbecher, C.I., Heinze, H.J., and Duzel, E. (2007). Ageing and early-stage Parkinson's disease affect separable neural mechanisms of mesolimbic reward processing. *Brain*, **130**(Pt 9), 2412–24.

Schultz, W. (2006). Behavioral theories and the neurophysiology of reward. *Annual Review of Psychology*, **57**, 87–115.

Schultz, W., Tremblay, L., and Hollerman, J.R. (2000). Reward processing in primate orbitofrontal cortex and basal ganglia. *Cereb Cortex*, **10**(3), 272–84.

Sinha, R., Fuse, T., Aubin, L.R., and O'Malley, S.S. (2000). Psychological stress, drug-related cues and cocaine craving. *Psychopharmacology*, **152**(2), 140–48.

Sinha, R., Garcia, M., Paliwal, P., Kreek, M.J., and Rounsaville, B.J. (2006). Stress-induced cocaine craving and hypothalamic-pituitary-adrenal responses are predictive of cocaine relapse outcomes. *Archives of General Psychiatry*, **63**(3), 324–31.

Stairs, D.J., Klein, E.D., and Bardo, M.T. (2006). Effects of environmental enrichment on extinction and reinstatement of amphetamine self-administration and sucrose-maintained responding. *Behavioural Pharmacology*, **17**(7), 597–604.

Taylor, J.R. and Horger, B.A. (1999). Enhanced responding for conditioned reward produced by intra-accumbens amphetamine is potentiated after cocaine sensitization. *Psychopharmacology (Berl)*, **142**(1), 31–40.

Tellegen, A. and Waller, N.G. (1997). Exploring personality through test construction: development of the multidimensional personality questionnaire. In S.R. Briggs and J.M. Cheek (eds), *Personality measures: development and evaluation* (Vol. 1). Greenwich: JAI Press.

Tobler, P.N., Fiorillo, C.D., and Schultz, W. (2005). Adaptive coding of reward value by dopamine neurons. *Science*, **307**(5715), 1642–45.

Tremblay, L., and Schultz, W. (1999). Relative reward preference in primate orbitofrontal cortex. *Nature*, **398**(6729), 704–708.

Verdejo-Garcia, A., Bechara, A., Recknor, E.C., and Perez-Garcia, M. (2006). Executive dysfunction in substance dependent individuals during drug use and abstinence: An examination of the behavioral, cognitive, and emotional correlates of addiction. *Journal of the International Neuropsychological Society*, **12**, 405–415.

Volkow, N.D. and Fowler, J.S. (2000). Addiction, a disease of compulsion and drive: involvement of the orbitofrontal cortex. *Cereb Cortex*, **10**(3), 318–25.

Volkow, N.D., Fowler, J.S., Wolf, A.P., Schlyer, D., Shiue, C.Y., Alpert, R. et al. (1990). Effects of chronic cocaine abuse on postsynaptic dopamine receptors. *Am J Psychiatry*, **147**(6), 719–24.

Volkow, N.D., Fowler, J.S., Wang, G.J., Hitzemann, R., Logan, J., Schlyer, D.J. et al. (1993). Decreased dopamine D2 receptor availability is associated with reduced frontal metabolism in cocaine abusers. *Synapse*, **14**(2), 169–77.

Volkow, N.D., Wang, G.J., Fowler, J.S., Logan, J., Gatley, S.J., Hitzemann, R. et al. (1997a). Decreased striatal dopaminergic responsiveness in detoxified cocaine-dependent subjects. *Nature*, **386**(6627), 830–33.

Volkow, N.D., Wang, G.J., Fischman, M.W., Foltin, R. W., Fowler, J.S., Abumrad, N. N. et al. (1997b). Relationship between subjective effects of cocaine and dopamine transporter occupancy. *Nature*, **386**(6627), 827–30.

Volkow, N.D., Fowler, J.S., Wang, G.J., Ding, Y. S., and Gatley, S.J. (2002a). Role of dopamine in the therapeutic and reinforcing effects of methylphenidate in humans: results from imaging studies. *Eur Neuropsychopharmacol*, **12**(6), 557–66.

Volkow, N.D., Wang, G.J., Fowler, J.S., Logan, J., Jayne, M., Franceschi, D. et al. (2002b). "Nonhedonic" food motivation in humans involves dopamine in the dorsal striatum and methylphenidate amplifies this effect. *Synapse,* **44**(3), 175–80.

Volkow, N.D., Fowler, J.S., Wang, G.J., and Swanson, J.M. (2004a). Dopamine in drug abuse and addiction: results from imaging studies and treatment implications. *Mol Psychiatry,* **9**(6), 557–69.

Volkow, N.D., Wang, G.J., Fowler, J.S., Telang, F., Maynard, L., Logan, J. et al. (2004b). Evidence that methylphenidate enhances the saliency of a mathematical task by increasing dopamine in the human brain. *Am J Psychiatry,* **161**(7), 1173–80.

Volkow, N.D., Wang, G.J., Begleiter, H., Porjesz, B., Fowler, J.S., Telang, F. et al. (2006a). High levels of dopamine D2 receptors in unaffected members of alcoholic families: possible protective factors. *Arch Gen Psychiatry,* **63**(9), 999–1008.

Volkow, N.D., Wang, G.J., Telang, F., Fowler, J.S., Logan, J., Childress, A.R. et al. (2006b). Cocaine cues and dopamine in dorsal striatum: mechanism of craving in cocaine addiction. *J Neurosci,* **26**(24), 6583–88.

Von Felsinger, J.M., Lasagna, L., and Beecher, H.K. (1955). Drug-induced mood changes in man. *II. Personality and reactions to drugs. J Am Med Assoc,* **157**(13), 1113–1119.

Washton, A.M., and Stone-Washton, N. (1993). Outpatient treatment of cocaine and crack addiction: a clinical perspective. *NIDA Res Monogr,* **135**, 15–30.

Watanabe, M. (1989). The appropriateness of behavioral responses coded in post-trial activity of primate prefrontal units. *Neurosci Lett,* **101**(1), 113–117.

Wilson, S.J., Sayette, M.A., and Fiez, J.A. (2004). Prefrontal responses to drug cues: a neurocognitive analysis. *Nat Neurosci,* **7**(3), 211–214.

Winkielman, P., Berridge, K.C., and Wilbarger, J.L. (2005). Unconscious affective reactions to masked happy versus angry faces influence consumption behavior and judgments of value. *Pers Soc Psychol Bull,* **31**(1), 121–35.

Wise, R.A. (2005). Forebrain substrates of reward and motivation. *J Comp Neurol,* **493**(1), 115–21.

Woicik, P.A., Moeller, S.J., Alia-Klein, N., Maloney, T., Lukasik, T. M., Yeliosof, O. et al. (2008). The Neuropsychology of Cocaine Addiction: Recent Cocaine Use Masks Impairment. *Neuropsychopharmacology.*

Woolverton, W.L. and Anderson, K.G. (2006). Effects of delay to reinforcement on the choice between cocaine and food in rhesus monkeys. *Psychopharmacology,* **186**(1), 99–106.

Wrase, J., Schlagenhauf, F., Kienast, T., Wustenberg, T., Bermpohl, F., Kahnt, T. et al. (2007). Dysfunction of reward processing correlates with alcohol craving in detoxified alcoholics. *Neuroimage,* **35**(2), 787–94.

Wyvell, C.L. and Berridge, K.C. (2001). Incentive sensitization by previous amphetamine exposure: increased cue-triggered "wanting" for sucrose reward. *J Neurosci,* **21**(19), 7831–40.

Yeung, N. and Sanfey, A. G. (2004). Independent coding of reward magnitude and valence in the human brain. *J Neurosci,* **24**(28), 6258–64.

Zijlstra, F., Veltman, D.J., Booij, J., van den Brink, W., and Franken, I. H. (2009). Neurobiological substrates of cue-elicited craving and anhedonia in recently abstinent opioid-dependent males. *Drug Alcohol Depend,* **99**(1–3), 183–92.

Zombeck, J.A., Chen, G.-T., Johnson, Z.V., Rosenberg, D.M., Craig, A.B., and Rhodes, J.S. (2008). Neuroanatomical specificity of conditioned responses to cocaine versus food in mice. *Physiology and Behavior,* **93**(3), 637–50.

Chapter 22

The neuropsychology of stimulant and opiate dependence: neuroimaging and neuropsychological studies

Karen D. Ersche

Abstract

Chronic use of stimulants and/or opiates has been associated with a wide range of cognitive deficits, involving domains of attention, inhibitory control, planning, decision making, learning, and memory. Although both stimulant and opiate users show marked impairment in various aspects of cognitive function, the impairment profile is distinctly different according to the substance of abuse. This chapter aims to provide an in-depth overview of the neuropsychology of stimulant and opiate dependence as informed by findings of recent neuropsychological and neuroimaging studies.

22.1 Introduction

According to United Nations' estimates, approximately 200 million people worldwide were consuming illegal psychoactive substances at the beginning of the millennium (United Nations Office on Drugs and Crime, 2003a). Although not everybody who takes drugs shows addictive behavior, such as compulsive drug-seeking or loss of control over drug intake, the damaging effects of repeated drug use are undisputed (United Nations Office on Drugs and Crime, 2003b). Such harm includes acute and chronic health problems, caused directly by drug use or indirectly through drug-related accidents (WHO, 2004). Furthermore, there is growing evidence that chronic drug use is associated with impaired cognitive function (see for review: Rogers and Robbins, 2001, 2003; Verdejo-Garcia et al., 2004), which may contribute to negative long-term consequences observed in chronic drug users.

The impact of chronic drug-use on cognition has received relatively little attention until recently. Contemporary theories on the neuropathology of drug addiction have highlighted the involvement of cognitive functions, such as memory, learning, attention, and inhibitory control in the development of drug dependence (Volkow et al., 2003; 2004). Advances in the psychometric assessment of neuropsychological functions and computer-based applications of test batteries (e.g. the Cambridge Neuropsychological Test Automated Battery (CANTAB; http://www.cantab.com) have facilitated research into cognitive impairments associated with drug dependence, and allowed comparisons to be drawn with cognitive profiles observed in other clinical populations. The development of paradigms capable of being applied in both animals and in humans has opened up new avenues, as drug users' behavior, observed clinically, can be modeled in animals, and findings in animals experimentally treated with drugs could be directly tested in humans (Robbins et al., 1994). Neuroimaging research, such as functional magnetic resonance imaging (fMRI) and positron emission tomography (PET), have provided vital insight into the neural substrates and neurochemical processes subserving cognition and have shed light on disrupted neural networks in chronic drug users (London et al., 2000; Volkow et al., 2004)

Comparisons of the cognitive profile associated with psychostimulants and narcotics is particularly interesting with regard to the different pharmacological actions and the distinct mechanisms of positive and negative reinforcement implicated in the development of stimulant and opiate dependence. This chapter will provide a concise overview of the neuropathology associated with chronic use of stimulants, such as amphetamines and cocaine, and opiates, such as heroin and methadone, review the cognitive systems and their dysregulation by these substances.

22.2 The use and misuse of stimulants and opiates

Stimulants and opiates are amongst the most commonly abused substances worldwide (United Nations Office on Drugs and Crime, 2007) but their psychoactive effects are distinctly different. Stimulants, such as amphetamines, methamphetamine, cocaine, or crack, produce an intensive state of arousal, paired with heightened levels of confidence and feelings of euphoria. Stimulant drugs have long been used for medical purposes; for example, as antidepressants associated with medical illness, as appetite suppressants for obese patients, as stimulants to increase alertness in narcolepsy, and for the treatment of attention deficit hyperactivity disorder (ADHD). Besides medical purposes, stimulants have been generally used in a variety of situations to improve performance; for example, for pilots to remain alert, soldiers to increase energy during combat, students to improve concentration while taking exams or in sports competitions. However, the largest consumer group of stimulants is young people who take stimulants recreationally (European Monitoring Centre for Drugs and Drug Addiction, 2006, 2007). Although chronic drug users are quite a heterogeneous group, amphetamine users have a number of characteristics that make them distinct from opiate users; for example, they tend to be younger than opiate users (Darke et al., 1998), exhibit a wider range of polysubstance use (Darke and Hall, 1995), are highly socially orientated (Vincent et al., 1999), and are less likely than opiate users to enter treatment programmes (Klee, H. and Morris, J., 1994). However, the greatest challenge to treatment services and prevention strategies are cocaine users, as this drug user group appears to be even more heterogeneous and more hidden than other groups of drug users (European Monitoring Centre for Drugs and Drug Addiction, 2007).

For example, cocaine is used recreationally by socially well integrated young people for limited periods of time, it is regularly taken by opiate and alcohol users enrolled in drug treatment programs, and heavily consumed amongst marginalized groups who are not seen by drug-treatment services. Cocaine is mainly sold on the black market in the form of white, crystalline powder or as rocks of "crack" cocaine. Cocaine is often snorted or rubbed into gums and, in marginalized groups, cocaine is injected or smoked. Amphetamines are sold in the form of amphetamine sulfate powder or as a putty-like paste known as "base" and can be taken in a number of ways, which determine the onset and intensity of the psychoactive effects. Metylamphetamine (or more commonly referred to as "methamphetamine," "meth," "ice," or "crystal") is a potent derivative of amphetamine with a particularly high risk for developing dependence and a high potential for health-related harm (Meredith et al., 2005). This may explain why methamphetamine users enroll in drug treatment much sooner than cocaine users in terms of the time they first used the drug (Castro et al., 2000). The abuse of methamphetamine, compared with other drugs of abuse, is also characterized by associations with high-risk sexual behaviors and HIV infections (Chesney et al., 1998; Semple et al., 2004).

Substances derived from the opium poppy are opiates. Opiate-like drugs have calming, relaxing effects by relieving anxiety and producing strong feelings of well-being and pleasure. Opiates also have analgesic effects and, in clinical practice, opioids are prescribed for the relief of pain, as a cough suppressant, and in gastrointestinal problems as a relief from diarrhea. Opiates have also been widely used for recreational purposes for several thousand years (Brownstein, 1993). Heroin has long been regarded as the drug of choice of songwriters and poets (Rauch, 2000); it is processed from morphine, and is known under the chemical name diacetylmorphine. Heroin can be smoked with tobacco, heated on tin foil, snorted, or injected. Methadone is a synthetically produced drug with morphine-like properties that is licensed for detoxification or maintenance treatment in opiate-dependent individuals. Methadone is usually prescribed in the form of syrup and taken orally. Due to its longer half-life compared to morphine-based drugs, administration once a day is sufficient to prevent opiate withdrawal for 24 hours (Kreek, 2000).

According to the British Crime Survey 2008/9 (Hoare, 2009), one in three people aged between 16 to 59 years living in the U.K. admit to having taken illicit drugs in their lives (37% of the population of England and Wales). Approximately half of them used Class A drugs such as heroin and cocaine (16%). The relatively low percentage of regular heroin users is surprising in light of the high addictive liability of heroin, but the figures clearly show that not everybody who takes heroin recreationally becomes addicted to it. In fact, only a quarter of people who have ever used heroin become addicted (Anthony and Helzer, 1995); but unfortunately, many who are addicted to opiates, and in particular those who are enrolled in methadone maintenance treatment, are highly stigmatized by members of society (Hunt et al., 1985; Latowsky and Kallen, E., 1997; Murphy and Irwin, 1992). While chronic stimulant abuse is not gender specific (Substance Abuse and Mental Health Services Administration, 2002), chronic heroin use is dominated by the male gender

(~70% are men) (Gossop et al., 1994; Powis et al., 1996). Male heroin users are also more likely to shift from inhaling ("chasing the dragon") to injecting heroin (Strang et al., 1999), and to use more additional substances, in particular alcohol and cannabis, compared to female heroin users (Bretteville-Jensen, 1999). Furthermore, chronic opiate users tend to have poorer general health than amphetamine users, which is often directly or indirectly caused by chronic heroin use, predisposing to infectious diseases, kidney problems, pneumonia, abscesses, and poor vision (Gordon, 2001; Isralowitz et al., 2005). Opiates are involved in the majority of deaths associated with illicit substance-use in Europe, including deaths caused directly through overdose or indirectly from organ damage caused by chronic opiate-use (EMCDDA, 2003). Although heroin is used in all social classes, chronic use is associated with a decrease in social-economic standing, employment in full-time higher paid occupations, and poor quality of life and well-being (Gordon, 2001; Hartnoll, 1994).

22.3 Neuropathology associated with chronic stimulant and opiate use

As most addictive substances, stimulants, and opiates cause their reinforcing effects by increasing dopamine in the midbrain dopamine system (Carboni et al., 2001; Di Chiara and Imperato, 1988). However, the pharmacological action by which stimulants and opiates increased dopaminergic neurotransmission is distinctly different.

Stimulant drugs, such as amphetamine and cocaine, acutely enhance dopamine neurotransmission, either by blockade of its re-uptake or by directly releasing it from presynaptic sites (Johanson and Fischman, 1989; Seiden et al., 1993, for review). In addition to dopamine, amphetamine and cocaine also affect levels of other neurotransmitters and differ from each other in their affinity for the individual monoaminergic transporters. Thus, whilst amphetamine has the highest affinity for dopamine and noradrenaline transporters, cocaine binds most strongly to serotonin (5-HT) transporter (White and Kalivas, 1998). Opiates, by contrast, exert their action mainly through μ-opioid receptors, indirectly increasing dopamine but decreasing noradrenaline levels. Several lines of investigation have indicated a mediation effect of 5-HT in opiate reinforcement, but at present, the mechanism is still unclear (Tao and Auerbach, 2002a, 2002b). In view of the distinct pharmacological actions and reinforcement mechanisms implicated in stimulant and opiate use (Bardo, 1998, for review), it may seem obvious that the neuropathology in chronic users of these substances differs significantly.

Growing evidence suggests that chronic stimulant-abuse results in long-lasting changes in dopamine neurotransmission, a neurotransmitter system critically implicated in motor, reward, and cognitive functions, thereby contributing to a wide range of behavior patterns (Cools and Robbins, 2004; Nieoullon, 2002; Robbins, 2005). Converging evidence from animal and human research indicates marked dopaminergic dysfunction as reflected by down-regulation of dopamine D1 and D2 receptors, glucose metabolism (London et al., 2004; Volkow et al., 1993 2001c; Wang et al., 2004) and perfusion (see for review: Baicy and London, 2007; Li et al., 2005) in both chronic amphetamine and cocaine users.

Neuroimaging studies using structural MRI have provided further evidence that abnormalities associated with chronic stimulant exposure are not only functional but also of a morphological nature; and it seems that the structural abnormalities are relatively specific to the stimulant of abuse.

For example, chronic amphetamine-abuse has been associated with profound reductions in gray matter in the cingulate, limbic, and paralimbic cortices and the inferior frontal gyrus (Thompson et al., 2004), while the neuropathology in chronic cocaine users involves predominantly cortical areas (Franklin et al., 2002; Lim et al., 2002; Matochik et al., 2003; Moeller et al., 2005). Although the toxic effects of amphetamines in humans are still a matter of debate, drug-induced changes in the dopamine system may be dose-dependent (Sung et al., 2007) and long-lasting (Johanson et al., 2006; McCann et al., 1998; Sekine et al., 2001; Volkow et al., 2001b). Yet, there is converging evidence from studies investigating brain glucose metabolism, brain metabolites, and dopamine transporter density that suggests recovery from some of the drug-induced dopaminergic alterations following protracted abstinence in amphetamine users (proton MRS: Nordahl et al., 2005; PET dopamine-ligand: Volkow et al., 2001b; FDG-PET: Wang et al., 2004). Chronic cocaine-exposure has been associated with a variety of medical complications (Benowitz, 1993), but neurotoxic effects have not yet been identified (Seiden and Kleven, 1988).

For opiates, there is evidence for marked changes in the density of μ-opioid receptors throughout the brain (Kling et al., 2000; Melichar et al., 2005). Although methadone is used as a substitute for heroin for the treatment of opiate-dependent individuals, the long-lasting effects between these two opiates differ. Thus, methadone administered in a maintenance regimen results in an up-regulation of μ-opioid receptors, which persists even after detoxification from opiates (Daglish and Nutt, 2003); conversely postmortem analyses of chronic heroin users have shown a down-regulation of μ-opioid receptors (Gabilondo et al., 1994). Regarding monoamines neurotransmission, chronic opiate use has been associated with reduced densities in noradrenaline (α2) and dopamine (D2) receptors (Gabilondo et al., 1994; Wang et al., 1997), but no evidence for neurotoxic effects on dopamine neurons has been identified (Kish et al., 2001). In particular, the effects on the dopamine system overall in opiate users are less pronounced than in stimulant users (Kish et al., 2001). Functional and structural abnormalities in opiate users are less specific than those observed in amphetamine users (Danos et al., 1998a, 1998b; Gerra et al., 1998; Lyoo et al., 2006; Rose et al., 1996; Pezawas et al., 1998).

In summary, neuropathological changes associated with chronic use of psychostimulants have been well documented for the midbrain dopamine system and the ascending dopamingergic pathways. Accordingly, structural and functional anomalies in areas of dopamine pathways, the corticostriatal loops, have been identified in chronic amphetamine and cocaine users, as measured by neuroimaging techniques. In contrast to the extensive research in psychostimulant users, the neuropathological changes in opiate users have been far less investigated to date. There is, however, substantial evidence showing that chronic opiate-use is associated with marked changes in the opioid system, while the dopamine system seems to be less affected. Abnormalities in brain structure and function appear to be less pronounced and less specific than in psychostimulant users. In light of differences in pharmacological actions of stimulants and opiates, and in the neuropathology associated with chronic use of these substances, it may be anticipated that cognitive function would be more severely impaired in chronic users of amphetamines and cocaine compared to chronic users of opiates.

22.4 The profile of cognitive deficits associated with stimulant and opiate dependence

Executive functions represent high-level, dissociable cognitive abilities such as planning, working memory, attentional set-shifting, and inhibition of prepotent responses, which are necessary for goal-directed behavior (Baddeley, 1986; Burgess, 1997). Executive dysfunction has generally been linked with a frontal lobe pathology (see for review: Elliott, 2003; Robbins, 1996), including chronic substance abuse (Rogers and Robbins, 2001). In the following sections, impairments in selected executive and memory domains in chronic users of stimulants and opiates are discussed.

22.5 Cognitive flexibility

Cognitive flexibility has been defined as "the ability to shift avenues of thought and action in order to perceive, process and respond to situations in different ways" (Eslinger and Grattan, 1993). *Cognitive stability*, by contrast, describes the ability to maintain a cognitive set in the face of distractions. Both cognitive flexibility and stability are antagonistic demands of cognitive function, which are mediated by the balance between striatal and prefrontal dopamine levels (see Cools, 2008 for review). Converging evidence from experimental studies in humans and animals indicates that enhanced dopaminergic neurotransmission in the striatum facilitates the switching between cognitive sets, whereas stimulation of dopamine receptors in the prefrontal cortex has the opposite effect.

The Wisconsin Card Sorting Test (WCST) (Grant and Berg, 1948) and the Intra-Dimensional/Extra-Dimensional (ID/ED) set-shifting task of the CANTAB test battery (Downes et al., 1989; Rogers et al., 2000a) both shown in Fig. 22.1, have been widely used to assess cognitive flexibility in laboratory settings. The latter paradigm specifically measures the ability to shift away from a previously relevant stimulus dimension towards a newly relevant dimension (i.e., extra-dimensional (ED)-shift), which is formally akin to a category shift on the WCST and has been associated with dorsolateral prefrontal cortex function (Konishi et al., 1998a; Rogers et al., 2000a). The ID/ED task, in particular, has proven suitable for translational medicine approach (Birrell and Brown, 2000; Dias et al., 1997). Studies with current amphetamine/methamphetamine users have shown marginal to severe impairment on cognitive flexibility (Ersche et al., 2006a; Ornstein et al., 2000; Simon et al., 2000), although these deficits were not evident in abstinent amphetamine/ methamphetamine users (Hoffman et al., 2006; Johanson et al., 2006). Interestingly, there is some evidence indicating that impaired cognitive flexibility in methamphetamine users

Tasks of Attentional Set-Shifting

(a) Wisconsin Card Sorting Test

(b) CANTAB 2D IDED-Task

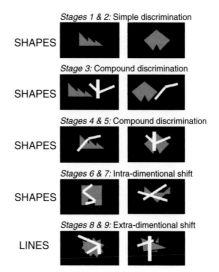

Fig. 22.1 (a) In the Wisconsin Card Sorting Test, participants are presented with a deck of cards showing stimuli that differ along the dimensions of color, shape, and number. Participants are asked to match each of the cards of the deck to one of the stimulus cards A–D displayed in front of them. Feedback informs the participant of the correctness of their choices. Successful matching requires the learning of a sorting rule and the adaptation of the matching strategy when the sorting rule changes. (b) In the CANTAB 2D-ID/ED task, participants are trained to discriminate stimuli that differ along the dimensions of shapes and lines. Feedback teaches the participant which stimulus is correct, and after six correct responses, the stimuli and/or rules are changed. Shapes remain the relevant dimension (i.e., shifts are intra-dimensional within the same dimension) until stage 8, when the new dimension, the white lines, become the relevant dimension (i.e., extra-dimensional shift).

is associated with male, but not female, users (Kim et al., 2005). This proposal finds support in research with healthy volunteers, showing that men release more dopamine in response to an amphetamine challenge than women (Munro et al., 2006). The implications of this gender difference in people who chronically use stimulant drugs are not yet fully understood (Dluzen and Liu, 2008). It is, however, conceivable that the enhanced response to stimulants in men makes them more susceptible than women to the neurotoxic effects of drugs such as methamphetamines (Dluzen et al., 2002; Myers et al., 2003).

Taken together, this may suggest that amphetamine exposure in male stimulant users acutely impairs the shifting of a mental set, while protracted abstinence from amphetamines may restore attentional set-shifting function. Compromised cognitive flexibility in abstinent methamphetamine users has been shown to be associated with decreased frontal white matter metabolism (Kim et al., 2005) and reduced grey matter density in the middle frontal cortex (Kim et al., 2006). The fact that task performance improves with protracted drug-abstinence (Kim et al., 2006), and may even reach normal levels (Hoffman et al., 2006; Johanson et al., 2006; Toomey et al., 2003), is interesting, given the relationship between performance and D2-receptor availability (Mehta et al., 1999, 2004; Volkow et al., 1998). One may speculate whether the improved task performance during protracted abstinence in amphetamine users is concomitant with recovery in dopamine transmission (Volkow et al., 2001b; Wang et al., 2004).

Cognitive flexibility in cocaine users has received much less attention, but the literature suggests an opposite profile of cognitive flexibility in cocaine users relative to amphetamine users. While current cocaine users do not show impairment in the WCST (Simon et al., 2002), performance is severely impaired during cocaine abstinence (Verdejo-Garcia et al., 2006). It is, however, important to bear in mind that more research is needed to support this proposal. In contrast to the findings in stimulant users, most studies in current and former opiate users did not identify impairments on cognitive flexibility, suggesting that chronic opiate consumption does not have an impact on attentional set-shifting (Ersche et al., 2006a; Pau et al., 2002; Rotheram-Fuller et al., 2004; Verdejo-Garcia et al., 2005). Given the pivotal role of dopamine in the modulation of cognitive flexibility, the observation that chronic opiate users are not measurably impaired in this domain reconciles well with the pharmacological profile of opiates, as they activate the dopamine system only indirectly.

The WCST and ID/ED tasks also assess the capacity to relearn a stimulus–reward association by inhibition of the previously reinforced dimension (i.e., reversal shift), which is subserved by orbitofrontal–striatal pathways (Dias et al., 1997; Rogers et al., 2000b). Deficits in response reversal are thought to reflect difficulties in adjusting one's actions according to changes in environmental contingencies (Rolls, 2000). In this regard it is important to note that current users of amphetamine, methamphetamine, or opiates were not measurably impaired on the reversal shift in the ID/ED task (Ersche et al., 2006a; Johanson et al., 2006; Ornstein et al., 2000).

The ability to adapt behavior to changing reward-contingencies is generally investigated with probabilistic response-reversal tasks (Cools et al., 2002; Hornak et al., 2004; Swainson et al., 2000), which involve the simultaneous presentation of two different stimuli. One stimulus is correct, and the other is wrong, which is indicated by positive and negative feedback, and participants are told to select the stimulus that is usually reinforced as being correct. Participants are also told that, at some time during the task, the other stimulus would become correct, and that when this happened, they should reverse their responses. In most cases, reversal tasks are of probabilistic nature, i.e., the computer provides false feedback on a minority of the trials (i.e., selecting the correct stimulus is then followed by false negative feedback). This has the advantage that participants' performance is attributable to the implementation of strategies rather than a reflection of motor disinhibition (Hornak et al., 2004).

In keeping with the unimpaired performance during reversal shifts on the WCST, amphetamine and opiate users showed no measurable impairments during probabilistic reversal-learning (Ersche et al., 2008). Chronic cocaine users, however, exhibited severe impairment in adjusting their responses to changes in reinforcement contingencies, as they continue to respond to the previously rewarded stimuli (Ersche et al., 2008; Fillmore and Rush, 2006). Importantly, this "sticky response" to the previously rewarded stimulus (response perseveration) was only seen in current users of cocaine, but not in the group of former drug users, suggesting that this impairment reflects a current effect of the drug. This perserverative pattern in responding seems similar to the reversal impairments observed in experimental monkeys following serotonin depletion in the prefrontal cortex (Clarke et al., 2004). It is thus conceivable that the pharmacological action of cocaine on the central serotonin system may account for cocaine users' inability to adjust their behavior during changing reinforcement-contingencies in the context of a probabilistic reversal-learning task.

It has to be acknowledged that some studies have reported increased perseverative responding on the WCST (i.e., responding to the previously correct stimulus dimension) in methadone-maintained opiate users (Darke et al., 2000; Lyvers and Yakimoff, 2003; Pirastu et al., 2006). However, response perseveration on the WCST has been associated with early methadone withdrawal (Lyvers and Yakimoff, 2003), co-morbid alcohol dependence, and previous heroin overdoses (Darke et al., 2000). In light of evidence indicating that the serotonin system is involved in opiate withdrawal (Akaoka and Aston-Jones, 1993), as well as in alcohol dependence (LeMarquand et al., 1994), it is likely that response preservation observed in opiate users is due to other factors and does not represent a characteristic behavioral correlate of opiate dependence. It is also of note that response reversal requires the inhibition of a previously rewarded response. Recent data indicates that the behavioral impairment profile on response inhibition tasks, such as the go/no-go task, is different in stimulant users than in opiate users, which will be explained in the next section.

In summary, accumulating evidence suggests that chronic abuse of amphetamines acutely impairs the shifting of a mental set, but performance seems to recover with protracted abstinence from amphetamines. The pharmacological actions of amphetamines on the dopamine system are likely to account for amphetamine users' impairment profile, and may explain why set shifting is not affected by chronic opiate abuse. The ability to reverse responding when reinforcement contingencies change seems to depend on serotonergic neurotransmission, and this ability is selectively impaired in chronic cocaine users.

22.6 Inhibitory control

A hallmark of drug dependence is the loss of control over substance intake, despite the negative consequences involved (American Psychiatric Association, 1994). Lack of inhibition has been regarded as a key element of drug addiction, including the suppression of emotional, cognitive, and behavioral responses (Goldstein and Volkow, 2002; Jentsch and Taylor, 1999). Inhibitory control can be investigated in the behavioral and cognitive domains.

22.6.1 Behavioral inhibition

Behavioral or motor response inhibition is defined as the process required to stop a planned movement (see Aron et al., 2004; Chamberlain and Sahakian, 2007) and is assessed using paradigms such as the go/no-go or stop/signal reaction time task (Dougherty

et al., 2003; Evenden et al., 2003). As shown in Fig. 22.2(a), in the go/no-go task, participants have to respond quickly to visual "go" cues but suppress the prepared response
whenever a "no-go" cue occurs on the computer screen. The index of behavioral inhibition is the number of false responses on "no-go" trials (i.e., commission errors), which
has been associated with activation in inferior frontal gyrus (Chikazoe et al., 2007; Konishi
et al., 1998b). Previous research suggests that cocaine users exhibit not only significant
inhibition failure by making more false responses on "no-go" trials than controls, but
also show significant inattention to "go" cues, as reflected in a higher rate of false misses
(i.e., omission errors) (Kaufman et al., 2003). Interestingly, attenuated error-related activation in the anterior cingulate cortex (ACC) was detected during go/no-go performance, suggesting disturbances in the processing of errors (Kaufman et al., 2003).
Alternatively, the attenuated error-related activation may also indicate that cocaine users
had difficulty differentiating target from non-target stimuli, since the ACC is thought to
play a key role in conflict and action monitoring (e.g. Carter et al., 1998; Gehring and
Knight, 2000). Remarkably, task-related activation in regions that have previously been
implicated in behavioral inhibition during go/no-go performance, such as the right inferior frontal gyrus, did not differ between cocaine users and controls. Thus, it is not clear
whether inhibition failure during go/no-go performance reflects attentional problems
and/or inefficient inhibitory control. Irrespective of the causes for the poor task performance, detailed analyses of cocaine users' performance suggest that they have little awareness of the errors they are making (Hester et al., 2007).

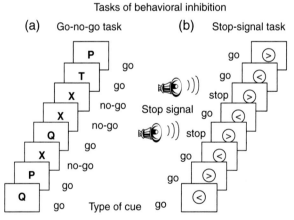

Fig. 22.2 (a) In the go/no-go task, participants are presented with a series of letters, and are
instructed to press a button as quickly and accurately as possible in response to any letter
presented except to the letter X. (b) In the stop/signal task, participants are presented with a
series of stimuli, and are instructed to press the button on the left of the response panel when
the arrow on the screen is pointing to the left, and to press the button on the right when the
arrow is pointing to the right. After a practice session of 16 "go" trials, participants are
instructed to withhold their responses when they hear a stop/signal (in 25% of trials a "beep"
sound—a 300-Hz tone).

Leland et al. (2008) have recently pointed out that successful inhibition of behavior in real life may not only depend on the ability to adequately control prepotent responses, but also on the capacity to timely detect situations that require response suppression. They used a cued "go/no-go" paradigm in abstinent methamphetamine users and healthy volunteers, which made it easier for participants to predict the occurrence of "no-go" trials. They found no behavioral differences in response inhibition performance between the two groups but significant group differences in the cue-related responses of the ACC. Methamphetamine users showed a direct relationship between cue-related activation in the ACC and improved response inhibition, a relationship that was not found in control volunteers. This finding is remarkable given that hypo-metabolism in the ACC in methamphetamine users has previously been linked with poor performance on a test of vigilance (London et al., 2005). It suggests that deficits in response inhibition are amenable to predictive signals that help methamphetamine users to prepare for the suppression of responses.

The stop/signal task, in contrast to the go/no-go task, does not involve switching between target and non-target stimuli but requires participants to respond quickly to "go" cues unless they hear a beep (in 25% of trials), which provides the signal to suppress this prepared motor response (see Fig. 2b). The stop/signal reaction time indexes the time that an individual needs to withhold the prepotent response, which is associated with the integrity of the right inferior frontal gyrus (Aron et al., 2004; Chamberlain and Sahakian, 2007; Rubia et al., 2003). Both methamphetamine and cocaine users have a significantly longer stopping process than controls, as reflected by a significantly longer stop/signal reaction time, indicating impairment in inhibitory control (Fillmore and Rush, 2002; Monterosso et al., 2005). It cannot be ruled out that poor inhibitory control might have predated drug-taking or even predisposed towards it (Nigg et al., 2004), but there are indications that exposure to stimulant drugs contributes to the behavioral disinhibited phenotype seen in chronic stimulant users. For example, prolonged stop/signal reaction time has shown to be associated with lifetime exposure to cocaine (Colzato et al. 2007) and with the previous amount of methamphetamine consumption (Monterosso et al., 2005). One may, therefore, speculate whether neuroadaptive changes underlie poor behavioral inhibition in chronic stimulant users. The neuropathology underlying behavioral disinhibition in stimulant users is currently not known. Functional and structural abnormalities have been identified in the prefrontal cortex in chronic users of methamphetamine (Thompson et al., 2004; Volkow et al., 2001a), which fuel speculation that disruptions in the neural network involving the inferior frontal gyrus may underlie the poor behavioral inhibitory control in chronic methamphetamine users (Monterosso et al., 2005). Functional neuroimaging research in cocaine users, however, suggests that hypo-function in ACC during stop/signal performance is not related to inhibitory control performance but rather with error monitoring and response regulation (Li et al., 2008).

In contrast to the accumulating evidence for response inhibition impairments in chronic psychostimulant users (e.g. Hester and Garavan, 2004; Hester et al., C. R., 2002; Kaufman et al., 2003; Monterosso et al., 2005), the majority of studies did not find behavioral inhibition deficits in opiate users (Fishbein et al., 2007; Forman et al., 2004; Lee et al., 2005; Verdejo-Garcia et al., 2007).

22.6.2 Cognitive inhibition

In the cognitive domain, inhibitory control is frequently assessed by the color-word Stroop test (Stroop, 1992), which requires participants to suppress a salient but conflicting stimulus property while identifying a less salient one (e.g. naming the word BLUE that is written in *red* ink requires more cognitive effort, so-called interference control, than naming the word BLUE when written in *blue* ink). Neuroimaging research has shown that the ACC is critically involved in the detection of the conflict between task-relevant and task-irrelevant stimulus properties during the color-word Stroop task (Bench et al., 1993; Leung et al., 2000; Pardo et al., 1990). Growing evidence indicates that cognitive control is compromised in both amphetamine (Salo et al., 2002, 2007, 2009; Simon, 2002) and opiate users (Brand et al., 2008; Fishbein et al., 2007; Mintzer and Stitzer, 2002; Prosser et al., 2006; Verdejo-Garcia et al., 2007). Poor interference control has been associated with decreased concentrations of N-acetylaspartate in the ACC in methamphetamine users (Salo et al., 2007; Taylor et al., 2004), which has been considered a marker of neuronal loss (Tsai and Coyle, 1995). This finding is in keeping with the structural and functional abnormalities in the ACC previously observed in methamphetamine users (Hwang et al., 2006; London et al., 2004, 2005; Nordahl et al., 2002; Thompson et al., 2004), elucidating the underpinnings of the impaired ability to effectively monitor situations of conflict in this drug user group (Salo et al., 2005). Some studies, however, did not find impaired interference control in recently abstinent methamphetamine users (Chang et al., 2002; Hoffman et al., 2006; Kalechstein et al., 2003), which may suggest partial recovery of brain function following abstinence from methamphetamine (Nordahl. et al., 2005; Wang et al., 2004).

Cognitive control using the color-word Stroop task has been widely used in cocaine-dependent individuals and, interestingly, the majority of these studies did not identify impairment in interference control in cocaine users (Bolla et al., 2004; Goldstein et al., 2001; Verdejo-Garcia and Perez-Garcia, 2007; Verdejo-Garcia et al., 2007; Woicik et al., 2008). Although task-related patterns of brain activation during Stroop performance revealed significant hypo-activation in the ACC in cocaine users, this was limited to the left hemisphere, while the right ACC was over-activated (Bolla, 2004). This pattern of brain activation suggests that cocaine users were able to use compensatory neural mechanisms to overcome deficient self-monitoring processes in the ACC during situations involving conflict. The mediating factors for successful functional compensation in cocaine users are not known. The observation that in cocaine, reduced N-acetylaspartate levels have mainly been reported in dorsolateral prefrontal cortex basal ganglia structures (Meyerhoff et al., 1999; Li et al., 1999), but not in ACC, may suggest differences in the neuropathology of ACC dysfunction between cocaine and amphetamine users.

Profound impairment in suppressing conflicting information on the standard color-word Stroop task has been identified in opiate users (Aragona and Carelli, 2006; Mintzer and Stitzer, 2002; Prosser et al., 2006; Verdejo-Garcia et al., 2007; Fishbein et al., 2007). The type of opiate used does not seem to influence performance on the Stoop task (Gruber et al., 2006; Verdejo-Garcia et al., 2005). Given the key role of the ACC in conflict monitoring, one may speculate that dysfunction in this area also accounts for the poor performance on the color-word Stroop test in opiate users. Indeed, there is now growing evidence suggesting that ACC function may be compromised in opiate users (Ersche et al., 2006; Forman et al., 2004; Lee. et al., 2005; Yucel et al., 2007). For example, opiate users showed attenuated error-related activation in the ACC during the go/no-go task (Forman et al., 2004) and lack a normal relationship between activation of the ACC and adaptive responding to negative feedback (Ersche et al., 2006), and to errors (Yucel et al., 2007). Reduced levels of the metabolite N-acetylaspartate have also been reported in chronic opiate users (Haselhorst et al., 2002; Yucel et al., 2007), but in contrast to meth-amphetamine users (Salo et al., 2007), these abnormalities were not associated with behavioral performance. At present, the nature of underlying biochemical abnormalities, such as the significant reductions in N-acetylaspartate in chronic drug-users, is still unclear. Given that the ACC has a high density of opioid receptors (see Vogt et al., 1995), and has been implicated in opioid analgesia (Casey et al., 2000; Petrovic et al., 2002), it seems conceivable that chronic exposure to opiate agonists, such as methadone and her-oin, modulates ACC function during cognitively challenging tasks, such as the Stroop task. Previous research has shown that task-related activation during the Stroop task overlaps with the neural network involved in processing of pain (Derbyshire et al., 1998) and opioid analgesia, respectively (Petrovic et al., 2002).

In summary, there is good clinical and experimental data in support of abnormal inhibitory control in individuals with stimulant and opiate dependence. However, rela-tively little is known about possible mechanisms of compensation that allow drug users to perform at a normal level under specific conditions.

22.7 **Sustained attention**

Sustained attention characterizes a state of "readiness to detect rarely and unpredictably occurring signals over prolonged periods of time" (Sarter et al., 2001) and has frequently been assessed by various versions of the continuous performance test (see Borgaro et al., 2003). In this test, participants are required to maintain vigilance and to react when target stimuli are presented but to avoid responding when distractors occur. Performance is usually assessed by the signal detection index (d'), which takes into account the number of missed targets and the number of false alarms. London et al. (2005) have recently shown that methamphetamine users made significantly more errors on an auditory ver-sion of the continuous performance test than non-drug-taking controls. Most impor-tantly, the authors found that d' was significantly smaller in methamphetamine users than in controls, providing evidence for impairments in methamphetamine users' ability to discriminate targets from non-targets. Poor test performance was further reflected in abnormal glucose metabolism in the ACC, insula, and orbitofrontal cortex at rest. Interestingly, compared with controls, glucose metabolism in the ACC was significantly reduced, and correlated negatively with the recent amount of methamphetamine used (London et al., 2004). Methamphetamine users with relatively elevated glucose metabolism at rest made significantly fewer errors during the task (London et al., 2005).

This may suggest that drug users with a smaller consumption of methamphetamine were able to compensate for an underlying neuropathology; a plausible proposal given that methamphetamine-induced neural damage in the frontal lobe, including the ACC, has shown to be dose-dependent (Oh et al., 2005; Sung et al., 2007). It is important to note that the aforementioned group differences on the continuous performance test only became apparent over a 30-min testing session (London et al., 2005) but not during a 15-min session (London et al., 2004), which suggests that methamphetamine users are, to some extent, able to compensate for the underlying neuropathology.

Although the length of the administered version of the continuous performance test is likely to determine the detection of deficits in sustained attention in stimulant users, the nature of the impairments identified is still unknown. It is important to acknowledge that not all studies find impairments in measures of signal detection (d') on the continuous performance test in stimulant users. For example, Levine et al. (2006) identified inattentiveness in stimulant users by increased numbers of omission errors and greater reaction time variability, although measures of discrimination targets and non-targets did not differ from controls. In light of the dose-dependent effects of methamphetamine in the ACC, one may speculate whether the type of stimulants used (i.e., amphetamine, methamphetamine, or cocaine) or the pattern of drug use (i.e., chronic or recreational use) might account for differences in performance profiles observed. Chronic cocaine use has also been associated with impairment in sustained attention (Gooding et al., 2008; Moeller et al., 2004, 2005), as reflected in lower d' and in an increased rate of commission errors. Poor attentional performance in cocaine users has been associated with widespread dysfunction in cortico-thalamic networks (Tomasi et al., 2007).

Although poor performance in the detection of targets has repeatedly been found in methadone-maintained opiate users (Forman et al., 2004; Mintzer and Stitzer, 2002), relatively little is known about the underlying neuropathology of these impairments in opiate users. Abnormalities in glucose metabolism and brain metabolites in the ACC of opiate users have been reported (Galynker et al., 2000; Yucel et al., 2007) and it is conceivable that opiate users need to compensate for ACC dysfunction in order to meet attentional demands. Functional MRI studies in opiate users have provided preliminary evidence for this assertion, as task-related under-activation of the ACC has been associated with deficits in the detection of targets (Forman et al., 2004). Normal task-related activation in the ACC, concomitant with additional recruitment of brain regions that are not typically activated by non-drug users, however, is associated with normal performance in opiate users (Yucel et al., 2007). Although attentional dysfunction has repeatedly been identified in laboratory settings (Forman et al., 2004; Mintzer and, 2002), driving ability (which requires sustained attention) is considered to be intact in chronic opiate users (Fishbain et al., 2003; Stout and Farrell, 2003). It may be that the compensatory recruitment of brain areas enables opiate users to drive safely without being involved in significantly more road accidents than non-drug users (see Fishbain et al., 2003). In summary, more research is needed to better understand the engagement of neural networks during forms of attentional processing in opiate-dependent individuals.

In summary, the ability to sustain attention to a task over a period of time is significantly impaired in both stimulant and opiate users. Hypo-activation in neural circuits involving the ACC have been associated with poor attentional functions in substance dependent individuals.

22.8 Strategic planning

The ability to "think ahead" and actively search for an appropriate solution is an essential part of goal-directed behavior, and is required in many daily activities (Owen, 1997). The Tower of London test (Owen et al., 1990; Shallice, 1982), or the more difficult version, the one-touch Tower of London (Owen et al., 1995), are widely used means to assess strategic planning in laboratory settings. Multiple lines of evidence indicate that planning performance on the Tower of London is subserved by a neural network, including the dorsolateral prefrontal cortex (Baker et al., 1996; Dagher et al., 2001; Manes et al., 2002). Both amphetamine and opiate users, regardless of current drug status, solved significantly fewer problems correctly on the one-touch Tower of London, and therefore needed more attempts in order to generate correct answers, compared to controls (Ersche et al., 2006a; Ornstein et al., 2000). This behavioral deficit occurred in the absence of latency differences between the groups and, as such, was not secondary to motor impulsivity (Ersche et al., 2006a). Whilst amphetamine and opiate users were equally impaired on planning problems of medium and high levels of difficulty, amphetamine users also struggled with generating solutions for the relatively easy three-move problems (Ersche et al., 2006a). The first stages of the Tower of London (i.e., one to three-move problems) require relatively little planning ability, as they can easily be solved by a visual matching-to-sample strategy (Owen, 1997). In light of accumulating evidence showing that basic visuo-spatial function, as assessed by the Rey–Osterrieth complex figure test (see Stern et al., 1994), is not impaired in amphetamine users (Chang et al., 2005; Hoffman et al., 2006; Kalechstein et al., 2003; Toomey et al., 2003), it is conceivable that the poor performance of amphetamine users at this low level of difficulty may reflect either an overconfident approach towards the solution or an inefficiency in concentrating on the task demands. High-level cognitive planning, as assessed on the Tower of London by planning problems requiring mental organization of four to six-sequences of moves, overlaps with different aspects of working memory (Owen, 1997; Robbins et al., 1998). Therefore, it may not be surprising that amphetamine and opiate users have also shown poor performance on tasks requiring complex spatial working memory function and visuo-spatial strategy generation (Ornstein et al., 2000). The marked impairment in solving planning problems on the Tower of London exemplifies the difficulty of drug users to mentally organize behavior to achieve a goal through a series of intermediate steps.

The fact that planning impairment was not only observed in current users of amphetamine and opiates, but also in a group of former drug users who had been drug abstinent for an average of eight years, may indicate that impairments do not simply reflect the current effect of the drug. Longitudinal studies are needed to settle the question whether neurocognitive impairment was caused by chronic drug exposure or predated drug-taking, or even represents a combination of both. Lack of planning and forethought has also been considered being a component of impulsive behavior (Dickman, 1990; Evenden, 1999). As a personality trait, non-planning is assessed by subscale of the Barratt Impulsiveness Scale (BIS-11) (Patton et al., 1995). Both chronic amphetamine users and opiate users not only report higher overall levels of impulsivity compared with non-drug using controls, they also score higher on the non-planning subscale of BIS-11 (Clark et al., 2006). In light of the poor performance during strategic planning, one may speculate whether this impairment may contribute to the impulsive behavior pattern frequently reported by chronic drug-users.

In summary, planning and strategic thinking require the integrity of prefrontal networks, and significant impairments in these abilities have been observed in chronic opiate-users, and to an even greater degree in chronic amphetamine users.

22.9 Decision making

The ability to make decisions is a key element in human behavior because the way people behave socially, financially, ecologically, and politically largely depends on this ability (Hastie, 2001; Mellers et al., 1998). Because decisions are usually made with a view to a favorable outcome, rewards provide the motivation to make decisions. Cognition is necessary to appraise the options and alternatives, assessing the means to achieve them, and evaluate the consequences involved with each choice (Ernst and Paulus, 2005; Hastie, 2001).

Neuropsychological studies have been investigating decision-making abilities in chronic drug-users with different experimental paradigms, providing evidence that decision-making performance differs between the type of substance used. For example, the Iowa Gambling Task (IGT) (Bechara et al., 1997), shown in Fig. 22.3(b), requires a series of card selections to be made concerning winning and losing monetary rewards. Optimal performance requires switching from selecting cards from high-gain/high-loss decks to low-gain/low-loss but more profitable decks. The main measure is the *net score*, which is calculated from the total number of cards selected from the two advantageous decks, minus the two disadvantageous decks, reflecting the decision-making strategy across the task. There are inconsistencies in drug users' decision-making strategies on the IGT across studies, and not all report the net score. Amongst those studies that report the net score, some did not find a measurable decision-making impairment in psychostimulant, opiate, and polydrug users (Adinoff et al., 2003; Bollaet al., 2003; Ernst, 2003; Mintzer and Stitzer, 2002; Mintzer et al., 2005), whereas others found significantly smaller but positive net scores in these groups of drug users compared with controls (Bechara et al., 2001; Grant, 2000; Pirastu et al., 2006), reflecting a disadvantageous decision-making strategy. It seems that only subgroups of polydrug users (Bechara et al., 2002) and subgroups of opiate users (Pirastu et al., 2006; Rotheram-Fuller et al., 2004) have negative net scores, indicating that these drug users preferably chose cards from the "risky decks." Negative net scores have also been identified in other clinical groups; for example, in suicide attempters, independently from their drug-using habits (Jollant, 2005), and in psychopathic individuals (Mitchell et al., 2002; van Honk et al., 2002). Interestingly, Vassileva et al. (2007) have recently shown significant differences in decision-making strategies between psychopathic and non-psychopathic opiate users. Whilst the psychopathic opiate users consistently selected cards from risky decks, the non-psychopathic opiate users successfully adjusted their decision-making strategy in the course of the task towards the advantageous decks. This selection strategy suggests difficulties in learning reward-contingencies, which at the beginning of the task had resulted in risky decisions. Taken together, accumulating evidence indicates that drug abuse per se does not mediate decision making on the IGT but it may act as a moderator, aggravating existing decision-making impairments.

One major drawback of the IGT is that volunteers need to learn reward–punishment associations over the course of the task, which means that individuals who are poor learners may develop a less successful decision-making strategy than good learners (Clark and Robbins, 2002). Consequently, the Cambridge Gamble Task (CGT) (Rogers et al., 1999a) and the Risk Task (Rogers et al., 1999b) have been developed to investigate

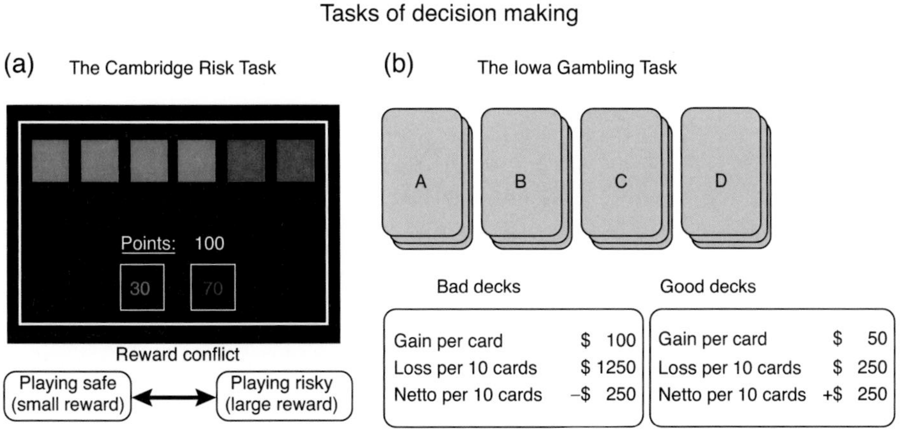

Tasks of decision making

Fig. 22.3 (a) The Risk Task requires participants to choose between two mutually exclusive options with different probabilities of reward and punishment. On each trial, an array of six boxes was presented on the screen, with a ratio of red and blue boxes that varied from trial to trial (5:1, 4:2, 3:3 boxes). Participants are told that the computer had hidden a yellow token, at random, behind one of the six boxes and they need to decide whether the token is hidden behind a red or blue box. Their decision on each trial is shaped by a fixed bet, associated with each alternative, regarding the magnitude of potential gain or loss (90:10, 80:20, 70:30; 60:40, 50:50 points). Feedback is provided by the way of gain or loss of points following each trial. Since the least likely option is always associated with the large reward value, participants are facing a reward–conflict situation. (b) In the Iowa Gambling Task, participants are presented with four card decks and asked to make series of card selections concerning winning and losing monetary rewards. Participants are not told that there are "safe" and "risky" decks. Over the course of the task, participants generally develop a preference for the "safe" decks (C and D) over the "risky" decks (A and B). The net score, which is calculated from the total number of cards selected from "safe" minus "risky" decks, reflects the decision-making strategy across the task.

decision making independently from learning. In the CGT, participants make choices between two mutually exclusive options and place bets on the expected outcome. Learning on the CGT is obviated by providing information about outcome probabilities and reward values on the screen, and by the fact that each trial is independent from its predecessor. The risk task is a variant of the CGT, which investigates decision making in a reward–conflict situation (see Fig. 22.3a). Research findings regarding decision making in chronic drug users, using either the CGT or the Risk Task, are strikingly similar to findings on the IGT. Chronic amphetamine users, but not opiate users, showed disadvantageous decision making (Rogers et al., 1999a). Amphetamine users overall selected the likely small reward option less frequently (i.e., in only 85% of trials) than opiate users (92%) and controls (95%), but showed no signs of impaired risk adjustment (Rogers et al., 1999a). In other words, although amphetamine users chose disadvantageously, they neither increased their gambles on the less favorable options nor did they significantly choose against the odds on the risky conditions. Disadvantageous decision-making strategy in amphetamine users on the CGT and risk task appears to be due to impairment in correctly estimating outcome probabilities and may not reflect a reward-seeking strategy per se. This proposal finds support from neuroimaging research, showing that methamphetamine users were not different regarding the sensitivity to positive or negative feedback, but showed disruptions in the neural network implicated in processing of feedback information, on the basis of which outcome probabilities were estimated (Paulus et al., 2002, 2003). Disadvantageous choices, particularly in amphetamine users, were also evident on the risk task (Ersche et al., 2005a). For example, in a neuroimaging study, amphetamine users selected the most favorable option in 72% of trials (opiate: 82%, and ex-drug: 79%, controls: 87%) (Ersche et al., 2005a). Although this difference was not statistically significant, the neuroimaging data revealed significant disturbance in the mediation of decision making by the prefrontal cortex in all three drug user groups. Chronic amphetamines or opiates users, regardless of whether they were currently using drugs, showed over-activation in the orbitofrontal cortex and under-activation in the dorsolateral prefrontal cortex. These findings are consistent with other neuroimaging studies in drug users (e.g. Bolla et al., 2003), showing abnormal brain activation during decision making, even before impairment becomes behaviorally measurable.

At present, the nature of impaired decision making in drug users is still unclear. There is some evidence that working-memory deficits adversely affect performance on the IGT (Bechara and Martin, 2004). Sub-optimal choices on the CGT and Risk Task, have been linked with the duration of amphetamine use (Rogers et al., 1999a) and the previous amount of daily cocaine use (Monterosso et al., 2001), which might indicate an adverse effect of chronic stimulant-use on probability estimations. Risky choices on the risk task have been associated with low intelligence in polydrug users (Fishbein et al., 2005), while risky reward-seeking on the IGT has been related to abnormalities in anticipatory skin conductance responses, prior to card selections from the "risky" decks (Bechara et al., 1997). Polydrug users who showed risky card selections on a discounting version of the

IGT had abnormal anticipatory skin conductance responses, reflecting a hypersensitivity to reward and a hyposensitivity to punishment (Bechara et al., 2002). This pattern of abnormal skin conductance responses has been interpreted as an inability to utilize ongoing feedback in guiding future decisions (Bechara et al., 2002).

Leland and Paulus (2005) investigated risky decision making in young people who had experiences with illicit stimulants. Volunteers had to quickly decide whether to accept a small but safe bet or to wait in prospect of a larger reward or penalty. Risky choices in young people, regardless of whether they were consuming stimulants, were associated with personality traits of sensation-seeking and motor impulsivity. They further found that, although young people with a history of stimulant use made riskier choices throughout the task than their drug-naïve counterparts, they showed normal responses to negative feedback (Leland and Paulus, 2005). The authors suggested that the increased risk-taking behavior in young stimulant users reflects a hypersensitivity to reward but normal sensitivity to punishment. This decision-making strategy stands in sharp contrast to the risky decision making observed in methadone-maintained opiate users. Although the overall decision-making performance in opiate users was not measurably impaired (Brand et al., 2008; Ersche et al., 2005a, 2005b; Rogers et al., 1999a), methadone-maintained opiate users were significantly more likely to make risky decisions when they had been unsuccessful on the previous trial (Ersche et al., 2005b). In other words, only those opiate users who were maintained on methadone were less inclined to "play safe" when they had lost on the previous trial; street heroin users, amphetamine users, and former drug users all showed normal responses to punishing feedback. Since the two opiate groups were matched on other descriptive variables collected, one possible explanation of this finding may be the type of the opiate used. Several possible explanations for the abnormal responses of methadone users have been proposed, including a down-regulation of noradrenaline, altering the perception of risk and a dysregulation in processing of punishment (Ersche et al., 2005b). Nevertheless, further research is warranted to elucidate the adverse influence of methadone on feedback processing. Recently, Brand et al. (2008) investigated behavioral adjustment following unfavorable, risky choices in a mixed group of abstinent and current opiate users, and also found that opiate users made insufficient use of feedback information to guide their ongoing behavior.

In summary, accumulating evidence has shown that chronic consumption of amphetamines and opiates is associated with difficulties in making decisions, which can involve negative consequences. Neuroimaging studies have provided strong evidence for neural network disruptions during decision making, even in the absence of detectable behavioral impairments on some paradigms (e.g., Bolla et al., 2003; Ersche et al., 2005a, 2006; Paulus et al., 2005). The quality of decision making in chronic amphetamine and opiate users may depend upon the cognitive demands that the decisional strategy requires. Cognitive deficits that adversely affect decisional choices have been shown to be associated with chronic amphetamine and opiate use, such as impaired learning of stimulus–reward associations, probability judgments, reflection, and feedback processing.

There are a variety of moderator variables, such as young age (Deakin et al., 2004), low intelligence quotient (Fishbein et al., 2005), affective instability (Jollant et al., 2005, 2007), low levels of cortisol (van Honk et al., 2003), or sensation-seeking (Leland and Paulus, 2005), which may exacerbate decision-making problems in individuals with substance use disorders.

22.10 Memory and learning

A substantial body of evidence has shown a wide range of learning and memory impairments in chronic amphetamine, methamphetamine, and cocaine users (Ersche et al., 2006a; Gonzalez et al., 2004; Hoffman et al., 2006; Kalechstein et al., 2003; Moon et al., 2007; Ornstein et al., 2000; Rippeth et al., 2004; Simon et al., 2002; Woods et al., 2005; Jovanovski et al., 2005; Simon et al., 2002; Ardila et al., S., 1991; Rosselli and Ardila, 1996; Scott et al., 2007). Memory impairment in chronic amphetamine users is related to self-reported severity of drug use (McKetin and Mattick, 1998) and correlate with the availability of dopamine transporters in the striatum (Volkow et al., 2001d). In cocaine users, verbal memory performance seems to be particularly impaired during early cocaine withdrawal (Kelley et al., 2005), and in amphetamine users, verbal memory improves following protracted drug abstinence (Wang et al., 2004). Woods et al. (2005) have shown that memory impairment in methamphetamine users is not necessarily due to mnemonic dysfunction but may result from inefficient strategies in encoding, organizing, and retrieving information. In contrast to the profound deficits in declarative memory, stimulant users seem to do better at tasks involving procedural learning and memory (Toomey et al., 2003; Van Gorp et al., 1999)

Impairment in memory function associated with chronic opiate users is less consistent in the literature, while a number of studies identified various aspects of memory impairment, such as word/pattern recognition, learning and recall of words/figures, episodic memory, paired associate learning, and retrieval (Amir and Bahri, 1994; Darke et al., 2000; Ersche et al., 2006a; Guerra et al., 1987; Ornstein et al., 2000; Papageorgiou et al., 2004; Pirastu et al., 2006; Prosser et al., 2006; Fishbein et al., 2007), others do not find memory deficits in opiate users (Davis et al., 2002, 2005; Papageorgiou et al., 2001; Rapeli et al., 2006; Rounsaville et al., 1982). The reasons for these inconsistencies are less clear but may be related to clinical differences between the samples, recentness of opiate use, or test sensitivity. Although most studies do not find associations with the amount of opiates consumed or the duration of use (Darke et al., 2000; Ersche et al., 2006a; Prosser, 2006; Rounsaville et al., 1982; Verdejo-Garcia et al., 2005), there is some evidence that methadone impairs episodic memory in a dose-dependent manner (Curran et al., 2001). For example, methadone-maintained opiate users showed significantly better episodic memory recall when they received placebo instead of their usual methadone treatment (Curran et al., 2001). It is not clear if the impairments were specific for methadone or reflect opiate-related impairment in general. By contrast, improved memory function has been reported in a within-subject comparison following two months of enrollment in methadone-maintenance treatment (Gruber et al., 2006). However, further validation would be welcome because this study lacked a placebo condition and did not control for potential practice effects.

22.11 General comments

Over recent years, neuropsychology has provided new insights into the neural basis of cognitive and behavioral problems associated with chronic drug use, including psychostimulants and opiates. Chronic abuse of these substances is associated with a wide range of cognitive deficits, including the domains of attention, inhibitory control, planning, decision making, learning, and memory, as summarized in Table 22.1. Although both stimulant and opiate users show marked impairment in various aspects of cognitive function, substance-specific differences are most pronounced in functions of inhibitory control and feedback processing. For example, while amphetamine users demonstrate profound deficits in suppressing planned actions (behavioral inhibition) and thoughts (cognitive inhibition), impairment in inhibitory control in opiate users appears to be limited to the cognitive domain. Cocaine dependence, however, seems to be associated with impairments in error monitoring and self-regulation; and, depending on the complexity of the situation, these deficits may lead to failure in inhibitory control. Chronic use of amphetamines has also shown to be associated with disturbances in the neural network implicated in feedback processing, which may cause difficulties predicting outcome probabilities. In opiate users, by contrast, the impairment in the processing of feedback seems to be specific to feedback of negative valence, such as errors and punishment. Compromised cognitive function in both substance user populations is reflected in abnormal patterns of brain activation, both at rest and during cognitive performance. Although this review did not discuss gender differences, there is accumulating evidence indicative of differences in brain structure and function between male and female stimulant users (Chang et al., 2005; Ersche et al., 2006a; Kim et al., 2005; Stout et al., 2005). Gender differences in brain function in chronic opiate users have received much less attention in research.

Despite the increasing knowledge of cognitive dysfunction in this population, cognitive abilities of drug users still play a peripheral role in clinical practice. Accumulating evidence has documented the moderating role of cognitive function on treatment retention and treatment efficacy, such that drug users with cognitive impairments are more likely to drop out of treatment and show less engagement in the treatment process (Aharonovich et al., 2003, 2006; Fals-Stewart and Lucente, 1994; Fals-Stewart and Schafer, 1992; Katz et al., 2005; Morgenstern and Bates, 1999; Teichner et al., 2002). In light of the growing need for improving treatment efficacy, in particular for psychostimulant users (de Lima et al., 2002; Shearer, James, 2007), addressing cognitive deficits within treatment settings may prove beneficial in many regards. For example, standardized cognitive status examination on admission would help to identify the individual's strengths and impairments, and provide valuable information for clinical decision making. Adjusting interventions to the cognitive abilities of drug users may not only be beneficial for the achievement of treatment goals, but could also improve communication and relationships between drug users and staff (Weinstein and Shaffer, 1993). Finally, improvement in cognitive function

Table 22.1 Overview of cognitive performance profiles associated with stimulant and opiate dependence, as reviewed in this chapter

Domains	Key Measures	Cognitive Profile		
		Methamphetamine Amphetamine	Cocaine Crack-cocaine	Methadone Heroin
Cognitive flexibility	set-shifting	✗✓	✗✓	✓
	response reversal	✓	✗	✓
Response inhibition	commission errors	✗	✗	✗✓
	interference control	✗	✓	✗
Sustained attention	discrimination index (d')	✗	✗	✗
Mental planning	strategic thinking	✗	—	✗
Decision making	probability discounting	✗	—	✓
	negative feedback	✓	—	✗
Memory	episodic memory	✗	✗	✗
	visuo-spatial memory	✗	✗	✗
	working memory	✗	✗	✗

✓unimpaired performance.
✗impaired performance.
✗✓inconsistent findings.
— not reported.

through neurocognitive training and remediation, as part of drug rehabilitation, may enhance treatment outcome in the long-term. The translation of neuropsychological knowledge into clinical practice will ideally become increasingly apparent in the coming years. Furthermore, understanding the neurobiological substrates underlying cognitive impairment in drug users may have the potential to guide therapeutic intervention in the future.

References

Adinoff, B., Devous, M. D., Cooper, D. B., Best, S. E., Chandler, P., Harris, T. et al. (2003). Resting regional cerebral blood flow and gambling task performance in cocaine-dependent subjects and healthy comparison subjects. *American Journal of Psychiatry*, 160, 1892–4.

Aharonovich, E., Nunes, E., and Hasin, D. (2003). Cognitive impairment, retention and abstinence among cocaine abusers in cognitive-behavioral treatment. *Drug and Alcohol Dependence*, 71, 207–11.

Aharonovich, E., Hasin, D. S., Brooks, A. C., Liu, X., Bisaga, A., and Nunes, E. V. (2006). Cognitive deficits predict low treatment retention in cocaine dependent patients. *Drug and Alcohol Dependence*, 81, 313–22.

Akaoka, H. and Aston-Jones, G. (1993). Indirect serotonergic agonists attenuate neuronal opiate withdrawal. *Neuroscience*, 54, 561–5.

American Psychiatric Association (1994). *Diagnostic and statistical manual of mental disorders*, 4th edn. Washington, DC, American Psychiatric Association.

Amir, T. and Bahri, T. (1994). Effect of substance-abuse on visuographic function. *Perceptual and Motor Skills,* **78,** 235–41.

Anthony, J. C. and Helzer, J. E. (1995). Epidemiology of drug independence. In M.T. Tsuang, M. Tohen, and G. E. Zahner (eds), *Textbook in psychiatric epidemiology* (pp. 361–406). New York: John Wiley and Sons Inc.

Aragona, B. J. and Carelli, R. M. (2006). Dynamic neuroplasticity and the automation of motivated behavior. *Learning and Memory,* **13,** 558–59.

Ardila, A., Rosselli, M., and Strumwasser, S. (1991). Neuropsychological deficits in chronic cocaine abusers. *International Journal of Neuroscience,* **57,** 73–9.

Aron, A. R., Robbins, T. W., and Poldrack, R. A. (2004). Inhibition and the right inferior frontal cortex. *Trends in Cognitive Sciences,* **8,** 170–7.

Baddeley, A. (1986). *Working Memory.* Oxford, UK: Clarendon Press.

Baicy, K. and London, E. D. (2007). Corticolimbic dysregulation and chronic methamphetamine abuse. *Addiction,* **102,** 5–15.

Baker, S. C., Rogers, R. D., Owen, A. M., Frith, C. D., Dolan, R. J., Frackowiak, R. S. J., and Robbins, T. W. (1996). Neural systems engaged by planning: a PET study of the Tower of London task. *Neuropsychologia,* **34,** 515–26.

Bardo, M. T. (1998). Neuropharmacological mechanisms of drug reward: beyond dopamine in the nucleus accumbens. *Critical Reviews in Neurobiology,* **12,** 37–67.

Bechara, A. and Martin, E. M. (2004). Impaired decision making related to working memory deficits in individuals with substance addictions. *Neuropsychology,* **18,** 152–62.

Bechara, A., Damasio, H., Tranel, D., and Damasio, A. R. (1997). Deciding advantageously before knowing the advantageous strategy. *Science,* **275,** 1293–5.

Bechara, A., Dolan, S., Denburg, N., Hindes, A., Anderson, S. W., and Nathan, P. E. (2001). Decision-making deficits, linked to a dysfunctional ventromedial prefrontal cortex, revealed in alcohol and stimulant abusers. *Neuropsychologia,* **39,** 376–89.

Bechara, A., Dolan, S., and Hindes, A. (2002). Decision-making and addiction (part II): myopia for the future or hypersensitivity to reward? *Neuropsychologia,* **40,** 1690–705.

Bench, C. J., Frith, C. D., Grasby, P. M., Friston, K. J., Paulesu, E., Frackowiak, R. S. J., and Dolan, R. J. (1993). Investigations of the functional anatomy of attention using the stroop test. *Neuropsychologia,* **31,** 907–22.

Benowitz, N. L. (1993). Clinical-pharmacology and toxicology of cocaine. *Pharmacology and Toxicology,* **72,** 3–12.

Birrell, J. M. and Brown, V. J. (2000). Medial frontal cortex mediates perceptual attentional set shifting in the rat. *Journal of Neuroscience,* **20,** 4320–24.

Bolla, K. I., Eldreth, D. A., London, E. D., Kiehl, K. A., Mouratidis, M., Contoreggi, C. et al. (2003). Orbitofrontal cortex dysfunction in abstinent cocaine abusers performing a decision-making task. *Neuroimage,* **19,** 1085–94.

Bolla, K., Ernst, M., Kiehl, K., Mouratidis, M., Eldreth, D., Contoreggi, C. et al. (2004). Prefrontal cortical dysfunction in abstinent cocaine abusers. *Journal of Neuropsychiatry,* **16,** 456–64.

Borgaro, S., Pogge, D. L., Deluca, V. A., Bilginer, L., Stokes, J., and Harvey, P. D. (2003). Convergence of different versions of the continuous performance test: clinical and scientific implications. *Journal of Clinical and Experimental Neuropsychology,* **25,** 283–92.

Brand, M., Roth-Bauer, M., Driessen, M., and Markowitsch, H. J. (2008). Executive functions and risky decision-making in patients with opiate dependence. *Drug and Alcohol Dependence,* **97,** 64–72.

Bretteville-Jensen, A. L. (1999). Gender, heroin consumption and economic behaviour. *Health Economics,* **8,** 379–89.

Brownstein, M. J. (1993). A brief history of opiates, opioid peptides, and opioid receptors. *Proceedings of the National Academy of Sciences*, **90**, 5391–3.

Burgess, P. W. (1997). Theory and methodology in executive function research. In P.Rabbitt (ed.), *Methodology of frontal and executive function*. Hove, East Sussex: Psychology Press.

Carboni, E., Spielewoy, C., Vacca, C., Nosten-Bertrand, M., Giros, B., and Di Chiara, G. (2001). Cocaine and amphetamine increase extracellular dopamine in the nucleus accumbens of mice lacking the dopamine transporter gene. *Journal of Neuroscience*, **21**, art–RC141.

Carter, C. S., Braver, T. S., Barch, D. M., Botvinick, M. M., Noll, D., and Cohen, J. D. (1998). Anterior cingulate cortex, error detection, and the online monitoring of performance. *Science*, **280**, 747–9.

Casey, K. L., Svensson, P., Morrow, T. J., Raz, J., Jone, C., and Minoshima, S. (2000). Selective opiate modulation of nociceptive processing in the human brain. *Journal of Neurophysiology*, **84**, 525–33.

Castro, F. G., Barrington, E. H., Walton, M. A., and Rawson, R. A. (2000). Cocaine and methamphetamine: Differential addiction rates. *Psychology of Addictive Behaviors*, **14**, 390–6.

Chamberlain, S. R. and Sahakian, B. J. (2007). The neuropsychiatry of impulsivity. *Current Opinion in Psychiatry*, **20**, 255–61.

Chang, L., Ernst, T., Speck, O., Patel, H., DeSilva, M., Leonido-Yee, M., and Miller, E. N. (2002). Perfusion MRI and computerized cognitive test abnormalities in abstinent methamphetamine users. *Psychiatry Research: Neuroimaging*, **114**, 65–79.

Chang, L., Cloak, C., Patterson, K., Grob, C., Miller, E. N., and Ernst, T. (2005). Enlarged striatum in abstinent methamphetamine abusers: A possible compensatory response. *Biological Psychiatry*, **57**, 967–74.

Chesney, M. A., Barrett, D. C., and Stall, R. (1998). Histories of substance use and risk behavior: Precursors to HIV seroconversion in homosexual men. *American Journal of Public Health*, **88**, 113–6.

Chikazoe, J., Konishi, S., Asari, T., Jimura, K., and Miyashita, Y. (2007). Activation of right inferior frontal gyrus during response inhibition across response modalities. *The Journal of Cognitive Neuroscience*, **19**, 69–80.

Clark, L. and Robbins, T. W. (2002). Decision-making deficits in drug addiction. *Trends in Cognitive Sciences*, **6**, 361–3.

Clark, L., Robbins, T. W., Ersche, K. D., and Sahakian, B. J. (2006). Reflection impulsivity in chronic and former substance users. *Biological Psychiatry*, **60**, 512–22.

Clarke, H. F., Dalley, J. W., Crofts, H. S., Robbins, T. W., and Roberts, A. C. (2004). Cognitive inflexibility after prefrontal serotonin depletion. *Science*, **304**, 878–80.

Colzato, L. S., Van den Wildenberg, W. P. M., and Hommel, B. (2007). Impaired inhibitory control in recreational cocaine users. *PLoS ONE*, **2**, e1143.

Cools, R. (2008). Role of dopamine in the motivational and cognitive control of behavior. *The Neuroscientist*, **14**, 381–95.

Cools, R. and Robbins, T. W. (2004). Chemistry of the adaptive mind. *Philosophical Transactions of the Royal Society of London Series A-Mathematical Physical and Engineering Sciences*, **362**, 2871–88.

Cools, R., Clark, L., Owen, A. M., and Robbins, T. W. (2002). Defining the neural mechanisms of probabilistic reversal learning using event-related functional magnetic resonance imaging. *Journal of Neuroscience*, **22**, 4563–7.

Curran, H. V., Kleckham, J., Bearn, J., Strang, J., and Wanigaratne, S. (2001). Effects of methadone on cognition, mood and craving in detoxifying opiate addicts: a dose-response study. *Psychopharmacology*, **154**, 153–60.

Dagher, A., Owen, A. M., Boecker, H., and Brooks, D. J. (2001). The role of the striatum and hippocampus in planning: a PET activation study in Parkinson's disease. *Brain*, **124**, 1020–32.

Daglish, M. R. C. and Nutt, D. J. (2003). Brain imaging studies in human addicts. *European Neuropsychopharmacology*, **13**, 453–8.

Danos, P., Kasper, S., Grunwald, F., Klemm, E., Krappel, C., Broich, K. et al. (1998a). Pathological regional blood flow in opiate-dependent patients during withdrawal: a HMPAO-SPECT study. *Neuropsychobiology*, 37, 194–9.

Danos, P., Van Roos, D., Kasper, S., Bromel, T., Broich, K., Krappel, C. et al. (1998b). Enlarged cerebrospinal fluid spaces in opiate-dependent male patients: a stereological CT study. *Neuropsychobiology*, 38, 80–3.

Darke, S. and Hall, W. (1995). Levels and correlates of polydrug use among heroin users and regular amphetamine users. *Drug and Alcohol Dependence*, 39, 231–5.

Darke, S., Sims, J., McDonald, S., and Wickes, W. (2000). Cognitive impairment among methadone maintenance patients. *Addiction*, 95, 687–95.

Davis, P. E., Liddiard, H., and McMillan, T. M. (2002). Neuropsychological deficits and opiate abuse. *Drug and Alcohol Dependence*, 67, 105–8.

de Lima, M. S., Soares, G. D., Reisser, A. A. P., and Farrell, M. (2002). Pharmacological treatment of cocaine dependence: a systematic review. *Addiction*, 97, 931–49.

Deakin, J. B., Aitken, M. R. F., Robbins, T. W., and Sahakian, B. J. (2004). Risk taking during decision-making in normal volunteers changes with age. *Journal of the International Neuroscience Society*, 10, 590–8.

Derbyshire, S. W. G., Vogt, B. A., and Jones, A. K. P. (1998). Pain and Stroop interference tasks activate separate processing modules in anterior cingulate cortex. *Experimental Brain Research*, 118, 52–60.

Di Chiara, G. and Imperato, A. (1988). Drugs abused by humans preferentially increase synaptic dopamine concentrations in the mesolimbic system of freely moving rats. *Proceedings of the National Academy of Sciences of the United States of America*, 85, 5274–8.

Dias, R., Robbins, T. W., and Roberts, A. C. (1997). Dissociable forms of inhibitory control within prefrontal cortex with an analog of the Wisconsin Card Sort Test: restriction to novel situations and independence from "'on-line'" processing. *Journal of Neuroscience*, 17, 9285–97.

Dickman, S. J. (1990). Functional and dysfunctional impulsivity—personality and cognitive correlates. *Journal of Personality and Social Psychology*, 58, 95–102.

Dluzen, D. E., Anderson, L. I., and Pilati, C. F. (2002). Methamphetamine-gonadal steroid hormonal interactions: Effects upon acute toxicity and striatal dopamine concentrations. *Neurotoxicology and Teratology*, 24, 267–73.

Dluzen, D. E. and Liu, B. (2008). Gender differences in methamphetamine use and responses: a review. *Gender Medicine*, 5, 24–35.

Dougherty, D. M., Bjork, J. M., Harper, R., Marsh, D. M., Moeller, F., Mathias, C. W., and Swann, A. C. (2003). Behavioral impulsivity paradigms: a comparison in hospitalized adolescents with disruptive behavior disorders. *Journal of Child Psychology and Psychiatry*, 44, 1145–57.

Downes, J. J., Roberts, A. C., Sahakian, B. J., Evenden, J. L., Morris, R. G., and Robbins, T. W. (1989). Impaired extra-dimensional shift performance in medicated and unmedicated Parkinson's disease: Evidence for a specific attentional dysfunction. *Neuropsychologia*, 27, 1329–43.

Elliott, R. (2003). Executive functions and their disorders. *British Medical Bulletin*, 65, 49–59.

EMCDDA (2003). *Annual report on the state of the drugs problem in the European Union 2003.* Luxembourg: Office for Official Publications of the European Communities.

Ernst, M., Grant, S. J., London, E. D., Contoreggi, C. S., Kimes, A. S., and Spurgeon, L. (2003). Decision making in adolescents with behavior disorders and adults with substance abuse. *American Journal of Psychiatry*, 160, 33–40.

Ernst, M. and Paulus, M. P. (2005). Neurobiology of decision making: a selective review from a neuro-cognitive and clinical perspective. *Biological Psychiatry*, 58, 597–604.

Ersche, K. D., Fletcher, P. C., Lewis, S. J. G., Clark, L., Stocks-Gee, G., London, M. et al. (2005a). Abnormal frontal activations related to decision-making in current and former amphetamine and opiate-dependent individuals. *Psychopharmacology*, 180, 612–23.

Ersche, K. D., Roiser, J. P., Clark, L., London, M., Robbins, T. W., and Sahakian, B. J. (2005b). Punishment induces risky decision-making in methadone-maintained opiate users but not in heroin users or healthy volunteers. *Neuropsychopharmacology, 30,* 2115–24.

Ersche, K. D., Clark, L., London, M., Robbins, T. W., and Sahakian, B. J. (2006a). Profile of executive and memory function associated with amphetamine and opiate dependence. *Neuropsychopharmacology, 31,* 1036–47.

Ersche, K. D., Fletcher, P. C., Roiser, J. P., Fryer, T. D., London, M., Robbins, T. W., and Sahakian, B. J. (2006b). Differences in orbitofrontal activation during decision-making between methadone-maintained opiate users, heroin users and healthy volunteers. *Psychopharmacology, 188,* 364–73.

Ersche, K. D., Roiser, J. P., Robbins, T. W., and Sahakian, B. J. (2008). Chronic cocaine but not chronic amphetamine-use is associated with perseverative responding in humans. *Psychopharmacology, 197,* 421–31.

Eslinger, P. J. and Grattan, L. M. (1993). Frontal lobe and frontal-striatal substrates for different forms of human cognitive flexibility. *Neuropsychologia, 31,* 17–28.

European Monitoring Centre for Drugs and Drug Addiction (2006). *Annual Report 2005/2006: the state of the drugs problem in Europe.* Lisbon: Office for Official Publications of the European Communities.

European Monitoring Centre for Drugs and Drug Addiction (2007). *Cocaine and crack cocaine: a growing public health problem.* Lisbon, Portugal: European Monitoring Centre for Drugs and Drug Addiction (EMCDDA).

Evenden, J. L. (1999). Varieties of impulsivity. *Psychopharmacology, 146,* 348–61.

Fals-Stewart, W. and Schafer, J. (1992). The relationship between length of stay in drug-free therapeutic communities and neurocognitive functioning. *Journal of Clinical Psychology, 48,* 539–43.

Fals-Stewart, W. and Lucente, S. (1994). The effect of cognitive rehabilitation on the neuropsychological status of patients in drug-abuse treatment who display neurocognitive impairment. *Rehabilitation Psychology, 39,* 75–94.

Fillmore, M. T. and Rush, C. R. (2002). Impaired inhibitory control of behavior in chronic cocaine users. *Drug and Alcohol Dependence, 66,* 265–73.

Fillmore, M. T. and Rush, C. R. (2006). Polydrug abusers display impaired discrimination-reversal learning in a model of behavioural control. *Journal of Psychopharmacology, 20,* 24–32.

Fishbain, D. A., Cutler, R. B., Rosomoff, H. L., and Rosomoff, R. S. (2003). Are opioid-dependent/tolerant patients impaired in driving-related skills? A structured evidence-based review. *Journal of Pain and Symptom Management, 25,* 559–77.

Fishbein, D., Hyde, C., Eldreth, D., London, E. D., Matochik, J., Ernst, M. et al. (2005). Cognitive performance and autonomic reactivity in abstinent drug abusers and nonusers. *Experimental and Clinical Psychopharmacology, 13,* 25–40.

Fishbein, D. H., Krupitsky, E., Flannery, B. A., Langevin, D. J., Bobashev, G., Verbitskaya, E. et al. (2007). Neurocognitive characterizations of Russian heroin addicts without a significant history of other drug use. *Drug and Alcohol Dependence, 90,* 25–38.

Forman, S. D., Dougherty, G. G., Casey, B. J., Siegle, G. J., Braver, T. S., Barch, D. M. et al. (2004). Opiate addicts lack error-dependent activation of rostral anterior cingulate. *Biological Psychiatry, 55,* 531–7.

Franklin, T. R., Acton, P. D., Maldjian, J. A., Gray, J. D., Croft, J. R., Dackis, C. A. et al. (2002). Decreased gray matter concentration in the insular, orbitofrontal, cingulate, and temporal cortices of cocaine patients. *Biological Psychiatry, 51,* 134–42.

Gabilondo, A. M., Meana, J. J., Barturen, F., Sastre, M., and Garciasevilla, J. A. (1994). Mu-opioid receptor and alpha(2)-adrenoceptor agonist binding- sites in the postmortem brain of heroin-addicts. *Psychopharmacology, 115,* 135–40.

Galynker, I. I., Watras-Ganz, S., Miner, C., Rosenthal, R. N., Jarlais, D. C. D., Richman, B. L., and London, E. (2000). Cerebral metabolism in opiate-dependent subjects: effects of methadone maintenance. *Mount Sinai Journal of Medicine*, **67**, 381–7.

Gehring, W. J. and Knight, R. T. (2000). Prefrontal-cingulate interactions in action monitoring. *Nature Neuroscience*, **3**, 516–20.

Gerra, G., Calbiani, B., Zaimovic, A., Sartori, R., Ugolotti, G., Ippolito, L. et al. (1998). Regional cerebral blood flow and comorbid diagnosis in abstinent opioid addicts. *Psychiatry Research: Neuroimaging*, **83**, 117–26.

Goldstein, R. Z. and Volkow, N. D. (2002). Drug addiction and its underlying neurobiological basis: Neuroimaging evidence for the involvement of the frontal cortex. *American Journal of Psychiatry*, **159**, 1642–52.

Goldstein, R. Z., Volkow, N. D., Wang, G. J., Fowler, J. S., and Rajaram, S. (2001). Addiction changes orbitofrontal gyrus function: involvement in response inhibition. *Neuroreport*, **12**, 2595–9.

Gonzalez, R., Rippeth, J. D., Carey, C. L., Heaton, R. K., Moore, D. J., Schweinsburg, B. C., Cherner, M., and Grant, I. (2004). Neurocognitive performance of methamphetamine users discordant for history of marijuana exposure. *Drug and Alcohol Dependence*, **76**, 181–90.

Gooding, D. C., Burroughs, S., and Boutros, N. N. (2008). Attentional deficits in cocaine-dependent patients: converging behavioral and electrophysiological evidence. *Psychiatry Research*, **160**, 145–54.

Gordon, S. M. (2001). *Heroin: challenge for the 21st century*. Wernersville, PA: Cardon Foundation.

Gossop, M., Griffiths, P., and Strang, J. (1994). Sex-differences in patterns of drug-taking behavior - a study at a london community drug team. *British Journal of Psychiatry*, **164**, 101–4.

Grant, D. A. and Berg, E. A. (1948). A behavioural analysis of degree of reinforcement and ease of shifting to new responses in a Weigl-type card-sorting problem. *Journal of Experimental Psychology*, **38**, 404–11.

Grant, S., Contoreggi, C., and London, E. D. (2000). Drug abusers show impaired performance in a laboratory test of decision making. *Neuropsychologia*, **38**, 1180–7.

Gruber, S. A., Silveri, M. M., Renshaw, P. F., Tzilos, G. K., Pollack, M., Kaufman, M. J., and Yurgelun-Todd, D. A. (2006). Methadone maintenance improves cognitive performance after two months of treatment. *Experimental and Clinical Psychopharmacology*, **14**, 157–64.

Guerra, D., Sole, A., Cami, J., and Tobena, A. (1987). Neuropsychological performance in opiate addicts after rapid detoxification. *Drug and Alcohol Dependence*, **20**, 261–70.

Hartnoll, R. L. (1994). Opiates—prevalence and demographic-factors. *Addiction*, **89**, 1377–83.

Haselhorst, R., Dursteler-MacFarland, K. M., Scheffler, K., Ladewig, D., Muller-Spahn, F., Stohler, R. et al. (2002). Frontocortical N-acetylaspartate reduction associated with long-term IV heroin use. *Neurology*, **58**, 305–7.

Hastie, R. (2001). Problems for judgment and decision making. *Annual Review of Psychology*, **52**, 653–83.

Hester, R. and Garavan, H. (2004). Executive dysfunction in cocaine addiction: evidence for discordant frontal, cingulate, and cerebellar activity. *Journal of Neuroscience*, **24**, 11017–22.

Hester, R., Simoes-Franklin, C., and Garavan, H. (2007). Post-error behavior in active cocaine users: Poor awareness of errors in the presence of intact performance adjustments. *Neuropsychopharmacology*, **32**, 1974–84.

Hoare, J. (2009). *Drug misuse declared in 2008/9: results from the British Crime Survey*. Home Office, Research Development and Statistics, London.

Hoffman, W. F., Moore, M., Templin, R., McFarland, B., Hitzemann, R. J., and Mitchell, S. H. (2006). Neuropsychological function and delay discounting in methamphetamine-dependent individuals. *Psychopharmacology*, **188**, 162–70.

Horn, N. R., Dolan, M., Elliott, R., Deakin, J. F. W., and Woodruff, P. W. R. (2003). Response inhibition and impulsivity: an fMRI study. *Neuropsychologia*, **41**, 1959–66.

Hornak, J., O'Doherty, J., Bramham, J., Rolls, E. T., Morris, R. G., Bullock, P. R., and Polkey, C. E. (2004). Reward-related reversal learning after surgical excisions in orbito-frontal or dorsolateral pre-frontal cortex in humans. *Journal of Cognitive Neuroscience*, 16, 463–78.

Hunt, D. E., Lipton, D. S., Goldsmith, D. S., Strug, D. L., and Spunt, B. (1985). It takes your heart - the image of methadone-maintenance in the addict world and its effect on recruitment into treatment. *International Journal of the Addictions*, 20, 1751–71.

Hwang, J., Lyoo, I. K., Kim, S. J., Sung, Y. H., Bae, S., Cho, S. N. et al. (2006). Decreased cerebral blood flow of the right anterior cingulate cortex in long-term and short-term abstinent methamphetamine users. *Drug and Alcohol Dependence*, 82, 177–81.

Isralowitz, R., Reznik, A., and Assa, V. (2005). Heroin addicts and vision problems: a prospective study. *Drugs-Education Prevention and Policy*, 12, 161–5.

Jentsch, J. D. and Taylor, J. R. (1999). Impulsivity resulting from frontostriatal dysfunction in drug abuse: implications for the control of behavior by reward- related stimuli. *Psychopharmacology*, 146, 373–90.

Johanson, C. E. and Fischman, M. W. (1989). The pharmacology of cocaine related to its abuse. *Pharmacological Reviews*, 41, 3–52.

Johanson, C. E., Frey, K. A., Lundahl, L. H., Keenan, P., Lockhart, N., Roll, J. et al. (2006). Cognitive function and nigrostriatal markers in abstinent methamphetamine abusers. *Psychopharmacology*, 185, 327–38.

Jollant, F., Bellivier, F., Leboyer, M., Astruc, B., Torres, S., Verdier, R. et al. (2005). Impaired decision making in suicide attempters. *American Journal of Psychiatry*, 162, 304–10.

Jollant, F., Guillaume, S., Jaussent, I., Castelnau, D., Malafosse, A., and Courtet, P. (2007). Impaired decision-making in suicide attempters may increase the risk of problems in affective relationships. *Journal of Affective Disorders*, 99, 59–62.

Jovanovski, D., Erb, S., and Zakzanis, K. K. (2005). Neurocognitive deficits in cocaine users: a quantitative review of the evidence. *Journal of Clinical and Experimental Neuropsychology*, 27, 189–204.

Kalechstein, A. D., Newton, T. F., and Green, M. (2003). Methamphetamine dependence is associated with neurocognitive impairment in the initial phases of abstinence. *Journal of Neuropsychiatry*, 15, 215–20.

Katz, E. C., King, S. D., Schwartz, R. P., Weintraub, E., Barksdale, W., Robinson, R., and Brown, B. S. (2005). Cognitive ability as a factor in engagement in drug abuse treatment. *American Journal of Drug and Alcohol Abuse*, 31, 359–69.

Kaufman, J. N., Ross, T. J., Stein, E. A., and Garavan, H. (2003). Cingulate hypoactivity in cocaine users during a go/no-go task as revealed by event-related functional magnetic resonance imaging. *Journal of Neuroscience*, 23, 7839–43.

Kelley, B. J., Yeager, K. R., Pepper, T. H., and Beversdorf, D. Q. (2005). Cognitive impairment in acute cocaine withdrawal. *Cognitive and Behavioral Neurology*, 18, 108–12.

Kim, S. J., Lyoo, I. K., Hwang, J., Sung, Y. H., Lee, H. Y., Lee, D. S. et al. (2005). Frontal glucose hypometabolism in abstinent methamphetamine users. *Neuropsychopharmacology*, 30, 1383–91.

Kim, S. J., Lyoo, I. K., Hwang, J., Chung, A., Sung, Y. H., Kim, J. et al. (2006). Prefrontal grey-matter changes in short-term and long-term abstinent methamphetamine abusers. *International Journal of Neuropsychopharmacology*, 9, 221–8.

Kish, S. J., Kalasinsky, K. S., Derkach, P., Schmunk, G. A., Guttman, M., Ang, L. et al. (2001). Striatal dopaminergic and serotonergic markers in human heroin users. *Neuropsychopharmacology*, 24, 561–7.

Klee, H. (1998). The love of speed: an analysis of the enduring attraction of amphetamine sulfate for British youth. *Journal of Drug Issues*, 28, 33–55.

Klee, H. and Morris, J. (1994). Factors that lead young amphetamine misusers to seek help - implications for drug prevention and harm reduction. *Drugs-Education Prevention and Policy*, 1, 289–97.

Kling, M. A., Carson, R. E., Borg, L., Zametkin, A., Matochik, J. A., Schluger, J. et al. (2000). Opioid receptor imaging with positron emission tomography and [F-18]cyclofoxy in long-term, methadone-treated former heroin addicts. *Journal of Pharmacology and Experimental Therapeutics*, 295, 1070–6.

Konishi, S., Nakajima, K., Uchida, I., Kameyama, M., Nakahara, K., Sekihara, K., and Miyashita, Y. (1998). Transient activation of inferior prefrontal cortex during cognitive set shifting. *Nature Neuroscience*, 1, 80–4.

Kreek, M. J. (2000). Methadone-related opioid agonist pharmacotherapy for heroin addiction—History, recent molecular and neurochemical research and future in mainstream medicine. *New Medications for Drug Abuse*, 909, 186–216.

Latowsky, M. and Kallen, E. (1997). Mainstreaming methadone maintenance treatment: the role of the family physician. *Canadian Medical Association Journal*, 157, 395–98.

Lee, T. M. C., Zhou, W. h., Luo, X. j., Yuen, K. S. L., Ruan, X. z., and Weng, X. c. (2005). Neural activity associated with cognitive regulation in heroin users: a fMRI study. *Neuroscience Letters*, 382, 211–6.

Leland, D. S. and Paulus, M. P. (2005). Increased risk-taking decision-making but not altered response to punishment in stimulant-using young adults. *Drug and Alcohol Dependence*, 78, 83–90.

Leland, D. S., Arce, E., Miller, D. A., and Paulus, M. P. (2008). Anterior cingulate cortex and benefit of predictive cueing on response inhibition in stimulant dependent individuals. *Biological Psychiatry*, 63, 184–90.

LeMarquand, D., Pihl, R. O., and Benkelfat, C. (1994). Serotonin and alcohol intake, abuse, and dependence: Clinical evidence. *Biological Psychiatry*, 36, 326–37.

Leung, H. C., Skudlarski, P., Gatenby, J. C., Peterson, B. S., and Gore, J. C. (2000). An event-related functional MRI study of the Stroop color word interference task. *Cerebral Cortex*, 10, 552–60.

Levine, A. J., Hardy, D. J., Miller, E., Castellon, S. A., Longshore, D., and Hinkin, C. H. (2006). The effect of recent stimulant use on sustained attention in HIV-Infected adults. *Journal of Clinical and Experimental Neuropsychology*, 28, 29–42.

Li, S. J., Wang, Y. K., Pankiewicz, J., and Stein, E. A. (1999). Neurochemical adaptation to cocaine abuse: Reduction of N-acetyl aspartate in thalamus of human cocaine abusers. *Biological Psychiatry*, 45, 1481–7.

Li, C. S. R., Kemp, K., Milivojevic, V., and Sinha, R. (2005). Neuroimaging study of sex differences in the neuropathology of cocaine abuse. *Gender Medicine*, 2, 174–82.

Li, C. S. R., Huang, C., Yan, P. S., Bhagwagar, Z., Milivojevic, V., and Sinha, R. (2008). Neural correlates of impulse control during stop signal inhibition in cocaine-dependent men. *Neuropsychopharmacology*, 33, 1798–806.

Lim, K. O., Choi, S. J., Pomara, N., Wolkin, A., and Rotrosen, J. P. (2002). Reduced frontal white matter integrity in cocaine dependence: a controlled diffusion tensor imaging study. *Biological Psychiatry*, 51, 890–5.

London, E. D., Ernst, M., Grant, S., Bonson, K., and Weinstein, A. (2000). Orbitofrontal cortex and human drug abuse: functional imaging. *Cerebral Cortex*, 10, 334–42.

London, E. D., Simon, S. L., Berman, S. M., Mandelkern, M. A., Lichtman, A. M., Bramen, J. et al. (2004). Mood disturbances and regional cerebral metabolic abnormalities in recently abstinent methamphetamine abusers. *Archives of General Psychiatry*, 61, 73–84.

London, E. D., Berman, S. M., Voytek, B., Simon, S. L., Mandelkern, M. A., Monterosso, J. et al. (2005). Cerebral metabolic dysfunction and impaired vigilance in recently abstinent methamphetamine abusers. *Biological Psychiatry*, 58, 770–8.

Lyoo, I. K., Pollack, M. H., Silveri, M. M., Ahn, K. H., Diaz, C. I., Hwang, J. et al. (2006). Prefrontal and temporal gray matter density decreases in opiate dependence. *Psychopharmacology*, 184, 139–44.

Lyvers, M. and Yakimoff, M. (2003). Neuropsychological correlates of opioid dependence and withdrawal. *Addictive Behaviors*, 28, 605–11.

Manes, F., Sahakian, B. J., Clark, L., Rogers, R. D., Antoun, N., Aitken, M., and Robbins, T. W. (2002). Decision-making processes following damage to the prefrontal cortex. *Brain*, 125, 624–39.

Matochik, J. A., London, E. D., Eldreth, D. A., Cadet, J. L., and Bolla, K. I. (2003). Frontal cortical tissue composition in abstinent cocaine abusers: a magnetic resonance imaging study. *Neuroimage*, 19, 1095–102.

McCann, U. D., Wong, D. F., Yokoi, F., Villemagne, V., Dannals, R. F., and Ricaurte, G. A. (1998). Reduced striatal dopamine transporter density in abstinent methamphetamine and methcathinone users: evidence from positron emission tomography studies with [C-11]WIN-35,428. *Journal of Neuroscience*, 18, 8417–22.

McKetin, R. and Mattick, R. P. (1998). Attention and memory in illicit amphetamine users: comparison with non-drug-using controls. *Drug and Alcohol Dependence*, 50, 181–4.

Mehta, M. A., Sahakian, B. J., McKenna, P. J., and Robbins, T. W. (1999). Systemic sulpiride in young adult volunteers simulates the profile of cognitive deficits in Parkinson's disease. *Psychopharmacology*, 146, 162–74.

Mehta, M. A., Manes, F. F., Magnolfi, G., Sahakian, B. J., and Robbins, T. W. (2004). Impaired set-shifting and dissociable effects on tests of spatial working memory following the dopamine D-2 receptor antagonist sulpiride in human volunteers. *Psychopharmacology*, 176, 331–42.

Melichar, J. K., Hume, S. P., Williams, T. M., Daglish, M. R. C., Taylor, L. G., Ahmad, R. et al. (2005). Using [C-11]diprenorphine to image opioid receptor occupancy by methadone in opioid addiction: Clinical and preclinical studies. *Journal of Pharmacology and Experimental Therapeutics*, 312, 309–15.

Mellers, B. A., Schwartz, A., and Cooke, A. D. J. (1998). Judgment and decision making. *Annual Review of Psychology*, 49, 447–77.

Meredith, C. W., Jaffe, C., ng-Lee, K., and Saxon, A. J. (2005). Implications of chronic methamphetamine use: a literature review. *Harvard Review of Psychiatry*, 13, 141–54.

Meyerhoff, D. J., Bloomer, C., Schuff, N., Ezekiel, F., Norman, D., Clark, W. et al. (1999). Cortical metabolite alterations in abstinent cocaine and cocaine/alcohol-dependent subjects: proton magnetic resonance spectroscopic imaging. *Addiction Biology*, 4, 405–19.

Mintzer, M. Z. and Stitzer, M. L. (2002). Cognitive impairment in methadone maintenance patients. *Drug and Alcohol Dependence*, 67, 41–51.

Mintzer, M. Z., Copersino, M. L., and Stitzer, M. L. (2005). Opioid abuse and cognitive performance. *Drug and Alcohol Dependence*, 78, 225–30.

Mitchell, D. G. V., Colledge, E., Leonard, A., and Blair, R. J. R. (2002). Risky decisions and response reversal: is there evidence of orbitofrontal cortex dysfunction in psychopathic individuals? *Neuropsychologia*, 40, 2013–22.

Moeller, F. G., Barratt, E. S., Fischer, C. J., Dougherty, D. M., Reilly, E. L., Mathias, C. W., and Swann, A. C. (2004). P300 event-related potential amplitude and impulsivity in cocaine-dependent subjects. *Neuropsychobiology*, 50, 167–73.

Moeller, F. G., Hasan, K. M., Steinberg, J. L., Kramer, L. A., Dougherty, D. M., Santos, R. M. et al. (2005). Reduced anterior corpus callosum white matter integrity is related to increased impulsivity and reduced discriminability in cocaine-dependent subjects: diffusion tensor imaging. *Neuropsychopharmacology*, 30, 610–7.

Monterosso, J., Ehrman, R., Napier, K. L., O'Brien, C. P., and Childress, A. R. (2001). Three decision-making tasks in cocaine-dependent patients: do they measure the same construct? *Addiction*, 96, 1825–37.

Monterosso, J. R., Aron, A. R., Cordova, X., Xu, J., and London, E. D. (2005). Deficits in response inhibition associated with chronic methamphetamine abuse. *Drug and Alcohol Dependence*, 79, 273–7.

Moon, M., Do, K. S., Park, J., and Kim, D. (2007). Memory impairment in methamphetamine dependent patients. *International Journal of Neuroscience*, 117, 1–9.

Morgenstern, J. and Bates, M. E. (1999). Effects of executive function impairment on change processes and substance use outcomes in 12-step treatment. *Journal of Studies on Alcohol*, 60, 846–55.

Munro, C. A., McCaul, M. E., Wong, D. F., Oswald, L. M., Zhou, Y., Brasic, J. et al.(2006). Sex differences in striatal dopamine release in healthy adults. *Biological Psychiatry*, 59, 966–74.

Murphy, S. and Irwin, J. (1992). Living with the dirty secret - problems of disclosure for methadone-maintenance clients. *Journal of Psychoactive Drugs*, **24**, 257–64.

Myers, R. E., Anderson, L. I., and Dluzen, D. E. (2003). Estrogen, but not testosterone, attenuates methamphetamine- evoked dopamine output from superfused striatal tissue of female and male mice. *Neuropharmacology*, **44**, 624–32.

Nieoullon, A. (2002). Dopamine and the regulation of cognition and attention. *Progress in Neurobiology*, **67**, 53–83.

Nigg, J. T., Glass, J. M., Wong, M. M., Poon, E., Jester, J. M., Fitzgerald, H. E. et al. (2004). Neuropsychological executive functioning in children at elevated risk for alcoholism: findings in early adolescence. *Journal of Abnormal Psychology*, **113**, 302–14.

Nordahl, T. E., Salo, R., Possin, K., Gibson, D. R., Flynn, N., Leamon, M. et al.(2002). Low N-acetyl-aspartate and high choline in the anterior cingulum of recently abstinent methamphetamine-dependent subjects: a preliminary proton MRS study. *Psychiatry Research: Neuroimaging*, **116**, 43–52.

Nordahl, T. E., Salo, R., Natsuaki, Y., Galloway, G. P., Waters, C., Moore, C. D. et al. (2005). Methamphetamine users in sustained abstinence: a proton magnetic resonance spectroscopy study. *Archives of General Psychiatry*, **62**, 444–52.

Oh, J. S., Lyoo, I. K., Sung, Y. H., Hwang, J., Kim, J., Chung, A. et al. (2005). Shape changes of the corpus callosum in abstinent methamphetamine users. *Neuroscience Letters*, **384**, 76–81.

Ornstein, T. J., Iddon, J. L., Baldacchino, A. M., Sahakian, B. J., London, M., Everitt, B. J., and Robbins, T. W. (2000). Profiles of cognitive dysfunction in chronic amphetamine and heroin abusers. *Neuropsychopharmacology*, **23**, 113–26.

Owen, A. M. (1997). Cognitive planning in humans: neuropsychological, neuroanatomical and neuropharmacological perspectives. *Progress in Neurobiology*, **53**, 431–50.

Owen, A. M., Downes, J. J., Sahakian, B. J., Polkey, C. E., and Robbins, T. W. (1990). Planning and spatial working memory following frontal-lobe lesions in man. *Neuropsychologia*, **28**, 1021–34.

Owen, A. M., Sahakian, B. J., Semple, J., Polkey, C. E., and Robbins, T. W. (1995). Visuo-spatial short-term recognition memory and learning after temporal lobe excisions, frontal lobe excisions or amygdalo-hippocampectomy in man. *Neuropsychologia*, **33**, 1–24.

Papageorgiou, C., Liappas, I., Asvestas, P., Vasios, C., Matsopoulos, G. K., Nikolaou, C. et al. (2001). Abnormal P600 in heroin addicts with prolonged abstinence elicited during a working memory test. *Neuroreport*, **12**, 1773–8.

Papageorgiou, C. C., Liappas, I. A., Ventouras, E. M., Nikolaou, C. C., Kitsonas, E. N., Uzunoglu, N. K., and Rabavilas, A. D. (2004). Long-term abstinence syndrome in heroin addicts: indices of P300 alterations associated with a short memory task. *Progress in Neuro-Psychopharmacology and Biological Psychiatry*, **28**, 1109–15.

Pardo, J. V., Pardo, P. J., Janer, K. W., and Raichle, M. E. (1990). The anterior cingulate cortex mediates processing selection in the Stroop attentional conflict paradigm. *Proceedings of the National Academy of Sciences*, **87**, 256–59.

Patton, J. H., Stanford, M. S., and Barratt, E. S. (1995). Factor structure of the Barratt impulsiveness scale. *Journal of Clinical Psychology*, **51**, 768–74.

Pau, C. W. H., Lee, T. M. C., and Chan, S. F. F. (2002). The impact of heroin on frontal executive functions. *Archives of Clinical Neuropsychology*, **17**, 663–70.

Paulus, M. P., Hozack, N. E., Zauscher, B. E., Frank, L., Brown, G. G., Braff, D. L., and Schuckit, M. A. (2002). Behavioral and functional neuroimaging evidence for prefrontal dysfunction in methamphetamine-dependent subjects. *Neuropsychopharmacology*, **26**, 53–63.

Paulus, M. P., Hozack, N., Frank, L., Brown, G. G., and Schuckit, M. A. (2003). Decision making by methamphetamine-dependent subjects is associated with error-rate-independent decrease in prefrontal and parietal activation. *Biological Psychiatry*, **53**, 65–74.

Paulus, M. P., Tapert, S. F., and Schuckit, M. A. (2005). Neural activation patterns of methamphetamine-dependent subjects during descision making predict relapse. *Archives of General Psychiatry*, **62**, 761–68.

Petrovic, P., Kalso, E., Petersson, K. M., and Ingvar, M. (2002). Placebo and opioid analgesia—imaging a shared neuronal network. *Science*, **295**, 1737–40.

Pezawas, L. M., Fischer, G., Diamant, K., Schneider, C., Schindler, S. D., Thurnher, M. et al. (1998). Cerebral CT findings in male opioid-dependent patients: stereological, planimetric and linear measurements. *Psychiatry Research: Neuroimaging*, **83**, 139–47.

Pirastu, R., Fais, R., Messina, M., Bini, V., Spiga, S., Falconieri, D., and Diana, M. (2006). Impaired decision-making in opiate-dependent subjects: effect of pharmacological therapies. *Drug and Alcohol Dependence*, **83**, 163–8.

Powis, B., Griffiths, P., Gossop, M., and Strang, J. (1996). The differences between male and female drug users: community samples of heroin and cocaine users compared. *Substance Use and Misuse*, **31**, 529–43.

Prosser, J., Cohen, L. J., Steinfeld, M., Eisenberg, D., London, E. D., and Galynker, I. I. (2006). Neuropsychological functioning in opiate-dependent subjects receiving and following methadone maintenance treatment. *Drug and Alcohol Dependence*, **84**, 240–47.

Rapeli, P., Kivisaari, R., Autti, T., Kahkonen, S., Puuskari, V., Jokela, O., and Kalska, H. (2006). Cognitive function during early abstinence from opioid dependence: a comparison to age, gender, and verbal intelligence matched controls. *BMC Psychiatry*, **6**, 9.

Rauch, L. (2000). The poet syndrome: opiates, psychosis and creativity. *Journal of Psychoactive Drugs*, **32**, 343–9.

Rippeth, J. D., Heaton, R. K., Carey, C. L., Marcotte, T. D., Moore, D. J., Gonzalez, R. et al. (2004). Methamphetamine dependence increases risk of neuropsychological impairment in HIV infected persons. *Journal of the International Neuropsychological Society*, **10**, 1–14.

Robbins, T. W. (1996). Dissociating executive functions of the prefrontal cortex. *Philosophical Transactions of the Royal Society of London Series B-Biological Sciences*, **351**, 1463–70.

Robbins, T. W. (2005). Chemistry of the mind: neurochemical modulation of prefrontal cortical function. *Journal of Comparative Neurology*, **493**, 140–6.

Robbins, T. W., James, M., Owen, A. M., Sahakian, B. J., Mcinnes, L., and Rabbitt, P. (1994). Cambridge neuropsychological test automated battery (Cantab)—a factor-analytic study of a large-sample of normal elderly volunteers. *Dementia*, **5**, 266–81.

Robbins, T. W., James, M., Owen, A. M., Sahakian, B. J., Lawrence, A. D., Mcinnes, L., and Rabbitt, P. M. A. (1998). A study of performance on tests from the CANTAB battery sensitive to frontal lobe dysfunction in a large sample of normal volunteers: implications for theories of executive functioning and cognitive aging. *Journal of the International Neuropsychological Society*, **4**, 474–90.

Rogers, R. D. and Robbins, T. W. (2001). Investigating the neurocognitive deficits associated with chronic drug misuse. *Current Opinion in Neurobiology*, **11**, 250–7.

Rogers, R. D. and Robbins, T. W. (2003). The neuropsychology of chronic drug abuse. In M.A.Ron and T. W. Robbins (eds), *Disorders of brain and mind: Vols 2* (pp. 447–67). Cambridge: Cambridge University Press.

Rogers, R. D., Everitt, B. J., Baldacchino, A., Blackshaw, A. J., Swainson, R., Wynne, K. et al. (1999a). Dissociable deficits in the decision-making cognition of chronic amphetamine abusers, opiate abusers, patients with focal damage to prefrontal cortex, and tryptophan-depleted normal volunteers: evidence for monoaminergic mechanisms. *Neuropsychopharmacology*, **20**, 322–39.

Rogers, R. D., Owen, A. M., Middleton, H. C., Williams, E. J., Pickard, J. D., Sahakian, B. J., and Robbins, T. W. (1999b). Choosing between small, likely rewards and large, unlikely rewards activates inferior and orbital prefrontal cortex. *Journal of Neuroscience*, **19**, 9029–38.

Rogers, R. D., Andrews, T. C., Grasby, P. M., Brooks, D. J., and Robbins, T. W. (2000a). Contrasting cortical and subcortical activations produced by attentional-set shifting and reversal learning in humans. *Journal of Cognitive Neuroscience*, 12, 142–62.

Rogers, R. D., Andrews, T. C., Grasby, P. M., Brooks, D. J., and Robbins, T. W. (2000b). Contrasting cortical and subcortical activations produced by attentional-set shifting and reversal learning in humans. *Journal of Cognitive Neuroscience*, 12, 142–62.

Rolls, E. T. (2000). The orbitofrontal cortex and reward. *Cerebral Cortex*, 10, 284–94.

Rose, J. S., Branchey, M., Buydens Branchey, L., Stapleton, J. M., Chasten, K., Werrell, A., and Maayan, M. L. (1996). Cerebral perfusion in early and late opiate withdrawal: A technetium-99m-HMPAO SPECT study. *Psychiatry Research: Neuroimaging*, 67, 39–47.

Rosselli, M. and Ardila, A. (1996). Cognitive effects of cocaine and polydrug abuse. *Journal of Clinical and Experimental Neuropsychology*, 18, 122–35.

Rotheram-Fuller, E., Shoptaw, S., Berman, S. M., and London, E. D. (2004). Impaired performance in a test of decision-making by opiate- dependent tobacco smokers. *Drug and Alcohol Dependence*, 73, 79–86.

Rounsaville, B. J., Jones, C., Novelly, R. A., and Kleber, H. (1982). Neuropsychological functioning in opiate addicts. *Journal of Nervous and Mental Disease*, 170, 209–16.

Rubia, K., Smith, A. B., Brammer, M. J., and Taylor, E. (2003). Right inferior prefrontal cortex mediates response inhibition while mesial prefrontal cortex is responsible for error detection. *Neuroimage*, 20, 351–8.

Salo, R., Nordahl, T. E., Possin, K., Leamon, M., Gibson, D. R., Galloway, G. P. et al. (2002). Preliminary evidence of reduced cognitive inhibition in methamphetamine-dependent individuals. *Psychiatry Research*, 111, 65–74.

Salo, R., Nordahl, T. E., Moore, C., Waters, C., Natsuaki, Y., Galloway, G. P. et al. (2005). A dissociation in attentional control: evidence from methamphetamine dependence. *Biological Psychiatry*, 57, 310–3.

Salo, R., Nordahl, T. E., Natsuaki, Y., Leamon, M. H., Galloway, G. P., Waters, C. et al. (2007). Attentional control and brain metabolite levels in methamphetamine abusers. *Biological Psychiatry*, 61, 1272–80.

Salo, R., Nordahl, T. E., Buonocore, M. H., Natsuaki, Y., Waters, C., Moore, C. D. et al. (2009). Cognitive control and white matter callosal microstructure in methamphetamine-dependent subjects: a diffusion tensor imaging study. *Biological psychiatry*, 65(2), 122–8. .

Sarter, M., Givens, B., and Bruno, J. P. (2001). The cognitive neuroscience of sustained attention: where top-down meets bottom-up. *Brain Research Reviews*, 35, 146–60.

Scott, J. C., Woods, S. P., Matt, G. E., Meyer, R. A., Heaton, R. K., Atkinson, J. H., and Grant, I. (2007). Neurocognitive effects of methamphetamine: a critical review and meta-analysis. *Neuropsychology Review*, 17, 275–97.

Seiden, S. L. and Kleven, M. S. (1988). Lack of toxic effects of cocaine on dopamine or serotonin neurons in the rat brain. In: D. Clouet, K. Asghar, and R. Brown (eds), *Mechanisms of cocaine abuse and toxicity* (pp. 276–89). Rockville, MD; USA: National Institute on Drug Abuse.

Seiden, L. S., Sabol, K. E., and Ricaurte, G. A. (1993). Amphetamine: effects on catecholamine systems and behavior. *Annual Review of Pharmacology and Toxicology*, 33, 639–76.

Sekine, Y., Iyo, M., Ouchi, Y., Matsunaga, T., Tsukada, H., Okada, H. et al. (2001). Methamphetamine-related psychiatric symptoms and reduced brain dopamine transporters studied with PET. *American Journal of Psychiatry*, 158, 1206–14.

Semple, S. J., Patterson, T. L., and Grant, I. (2004). The context of sexual risk behavior among heterosexual methamphetamine users. *Addictive Behaviors*, 29, 807–10.

Shallice, T. (1982). Specific impairments of planning. *Philosophical Transactions of the Royal Society of London Series B-Biological Sciences*, 298, 199–209.

Shearer, J. (2007). Psychosocial approaches to psychostimulant dependence: a systematic review. *Journal of Substance Abuse Treatment, 32,* 41–52.

Simon, S. L., Domier, C., Carnell, J., Brethen, P., Rawson, R., and Ling, W. (2000). Cognitive impairment in individuals currently using methamphetamine. *American Journal on Addictions, 9,* 222–31.

Simon, S. L., Domier, C. P., Sim, T., Richardson, K., Rawson, R. A., and Ling, W. (2002). Cognitive performance of current methamphetamine and cocaine abusers. *Journal of Addictive Diseases, 21,* 61–74.

Stern, R. A., Singer, E. A., Duke, L. M., Singer, N. G., Morey, C. E., Daughtrey, E. W., and Kaplan, E. (1994). The Boston qualitative scoring system for the rey-osterrieth complex figure—description and interrater reliability. *Clinical Neuropsychologist, 8,* 309–22.

Stout, P. R. and Farrell, L. J. (2003). Opioids—effects on human performance and behavior. *Forensic Science Review, 15,* 30–59.

Stout, J. C., Rock, S. L., Campbell, M. C., Busemeyer, J. R., and Finn, P. R. (2005). Psychological processes underlying risky decisions in drug abusers. *Addictive Behaviors, 19,* 148–57.

Strang, J., Griffiths, P., Powis, B., and Gossop, M. (1999). Heroin chasers and heroin injectors: Differences observed in a community sample in London, UK. *American Journal on Addictions, 8,* 148–60.

Stroop, J. R. (1992). Studies of interference in serial verbal reactions (Reprinted from Journal Experimental-Psychology, Vol. 18, Pg 643–662, 1935). *Journal of Experimental Psychology-General, 121,* 15–23.

Substance Abuse and Mental Health Services Administration (2002). *National survey on drug use and health.* Rockville, MD: Office of Applied Studies.

Sung, Y. H., Cho, S. C., Hwang, J., Kim, S. J., Kim, H., Bae, S. et al. (2007). Relationship between N-acetyl-aspartate in gray and white matter of abstinent methamphetamine abusers and their history of drug abuse: a proton magnetic resonance spectroscopy study. *Drug and Alcohol Dependence, 88,* 28–35.

Swainson, R., Rogers, R. D., Sahakian, B. J., Summers, B. A., Polkey, C. E., and Robbins, T. W. (2000). Probabilistic learning and reversal deficits in patients with Parkinson's disease or frontal or temporal lobe lesions: possible adverse effects of dopaminergic medication. *Neuropsychologia, 38,* 596–612.

Tao, R. and Auerbach, S. B. (2002a). GABAergic and glutamatergic afferents in the dorsal raphe nucleus mediate morphine-induced increases in serotonin efflux in the rat central nervous system. *Journal of Pharmacology and Experimental Therapeutics, 303,* 704–10.

Tao, R. and Auerbach, S. B. (2002b). Opioid receptor subtypes differentially modulate serotonin efflux in the rat central nervous system. *Journal of Pharmacology and Experimental Therapeutics, 303,* 549–56.

Taylor, M. J., Letendre, S. L., Schweinsburg, B. C., Alhassoon, O. M., Brown, G. G., Gongvatana, A., and Grant, I. (2004). Hepatitis C virus infection is associated with reduced white matter N-acetylaspartate in abstinent methamphetamine users. *Journal of the International Neuropsychological Society, 10,* 110–3.

Teichner, G., Horner, M. D., Roitzsch, J. C., Herron, J., and Thevos, A. (2002). Substance abuse treatment outcomes for cognitively impaired and intact outpatients. *Addictive Behaviors, 27,* 751–63.

Thompson, P. M., Hayashi, K. M., Simon, S. L., Geaga, J. A., Hong, M. S., Sui, Y. H. et al. (2004). Structural abnormalities in the brains of human subjects who use methamphetamine. *Journal of Neuroscience, 24,* 6028–36.

Tomasi, D., Goldstein, R. Z., Telang, F., Maloney, T., Alia-Klein, N., Caparelli, E. C., and Volkow, N. D. (2007). Thalamo-cortical dysfunction in cocaine abusers: Implications in attention and perception. *Psychiatry Research-Neuroimaging, 155,* 189–201.

Toomey, R., Lyons, M. J., Eisen, S. A., Xian, H., Chantarujikapong, S., Seidman, L. J. et al.(2003). A twin study of the neuropsychological consequences of stimulant abuse. *Archives of General Psychiatry, 60,* 303–10.

Tsai, G. and Coyle, J. T. (1995). N-Acetylaspartate in neuropsychiatric disorders. *Progress in Neurobiology*, 46, 531–40.

United Nations Office on Drugs and Crime (2003a). *Global illicit drug trends 2003*. New York, NY: United Nations Office on Drugs and Crime (UNODC).

United Nations Office on Drugs and Crime (2003b). *World drug report 2004*. (Vol. 1: Analysis) Vienna, AU: United Nations Office on Drugs and Crime (UNODC).

United Nations Office on Drugs and Crime (2007). *World drug report 2007*. New York, NY: United Nations Office on Drugs and Crime (UNODC).

Van Gorp, W. G., Wilkins, J. N., Hinkin, C. H., Moore, L. H., Hull, J., Horner, M. D., and Plotkin, D. (1999). Declarative and procedural memory functioning in abstinent cocaine abusers. *Archives of General Psychiatry*, 56, 85–9.

van Honk, J., Hermans, E. J., Putman, P., Montague, B., and Schutter, D. J. L. G. (2002). Defective somatic markers in sub-clinical psychopathy. *Neuroreport*, 13, 1025–27.

van Honk, J., Schutter, D. J. L. G., Hermans, E. J., and Putman, P. (2003). Low cortisol levels and the balance between punishment sensitivity and reward dependency. *Neuroreport*, 14, 1993–6.

Vassileva, J., Petkova, P., Georgiev, S., Martin, E. M., Tersiyski, R., Raycheva, M. et al. (2007). Impaired decision-making in psychopathic heroin addicts. *Drug and Alcohol Dependence*, 86, 287–9.

Verdejo-Garcia, A. and Perez-Garcia, M. (2007). Profile of executive deficits in cocaine and heroin polysubstance users: common and differential effects on separate executive components. *Psychopharmacology*, 190, 517–30.

Verdejo-Garcia, A., Lopez-Torrecillas, F., Gimenez, C. O., and Perez-Garcia, M. (2004). Clinical implications and methodological challenges in the study of the neuropsychological correlates of cannabis, stimulant, and opioid abuse. *Neuropsychology Review*, 14, 1–41.

Verdejo-Garcia, A., Toribio, I., Orozco, C., Puente, K. L., and Perez-Garcia, M. (2005). Neuropsychological functioning in methadone maintenance patients versus abstinent heroin abusers. *Drug and Alcohol Dependence*, 78, 238–88.

Verdejo-Garcia, A., Bechara, A., Recknor, E. C., and Perez-Garcia, M. (2006). Executive dysfunction in substance dependent individuals during drug use and abstinence: an examination of the behavioral, cognitive and emotional correlates of addiction. *Journal of the International Neuropsychological Society*, 12, 405–15.

Verdejo-Garcia, A. J., Perales, J. C., and Perez-Garcia, M. (2007). Cognitive impulsivity in cocaine and heroin polysubstance abusers. *Addictive Behaviors*, 32, 950–66.

Vincent, N., Shoobridge, J., Ask, A., Allsop, S., and Ali, R. (1999). Characteristics of amphetamine users seeking information, help and treatment in Adelaide, South Australia. *Drug and Alcohol Review*, 18, 63–73.

Vogt, B. A., Wiley, R. G., and Jensen, E. L. (1995). Localization of mu-opioid and delta-opioid receptors to anterior cingulate afferents and projection neurons and input- output model of mu regulation. *Experimental Neurology*, 135, 83–92.

Volkow, N. D., Fowler, J. S., Wang, G. J., Hitzemann, R., Logan, J., Schlyer, D. J. et al. (1993). Decreased Dopamine-D(2) Receptor Availability Is Associated with Reduced Frontal Metabolism in Cocaine Abusers. *Synapse*, 14, 169–77.

Volkow, N. D., Gur, R. C., Wang, G. J., Fowler, J. S., Moberg, P. J., Ding, Y. S. et al. (1998). Association Between Decline in Brain Dopamine Activity With Age and Cognitive and Motor Impairment in Healthy Individuals. *American Journal of Psychiatry*, 155, 344–49.

Volkow, N. D., Chang, L., Wang, G. J., Fowler, J. S., Ding, Y. S., Sedler, M. et al. (2001a). Low level of brain dopamine D-2 receptors in methamphetamine abusers: Association with metabolism in the orbitofrontal cortex. *American Journal of Psychiatry*, 158, 2015–21.

Volkow, N. D., Chang, L., Wang, G. J., Fowler, J. S., Franceschi, D., Sedler, M. et al. (2001b). Loss of dopamine transporters in methamphetamine abusers recovers with protracted abstinence. *Journal of Neuroscience*, 21, 9414–18.

Volkow, N. D., Chang, L., Wang, G. J., Fowler, J. S., Franceschi, D., Sedler, M. J. et al. (2001c). Higher cortical and lower subcortical metabolism in detoxified methamphetamine abusers. *American Journal of Psychiatry*, **158**, 383–89.

Volkow, N. D., Chang, L., Wang, G. J., Fowler, J. S., Leonido-Yee, M., Franceschi, D. et al. (2001d). Association of dopamine transporter reduction with psychomotor impairment in methamphetamine abusers. *American Journal of Psychiatry*, **158**, 377–82.

Volkow, N. D., Fowler, J. S., and Wang, G. J. (2003). The addicted human brain: insights from imaging studies. *Journal of Clinical Investigation*, **111**, 1444–51.

Volkow, N. D., Fowler, J. S., and Wang, G. J. (2004). The addicted human brain viewed in the light of imaging studies: brain circuits and treatment strategies. *Neuropharmacology*, **47**, 3–13.

Wang, G. J., Volkow, N. D., Fowler, J. S., Logan, J., Abumrad, N. N., Hitzemann, R. J. et al. (1997). Dopamine D-2 receptor availability in opiate-dependent subjects before and after naloxone-precipitated withdrawal. *Neuropsychopharmacology*, **16**, 174–82.

Wang, G. J., Volkow, N. D., Chang, L., Miller, E., Sedler, M., Hitzemann, R. et al. (2004). Partial recovery of brain metabolism in methamphetamine abusers after protracted abstinence. *American Journal of Psychiatry*, **161**, 242–8.

Weinstein, C. S. and Shaffer, H. J. (1993). Neurocognitive aspects of substance-abuse treatment—a psychotherapists primer. *Psychotherapy*, **30**, 317–33.

White, F. J. and Kalivas, P. W. (1998). Neuroadaptations involved in amphetamine and cocaine addiction. *Drug and Alcohol Dependence*, **51**, 141–53.

WHO (2004). *Neuroscience of psychoactive substance use and dependence*. Geneva, CH: WHO Publications.

Woicik, P. A., Moeller, S. J., Alia-Klein, N., Maloney, T., Lukasik, T. M., Yeliosof, O. et al. (2008). The neuropsychology of cocaine addiction: recent cocaine use masks impairment. *Neuropsychopharmacology*, **34**(5), 1360.

Woods, S. P., Rippeth, J. D., Conover, E., Gongvatana, A., Gonzalez, R., Carey, C. L. et al. (2005). Deficient strategic control of verbal encoding and retrieval in individuals with methamphetamine dependence. *Neuropsychology*, **19**, 35–43.

Yucel, M., Lubman, D. I., Harrison, B. J., Fornito, A., Allen, N. B., Wellard, R. M. et al. (2007). A combined spectroscopic and functional MRI investigation of the dorsal anterior cingulate region in opiate addiction. *Mol Psychiatry*, **12**, 691–702.

Chapter 23

Depression and resilience: insights from cognitive, neuroimaging, and psychopharmacological studies

Barbara J. Sahakian and Sharon Morein-Zamir

Abstract

Depressive disorders are amongst the leading causes of disability worldwide. Cognitive abnormalities are core to depression, as evidenced by the daily life experiences of patients with mood disorders, and are integral to diagnostic criteria. Indeed, these cognitive problems may impair performance of everyday functioning. For example, negative attentional bias and abnormal response to negative feedback are core cognitive characteristics in depression and are likely contributors to negative impact on quality of life in depressed patients. The results from cognition, neuroimaging, and psychopharmacological studies indicate that general underlying processes, such as negative attentional bias and abnormal response to negative or error feedback, are core cognitive impairments in major depressive disorder (MDD) which may account for broad-ranging cognitive deficits. Furthermore, results from functional imaging studies in unmedicated MDD patients, suggest that disrupted top-down control by the prefrontal cortex of the amygdala underlies the hypersensitivity to negative feedback in MDD. Additional findings indicate a role of serotonin and, more recently, dopamine, in the modulation of performance on tests of attentional bias and response to error feedback. Examining these processes in healthy individuals, such as the presence and maintenance of positive affective biases and the ability to exert cognitive control over an emotional response, provide an opportunity to gauge markers of resilience. It is concluded that negative attentional bias and abnormal response to negative or error feedback may be useful cognitive biomarkers in early detection of symptoms and monitoring of relapse in depression, and in assessing the efficacy of current and novel pharmacological and psychological treatments.

23.1 **Introduction**

The symptoms of depression include persistent low mood, feelings of helplessness, hope-lessness, or worthlessness, and anhedonia, or the inability to experience pleasure. Mood is influenced by a complex interaction of genetic, social, environmental, and other fac-tors, such as substance abuse. Depression is further characterized by dysfunctional atti-tudes and negative automatic thoughts or ruminations. Psychiatric diagnostic criteria distinguish patients who experience only depressive episodes (unipolar depression or major depressive disorder, MDD) from patients who experience depressive episodes but also manic ones (bipolar disorder, BD). The symptoms of mania, on the other hand, include euphoria, over-activity, distractibility, socially inappropriate behavior, increased appetite, and impaired insight (American Psychiatric Association, 2000). Thus, the emo-tional states of patients with depression and mania can be considered to represent two polar extremes on a mood spectrum. The states manifested in depression and mania are pathological in that they are extreme, disrupt quality of life, and are persistent and often recurrent (Chamberlain and Sahakian, 2004; Robinson and Sahakian, 2008). In this chapter, we examine not only depression in MDD, but also contrast it with the, at times similar but at times diametrically opposed, symptoms of other disorders, such as BD, to achieve better insight. Moreover, this aim is strengthened by also examining resilience in healthy individuals, i.e., how can mood remain normal despite factors such as adverse life events. Research on resilience has focused on determining the protective factors that allow some individuals to have more positive outcomes, despite being exposed to a variety of stressors.

MDD is the most common of all psychiatric disorders, with a lifetime risk of 7–12% in men and 20–25% in women (Kessler et al., 2005; Weissman et al., 1996). An estimated 6% of children aged 9–17 are affected by depression. This leads to an estimate of 50.8 mil-lion people worldwide affected by depression and 14.1 million affected by bipolar disor-der. It is not surprising, therefore, that depression is the leading cause of disability and bipolar disorder ranked number six, with MDD also ranking as the leading cause of years of life lived with disability (WHO, 2001). These disorders not only impact the sufferers, but also their families and care-takers (Beddington et al., 2008). Mood disorders are also costly to the economy, with the economic burden estimated at approximately $44 billion dollars in the USA in one year (Greenberg et al., 2003). Total cost of treatment for depres-sion in the UK alone is about £230 million pounds (McCrone et al., 2008). Antidepressants, which potentiate monoamine and primarily serotonin (5-HT) neurotransmission as well as psychological cognitive therapy, are the first-line treatments for major depression (Academy of Medical Sciences Report, 2008; DeRubeis et al., 2008; Nutt, 2002).

23.1.1 **Cognition in depression**

Individuals with depression suffer from cognitive impairment across a broad range of domains (Chamberlain and Sahakian, 2004, 2005; Taylor Tavares et al., 2003). In fact, the DSM-IV criteria for major depressive episode and manic episode include cognitive symp-toms. For depression, the criteria include diminished ability to think or concentrate, or indecisiveness nearly everyday. This impaired cognition can affect daily functioning in some depressed patients (Jeager et al., 2006). In severely ill patients, cognitive deficits may also be expected to impair ability to engage with psychological treatment (Murphy et al., 1998, 1999). In fact, cognitive difficulties may impact on the ability to perform successfully at work and, therefore, may prove the biggest barrier for rehabilitation, as is the case for schizophrenia (Goldberg et al., 1993; Taylor Tavares et al., 2007; Zarate et al., 2000).

Neuropsychological testing has confirmed marked deficits across a broad range of cognitive functions. Cognitive impairments are frequently found to disappear on remission from depression, suggesting that mood interacts with the ability to perform some cognitive tasks. Nonetheless, cognitive deficits persist in some patients, even in remission and when controlling for residual mood symptoms (e.g., Clark et al., 2002; Rubinsztein et al., 2000; see also Abas et al., 1990). Particularly in BD, cognitive symptoms may be the most sensitive indicators of incomplete remission and may, in addition, pose a barrier to effective rehabilitation (Murphy et al., 1998; Rogers et al., 2003; Roiser et al., 2003). Cognitive impairment in depression also appears to become greater with age, relative to controls (Beats et al., 1996; Elliott et al., 1996; Purcell et al., 1997; Sweeney et al., 2000). This may be mediated by the number of episodes and duration of depression (Kessing, 1998).

Cognitive functions impaired in MDD include attention, memory functions, psychomotor abilities, and executive control, where executive control encompass higher level cognitive functions involved in the flexible organization of behavior, including working memory, forward planning, and behavioral inhibition. Specifically, impairments are seen on a wide array of neuropsychological tests of executive function, including cognitive flexibility, planning, spatial working memory, and tests of visual memory, such as delayed matching to sample, which are subserved by neurocircuitry involving the frontal lobes and hippocampal formation, respectively (Beats et al., 1996; Purcell et al., 1997; Taylor Tavares et al., 2003). DSM-IV criteria for mania also include cognitive symptoms including distractibility, and excessive involvement in pleasurable activities that have a high potential for painful consequences. As expected, numerous studies of bipolar patients in the *manic* phase of their illness also found broad neuropsychological impairments in standard tests of memory, executive function, and attention (Clark and Sahakian, 2008). More importantly, *depressed* bipolar patients were also found to be impaired on tests of memory and executive functioning, such as cognitive flexibility and decision making (Martinez-Aran et al., 2004; Rubinsztein et al., 2006).

Based on the somewhat similar deficits in tests of memory and planning between MDD and depressed BD, it has been argued that similar, rather than opposite, processes are involved in both, despite markedly different clinical presentations (Johnson and Magaro, 1987).Some studies have reported comparable impairments in patients with BD in depressed state, relative to patients with MDD (Kessing, 1998; Sweeney et al., 2000). Yet other studies have found worse performance on measures of memory, and executive and attentional functions in medicated depressed BD, compared to MDD individuals (Borkowska and Rybakowski, 2001; Wolfe et al., 1987). When considering this evidence, it is also important to note that medication regimes in BD and MDD differ considerably. Whereas serotonin selective reuptake inhibitors (SSRIs) are typical for MDD, the usual treatment for BD includes mood stabilizers, antipsychotics, or both. Taylor Tavares and colleagues compared unmedicated MDD and depressed BD patients to address this issue. The two groups scored similarly on the scales of depressive symptomology, anxiety, and mania, and had been off medication for a substantial and comparable length of time. Their results suggested that the unmedicated depressed BD subjects demonstrated generally intact performance compared to controls in a wide range of neuropsychological domains, including memory function, executive function, and decision making. Unmedicated MDD patients displayed a number of impairments, primarily in executive functioning, such as spatial working memory, cognitive flexibility, and decision making (Taylor Tavares et al., 2007).

23.1.2 Abnormal neural networks in depression

Despite the widespread cognitive impairments, there are specific neural substrates that appear key to MDD and BD. Neuroanatomical, neuroimaging, and neuropsychological studies in brain-damaged patient research have revealed differences between "hot" and "cold" processing, though they are not completely distinct and many tasks involve both (see Roiser et al 2003). Cold, or emotion-independent processing, is believed to utilize neuroanatomical loops involving the dorsolateral prefrontal cortex (PFC). Hot, or emotion-dependent processing, is involved in tasks using affective material or that produce an emotional response. Hot processing is thought to utilize the limbic-cortical-striatal-pallidal-thalamic circuits formed by connections between the orbital and medial PFC, amygdala, hippocampus, ventromedial striatum, several thalamic nuclei, and ventral pallidum (Drevets et al., 2008a; Mayberg, 2002; Ongur et al., 2003). The orbital and medial PFC are further associated with two extended cortical circuits. One circuit codes the affective characteristics of stimuli, involving the orbito-prefrontal network and sensory association areas. The other circuit is involved in interoceptive functions, such as mood and emotion, and involves the medial prefrontal network, the dorsomedial and dorsolateral PFC, the cingulate gyrus, as well as visceral control structures such as the hypothalamus (Drevets et al., 2008a). Impairments in these hot processing circuits may, directly or indirectly, adversely influence emotional, motivational, cognitive, and behavioral manifestations of mood disorders (Kyte et al., 2005). The affective circuits are especially modulated by monoamine neurotransmitters, such as serotonin and dopamine (Phillips et al., 2003a). Though serotonin has long been implicated as playing an important role in depression, in recent years there has been an increasing focus on dopamine as well. Mood disorders have also been associated with abnormalities in glutamine and gamma-aminobutyric acid (GABA), as well as additional neurotransmitters such as noradrenaline, acetylcholine, glucocorticoids, and peptides (e.g., corticotrophin releasing factor) (Drevets et al., 2008a).

There is considerable evidence for structural and functional neuroanatomical or neuropathological changes in regions important for emotion processing in depressed patients. For example, postmortem studies on depressed patients have found reduced cell numbers and density in the amygdala (Bowley et al., 2002), the subgenual anterior cingulate gyrus, and orbitofrontal cortex (Cotter et al., 2001; Drevets et al., 1998; Ongur et al., 1998), and the dorsolateral PFC (Rajkowska et al., 1999, 2001). Similarly, in patients with BD, reduced cell number and density was found in PFC, subgenual anterior cingulate gyrus, and hippocampus (Rajkowska et al., 2001). Structural neuroimaging methods have also reported volume reductions in a wide array of brain structures in MDD, including the orbitofrontal cortex, the putamen, and caudate nucleus, and the amygdala and hippocampus, (e.g., Bremner et al., 2000, 2002; Campbell, et al., 2004; Drevets et al., 2008a; Videbech and Ravnkilde, 2004). Hippocampal volume reductions appear to increase with increasing number of episodes and duration of illness (Bell-McGinty et al., 2002; MacQueen et al., 2003). Though structural differences have also been noted in bipolar patients in areas such as the PFC, the caudate, the temporal lobes, and the amygdala, it remains unclear whether the brain abnormalities are associated with the depressive, euthymic, or manic phases of the disorder (Phillips et al., 2003b).

Brain-imaging techniques have also provided insight into the underlying neurochemistry of mood disorders. For example positron emission tomography (PET) imaging studies have used receptor-selective tracers to examine the binding potential (BP) of various neurotransmitters, and have demonstrated abnormal receptor densities of serotonin and dopamine in depressed individuals. For instance, unmedicated MDD patients, who were compared to healthy controls, showed a 41% reduction in 5-HT1A binding potential in the raphe nucleus, the source of the ascending serotonin projection, coupled with a 27% reduction in BP in the medial temporal lobe, incorporating hippocampus and amygdala (Drevets, 1999). More recently, unmedicated MDD patients were also found to have reduced dopamine D1 receptor binding in the left middle caudate, which correlated negatively with illness duration, and which is the target of afferent neural projections from the orbitofrontal and anterior cingulate cortices (Cannon et al., 2009; see also Dougherty et al., 2006).

Importantly, a region of the PFC has been highlighted in numerous positron emission tomography (PET) studies, using cerebral blood flow and rate of glucose metabolism, as a key area to be both structurally and functionally abnormal in depression (Drevets et al., 1997). Specifically, metabolic activity in the subgenual PFC, which lies in the ventromedial prefrontal cortex (VMPFC), was found to be overactive during periods of unipolar and bipolar depression, when the metabolic data was corrected for volumetric deficits (Drevets et al., 2008a, 2008b). The subgenual PFC (Brodmann's Area, BA 25/24) appears to be involved in emotional experience, regulation, and processing (Ressler and Mayberg, 2007). The rostral anterior cingulate has been further highlighted by Mayberg and colleagues as a key area in response to treatment in depression, with their studies also identifying functional *hyperactivity* in the subgenual cingulate during depression (Mayberg, 2003). Specifically, the rostral anterior cingulate metabolism predicted antidepressant psychopharmacological treatment response, whereby higher pretreatment metabolism correlated with eventual improvement (Mayberg et al., 1997; Saxena et al., 2003). When comparing to controls, responders were differentiated as initially hypermetabolic in the rostral anterior cingulate, whereas nonresponders were hypometabolic (Mayberg et al., 1997). Additional studies have compared metabolism in the same depressed individuals, before and after treatment. The metabolism in this area, along with that in related neural circuitry, decreased upon recovery from depression following pharmacological treatment, as well as cognitive behavioral therapy (CBT) (e.g., Kennedy et al., 2001, 2007; see also Ressler and Mayberg, 2007). Interestingly, subjects who were randomized to placebo, but also showed a natural recovery from symptoms of depression, also had decreased activity in the subgenual cingulate, compared to their initial baseline. Thus, it has been proposed that the rostral cingulate area plays a critical role in abnormal mood states, serving as a facilitator of interactions between limbic and frontal brain regions (Kennedy et al., 2001), and that it may be used as a potential predictor of treatment response (Mayberg, 1997). Accordingly, chronic deep brain stimulation (DBS) to the subgenual cingulate cortex can reduce depression symptoms in patients with severe refractory depression (Lozano et al., 2008; Mayberg et al., 2005).

23.2 Exploring two core cognitive features in depression

Attentional biases and an abnormal response to negative feedback in depression have been proposed to be core cognitive features that relate to the symptomatology, e.g., dysfunctional attitudes, negative automatic thoughts, and anhedonia. Therefore it would be expected that these must be effectively treated for patients to have complete recovery and rehabilitation. Distortions of cognitive processing by affective factors are at the core of many influential theories of depression. Both an emotional processing bias and abnormal response to negative feedback are consistent with clinical accounts, such as Beck's cognitive theory of depression (Beck, 1967, 1976). A negative processing bias is consistent with the dysfunctional negative schemas that are used to interpret incoming experience. The distorted thought process and an automatic tendency to distort environmental information in a negative manner play a role in the development and maintenance of the affective, physiological, and behavioral components of depression (Robinson and Sahakian, 2008). Consistent with the abnormal response to negative feedback account, research in the area of social cognition has likewise suggested that depressed individuals often magnify the significance of failure and have difficulty suppressing failure-related thoughts (Conway et al., 1991; Gotlib, 1983). Such negative cognitions are an important target for treatment in CBT for depression and anxiety (see Salkovskis, 1997).

23.2.1 Cognitive biases to sad stimuli

The approach of studying emotional biases has the advantage of explicitly linking mood and cognition in a manner that can be related to cognitive behavioral theories of depression, on which treatment strategies have been based. Thus, patients with depression may be differentially sensitive to negatively toned information and process it more effectively. Previous evidence has suggested that patients with depression are more likely to recall negative autobiographical memories, and when they do recall positive experiences, they are lacking in detail (Brittlebank et al., 1993). This could reinforce depressed mood and contribute to the maintenance of the disorder (Elliott et al., 2002)

The affective go/no-go task was developed to address processing of emotional stimuli within the context of inhibitory control. The use of words as emotional stimuli has the ability to trigger the patients' own semantic network of negative automatic thoughts (Elliott et al., 2000). In this task, participants are presented with word blocks, each contained affectively valenced words. The words are presented one at a time on a computer screen and the participants are instructed to respond to each word by pressing a button to one category of words (e.g., happy words, such as joyful, success, and confident) and to refrain from pressing to another category of words (e.g., sad words, such as gloomy, hopeless, and failure), where each category is presented half of the time in an unpredictable order. On different blocks, the instructions are reversed, so at times participants must respond to the sad words and withhold responding to happy words. The task assesses attentional processing bias as the speed of responding to the target emotional stimuli, and at the same time assesses inhibitory control as refraining from having attention grabbed by distracting emotional stimuli.

In an initial study, medicated MDD patients, diagnosed according to DSM-IV criteria, with mild to moderate depression severity were compared to age, verbal-IQ, and gender-matched healthy controls (Murphy et al., 1999). The patients were slower to respond to happy compared to sad word targets. The healthy controls, on the other hand, had similar response latencies for sad and happy targets. This study also included a group of matched BD manic-episode patients. As opposed to the other two groups, the manic patients were faster to respond to happy compared to sad word targets. Likewise, the manic patients made considerably more commission errors, pressing rather than withholding, and omission errors, withholding rather than pressing, suggesting they were also impaired in inhibiting responses to irrelevant stimuli. The contrasting patterns of affective processing in the depressed and manic groups are consistent with their respective clinical descriptions. When examining an affective bias in depressed bipolar patients and in bipolar patients in remission, an attentional bias was not evident on the affective go/no-go task (Rubinsztein et al., 2000, 2006).

Following up on these results, the affective go/no-go task was examined in a group of unmedicated MDD patients to ascertain the possible role of medication (Erickson et al., 2005). Again, participants with MDD required more time to respond to happy than to sad words. Additionally, they made more omission errors when responding to happy than to sad words. Taken together, the results suggest a perseveration of a mood-congruent processing bias, within the context of an attention deficit, regardless of pharmacological treatment. Importantly, in this and later studies, the healthy participants required more time to respond to sad than to happy words and made more omission/target errors when responding to sad words. This positive bias may confer resilience against the psychological impact of negative life events. Presently, the extent, consistency over time, and role of individual differences in mood-congruent biases in healthy people remains to be elucidated.

Neuroimaging studies have adapted the affective go/no-go task to the functional magnetic resonance imaging (fMRI) environment to examine the neural correlates of affective processing in adult healthy, depressed, and manic groups. These studies have added neutral–neutral blocks as baseline, in addition to neutral–sad and neutral–happy blocks, where neutral words act as targets or distractors. An initial study on healthy volunteers found activations in the subgenual cingulate region in response to emotional compared to neutral targets (Elliott et al., 2000), in the same region previously reported as abnormal in MDD and BD groups (Drevets et al., 1997). In addition, the hippocampal gyri and the insula were also activated for emotional compared to neutral targets. There was increased ventral anterior cingulate activation (although dorsal to the subgenual region) for happy relative to sad targets, and there were no differential neural responses reflecting differences in the emotional valence of distractors.

When compared to the healthy group, a group of medicated depressed patients showed attenuated neural response to emotional, relative to neutral, targets in cortical and subcortical structures, including the medial PFC, extending from rostral ventral cingulate (BA 32/24) to the medial PFC (BA 9/10), as well as posterior orbitofrontal cortices, the insula, and thalamus (Elliott et al., 2002). The attenuation was more pronounced for happy than sad targets. The attenuation to emotional responses in the ventral anterior cingulate adjacent to the subgenual region, suggests that a functional abnormality here might mediate emotional modulation of cognitive processing (see Fig. 23.1). Additionally, there was an elevated response, specific to sad targets, in depressed individuals, in rostral anterior cingulate, extending to anterior medial PFC. This region also responded more strongly to happy targets in the healthy volunteers. Moreover, unlike the healthy volunteers, depressed patients showed a differential neural response to emotional, particularly sad, distractors in the right, lateral, orbitofrontal cortex (BA 11/47) suggesting attention is "grabbed" by sad distractors in depression. This latter finding is consistent with behavioral evidence from first-episode depressed adolescents, where attention is captured by sad distractors in depression (Kyte et al., 2005).

Elliott and colleagues (2004) also scanned a group of medicated manic patients on the affective go/no-go task. They found that, compared to the group of healthy controls, attention is grabbed by happy distractors in mania patients, as these patients showed enhanced responses to happy distractors in bilateral dorsolateral PFC (BA 46) and subgenual cingulate, extending to medial orbitofrontal cortex (BA 10). Mania patients also showed an enhanced response to sad relative to neutral distractors in right dorsolateral (BA 9/46) and ventrolateral (BA 44/45) PFC. Additionally, the manic patients showed enhanced response of the left ventrolateral region to emotional relative to neutral targets (Elliott et al., 2004).

Taken together, the results for processing biases to happy and sad stimuli are largely congruent with symptomology. Depressed patients show a bias to sad stimuli, which is not related to medication. This bias appears to be evident, even in first-episode depression in adolescence. Manic patients show an exaggerated bias to happy stimuli, compared to healthy volunteers. Thus, the affective go/no-go task may prove useful in detecting at-risk populations and for assessing treatment efficacy in mania and depression. The bias to happy stimuli often observed in healthy volunteers may be indicative of resilience against depression.

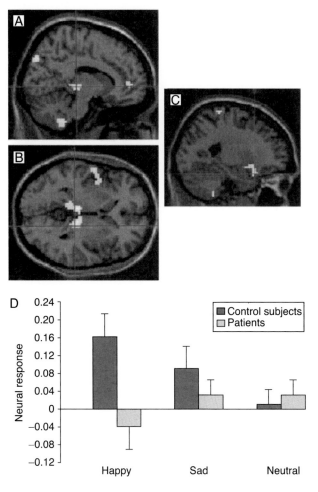

Fig. 23.1 Regions where attenuated neural response to emotional compared with neutral targets was seen in patients (n = 10) relative to control subjects (n = 11). Significantly attenuated neural response in the ventral cingulate (A), pulvinar (B), and inferior frontal gyrus (C) is shown superimposed on a standard structural magnetic resonance image template. (D) Relative adjusted neural response (no units) in ventral cingulate to different types of targets in patients (n = 10) and controls (n = 11), with matched distractor types. Error bars represent SE. Similar patterns of response are seen in the thalamus, posterior orbitofrontal cortex, and insula.

Reproduced from Elliott et al., 2002, *Archives of General Psychiatry*; 59:597–604. Copyright © American Medical Association, 2002.

23.2.2 Oversensitivity to negative feedback

In one study, compared with age- and IQ-matched controls, 93% of depressed patients showed some degree of impairment, and most of these were impaired across several cognitive domains (Elliott et al., 1996). Following the observations of catastrophic reactions to perceived failure, Sahakian and colleagues questioned whether the observed cognitive deficits in depression could be explained by some general underlying process (Beats et al., 1996). The notion of "abnormal response to negative feedback" in depressed individuals is of a fundamental impairment of cognition, which could potentially represent an important link between negative affect and many of the cognitive impairments associated with depression (Elliott et al., 1996). Preliminary evidence supporting this notion was found in two computerized tests from the Cambridge Neuropsychological Test Automated Battery (CANTAB)—Simultaneous and Delayed Matching-to-Sample (SDMTS) and the one-touch Tower of London (TOL)—where failure on one problem led to disproportionate increases in the probability of failure on the immediately subsequent problem in depressed patients (see Fig. 23.2). This suggested that negative feedback had an abnormal detrimental effect on subsequent performance in depression (Elliott et al., 1997a). Additional studies established that this abnormal response to negative feedback appears to be *specific* to depression, as it was not found in other clinical groups such as patients with Parkinson's disease, schizophrenia, or neurosurgical lesions of frontal or temporal lobes (Elliott et al., 1997a).

Nevertheless, the results from the initial studies were only suggestive and it remained unclear to what extent the "abnormal response" observed in depressed patients was due to impairment in processing the information qualities or the affective qualities of the feedback. The probabilistic reversal learning task with misleading negative feedback was thus employed to determine whether depressed patients are specifically impaired in their ability to use the information conveyed by negative feedback to facilitate task performance. The probabilistic reversal task requires that individuals learn in situations where the feedback provided is unclear and potentially inconsistent (Swainson et al., 2000). In this way, the task resembles everyday learning. In an initial stage participants must chose between two visual stimuli and learn which is the "correct" one. They are told to always select the stimulus that is *usually* correct, but also that at some point the rule may change so that the other stimulus is now usually correct. Crucially, only 80% of responses to the "correct" stimulus resulted in positive feedback, while 20% of correct responses resulted in negative feedback. Likewise, only 80% of responses to the "incorrect" stimulus resulted in negative feedback. The feedback comprises both a verbal message on the computer

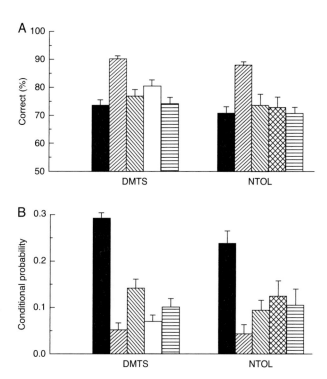

Fig. 23.2 The percentage of problems solved correctly (A) and conditional probabilities of failing problem x+1 having just failed problem x (B) on the DMTS and one touch tower tests for depressed patients, controls, patients with Parkinson's disease, neurosurgical patients, and patients with schizophrenia. Bars represent SEM.

Reproduced from Elliott et al., 1997, *Journal of Neurology, Neurosurgery and Psychiatry*; 63:74–82. Copyright © BMJ Publishing Group Ltd., 1997.

screen, as well as an accompanying sound. In the second stage, the contingencies are reversed, so that the previous "incorrect" stimulus now becomes "correct."

When medicated depressed patients performed the probabilistic reversal task, they showed intact levels of rule acquisition and normal levels of response perseveration when the rule actually reversed. However, the patients were impaired in their ability to maintain response set in the face of the intermittent misleading negative feedback (Murphy et al., 2003). They were significantly more likely than controls to switch their response to the "incorrect" stimulus following the imperfect negative feedback for the "correct" stimulus in both stages of the task (Murphy et al., 2003). The impairment in depressed individuals in the task was distinct from that found in additional patient groups, such Huntington's disease (Lawrence et al., 1998), Parkinson's disease, and those with damage to the frontal or temporal lobes (Swainson et al., 2000). At the same time, depressed patients were unimpaired in their ability to use accurate negative feedback to facilitate their performance in an additional working memory test, suggesting that, when the negative feedback was both accurate and informative, they were as likely, and not more so, as healthy individuals to utilize the feedback (Murphy et al., 2003).

Taylor Tavares and colleagues (2008) examined the neural mechanism by which the normal processing of feedback is dysfunctional in depressed individuals, using fMRI. They studied unmedicated depressed participants to distinguish the neural activity related to the processing of negative feedback from the neural activity related to behavioral reversal, which previously appeared unimpaired behaviorally in depressed patients. Investigating unmedicated participants was particularly important, as feedback processing is known to be modulated by antidepressant drugs (Chamberlain et al., 2006), and the hemodynamic parameters that compose the fMRI signal may be altered by the psychotropic drug effects (see below for further details). This study employed a variant of the probabilistic reversal learning task adapted for event-related fMRI (Cools et al., 2002), enabling the implementation of multiple discrimination stages and therefore numerous reversals across sessions. A rule reversal occurred every 10–15 correct responses, and misleading negative feedback (probabilistic errors) was presented in a pseudo-random sequence on approximately 20% of trials, resulting in 0–4 probabilistic errors per discrimination stage. Abstract visual stimuli were used to limit rule verbalization, and positive and negative feedback were happy, green, smiley and sad, red faces, respectively.

As evidenced in the medicated depressed patients, the unmedicated patients also demonstrated oversensitivity to negative feedback by being more likely to switch their response, than healthy controls, after misleading negative feedback (see Fig. 23.3). Other types of errors did not differ across groups, suggesting the results did not merely reflect an increase in incorrect responses. When examining the neural correlates, the controls recruited the bilateral ventrolateral PFC and dorsomedial PFC regions of interest on trials in which misleading negative feedback triggered reversal, compared to trials in which misleading negative feedback did not precipitate reversal (see also: Cools et al., 2002; Evers et al., 2005). In contrast, the depressed group failed to recruit the ventrolateral PFC and dorsomedial PFC on trials where negative feedback triggered reversal. The fMRI data confirmed that this network was also recruited during appropriate reversal switches in the healthy controls. Thus, there was greater dorsomedial PFC activation in healthy participants following negative feedback, compared to depressed participants. There was also greater ventrolateral PFC activation in healthy participants following misleading negative feedback that resulted in a response switch, compared to depressed participants.

Importantly, there was also greater right amygdala "deactivation" in the healthy controls during negative-feedback trials, compared to depressed individuals. The greater the "deactivation" of right amygdala to all negative feedback, the less likely healthy controls were to switch following misleading negative feedback. This correlation was absent in the depressed individuals (see Fig. 23.4). Thus, the reduced amygdala activity in healthy controls during receipt of negative feedback was directly predictive of their ability to suppress

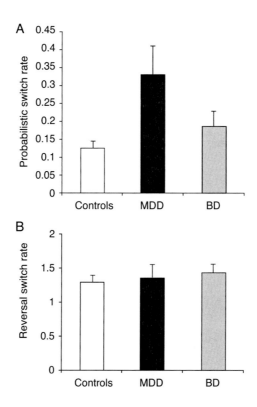

Fig. 23.3 Subjects with Major Depressive Disorder (MDD) were oversensitive to misleading negative feedback. (A) The probabilistic switch rate (the number of reversals after misleading negative feedback/total number of probabilistic errors) was increased in the MDD group compared to healthy controls, and tended to be higher in the MDD subjects than in the subjects with bipolar disorder (BD), who displayed a similar degree of depression. (B) There were no differences between the three groups in the reversal switch rate (the number of reversal errors/total number of rule reversals). Error bars depict standard error of the mean.

Reproduced from Taylor Tavares et al., *NeuroImage* 2008; 42:1118–26. Copyright © Elsevier, 2008.

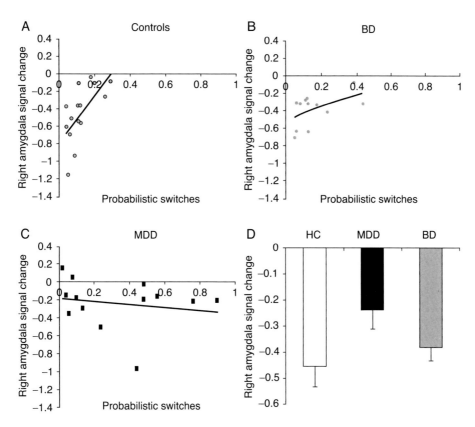

Fig. 23.4 Scatter graphs depicting the relationship between the signal change in the right amygdala during receipt of negative feedback (minus the correct response baseline) and the probabilistic switch rate. The probabilistic switch rate was calculated from the total number of response reversals after misleading negative feedback, divided by the total number of trials where misleading negative feedback was presented. (A) The correlation between the amygdala response to negative feedback and the probabilistic switch ratewas significant in the healthy control (HC) group (r = 0.63, p = 0.011) and (B) was apparent at trend level in the bipolar depressed group (BD) (r = 0.50, p = 0.096). (C) There was no significant association between right amygdala response and probabilistic switch rate in the major depressive disorder (MDD) group (r = −0.16, p = 0.59), and the correlation between HC and MDD groups differed significantly (Fisher's r to z: z = 2.13 p = 0.033). (D) For the all negative feedback contrast there was less of a reduction in right amygdala activity in the MDD group compared to the HC group (p = 0.05). Error bars depict standard error of the mean.

Reproduced from Taylor Tavares et al., *NeuroImage* 2008; 42:1118–26. Copyright © Elsevier, 2008.

the reversal in response to misleading negative feedback. This amygdala effect was attenuated in the depressed group and was not associated with behavioral performance.

Taylor Tavares and colleagues (2008) also examined the abnormal response to negative feedback and its neural correlates in a group of unmedicated depressed patients with bipolar disorder. When the patients with bipolar disorder, who displayed a similar degree of depression compared to the MDD patients, were tested on the reversal task, there were no significant differences in behavioral performance, as compared with healthy control subjects. Moreover, there were also no significant differences in the patterns of neural activity between the bipolar patients and the healthy controls, with the patients showing increased activity in dorsal and lateral PFC, and a negative correlation between amygdala activation and the suppression of a reversal in response to misleading negative feedback (Taylor Tavares et al., 2008).

In sum, depressed subjects, but not bipolar disorder subjects, showed attenuated PFC responses during reversal shifting and additionally failed to deactivate the amygdala in response to misleading feedback relative to positive feedback. This latter response was predictive of healthy subjects' capacity to ignore immediate misleading feedback. This effect has implications for resilience to stressful uncontrollable situations (e.g. learned helplessness), as the suppression of amygdala response appears adaptive in healthy individuals. The increased activity in PFC in healthy controls may be associated with attempts to exert cognitive control over an emotional response. This is consistent with recent work that has suggested that lateral and medial PFC may implement top-down control over amygdala activation in situations where subjects must inhibit or reappraise emotional responses to negatively valenced stimuli (Ochsner et al., 2002; Pezawas et al., 2005; Phelps and LeDoux, 2005). The data also suggest complementary mechanisms in PFC and limbic circuitry for utilizing trial-by-trial feedback to optimize task performance. In sum, this functional neuroimaging study in unmedicated depressed patients demonstrated disrupted top-down control by the PFC of the amygdala that leads to the hypersensitivity to negative feedback found in major depressive disorder. Notably, abnormalities in response to misleading negative feedback appeared specific to unipolar depressive illness, as they did not extend to BD subjects who scored similarly on depression severity ratings.

Converging evidence for the specificity of sensitivity to negative feedback in MDD was also found using a very different decision-making task. In the Cambridge Gamble Task, participants are presented with a display of 10 boxes, colored red or blue. They are instructed that the computer has hidden a token inside one of the boxes. The ratio of red:blue boxes varies across trials from 6:4, 7:3, 8:2, to 9:1. On each trial, the participants must first decide whether the token is hidden in a red or blue box and must then stake a percentage of their current points on their choice. After betting, the location of the token is revealed, and the bet is added or deducted from their total score, as appropriate. Notably, unmedicated MDD patients, unlike unmedicated depressed BD patient, were more sensitive to loss on this task, resulting in poorer quality decision making the trial following a loss but not a win (Taylor Tavares et al., 2007). In MDD patients, there was also a correlation between hypersensitivity to loss on the gambling task and anhedonia ratings, so that patients with increased sensitivity to loss also had higher scores of anhedonia. This in turn suggests that an inability to feel pleasure may underlie the oversensitivity to negative feedback. As such, anhedonia appears to reflect both a blunting of positive-reinforcement processing, as well as an inability to use negative feedback to improve task performance (Clark et al., 2009).

To conclude, oversensitivity to negative feedback may be core and specific to the diagnosis of MDD, as it is not typically found in either manic or depressed BD patients. Pharmacological and psychological treatments that target this oversensitivity are likely to be more effective, both in initial treatment and in preventing relapse of depression in MDD.

23.3 The role of serotonin in the core cognitive features

As noted above, many neurotransmitters are likely involved in the abnormal mood and cognition in depression. Of these, serotonin (5-hydroxytryptamine or 5-HT) has received the most attention due to its role in the regulation of emotional behavior, and its implication in the pathophysiology of depression (Schatzberg et al., 2002). The "indoleamine hypothesis" and the "serotonin hypothesis" posit that depression is associated with reduced levels of serotonin or, alternatively, abnormal numbers or sensitivity of serotonin receptors in relevant neural regions (Clark and Sahakian, 2006; Coppen et al., 1972; Yatham et al., 2000). Considerable evidence supports the key role of serotonin in depression. Serotonin selective reuptake inhibitors (SSRIs), that increase levels of serotonin in the synapse, are effective antidepressant agents and are currently the drug of choice in treating depression (Ackerman et al., 2002; Cowen, 1990). Likewise, reducing brain serotonin via tryptophan depletion (see below) in recovered depressives reinstates depressed mood (Delgado et al., 1990; Smith et al., 1997). There is also evidence for a role of the serotonin transporter polymorphism in affective disorders and in treatment response to SSRIs (e.g., Furlong et al., 1999; Serretti et al., 2005; Zanardi et al., 2001). To probe the role of serotonin in cognition and emotion in healthy volunteers and patients, pharmacological and dietary manipulations can be used. Specifically, it would be expected that biases to affective stimuli and oversensitivity to negative feedback would be sensitive to such serotonergic manipulations. Interestingly, administration of a single dose of the SSRI citalopram was found to increase sensitivity to misleading negative feedback in healthy volunteers, relative to a comparable group who received placebo. Thus, the SSRI led to an increased likelihood to shift responding away from the correct stimulus, similar to the effects seen in MDD (Chamberlain et al., 2006). The authors interpreted this finding as possibly resulting from presynaptic autoreceptor feedback effects leading to temporary reduction in serotonin function following acute dosing, or, alternatively, resulting from supraoptimal PFC serotonin availability (Chamberlain et al., 2006). The same study found that atomoxetine (a selective noradrenaline reuptake inhibitor) had no such effect.

Acute tryptophan depletion (ATD) has also proved an instructive experimental tool in studying how serotonin modulates mood, emotional processing, and cognition in patients, healthy volunteers, and in animals (Bell et al., 2005). Given that the synthesis of serotonin depends on the availability of its amino acid precursor, L-tryptophan, ATD entails the ingestion of an amino acid mixture selectively lacking tryptophan. In addition to a decrease in plasma tryptophan stores, the amino acid load results in competition for the active transport system that the amino acids share for entry across the blood–brain barrier, resulting in a robust lowering of serotonin availability in the brain (Carpenter et al., 1998; Williams et al., 1999). Ingestion of an amino acid drink lacking tryptophan, compared to a balanced drink, produces a 70–90% reduction in plasma tryptophan approximately 6 h following administration (Hood et al., 2005).

As noted above, reducing brain serotonin via ATD in a proportion of recovered depressives reinstated a temporary depressed mood (Booij et al., 2005; Delgado et al., 1990; Smith et al., 1997). This effect appears to be most marked in patients maintained on SSRIs, though mood change in unmedicated remitted major depressive disorder patients has also been reported (Neumeister et al., 2004). Healthy volunteers, without a history of affective illness, rarely show ATD induction of negative mood (Bell et al., 2005; Robinson and Sahakian, 2008). Nevertheless, numerous studies have reported that ATD in healthy humans impairs performance on neuropsychological tasks that have an emotional component and on some of the cognitive functions impaired in depression, though ATD is not associated with global impairments of executive functions, such as planning (e.g., Murphy et al., 2002; Robinson and Sahakian, 2009). For example, it has been reported that ATD impaired decision making on gambling games (Rogers et al., 1999, 2003), attenuated motivation on a reinforced speeded reaction-time task (Cools et al., 2005; Roiser et al., 2006), and impaired episodic long- but not short-term memory (Riedel et al., 1999), as well as recognition of emotional expressions (Harmer, 2008).

Several studies have also examined the effect of ATD on probabilistic reversal learning in healthy humans in order to establish a link between cognitive dysfunction and altered serotonin metabolism in depressive illness. An initial double-blind, placebo-controlled, counterbalanced, cross-over design study found an association between ATD and a general slowing of responses in the probability reversal task in the first session, but a specific deficit in reversing the acquired rule was not observed (Murphy et al., 2002). A similar effect on behavior was noted in a subsequent study that examined the effects of ATD on the blood oxygenation level-dependent (BOLD) response in healthy males during probabilistic reversal learning (Evers et al., 2005). Consistent with previous findings (Cools et al., 2002), behavioral reversal was accompanied by significant signal change in the right ventrolateral and dorsomedial PFC. During negative feedback, ATD led to increased task-related BOLD response in the dorsomedial PFC, but not ventrolateral PFC. The ATD-induced effect in the dorsomedial PFC was not restricted to errors that preceded a behavioral switch, but extended to trials where subjects received negative feedback and did not change their behavior. The increased BOLD signal in the dorsomedial PFC was taken to reflect enhanced processing of aversive signals in ATD, or error feedback, leading to enhanced response conflict on both switch and nonswitch trials. This interpretation was strengthened by a subsequent finding that serotonin depletion selectively enhanced reversal learning from punishment cues (Cools et al., 2008). Hence, ATD appeared to improve the ability of healthy participants to predict whether a stimulus was likely to predict punishment, while having no effect on reward prediction.

The role of serotonin has also been investigated in affective processing using the affective go/no-go task. Relative to placebo, healthy female volunteers performing the task during ATD demonstrated increased response times for happy targets, possibly due to heightened interference from sad distractors (Murphy et al., 2002). Latencies for sad targets, however, were similar following the two treatments, suggesting that, in healthy adults, ATD reduced the bias for happy stimuli, possibly via a reduction in resilience. Though ATD did not influence depressive symptomatology or subjective ratings of mood, the findings parallel the increased reaction times for happy, but not sad, targets found in depressed individuals (Murphy et al., 2002). Similarly, in a subsequent fMRI study on affective bias, though healthy participants did not experience significant mood change, emotional information processing was substantially modified following ATD (Roiser et al., 2008). A highly significant attentional bias toward positive distractors, evident under placebo, was attenuated following tryptophan depletion, and this change was associated with increased BOLD responses to emotionally valenced words, as compared to neutral words, in the ventral striatum, hippocampal complex, insula, and ventrolateral PFC. ATD also increased BOLD response to negative relative to positive words in the STG and posterior cingulate cortex, which have also consistently been implicated in unipolar depression. Increased hemodynamic responses during the processing of emotional words were also noted in several subcortical structures, such as the amygdala, caudate, and parahippocampal gyrus. Participants who became more anxious following tryptophan depletion also showed increased BOLD response in the caudate to negative relative to positive distractors. Notably, BOLD response to emotional words was increased following tryptophan depletion in the same region. The findings also replicated the results of healthy controls without ATD, as responding to emotional relative to neutral words resulted in increased BOLD response in the pregenual ACC region as was previously found in healthy humans (Elliott et al., 2000). The increased neural responses in ventromedial prefrontal and subcortical areas to emotional stimuli were also similar to aberrant neural responses seen in MDD (Elliott et al., 2002).

Though ATD produces changes in emotional processing similar to those seen in acute depression, it has recently been demonstrated to be independent from changes in mood, indicating ATD does not mediate mood (Robinson and Sahakian, 2009). Mood induction to positive, negative, or neutral mood did not influence the affective bias, whether participants were on placebo or following ATD. At the same time, the positive bias found under placebo was abolished following ATD, but only in female participants, suggesting women are more susceptible to the effects of serotonin fluctuation than men. This may, in part, underlie the increased incidence of depression in women and possibly confers some element of resilience to men. Such results suggest that objective measurements of emotional bias measurements may be more sensitive to manipulations of serotonin function than subjective self-reported mood (Chamberlain and Sahakian, 2004; Harmer, 2008).

The influence of serotonin on affective disorders is also likely to be modulated by genetic factors, one of which is the serotonin transporter polymorphism (e.g., Furlong et al., 1999;

Zanardi et al., 2001). The serotonin transporter linked polymorphic region (*5-HTTLPR*) has repeatedly been implicated in gene by environment interactions for disorders of emotional dysregulation and has been associated with increased risk for affective disorders (Canli and Lesch, 2007). Individuals with one or two copies of the short allele of the 5-HT T promoter polymorphism exhibited more depressive symptoms, diagnosable depression, and suicidality in relation to stressful life events than individuals homozygous for the long allele (Caspi et al., 2003). Carriers of the risk-conferring *5-HTTLPR* polymorphism have reduced gray matter volume in the perigenulate region surrounding subgenual PFC, as well as in the amygdala (Ressler and Mayberg, 2007). Likewise, this polymorphism has been associated with greater vulnerability to mood change following serotonin depletion. For example, women homozygous for the s allele at the 5-HT transporter linked polymorphic region (5-HTTLPR) were vulnerable to mood change following ATD, while those homozygous for the l allele did not show mood change (Neumeister et al., 2002). An investigation of the effect of ATD on affective bias in healthy volunteers of ll and ss genotypes at the 5-HTTLPR, however, did not find any differences between them (Roiser et al., 2007). Polymorphism in the serotonin transporter gene did however play a role in affective bias in ecstasy users (3,4-methylenedioxymethamphetamine or MDMA) (Roiser et al., 2005a). Numerous lines of evidence indicate MDMA involvement in serotonin dysregulation (Hatzidimitriou et al., 1999; McCann et al., 1998; Reneman et al., 2006; Ricaurte and McCann, 2001). Ecstasy use altered performance on the Affective Go/No-Go test but only for individuals carrying the s allele (ss and ls genotype). This dovetailed with the finding that *ss* MDMA users had the highest depression ratings (Roiser et al., 2005a).

In sum, reducing brain serotonin in healthy volunteers broadly resembles findings seen in MDD. Reduced positive bias and, at times, an enhanced negative bias are apparent following ATD, even in the absence of overt changes in mood. Furthermore ATD leads to increased BOLD response to emotional stimuli in many structures implicated in unipolar depression, as well as to increased responses to specifically negative stimuli in areas implicated in the processing of emotionally valenced verbal information. These data suggest a neural mechanism by which hypofunction of the serotonergic system, such as hypothesized to exist in MDD, may result in a maladaptive bias toward negative stimuli. Taken as a whole, the results support a critical role for serotonin in affective processing and sensitivity to negative feedback, as well as demonstrate the possible link between reduced serotonin and the neuropsychology of depression. The data also point to the importance of serotonin in mediating resilience against negative stimuli in never-depressed individuals.

Given the importance of dopamine systems in motivating behavior, the role of dopamine in affective processing has also been investigated in both healthy and depressed individuals, though less extensively (Nutt, 2006). Of the two major dopamine forebrain projections, the mesocorticolimbic system, which innervates limbic structures, such as the nucleus accumbens, amygdala and ventral hippocampus, and the PFC, supports a variety of behavioral functions related to motivation and reward (Robbins, 2000). Thus, an obvious prediction is that dopamine hypofunction could mediate both the inability to experience pleasure (anhedonia) and the loss of motivation seen in MDD.

Conceptually similar to ATD, acute phenylalanine and tyrosine depletion (APTD) involves providing an unbalanced amino acid drink lacking in tyrosine and phenylalanine selectively lowers dopamine synthesis in humans (for review see Booij, Van der Does, and Riedel, 2003). Another method examines dopamine and noradrenaline depletion by oral administration of alpha-mehtylparatyrosine (AMPT), a competitive inhibitor of the rate-limiting enzyme in catecholamine synthesis tyrosine hydroxylase. This latter method has resulted in increased depressive and anhedonic symptoms from MDD patients in remission (e.g., Hasler et al., 2008).

A study using APTD found that, when performing the affective go/no-go task, a group of healthy participants on placebo demonstrated a happy latency bias, while in contrast the group on APTD demonstrated a sad latency bias (McLean et al., 2004). APTD in recovered depressed individuals did not result in a marked lowering of mood, nor did it influence performance in the reversal learning task, including responses to negative feedback (Roiser et al., 2005b). In the affective go/no-go task, whilst there was a positive bias following placebo in these recovered patients, there was a trend towards a negative affective bias following APTD. More recently, Hasler and colleagues utilized AMPT for catecholamine depletion, in both healthy females and those with MDD in remission (Hasler et al., 2009). They found that the dopamine and noradrenaline depletion resulted in a selective impairment in probability reversal, which did not differ between the patients and controls, but did correlate with metabolism in the perigenual ACC. Thus, though serotonin is likely a primary neuromodulator involved in mood disorders, through its various effects in affective processing (e.g., Robinson and Sahakian, 2008; Robinson et al., 2009), additional neurotransmitters likely play significant roles as well. The recent interest in dopamine and noradrenaline functionality in depression is likely to continue to yield new insights. Future research will undoubtedly further examine not only the role of additional neurotransmitters such acetylcholine, glutamate, and GABA in mood and cognition in depression and resilience, but also the interactions between them all as well as with the glucocorticoid system (e.g., McAllister-Williams et al., 2007).

23.4 Conclusion

The results discussed in this chapter suggest that general underlying processes, such as negative attentional bias and abnormal response to negative feedback, are core cognitive characteristics in MDD. The latter of which may also be able to account in part for some impairments in performance, with the broad-ranging impairments in cognition resulting from altered brain function. The evidence suggests that disrupted top-down control of the amygdala by the prefrontal cortex underlies the hypersensitivity to negative feedback in MDD. Thus, improvement of MDD following SSRI treatment may be enhanced by psychological therapy, such as cognitive behavioral therapy (CBT), which provides patients with top-down cognitive control over their depressive symptoms (Robinson and Sahakian, 2009). This combination, which promotes adaptive learning, including within a social context, may improve efficacy, reduce relapse and reduce the delay in improvement following SSRI treatment. From a pharmacological standpoint, performance on the affective go/no-go task and the probabilistic reversal learning task is modulated by serotonergic and catecholaminergic function. Thus, these tests may prove useful in the early detection of symptoms. In this context, objective yet inexpensive measures of these core cognitive features in depression are likely to prove more sensitive than subjective rating scales, especially when taken together within a general neurocognitive profile. Moreover, such research allows for determining the relationship between core cognitive deficits, psychiatric and behavioral symptoms, genetic factors, and underlying brain mechanisms. Future research may examine the markers of resilience in greater detail, such as the presence and maintenance of positive affective biases in healthy individuals and the ability to exert cognitive control over an emotional response. This may be particularly pertinent to those at risk, due to genetic and social/environmental factors (Beddington et al., 2008). Thus, in individuals where genetic factors contribute to lesser resilience, treatments may target those neurochemical systems believed to be associated with the genotype. Such an approach may be particularly useful with the likely availability of multiple antidepressant agents, which could be used in combination. Likewise, in future, information about resilience may be combined with genetic and personality factors to inform the optimal treatment for each individual. By drawing together cognitive, neuroanatomical, neurofunctional, and pharmacological tiers of research, better treatment targets and directions for future investigation can be identified. This in turn will allow for the identification of people at risk, minimization of relapse, and maximization of long-term beneficial outcomes for those suffering from depression.

Acknowledgments

This research work was funded by the Wellcome Trust and the Medical Research Council. Dr. Sharon Morein-Zamir is funded by the Wellcome Trust (076274/Z/04/Z). The University of Cambridge and the Behavioural and Clinical Neuroscience Institute is jointly funded by The Medical Research Council and Wellcome Trust.

References

Abas, M. A., Sahakian, B. J., and Levy, R. (1990). Neuropsychological deficits and CT scan changes in elderly depressives. *Psychological Medicine,* 20(3), 507–20.

Ackerman, D. L., Unutzer, J., Greenland, S., and Gitlin, M. (2002). Inpatient treatment of depression and associated hospital charges. *Pharmacoepidemiol Drug Saf,* 11(3), 219–27.

APA. (2000). *Diagnostic and statistical manual—IV (text revision).* Washington, DC: American Psychiatric Associations.

Beats, B. C., Sahakian, B. J., and Levy, R. (1996). Cognitive performance in tests sensitive to frontal lobe dysfunction in the elderly depressed. *Psychological Medicine,* 26(3), 591–603.

Beck, A. T. (1967). *Depression: clinical experimental and theoretical aspects.* New York: Harper and Row.

Beck, A. T. (1976). *Cognitive therapy and the emotional disorders.* New York: International Universities Press.

Beddington, J., Cooper, C. L., Field, J., Goswami, U., Huppert, F. A., Jenkins, R. et al. (2008). The mental wealth of nations. *Nature,* 455(7216), 1057–60.

Bell, C. J., Hood, S. D., and Nutt, D. J. (2005). Acute tryptophan depletion. Part II: clinical effects and implications. *Australian and New Zealand Journal of Psychiatry,* 39(7), 565–74.

Bell-McGinty, S., Butters, M. A., Meltzer, C. C., Greer, P. J., Reynolds, C. F., 3rd, and Becker, J. T. (2002). Brain morphometric abnormalities in geriatric depression: long-term neurobiological effects of illness duration. *American Journal of Psychiatry*, **159**(8), 1424–27.

Booij, L., Van der Does, A. J., and Riedel, W. J. (2003). Monoamine depletion in psychiatric and healthy populations: review. *Molecular Psychiatry*, **8**(12), 951–73.

Booij, L., Van der Does, A. J., Haffmans, P. M., Riedel, W. J., Fekkes, D., and Blom, M. J. (2005). The effects of high-dose and low-dose tryptophan depletion on mood and cognitive functions of remitted depressed patients. *Journal of Psychopharmacology*, **19**(3), 267–75.

Borkowska, A. and Rybakowski, J. K. (2001). Neuropsychological frontal lobe tests indicate that bipolar depressed patients are more impaired than unipolar. *Bipolar Disorder*, **3**(2), 88–94.

Bowley, M. P., Drevets, W. C., Ongur, D., and Price, J. L. (2002). Low glial numbers in the amygdala in major depressive disorder. *Biological Psychiatry*, **52**(5), 404–12.

Bremner, J. D., Narayan, M., Anderson, E. R., Staib, L. H., Miller, H. L., and Charney, D. S. (2000). Hippocampal volume reduction in major depression. *American Journal of Psychiatry*, **157**(1), 115–118.

Bremner, J. D., Vythilingam, M., Vermetten, E., Nazeer, A., Adil, J., Khan, S. et al. (2002). Reduced volume of orbitofrontal cortex in major depression. *Biological Psychiatry*, **51**(4), 273–79.

Brittlebank, A. D., Scott, J., Williams, J. M., and Ferrier, I. N. (1993). Autobiographical memory in depression: state or trait marker? *British Journal of Psychiatry*, **162**, 118–21.

Campbell, S., Marriott, M., Nahmias, C., and MacQueen, G. M. (2004). Lower hippocampal volume in patients suffering from depression: a meta-analysis. *American Journal of Psychiatry*, **161**(4), 598–607.

Canli, T. and Lesch, K. P. (2007). Long story short: the serotonin transporter in emotion regulation and social cognition. *Nature Neuroscience*, **10**(9), 1103–109.

Cannon, D. M., Klaver, J. M., Peck, S. A., Rallis-Voak, d., Erickson, K., and Drevets, W. C. (2009). Dopamine Type-1 Receptor Binding in Major Depressive Disorder Assessed Using Positron Emission Tomography and [11C]NNC-112. *Neuropsychopharmacology*, **34**, 1277–87.

Carpenter, L. L., Anderson, G. M., Pelton, G. H., Gudin, J. A., Kirwin, P. D., Price, L. H. et al. (1998). Tryptophan depletion during continuous CSF sampling in healthy human subjects. *Neuropsychopharmacology*, **19**(1), 26–35.

Caspi, A., Sugden, K., Moffitt, T. E., Taylor, A., Craig, I. W., Harrington, H. et al. (2003). Influence of life stress on depression: moderation by a polymorphism in the 5-HTT gene. *Science*, **301**(5631), 386–89.

Chamberlain, S. R. and Sahakian, B. J. (2004). Cognition in mania and depression: psychological models and clinical implications. *Current Psychiatry Report*, **6**(6), 451–58.

Chamberlain, S. R. and Sahakian, B. J. (2005). Nueropsychological assessment of mood disorders. *Clinical Neuropsychiatry*, **2**(3), 137–48.

Chamberlain, S. R., Muller, U., Blackwell, A. D., Clark, L., Robbins, T. W., and Sahakian, B. J. (2006). Neurochemical modulation of response inhibition and probabilistic learning in humans. *Science*, **311**(5762), 861–63.

Clark, L., Iversen, S. D., and Goodwin, G. M. (2002). Sustained attention deficit in bipolar disorder. *Br J Psychiatry*, **180**, 313–19.

Clark, L., Chamberlain, S. R., and Sahakian, B. J. (2009). Neruocognitive mechanisms in depression: implications for treatment. *Annual Review of Neuroscience*, **32**, 57–74.

Clark, L. and Sahakian, B. J. (2006). *Neuropsychological and biological approaches to understanding bipolar disorder*. Oxford University Press.

Clark, L. and Sahakian, B. J. (2008). Cognitive neuroscience and brain imaging in bipolar disorder. *Dialogues in Clinical Neuroscience*, **10**(2), 153–63.

Conway, M., Howell, A., and Giannopoulos, C. (1991). Dysphoria and thought suppression. *Cognitive Therapy and Research*, **15**, 153–66.

Cools, R., Clark, L., Owen, A. M., and Robbins, T. W. (2002). Defining the neural mechanisms of probabilistic reversal learning using event-related functional magnetic resonance imaging. *J Neuroscience*, 22(11), 4563–67.

Cools, R., Blackwell, A., Clark, L., Menzies, L., Cox, S., and Robbins, T. W. (2005). Tryptophan depletion disrupts the motivational guidance of goal-directed behavior as a function of trait impulsivity. *Neuropsychopharmacology*, 30(7), 1362–73.

Cools, R., Robinson, O.J., and Sahakian, B. (2008). Acute tryptophan depletion in healthy volunteers enhances punishment prediction but does not affect reward prediction. *Neuropsychopharmacology*, 33(9), 2291–99.

Coppen, A., Prange, A. J., Jr., Whybrow, P. C., and Noguera, R. (1972). Abnormalities of indoleamines in affective disorders. *Archives of General Psychiatry*, 26(5), 474–78.

Cotter, D., Mackay, D., Landau, S., Kerwin, R., and Everall, I. (2001). Reduced glial cell density and neuronal size in the anterior cingulate cortex in major depressive disorder. *Archives of General Psychiatry*, 58(6), 545–53.

Cowen, P. J. (1990). A role for 5-HT in the action of antidepressant drugs. *Pharmacological Therapy*, 46, 43–51.

Delgado, P. L., Charney, D. S., Price, L. H., Aghajanian, G. K., Landis, H., and Heninger, G. R. (1990). Serotonin function and the mechanism of antidepressant action. Reversal of antidepressant-induced remission by rapid depletion of plasma tryptophan. *Archives of General Psychiatry*, 47(5), 411–18.

DeRubeis, R. J., Siegle, G. J., and Hollon, S. D. (2008). Cognitive therapy versus medication for depression: treatment outcomes and neural mechanisms. *Nature Review Neuroscience*, 9(10), 788–96.

Dougherty, D. D., Bonab, A. A., Ottowitz, W. E., Livini, E., Alpert, N. M., Rauch S. L. et al. (2006). Decreased striatal D1 binding as measured using PET and [11C]SCH 23, 390 in patients with major depression with anger attacks. *Depression and Anxiety*, 23(3), 175–7.

Drevets, W. C. (1999). Prefrontal cortical-amygdalar metabolism in major depression. *Annals of the NY Academy of Science*, 877, 614–37.

Drevets, W. C., Price, J. L., Simpson, J. R., Jr., Todd, R. D., Reich, T., Vannier, M. et al. (1997). Subgenual prefrontal cortex abnormalities in mood disorders. *Nature*, 386(6627), 824–27.

Drevets, W. C., Ongur, D., and Price, J. L. (1998). Neuroimaging abnormalities in the subgenual prefrontal cortex: implications for the pathophysiology of familial mood disorders. *Molecular Psychiatry*, 3(3), 220–26, 190–21.

Drevets, W. C., Price, J. L., and Furey, M. L. (2008a). Brain structural and functional abnormalities in mood disorders: implications for neurocircuitry models of depression. *Brain Structure and Function*, 213(1-2), 93–118.

Drevets, W. C., Savitz, J., and Trimble, M. (2008b). The subgenual anterior cingulate cortex in mood disorders. *CNS Spectrums*, 13(8), 663–81.

Elliott, R., Sahakian, B. J., McKay, A. P., Herrod, J. J., Robbins, T. W., and Paykel, E. S. (1996). Neuropsychological impairments in unipolar depression: the influence of perceived failure on subsequent performance. *Psychological Medicine*, 26(5), 975–89.

Elliott, R., Sahakian, B. J., Herrod, J. J., Robbins, T. W., and Paykel, E. S. (1997a). Abnormal response to negative feedback in unipolar depression: evidence for a diagnosis specific impairment. *Journal of Neurology Neurosurgery Psychiatry*, 63(1), 74–82.

Elliott, R., Baker, S. C., Rogers, R. D., O'Leary, D. A., Paykel, E. S., Frith, C. D. et al. (1997b). Prefrontal dysfunction in depressed patients performing a complex planning task: a study using positron emission tomography. *Psychological Medicine*, 27(4), 931–42.

Elliott, R., Rubinsztein, J. S., Sahakian, B. J., and Dolan, R. J. (2000). Selective attention to emotional stimuli in a verbal go/no-go task: an fMRI study. *Neuroreport*, 11(8), 1739–44.

Elliott, R., Rubinsztein, J. S., Sahakian, B. J., and Dolan, R. J. (2002). The neural basis of mood-congruent processing biases in depression. *Archives of General Psychiatry*, 59(7), 597–604.

Elliott, R., Ogilvie, A., Rubinsztein, J. S., Calderon, G., Dolan, R. J., and Sahakian, B. J. (2004). Abnormal ventral frontal response during performance of an affective go/no go task in patients with mania. *Biological Psychiatry*, **55**(12), 1163–70.

Erickson, K., Drevets, W. C., Clark, L., Cannon, D. M., Bain, E. E., Zarate, C. A., Jr. et al. (2005). Mood-congruent bias in affective go/no-go performance of unmedicated patients with major depressive disorder. *American Journal of Psychiatry*, **162**(11), 2171–73.

Evers, E. A., Cools, R., Clark, L., van der Veen, F. M., Jolles, J., Sahakian, B. J. et al. (2005). Serotonergic modulation of prefrontal cortex during negative feedback in probabilistic reversal learning. *Neuropsychopharmacology*, **30**(6), 1138–47.

Furlong, R. A., Rubinsztein, J. S., Ho, L., Walsh, C., Coleman, T. A., Muir, W. J. et al. (1999). Analysis and metaanalysis of two polymorphisms within the tyrosine hydroxylase gene in bipolar and unipolar affective disorders. *American Journal of Medical Genetics*, **88**(1), 88–94.

Goldberg, T. E., Gold, J. M., Greenberg, R., Griffin, S., Schulz, S. C., Pickar, D. et al. (1993). Contrasts between patients with affective disorders and patients with schizophrenia on a neuropsychological test battery. *American Journal of Psychiatry*, **150**(9), 1355–62.

Gotlib, I. H. (1983). Perception and recall of interpersonal feedback: negative bias in depression. *Cognitive Therapy and Research*, 7, 399–412.

Greenberg, P. E., Kessler, R. C., Birnbaum, H. G., Leong, S. A., Lowe, S. W., Berglund, P. A. et al. (2003). The economic burden of depression in the United States: how did it change between 1990 and 2000? *Journal of Clinical Psychiatry*, **64**(12), 1465–75.

Harmer, C. J. (2008). Serotonin and emotional processing: Does it help explain antidepressant drug action? *Neuropharmacology*, 55, 1023–28.

Hasler, G., Fromm, S., Carlson, P. J., Luckenbaugh, D. A., Waldeck, T., Geraci, M. et al. (2008). Neural response to catecholamine depletion in unmedicated subjects with major depressive disorder in remission and healthy subjects. *Archives of General Psychiatry*, **65**(5), 521–31.

Hasler, G., Mondillo, K., Drevets, W. C., and Blair, J. R. (2009). Impairments of probabilistic response reversal and passive avoidance following catecholamine depletion. *Neuropsychopharmacology*, **34**(13), 2691–8.

Hatzidimitriou, G., McCann, U. D., and Ricaurte, G. A. (1999). Altered serotonin innervation patterns in the forebrain of monkeys treated with (+/-)3,4-methylenedioxymethamphetamine seven years previously: factors influencing abnormal recovery. *Journal of Neuroscience*, **19**(12), 5096–107.

Hood, S. D., Bell, C. J., and Nutt, D. J. (2005). Acute tryptophan depletion. Part I: rationale and methodology. *Australian and New Zealand Journal of Psychiatry*, **39**(7), 558–64.

Horn, G. (2008). *Brain Science, addiction and drugs*. The Academy of Medical Sciences.

Jaeger, J., Berns, S., Uzelac, S., and Davis-Conway, S. (2006). Neurocognitive deficits and disability in major depressive disorder. *Psychiatric Research*, **145**(1), 39–48.

Johnson, M. H. and Magaro, P. A. (1987). Effects of mood and severity on memory processes in depression and mania. *Psychological Bulletin*, **101**(1), 28–40.

Kennedy, S. H., Evans, K. R., Kruger, S., Mayberg, H. S., Meyer, J. H., McCann, S. et al. (2001). Changes in regional brain glucose metabolism measured with positron emission tomography after paroxetine treatment of major depression. *American Journal of Psychiatry*, **158**(6), 899–905.

Kennedy, S. H., Konarski, J. Z., Segal, Z. V., Lau, M. A., Bieling, P. J., McIntyre, R. S. et al. (2007). Differences in brain glucose metabolism between responders to CBT and venlafaxine in a 16-week randomized controlled trial. *American Journal of Psychiatry*, **164**(5), 778–88.

Kessing, L. V. (1998). Cognitive impairment in the euthymic phase of affective disorder. *Psychological Medicine*, **28**(5), 1027–38.

Kessler, R. C., Chiu, W. T., Demler, O., Merikangas, K. R., and Walters, E. E. (2005). Prevalence, severity, and comorbidity of 12-month DSM-IV disorders in the National Comorbidity Survey Replication. *Archives of General Psychiatry*, **62**(6), 617–27.

Kyte, Z. A., Goodyer, I. M., and **Sahakian, B. J.** (2005). Selected executive skills in adolescents with recent first episode major depression. *Journal of Child Psychology and Psychiatry and Allied Disciplines,* **46**(9), 995–1005.

Lawrence, A. D., Hodges, J. R., Rosser, A. E., Kershaw, A., ffrench-Constant, C., Rubinsztein, D. C. et al. (1998). Evidence for specific cognitive deficits in preclinical Huntington's disease. *Brain,* **121** (Pt 7), 1329–41.

Lozano, A. M., Mayberg, H. S., Giacobbe, P., Hamani, C., Craddock, R. C., and Kennedy, S. H. (2008). Subcallosal cingulate gyrus deep brain stimulation for treatment-resistant depression. *Biological Psychiatry,* **64**(6), 461–67.

MacQueen, G. M., Campbell, S., McEwen, B. S., Macdonald, K., Amano, S., Joffe, R. T. et al. (2003). Course of illness, hippocampal function, and hippocampal volume in major depression. *Proceedings of the National Academy of Science USA,* **100**(3), 1387–92.

Martinez-Aran, A., Vieta, E., Colom, F., Torrent, C., Sanchez-Moreno, J., Reinares, M. et al. (2004). Cognitive impairment in euthymic bipolar patients: implications for clinical and functional outcome. *Bipolar Disorder,* **6**(3), 224–32.

Mayberg, H. S. (1997). Limbic-cortical dysregulation: a proposed model of depression. *Journal of Neuropsychiatry and Clinical Neuroscience,* **9**(3), 471–81.

Mayberg, H. (2002). Depression, II: localization of pathophysiology. *American Journal of Psychiatry,* **159**(12), 1979.

Mayberg, H. S. (2003). Positron emission tomography imaging in depression: a neural systems perspective. *Neuroimaging Clin North America,* **13**(4), 805–815.

Mayberg, H. S., Brannan, S. K., Mahurin, R. K., Jerabek, P. A., Brickman, J. S., Tekell, J. L. et al. (1997). Cingulate function in depression: a potential predictor of treatment response. *Neuroreport,* **8**(4), 1057–61.

Mayberg, H. S., Lozano, A. M., Voon, V., McNeely, H. E., Seminowicz, D., Hamani, C. et al. (2005). Deep brain stimulation for treatment-resistant depression. *Neuron,* **45**(5), 651–60.

McAllister-Williams, R. H., Massey, A. E., and Fairchild, G. (2007). Repeated cortisol administration attenuates the EEG response to buspirone in healthy volunteers: evidence for desensitization of the 5-HT1A autoreceptor. *Journal of Psychopharmacology,* **21**(8), 826–32.

McCann, U. D., Szabo, Z., Scheffel, U., Dannals, R. F., and Ricaurte, G. A. (1998). Positron emission tomographic evidence of toxic effect of MDMA ("Ecstasy") on brain serotonin neurons in human beings. *Lancet,* **352**(9138), 1433–37.

McCrone, P., Dhanasiri, S., Patel, A., Knapp, M., and Lawton-Smith, S. (2008). *Paying the Price: The Cost of Mental Health Care in England to 2026.* http://www.kingsfund.org.uk/publications/the_kings_fund_publications/paying_the_price.html: Accessed April 1 2009 London: King's Fund.

McLean, A., Rubinsztein, J. S., Robbins, T. W., and **Sahakian, B. J.** (2004). The effects of tyrosine depletion in normal healthy volunteers: implications for unipolar depression. *Psychopharmacology (Berl),* **171**(3), 286–97.

Murphy, F. C., **Sahakian, B. J.**, and O'Carroll, R. E. (1998). Cognitive impairment in depression: psychological models and clinical issues. In D. Ebert and K. P. Ebmeier (Eds.), *New models for depression. Adv Biological Psychiatry* (pp. 1–33). Basel: Karger.

Murphy, F. C., **Sahakian, B. J.**, Rubinsztein, J. S., Michael, A., Rogers, R. D., Robbins, T. W. et al. (1999). Emotional bias and inhibitory control processes in mania and depression. *Psychological Medicine,* **29**(6), 1307–21.

Murphy, F. C., Smith, K. A., Cowen, P. J., Robbins, T. W., and **Sahakian, B. J.** (2002). The effects of tryptophan depletion on cognitive and affective processing in healthy volunteers. *Psychopharmacology (Berl),* **163**(1), 42–53.

Murphy, F. C., Michael, A., Robbins, T. W., and Sahakian, B. J. (2003). Neuropsychological impairment in patients with major depressive disorder: the effects of feedback on task performance. *Psychological Medicine,* **33**(3), 455–67.

Neumeister, A., Konstantinidis, A., Stastny, J., Schwarz, M.J., Vitouch, O., Willeit, M. et al. (2002). Association between serotonin transporter gene promoter polymorphism (5HTTLPR) and behavioral responses to tryptophan depletion in healthy women with and without family history of depression. *Archives of General Psychiatry,* **59**, 613–20.

Neumeister, A., Nugent, A. C., Waldeck, T., Geraci, M., Schwarz, M., Bonne, O. et al. (2004). Neural and behavioral responses to tryptophan depletion in unmedicated patients with remitted major depressive disorder and controls. *Archives of General Psychiatry,* **61**(8), 765–73.

Nutt, D. J. (2002). The neuropharmacology of serotonin and noradrenaline in depression. *International Clinical Psycopharmacology,* **17** Suppl 1, S1–12.

Nutt, D. J. (2006). The role of dopamine and norepinephrine in depression and antidepressant treatment. *Journal of Clinical Psychiatry,* **67**, 3–8.

Ochsner, K. N., Bunge, S. A., Gross, J. J., and Gabrieli, J. D. (2002). Rethinking feelings: an FMRI study of the cognitive regulation of emotion. *Journal of Cognitive Neuroscience,* **14**(8), 1215–29.

Ongur, D., Drevets, W. C., and Price, J. L. (1998). Glial reduction in the subgenual prefrontal cortex in mood disorders. *Proceedings of the National Academy of Science USA,* **95**(22), 13290–95.

Ongur, D., Ferry, A. T., and Price, J. L. (2003). Architectonic subdivision of the human orbital and medial prefrontal cortex. *Journal of Comparitive Neurology,* **460**(3), 425–49.

Pezawas, L., Meyer-Lindenberg, A., Drabant, E. M., Verchinski, B. A., Munoz, K. E., Kolachana, B. S. et al. (2005). 5-HTTLPR polymorphism impacts human cingulate-amygdala interactions: a genetic susceptibility mechanism for depression. *Nature Neuroscience,* **8**(6), 828–34.

Phelps, E. A., and LeDoux, J. E. (2005). Contributions of the amygdala to emotion processing: from animal models to human behavior. *Neuron,* **48**(2), 175–87.

Phillips, M. L., Drevets, W. C., Rauch, S. L., and Lane, R. (2003a). Neurobiology of emotion perception I: The neural basis of normal emotion perception. *Biological Psychiatry,* **54**, 504–14.

Phillips, M. L., Drevets, W. C., Rauch, S. L., and Lane, R. (2003b). Neurobiology of emotion perception II: Implications for major psychiatric disorders. *Biological Psychiatry,* **54**(5), 515–28.

Purcell, R., Maruff, P., Kyrios, M., and Pantelis, C. (1997). Neuropsychological function in young patients with unipolar major depression. *Psychological Medicine,* **27**(6), 1277–85.

Rajkowska, G., Miguel-Hidalgo, J. J., Wei, J., Dilley, G., Pittman, S. D., Meltzer, H. Y. et al. (1999). Morphometric evidence for neuronal and glial prefrontal cell pathology in major depression. *Biological Psychiatry,* **45**(9), 1085–98.

Rajkowska, G., Halaris, A., and Selemon, L. D. (2001). Reductions in neuronal and glial density characterize the dorsolateral prefrontal cortex in bipolar disorder. *Biological Psychiatry,* **49**(9), 741–52.

Reneman, L., de Win, M. M., van den Brink, W., Booij, J., and den Heeten, G. J. (2006). Neuroimaging findings with MDMA/ecstasy: technical aspects, conceptual issues and future prospects. *Journal of Psychopharmacology,* **20**(2), 164–75.

Ressler, K. J. and Mayberg, H. S. (2007). Targeting abnormal neural circuits in mood and anxiety disorders: from the laboratory to the clinic. *Nature Neuroscience,* **10**(9), 1116–24.

Ricaurte, G. A. and McCann, U. D. (2001). Assessing long-term effects of MDMA (ecstasy). *Lancet,* **358**(9296), 1831–32.

Riedel, W. J., Klaassen, T., Deutz, N. E., van Someren, A., and van Praag, H. M. (1999). Tryptophan depletion in normal volunteers produces selective impairment in memory consolidation. *Psychopharmacology (Berl),* **141**(4), 362–69.

Robbins, T. W. (2000). Chemical neuromodulation of frontalexecutive functions in humans and other animals. *Experimental Brain Research*, **133**, 130–38.

Robinson, O. and Sahakian, B. J. (2008). Recurrence in major depressive disorder: a neurocognitive perspective. *Psychological Medicine*, **38**, 315–18.

Robinson, O. and Sahakian, B. J. (2009). A double dissociation in the roles of serotonin and mood in healthy subjects. *Biological Psychiatry*, **65**(1), 89–92.

Robinson, O., Cools, R., Crockett, M., and Sahakian, B. (2009). Mood state moderates the role of serotonin in cognitive biases. *Journal of Psychopharmacology*, **24**(4), 573–83.

Rogers, R. D., Blackshaw, A. J., Middleton, H. C., Matthews, K., Hawtin, K., Crowley, C. et al. (1999). Tryptophan depletion impairs stimulus-reward learning while methylphenidate disrupts attentional control in healthy young adults: implications for the monoaminergic basis of impulsive behavior. *Psychopharmacology (Berl)*, **146**(4), 482–91.

Rogers, R. D., Tunbridge, E. M., Bhagwagar, Z., Drevets, W. C., Sahakian, B. J., and Carter, C. S. (2003). Tryptophan depletion alters the decision making of healthy volunteers through altered processing of reward cues. *Neuropsychopharmacology*, **28**(1), 153–62.

Roiser, J. P., Rubinsztein, J. S., and Sahakian, B. J. (2003). Cognition in depression. *Psychiatry*, **2**, 43–47.

Roiser, J. P., Cook, L. J., Cooper, J. D., Rubinsztein, D. C., and Sahakian, B. J. (2005a). Association of a functional polymorphism in the serotonin transporter gene with abnormal emotional processing in ecstasy users. *American Journal of Psychiatry*, **162**(3), 609–12.

Roiser, J. P., McLean, A., Ogilvie, A. D., Blackwell, A. D., Bamber, D. J., Goodyer, I. et al. (2005b). The subjective and cognitive effects of acute phenylalanine and tyrosine depletion in patients recovered from depression. *Neuropsychopharmacology*, **30**(4), 775–85.

Roiser, J. P., Blackwell, A. D., Cools, R., Clark, L., Rubinsztein, D. C., Robbins, T. W. et al. (2006). Serotonin transporter polymorphism mediates vulnerability to loss of incentive motivation following acute tryptophan depletion. *Neuropsychopharmacology*, **31**(10), 2264–72.

Roiser, J. P., Muller, U., Clark, L., and Sahakian, B. J. (2007). The effects of acute tryptophan depletion and serotonin transporter polymorphism on emotional processing in memory and attention. *International Journal of Neuropsychopharmacology*, **10**(4), 449–61.

Roiser, J. P., Levy, J., Fromm, S. J., Wang, H., Hasler, G., Sahakian, B. J. et al. (2008). The effect of acute tryptophan depletion on the neural correlates of emotional processing in healthy volunteers. *Neuropsychopharmacology*, **33**(8), 1992–2006.

Rubinsztein, J. S., Michael, A., Paykel, E. S., and Sahakian, B. J. (2000). Cognitive impairment in remission in bipolar affective disorder. *Psychological Medicine*, **30**(5), 1025–36.

Rubinsztein, J. S., Michael, A., Underwood, B. R., Tempest, M., and Sahakian, B. J. (2006). Impaired cognition and decision making in bipolar depression but no "affective bias" evident. *Psychological Medicine*, **36**(5), 629–39.

Salkovskis, P. M. (1996). *Frontiers of Cognitive Therapy*. New York: Guilford Press.

Saxena, S., Brody, A. L., Ho, M. L., Zohrabi, N., Maidment, K. M., and Baxter, L. R., Jr. (2003). Differential brain metabolic predictors of response to paroxetine in obsessive-compulsive disorder versus major depression. *American Journal of Psychiatry*, **160**(3), 522–32.

Schatzberg, A. F., Garlow, S. J., and Nemeroff, C. B. (2002). Molecular and cellular mechanisms in depression. In K. L. Davis, D. S. Charneym, J. T. Coyle and C. B. Nemeroff (eds), *Neuropsychopharmacology. the fifth generation of progress* (pp. 1039–50). Philadelphia: Lippincott, Williams and Wilkins.

Serretti, A., Benedetti, F., Zanardi, R., and Smeraldi, E. (2005). The influence of Serotonin Transporter Promoter Polymorphism (SERTPR) and other polymorphisms of the serotonin pathway on the efficacy of antidepressant treatments. *Progress in Neuropsychopharmacol Biological Psychiatry*, **29**(6), 1074–84.

Smith, K. A., Fairburn, C. G., and Cowen, P. J. (1997). Relapse of depression after rapid depletion of tryptophan. *Lancet,* 349(9056), 915–19.

Swainson, R., Rogers, R. D., Sahakian, B. J., Summers, B. A., Polkey, C. E., and Robbins, T. W. (2000). Probabilistic learning and reversal deficits in patients with Parkinson's disease or frontal or temporal lobe lesions: possible adverse effects of dopaminergic medication. *Neuropsychologia,* 38(5), 596–612.

Sweeney, J. A., Kmiec, J. A., and Kupfer, D. J. (2000). Neuropsychologic impairments in bipolar and uni-polar mood disorders on the CANTAB neurocognitive battery. *Biological Psychiatry,* 48(7), 674–84.

Taylor Tavares, J. V., Drevets, W. C., and Sahakian, B. J. (2003). Cognition in mania and depression. *Psychological Medicine,* 33(6), 959–67.

Taylor Tavares, J. V., Clark, L., Cannon, D. M., Erickson, K., Drevets, W. C., and Sahakian, B. J. (2007). Distinct profiles of neurocognitive function in unmedicated unipolar depression and bipo-lar II depression. *Biological Psychiatry,* 62(8), 917–24.

Taylor Tavares, J. V., Clark, L., Furey, M. L., Williams, G. B., Sahakian, B. J., and Drevets, W. C. (2008). Neural basis of abnormal response to negative feedback in unmedicated mood disorders. *Neuroimage,* 42(3), 1118–26.

Videbech, P. and Ravnkilde, B. (2004). Hippocampal volume and depression: a meta-analysis of MRI studies. *American Journal of Psychiatry,* 161(11), 1957–66.

Vrshek-Schallhorn, S., Wahlstrom, D., Benolkin, K., White, T., and Luciana, M. (2006). Affective bias and response modulation following tyrosine depletion in healthy adults. *Neuropsychopharmacology,* 31(11), 2523–36.

Weissman, M. M., Bland, R. C., Canino, G. J., Faravelli, C., Greenwald, S., Hwu, H. G. et al. (1996). Cross-national epidemiology of major depression and bipolar disorder. *Jama,* 276(4), 293–99.

WHO (2001). *The World Health report: mental health: new understanding, new hope:* www.who.int. Accessed April 1 2009.

Williams, W. A., Shoaf, S. E., Hommer, D., Rawlings, R., and Linnoila, M. (1999). Effects of acute tryptophan depletion on plasma and cerebrospinal fluid tryptophan and 5-hydroxyindoleacetic acid in normal volunteers. *Journal of Neurochemistry,* 72(4), 1641–47.

Wolfe, J., Granholm, E., Butters, N., Saunders, E., and Janowsky, D. (1987). Verbal memory deficits associated with major affective disorders: a comparison of unipolar and bipolar patients. *Journal of Affective Disorders,* 13(1), 83–92.

Yatham, L. N., Liddle, P. F., Shiah, I. S., Scarrow, G., Lam, R. W., Adam, M. J. et al. (2000). Brain serotonin2 receptors in major depression: a positron emission tomography study. *Archives of General Psychiatry,* 57(9), 850–58.

Zanardi, R., Serretti, A., Rossini, D., Franchini, L., Cusin, C., Lattuada, E. et al. (2001). Factors affect-ing fluvoxamine antidepressant activity: influence of pindolol and 5-HTTLPR in delusional and nondelusional depression. *Biological Psychiatry,* 50(5), 323–30.

Zarate, C. A., Jr., Tohen, M., Land, M., and Cavanagh, S. (2000). Functional impairment and cognition in bipolar disorder. *Psychiatric Quarterly,* 71(4), 309–29.

Author Index

Subject Index

Printed and bound by CPI Group (UK) Ltd, Croydon, CR0 4YY